PRINCIPLES OF HEALTH
Nursing

PRINCIPLES OF HEALTH
Nursing

Editor
Patricia Stanfill Edens, MS, MBA, PhD, RN, LFACHE

SALEM PRESS
A Division of EBSCO Information Services, Inc.
Ipswich, Massachusetts

GREY HOUSE PUBLISHING

Cover photo: iStock by Getty Images

Copyright © 2021, by Salem Press, A Division of EBSCO Information Services, Inc., and Grey House Publishing, Inc.

Principles of Health: Nursing, published by Grey House Publishing, Inc., Amenia, NY, under exclusive license from EBSCO Information Services, Inc.

All rights reserved. No part of this work may be used or reproduced in any manner whatsoever or transmitted in any form or by any means, electronic or mechanical, including photocopy, recording, or any information storage and retrieval system, without written permission from the copyright owner. For permissions requests, contact proprietarypublishing@ebsco.com.

For information contact Grey House Publishing/Salem Press, 4919 Route 22, PO Box 56, Amenia, NY 12501.

∞ The paper used in these volumes conforms to the American National Standard for Permanence of Paper for Printed Library Materials, Z39.48 1992 (R2009).

Publisher's Cataloging-In-Publication Data
(Prepared by The Donohue Group, Inc.)

Names: Edens, Patricia Stanfill, editor.
Title: Principles of health. Nursing / editor, Patricia Stanfill Edens, MS, MBA, PhD, RN, LFACHE.
Other Titles: Nursing
Description: Ipswich, Massachusetts : Salem Press, a division of EBSCO Information Services, Inc. ; Amenia, NY : Grey House Publishing, [2021] | Includes bibliographical references and index.
Identifiers: ISBN 9781642657685
Subjects: LCSH: Nursing—Vocational guidance. | LCGFT: Reference works.
Classification: LCC RT82 .P75 2021 | DDC 610.73023—dc23

FIRST PRINTING
PRINTED IN THE UNITED STATES OF AMERICA

Contents

Publisher's Note vii
Introduction ix
Contributors xi

What Is Nursing?
Nursing: Its History and Evolution 3
Roles on the Healthcare Team 9
Nursing Concepts 12
Nursing Process 15
Ethics of Nursing 17
Autonomy and Physician Orders 19
Scope of Nursing Practice 21
Informed Consent 23
Clinical Research Trials 25

Nursing Theory
Nursing Theory 31
Metaparadigm Concepts in Nursing 33
Grand Theories 35
Middle-Range Theories 38
Practice-Level Theories 40

Nursing Theorists
Florence Nightingale 45
Hildegard Peplau 47
Faye Abdellah 49
Ida Jean Orlando 51
Dorothea Orem 53
Imogene King 55
Betty Neuman 57
Callista Roy 58
Jean Watson 60
Abraham Maslow 62
Katharine Kolbaca and Kristen M. Swanson 65
Nola Pender 67

Becoming a Nurse
Selecting the Right Program and Finding
   the Right College 71
Learning Styles and Study Skills 75
Cover Letter and Resume Writing 80
Interviewing 83
Career and Personnel Testing 87
College and Nursing Entrance Examinations . . . 92

Succeeding at Work 95
Nursing Certifications and Degrees: Licensed
   Practical Nurse and Registered Nurse 102
Advanced Practice Nurses 104
Licensure and Certification 107
Professional Nursing Organizations and
   Certification 109
Magnet Recognition Program in Nursing 111
Nurse-Patient Ratio 113
Models of Nursing Care 115

Skills Needed in Nursing
Leadership 119
Leadership Skills 121
Volunteering and Community Service 124
Time Management 127
Communicating Effectively: Interpersonal
   Communication, Skills, and Technology 131
Writing Skills 140
Public Speaking 142
Networking 146

Nursing Specialties
Staff Nurse and Primary Care Nurse 151
Nursing Administrator 152
Medical-Surgical Nurses and Perioperative
   Nurses 154
Obstetric and Neonatal Nurses 157
Perinatology 159
Pediatrics 162
Gerontological Nursing 170
Critical Care Nursing 173
Clinical Nurse Specialist (CNS) 176
Doctor's Office, Clinic Nurses, and Physician
   Assistants (PAs) 177
Nurse Practitioner (NP) 179
Nurse Anesthetist 181
Home Health Nurse and Public Health Nurse . . 184
Occupational Health 187
Transitional Care 189
Wound, Ostomy, and Continence (WOC)
   Nurse 191
Telehealth Nursing 192
Palliative Care and Hospice Nursing 194

Travel Nurse 198
Clinical Research Nurse 199
Case Management/Utilization Management
   and Care Navigation................... 201
Educators—Academic and Vocational
   Programs............................. 203
Continuing Education Coordinator and
   Patient Educator 205

Specific Nursing Care
Dying, Death, and Grief 211
Pain Management........................ 217
National Institutes of Health (NIH) 221
Health Promotion....................... 226
Diet-Based Therapies 230
Exercise-Based Therapies................. 232
Education and Training of CAM Practitioners.. 237
Integrative Medicine..................... 242
Internet Medicine....................... 246
Internet and Health Information 250
Office of Cancer Complementary and
   Alternative Medicine (OCCAM).......... 252
Office of Dietary Supplements (ODS) 253
Self-Care 255

Spirituality and CAM 257
Relaxation Response..................... 260
Relaxation Therapies 262
Meditation 267
Transcendental Meditation (TM) 270
Mind-Body Medicine 273
Guided Imagery 275
Natural Treatments for Stress............... 276
Natural Treatments for Well-Being........... 280
Therapeutic Touch (TT)................... 282
Reiki 285
Rolfing 289
Art Therapy 290
Music Therapy 293
Biofeedback 297
Nursing Care Plan 301
Genetic Counseling...................... 303
Robotics in Healthcare 307
Bioinformatics.......................... 312
Popular Health Movement 314

Nursing Terminology 317
General Bibliography and Further Reading.... 319
Index................................. 347

Publisher's Note

Salem Press is pleased to add *Principles of Health: Nursing* as the fifth title of our growing *Principles of Health* series. Other titles in this series include *Diabetes, Anxiety & Stress, Pain Management,* and *Obesity*.

This new title introduces students and researchers to the fundamentals of nursing, using easy to understand language that provides a solid background as a deeper understanding and appreciation of this crucial profession. The 104 entries are arranged into seven broad categories:
- What is Nursing?
- Nursing Theory
- Nursing Theorists
- Becoming a Nurse
- Skills Needed in Nursing
- Nursing Specialties
- Specific Nursing Care

Entries are far reaching and include the background and evolution of the profession, as well as where a career in nursing can lead today—LPN, Perioperative Nurse, Clinical Research Nurse, Neonatal Nurse, Palliative Nurse—the options are endless.

In addition to nursing career options, this work includes valuable information about training to become a nurse, what skills you will need, what you can expect from different nursing specialties, and the different environments your work will take you.

Each entry includes an Abstract that provides a brief, concrete summary of the topic and its significance, followed by a detailed essay that provides extensive background to the topic and explains its significance to the field of nursing. Photos and illustrations enhance many of the entries, and a list of Further Reading for those who wish to pursue the topic in more depth appears at the end of each entry.

In addition, *Principles of Health: Nursing* includes the following helpful back matter:
- A list of Nursing Terminology defines key and specialized terms used throughout the book and in the profession at large;
- A comprehensive General Bibliography and Further Reading comprises all the works that the authors drew upon in writing their essays, as well as subjects for further study;
- A Subject Index offers multiple points of entry for the reader.

Salem Press extends its appreciation to all individuals involved in the development and production of this work, especially volume editor Patricia Stanfill Edens, who also contributed a number of articles and a comprehensive introduction to this work. All of the entries have been written by experts in the field of nursing. Their names and affiliations follow this note.

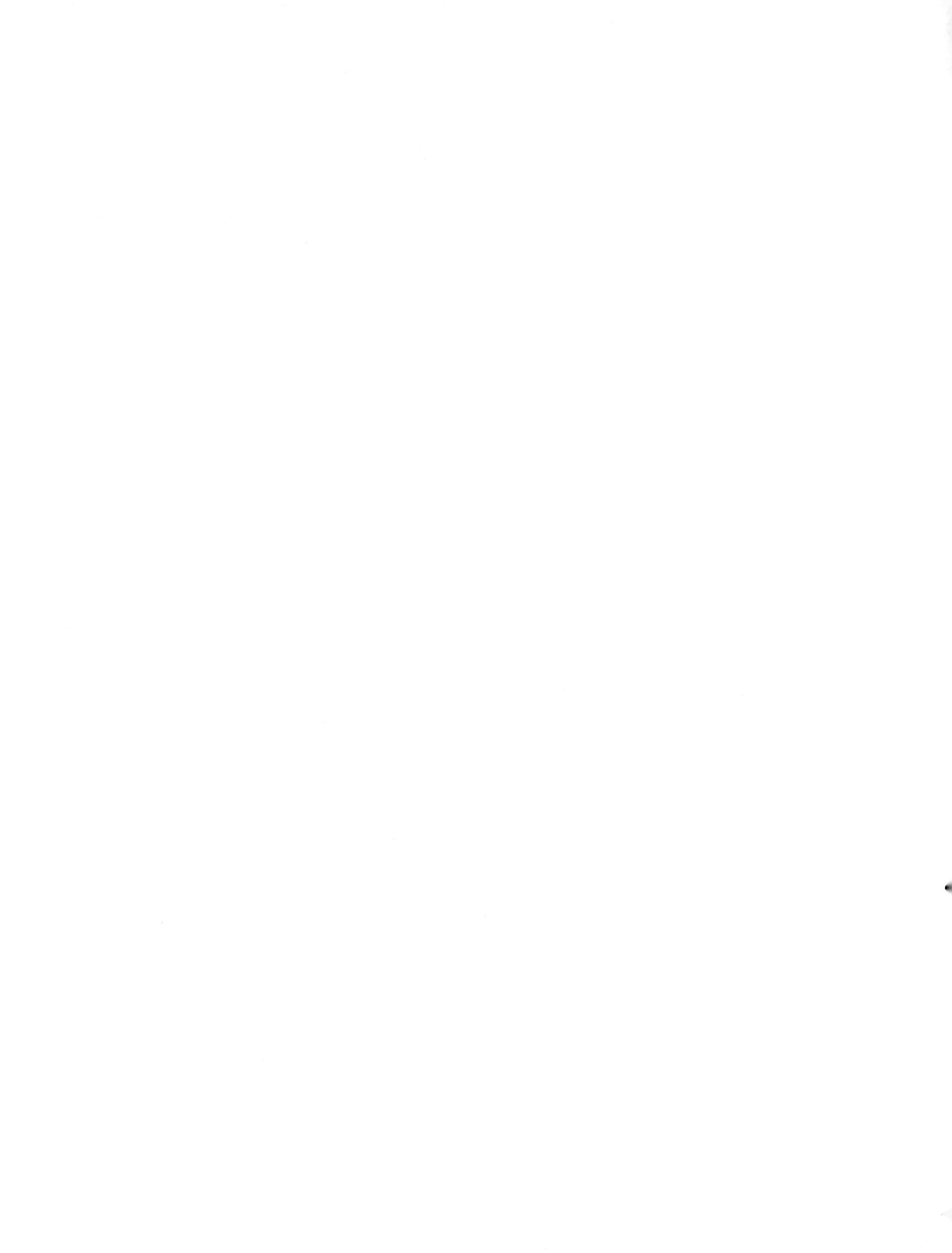

Introduction

I'm often asked why I chose nursing as my career. It seemed a natural choice, based on early years of caring for others—babysitting, teaching children how to swim, working as a volunteer in my church nursery. Nursing is all about caring for others, whether patients, their family and caregivers, students, co-workers, direct reports, and so many others that nurses interact with on a daily basis. Nurses literally help save lives and provide comfort to those in need.

Although caring for others is usually the common denominator for people choosing nursing as a career, there are a variety of specific motivators. Are there family members with a chronic or terminal illness? Do family and friends in nursing sing the praises of the profession? Do you have skills and characteristics that would make for a good nurse? Are you looking for a challenge, or long term job security? Do you simply want to make a difference in people's lives? Understanding why you are considering a career in nursing is the first step in making this monumental decision. This volume provides information that will allow you to better understand the profession, education needed to become a nurse, skills and knowledge necessary to succeed, and nursing specialties and specific nursing care components. Making a decision, especially about a career, is easier when you are equipped with as much information as possible.

Nursing is the largest healthcare profession in the United States today. More than 3 million nurses practice in a variety of settings. Many nurses work in a hospital, which offers opportunity for both general nursing, and working in specialty units such as intensive care units, operating rooms, and neonatal intensive care units. Outside of the hospital setting, however, there are many options for nurses, depending on their skills and education. For example, home health nurses work collaboratively with physicians and family members to provide care for the patient in the home setting. Faculty member nurses work to educate students in nursing programs across the country. Nurse practitioners, nurse anesthetists and clinical nurse specialists can work with physicians and surgeons, assume full responsibility for a group of patients, provide anesthesia during a surgical procedure, or provide nursing orientation to new employees. Public health nurses work in the community or in schools to better provide for a group of diversely advantaged people.

Once you have decided to become a nurse, the next important decision is selecting the right program to meet your career goals, personal goals, and financial resources. To be accepted into a nursing program requires good grades, evidence of community activities that demonstrate your commitment to others, and the ability to learn challenging information and that you can successfully impart to patients under your care. Most college-based nursing programs require good ACT or SAT scores, plus high marks on other tests that determine aptitude for the nursing curriculum.

Different nursing specialties require different education paths. For example, if you are interested in becoming a registered nurse, there are three program choices: bachelor's degree in nursing (BSN); associate's degree in nursing (ADN); diploma in nursing. A BSN, usually requiring 4 to 5 years of schooling, opens the most opportunities for advancement and is often needed to pursue advanced practice degrees such as a master's of science in nursing (MSN) or a doctorate. An associate's degree is most often a two-year program in a community college, but allows graduates of the program (like BSN graduates) to take the NCLEX-RN examination to become a registered nurse. Diploma programs in nursing are two to three-year programs that do not confer a college degree, often based in hospitals. Some diploma programs are, however, affiliated with local colleges and grant college credit. Like those with a BSN or ADN, the diploma nurse must successfully pass NCLEX-RN exam to receive a nursing license. Diploma programs have dwindled dramatically in the last 60 years. Today, diploma nurses make up 10 percent of nursing program admissions, and most hospitals prefer a BSN or ADN degree. Scholarships and grants for both college and diploma programs are available to assist with the cost of schooling.

In addition to nursing programs leading to the RN designation, the Licensed Practical Nurse (LPN) or Licensed Vocational Nurse (LVN) is a 12 to 18-month program often provided by vocational career centers or community colleges. The cost of the program is often much less than that of a BSN or ADN program and offers a faster path to employment. Some states, such as Tennessee, provide two years of community college free for LPN and LVN programs. The LPN/LVN must also take the NCLEX-PN certification examination at the completion of the program to be granted a license to practice nursing. The LPN and LVN works under the supervision of an RN in most settings. Job options for practical nurses are more limited than for registered nurses, but hospitals, nursing homes, physician offices and other settings are all potential practice sites.

Regardless of the program you select, it is smart to be as sure as possible that nursing is the career you want to pursue. Because much of the nursing curriculum is unique to the profession, transferring to another major may result in lost credits or student loan money. To help you decide, many colleges, hospitals, and physician offices will allow students to shadow or follow a nurse to understand day to day expectations.

The good news about a nursing career is that completing a nursing program almost guarantees you an immediate job with a good salary. Nursing shortages often always exist, leading to competition for new graduates, sign on bonuses, and better-than-average starting salaries. Hours of work vary with the job, but most hospitals offer three 12-hour shifts per week for a full salary, leaving four days a week to go back to school, care for your family or enjoy personal time. It's likely that weekends or nights will be part of your shifts, but days off, vacation policies, and salary usually make up for this. Most employers will pay for you to go back to school to further your nursing career, or support the pursuit of an advanced degree depending on the facilities' needs in return for you to stay in your position for a designated time. Working in a physician office, as many LPN/LVNs often do, usually pays less than a hospital, but will likely not include weekend or night work. The LPN/LVN program may be an option for the older adult seeking a career change without having the time or resources for an RN program.

Principles of Health: Nursing is designed to help you learn about the profession, help you make an educated decision about a nursing career, and understand the role of nurses in today's health care. All nurses make a difference in peoples' lives whether they choose that path right out of high school or as a second career. From birth to death, nurses are at our side.

Nursing was an excellent choice for me and opened many doors over the years. I began as a staff nurse, transitioned to teaching in a nursing program, and moved into management before retiring. Now, my nursing background allows me to do consulting and writing. I hope *Principles of Health: Nursing* encourages and educates as you consider a nursing career. There is no better choice if you want to make a difference in, or even save, peoples' lives.

—Patricia Stanfill Edens,
MS, MBA, PhD, RN, LFACHE

Contributors

Deborah A. Appello
Brick, NJ

Mihaela Avramut
*Verlan Medical Communications;
    American Medical Writers Association*

Thomas E. Baker
Florida International University

Carol A. Beehler
Independent Scholar

Dawn M. Bielawski
Wayne State University

Steven Bratman
Fort Collins, CO

Courtney Brogle
The U.S. Sun

Eric Bullard
Independent Scholar

Cait Caffrey
Independent Scholar

Josephine Campbell
Northeast Editing

Christine M. Carroll
American Medical Writers Association

Rosalyn Carson-DeWitt
Everyday Health

Robert S. Cavera
Mount Sinai South Nassau

Philip Cheng
Henry Ford Health System

Maryalice Citera
SUNY New Paltz

Patrick G. Cooper
EBSCO Information Services

Barbara Williams Cosentino
New York, NY

Everett J. Delahanty Jr.
Independent Scholar

Joseph Dewey
University of Pittsburgh

Mark Dziak
Northeast Editing

Patricia Stanfill Edens
Medical Writer

Renée Euchner
American Medical Writers Association

Merrill Evans
Tucson, AZ

C. Richard Falcon
Roberts and Raymond Associates, Philadelpha

L. Fleming Fallon, Jr.
Bowling Green State University

Fernando J. Ferrer
Carlsbad, CA

Lenela Glass-Godwin
Texas A&M University

Kimberly Glazier
Icahn School of Medicine at Mount Sinai

Carly A. Gray
Yale University

Christina Hamme Peterson
Rider University

Contributors

Angela Harmon
Independent Scholar

Robert A. Hock
University of South Carolina

David Hutto
Tetrascribe

Bruce E. Johansen
University of Nebraska, Omaha

Pamela Jones
Independent Scholar

Olivia Poteete Kerstens
Independent Scholar

M. Barbara Klyde
House Call Physicians

Marylane Wade Koch
University of Memphis, Loewenberg School of Nursing

Bill Kte'pi
Independent Scholar

Dawn Laney
Emory University

Stefan Leonte
Independent Scholar

Barb Lightner
Independent Scholar

Martha O. Loustaunau
New Mexico State University

Rebecca Lovell Scott
Independent Scholar, Sandwich, Massachusetts

Marianne M. Madsen
University of Utah

Christina Maher
Independent Scholar

Nancy Farm Mannikko
Centers for Disease Control and Prevention

Mary E. Markland
Oregon State University

Geraldine Marrocco
Yale University School of Nursing

Karen A. Mattern
Visiting Nurse Association Home Health Services

Paul Moglia
Mount Sinai South Nassau

Elizabeth Mohn
Northeast Editing

David A. Olle
Eastshire Communications Inner Medicine Publishing

Beverly B. Palmer
California State University

Crystal L. Park
University of Connecticut

Joseph G. Pelliccia
Bates College

Jane Piland-Baker
Independent Scholar

Nancy A. Piotrowski
University of California, Berkeley

Marie President
Sequoia Medical Associates

Debra S. Preston
Independent Scholar

Brian Randall
EBSCO Information Services

Elizabeth Rholetter Purdy
Independent Scholar

Bernadette Riley
New York Institute of Technology

Gina Riley
Hunter College

Andrew Schenker
Independent Scholar

Sharon W. Stark
Monmouth University

Janine Ungvarsky
Independent Scholar

Peter J. Waddell
University of South Carolina

Allyson Washburn
National University

Debra Wood
Orlando, FL

Robin L. Wulffson
American Medical Writers Association

Ling-Yi Zhou
University of St. Francis

WHAT IS NURSING?

The nine articles in this section provide a general overview of the history of nursing and how the profession has evolved over the years. Coverage includes how nurses fit into healthcare teams, general nursing processes, and challenging issues that nurses are likely to encounter, like ethical decisions and informed consent. Also discussed in this section is the balance between the autonomy of nurses vs. following doctor's orders, and a nurse's role in clinical trials.

<ul>
<li>Nursing: Its History and Evolution . . . . 3</li>
<li>Roles on the Healthcare Team . . . . 9</li>
<li>Nursing Concepts . . . . 12</li>
<li>Nursing Process . . . . 15</li>
<li>Ethics of Nursing . . . . 17</li>
<li>Autonomy and Physician Orders . . . . 19</li>
<li>Scope of Nursing Practice . . . . 21</li>
<li>Informed Consent . . . . 23</li>
<li>Clinical Research Trials . . . . 25</li>
</ul>

Nursing: Its History and Evolution

ABSTRACT

Nursing is a helping profession that focuses on the care of the sick and disabled and on the maintenance of the health and well-being of all individuals. Understanding the evolution of nursing is part of the decision-making process for entering the profession.

THE ROLE OF NURSING

Nursing and medicine are codependent and there are many ways they interrelate. While some people think that nursing began with Florence Nightingale (1820–1910), nursing is as old as medicine itself. Throughout history, there have been periods when the two fields functioned interdependently and times when they were practiced separately from each other. It seems likely that the role of the mother-nurse would have preceded the magician-priest or medicine man. Even the seeds of medical knowledge were sown by the natural remedies used by the mother.

Nurses may become involved in many areas of healthcare, including the administration of diagnostic tests, the performance of physical examinations, and assistance during surgical procedures. Nurses do not just work in hospitals. There are a variety of sites that employ nurses, including physician offices, schools, pharmaceutical companies, and others. Advanced practice nurses may practice remotely from a physician and provide primary care for a population of patients. Nurse midwives, nurses with advanced training, may deliver babies. Nurse anesthetists put patients to sleep during surgery and other procedures under the license of an anesthesiologist, a doctor with special training to put patients to sleep during surgery, and other procedures.

Over the course of human history, the words "nurse" and "nursing" have had many meanings, and the connotations have changed as tribes became highly developed and sophisticated nations. The word "nurse" comes from the Latin *nutrix*, which means "nursing mother." The word "nursing" originated from the Latin *nutrire*, meaning "to nourish." The word "nurse" as a noun was first used in the English language in the thirteenth century, being spelled "norrice," then evolving to "nurice" or "nourice," and finally to the present "nurse." The word "nurse" as a verb meant to suckle and to nourish. The meanings of both the noun and the verb have expanded to include more and more functions related to the care of all human beings. In the sixteenth century, the meaning of the noun included "a person, but usually a woman, who waits upon or tends the sick." By the nineteenth century, the meaning of the verb included "the training of those who tend the sick and the carrying out of such duties under the supervision of a physician."

With the origin of nursing as mother care came the idea that nursing was a woman's role. Suckling and nurturing were associated with maternal instincts. Ill or helpless children were also cared for by their mothers. The image of the nurse as a loving and caring mother remains popular. The true spirit of nursing, however, has no gender barriers. History has seen both men and women respond to the needs of the sick.

The role of the nurse has certainly expanded from that of the mother in the home, nourishing infants and caring for young children. Care of the sick, infirm, helpless, elderly, and handicapped and the promotion of health have become vital aspects of nursing as a whole. In history, the role of nursing developed with the culture and society of a given age. Tribal women practiced nursing as they cared for the members of their own tribes. As tribes developed into civilizations, nursing began to be practiced outside the home. As cultures developed, nursing care became more complex, and qualities other than a nurturing instinct were needed to do the work of a nurse. Members of religious orders, primarily those composed of women, responded by devoting their lives to study, service, and self-sacrifice in caring for the needs of the sick. These individuals were among the educated people of their time, and they helped set the stage for nursing to become an art and a science.

It was not until the nineteenth century that the basis of nursing as a profession was established. The beliefs and examples of Florence Nightingale laid that foundation. Nightingale was born in Italy in 1820, but she grew up in England. Unlike many of the children of her time, she was educated by governesses and by her father. Against the wishes of her family, she trained to be a nurse at the age of thirty-one. Amid enormous difficulties and prejudices, she organized and managed the nursing care for a military hospital in Turkey during the Crimean War. She returned to England after the war, where she established a school, the Nightingale Training School for Nurses, to train nurses. Again, she encountered great opposition, as nurses were considered little more than housemaids by the physicians of the time. Because of her efforts, the status of nurses was raised to a respected occupation, and the basis for professional nursing in general was established.

Nightingale's contributions are noteworthy. She recognized that nutrition is an important part of nursing care. She instituted occupational and recreational therapy for the sick and identified the personal needs of the patient and the role of the nurse in meeting those needs. Nightingale established standards for hospital management and a system of nursing education, making nursing a respected occupation for women. She recognized the two components of nursing: promoting health and treating illness. Nightingale believed that nursing is separate and distinct from medicine as a profession.

Nightingale's methods and the response of nursing to American Civil War casualties in the 1860s pointed out the need for nursing education in the United States. Schools of nursing were established, based on the values of Nightingale, but they operated more like apprenticeships than educational programs. The schools were also controlled by hospital administrators and physicians.

In 1896, nurses in the United States banded together to seek standardization of educational programs, to establish laws to ensure the competency of nurses, and to promote the general welfare of nurses. The outcome of their efforts was the American Nurses Association. In 1900, the first nursing journal, the *American Journal of Nursing*, was founded.

The effects of World War II also made clear the need to base schools of nursing on educational objectives. Many women had responded to the need for nurses during the war. A great expansion in medical knowledge and technology had taken place, and the roles of nurses were expanding as well. Nursing programs developed in colleges and universities and offered degrees in nursing to both women and men.

While there were impressive changes in the expectations and styles with which nursing care has been delivered from ancient times into the twenty-first century, the role and function of the nurse have been and continue to be diverse.

The nurse is a caregiver, providing care to patients based on knowledge and skill. Consideration is given to physical, emotional, psychological, socioeconomic, and spiritual needs. The role of the nurse-caregiver is holistic and integrated into all other roles that the nurse fulfills, thus maintaining and promoting health and well-being.

The nurse is a communicator. Using effective and therapeutic communication skills, the nurse strives to establish relationships to assist patients of all ages to manage and become responsible for their own health needs. In this way, the nurse is also a teacher who assists patients and families to meet their learning needs. Individualized teaching plans are developed and used to accomplish set goals.

The nurse is a leader. Based on the self-confidence gained from a nursing education and experience, the nurse is able to be assertive in meeting the needs of patients. The nurse facilitates change to improve care for patients, whether individually or in general. The nurse is also an advocate. Based on the belief that patients have a right to make their own decisions about health and life, the nurse strives to protect their human and legal rights in making those choices.

The nurse is a counselor. By effectively using communication skills, the nurse provides information, listens, facilitates problem-solving and decision-making abilities, and makes appropriate referrals for patients.

Finally, the nurse is a planner, a task that calls forth qualities far beyond nurturing and caring. In an age confronted with controversial topics such as abortion, organ transplants, the allocation of limited resources, and medical research, the role of nurses will continue to expand to meet these challenges in the spirit that allowed nursing to evolve and become a respected profession.

SCIENCE AND PROFESSION

While the nurse-mother of ancient times functioned within a very limited framework, the modern nurse has the choice of many careers within the nursing role. The knowledge explosion of the last century created many job specialties from which nurses can choose a career. The clinical nurse specialist is a nurse with experience, education, or an advanced degree in a specialized area of nursing. Some examples are enterostomal therapy, geriatrics, infection control, oncology, orthopedics, emergency room care, operating room care, intensive and coronary care, quality assurance, and community health. Nurses who function in such specialties carry out direct patient care; teach patients, families, and staff members; act as consultants; and sometimes conduct research to improve methods of care.

The nurse practitioner is a nurse with an advanced degree who is certified to work in a specific aspect of patient care. Nurse practitioners work in a variety of settings or in independent practice. They perform health assessments and give primary care to their patients.

The nurse anesthetist is a nurse who has also successfully completed a course of study in anesthesia. Nurse anesthetists make preoperative visits and assess patients prior to surgery, administer and monitor anesthesia during surgery, and evaluate the postoperative condition of patients.

The nurse midwife is a nurse who has successfully completed a midwifery program. The nurse midwife provides prenatal care to expectant mothers, delivers babies, and provides postnatal care after the birth.

The nurse administrator functions at various levels of management in the healthcare field. Depending on the position held, advanced education may be in business or hospital administration. The administrator is directly responsible for the operation and management of resources and is indirectly responsible for the personnel who give patient care.

The nurse educator is a nurse, usually with a master's degree, who teaches or instructs in clinical or educational settings. This nurse can teach both theory and clinical skills.

The nurse researcher usually has an advanced degree and conducts special studies that involve the collection and evaluation of data in order to report on and promote the improvement of nursing care and education.

Regardless of role, nurses must have compassion, concern for others, a willingness to be an advocate for patients in their care, and a willingness to learn. Nursing is a complex field but offers an incredible number of opportunities to those strong enough to pursue them.

DUTIES AND PROCEDURES

Creativity and education are the keys to keeping pace with continued changes and progress in the nursing profession. Nurses are expected to play many roles, function in a variety of settings, and strive for excellence in the performance of their duties. A service must be provided that contributes to the health and well-being of people. The following examples of nursing—an operating room nurse and a home health nurse—provide a limited portrait of how nurses function and what roles they play in medical care. As care specialties evolve, nurses must also expand their knowledge and skills to keep up with advances in medicine.

Operating room nurses function both directly and indirectly in patient care and render services in a number of ways. Operating room nurses, usually known as circulating nurses, briefly interview patients upon their arrival at the operating room. They accompany patients to specific surgery rooms and assist in preparing them for surgical procedures. They are responsible for seeing that surgeons correctly identify patients prior to anesthesia. They are also directly attentive to patients when anesthesia is first administered.

Circulating nurses perform the presurgical scrub, which is a cleansing of the skin with a specified solution for a given number of minutes. It is their overall responsibility to monitor aseptic (sterile) techniques in certain areas of the operating room and to deal with the situation immediately if aseptic techniques are broken. They count the surgical sponges with surgical technologists before the first incision is made, throughout the procedure as necessary, and again before the incision is closed. They secure needed items requested by surgical technologists, surgeons, or anesthesia personnel: medications, blood, additional sterile instruments, or more sponges. At times, they prepare and assist with the operation of equipment used for surgeries, such as lasers, insufflators (used for laparoscopic surgery), and blood saver and reinfuser machines. They arrange for the transportation of specimens to the laboratory. They may also be instrumental in sending communications to waiting family members when the surgery takes longer than anticipated. When the surgery is completed, they accompany patients to the recovery room with the anesthesia personnel.

Home health nurses, on the other hand, function in a very different manner. This type of nurse usually works for a private home health services agency, or as part of an outreach program for home services through a hospital. Referrals come to the agency or program via the physician, through the physician's office, by way of the social services department in a hospital, or by an individual requesting skilled services through the physician.

The following scenario is an example of a patient whom a home health nurse may be requested to see: a seventy-six-year-old man who was hospitalized with a recent diagnosis of diabetes mellitus, for which he is now insulin-dependent. He also has an open wound on his right ankle. The number of days allowed for hospitalization for his diagnosis has expired, but he still needs help using a glucometer to take his blood sugar readings and assistance with drawing up his insulin. He still has questions about how to manage his diabetes, especially the dietary parameters. He is unable to manage the wound care on his right ankle. His wife is willing to assist him, but she has no knowledge about diabetes or wound care.

The home health nurse performs the following assessments on the initial visit: general physical condition, the patient's level of knowledge and understanding and his ability to manage his diabetic condition, all medications used, and the patient's understanding of the actions, side effects, and interactions of these medications. An assessment is made of the home setting in general: the patient's safety, the support system, and any special needs, such as assistive devices. If services such as physical therapy, speech therapy, or occupational therapy are needed, the nurse makes these referrals. If the patient requires additional in-home services, a referral to a medical social worker is made. Wound care is performed, and the nurse will then set up a plan of care, with the patient's input, for follow-up visits. Guidelines requested by the physician, as well as approval needed by health insurance companies covering the cost for home health services, will be taken into consideration when planning ongoing visits. If the home health agency has a nurse who is

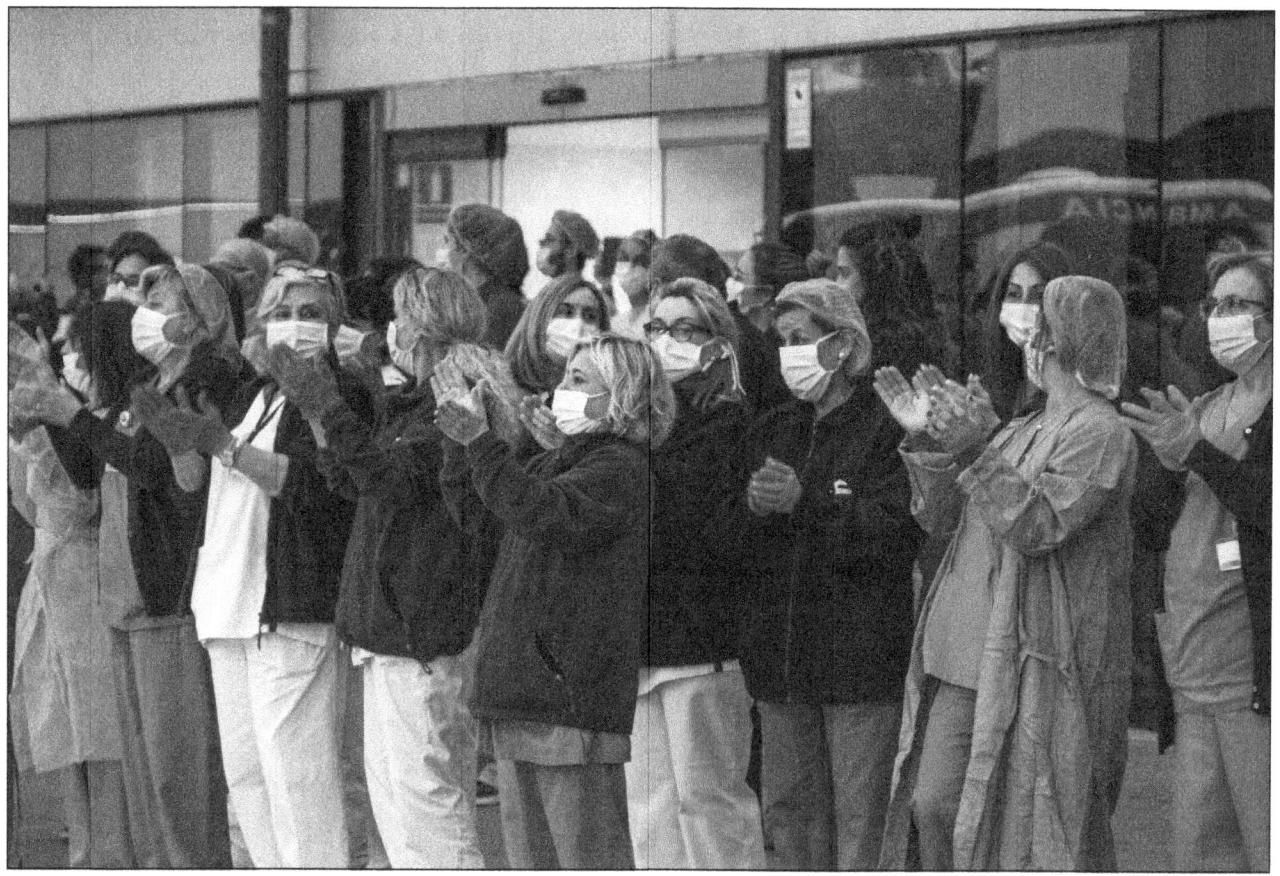

An appreciation for care workers event. Nursing will continue to meet the challenge to improve the quality of health care around the world. (mediamasmedia via iStock)

a diabetic specialist, the nurse can either consult with that specialist about the care of this patient or have the diabetic specialist make a home visit.

PERSPECTIVE AND PROSPECTS

From the beginning of time, nursing and the role of the nurse have been defined by the people and the society of a particular age. Nursing as it is known today is still influenced by what occurred over the centuries.

In primitive times, people believed that illness was supernatural, caused by evil gods. The roles of the physician and the nurse were separate and unrelated. The physician was a medicine man, sometimes called a shaman or a witch doctor, who treated disease by ritualistic chants, by fear or shock techniques, or by boring holes into a person's skull with a sharp stone to allow the evil spirit or demon an escape. The nurse, on the other hand, was usually the mother who tended to family members and provided for their physical needs, using herbal remedies when they were ill.

As tribes evolved, the centers for medical care were temples. Some tribes believed that illness was caused by sin and the displeasure of gods. The physician of this age was a priest and was held in high regard. The nurse was a woman, seen as a slave, who performed menial tasks ordered by the priest-physician.

Living in the same era were Hebrew tribes who used the Ten Commandments and the Mosaic Health Code to develop standards for ethical human relationships, mental health treatment, and disease control. Nurses visited the sick in their homes, practiced as midwives, and provided for the physical and spiritual needs of family members who cared for the ill. These nurses provided a family-centered approach to care.

With the advent of Christianity, the value of the individual was emphasized, and the responsibility for recognizing the needs of each individual emerged. Nursing gained an elevated position in society. A spiritual foundation for nursing was established as well. The first organized visiting of the sick was done by deaconesses and Christian Roman matrons of the time. Members of male religious orders also cared for the sick and buried the dead.

During the time of the Crusades, there were both male and female nursing orders, and nursing at this time was a respected vocation. Men usually belonged to military nursing orders, who cared for the sick, on one hand, and defended the hospital when it was under attack, on the other. In medieval times, hospitals became a place to keep, not cure, patients. There were no methods of infection control. Nursing care was largely custodial, and the practice of accepting individuals of low character to supplement inadequate nursing staffs became common.

The worst era in nursing history was probably from 1500 to 1860. Nursing at this time was not a respected profession. Women who had committed a crime were sent into nursing as an alternative to serving a jail term. Nurses received poor wages and worked long hours under deplorable conditions. Changes in the Reformation and the Renaissance did little or nothing to improve the care of the sick. The attitude prevailed that nursing was a religious and not an intellectual occupation. Charles Dickens quite aptly portrayed the nurse and nursing conditions of the time through his caricatures of Sairey Gamp and Betsey Prig in *Martin Chuzzlewit* (1843–1844).

It was not until the middle of the nineteenth century that this situation began to change. Through Nightingale's efforts, nursing became a respected occupation once more, the quality of nursing care improved tremendously, and the foundation was laid for modern nursing education.

By 2018, the issue of quality patient care in the nursing field had been brought to the forefront once more when advocates, particularly nursing unions, in the state of Massachusetts began strongly pushing for a legal limit to the number of patients that can be assigned to each nurse within the period of a shift. Those in favor of such a measure, which had been in place in California since the early twenty-first century, argued that setting a limit on the number of patients allows for improved treatment results. On the other hand, some medical professionals and groups have expressed concern that setting these limits would require hiring additional staff and cutting costs in other crucial areas.

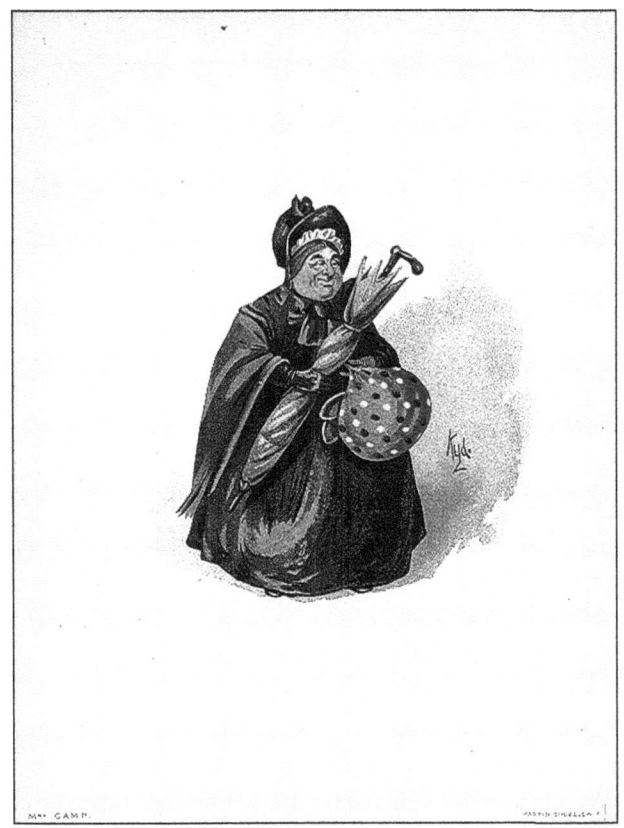

Dickens's Sairey Gamp character became a notorious stereotype of untrained and incompetent nurses of the early Victorian era, before the reforms of campaigners like Florence Nightingale. (Wikimedia Commons)

As innovations in healthcare have an impact on nursing, nurses' roles will continue to expand in the future. Nursing can also be a background from which both men and women begin to bridge gaps of service where other affiliations are needed: computer science, medical-legal issues, health insurance agencies, and bioethics, to name a few. The words of Florence Nightingale still echo as a challenge to the nursing profession:

> *May the methods by which every infant, every human being will have the best chance of health, the methods by which every sick person will have the best chance of recovery, be learned and practiced! Hospitals are only an intermediate state of civilization never intended, at all events, to take in the whole sick population.*

Nursing will continue to meet this challenge to improve the quality of healthcare around the world.

—*Karen A. Mattern*

Further Reading

Black, Beth Perry. *Professional Nursing: Concepts and Challenges*. 7th ed., Elsevier, 2014

Brown, Di, et al. *Lewis's Medical-Surgical Nursing: Assessment and Management of Clinical Problems*. 4th ed., Mosby, 2015.

Delaune, Sue C., and Patricia K. Ladner, editors. *Fundamentals of Nursing: Standards and Practices*. 4th ed., Delmar Thomson, 2011.

Dolan, Josephine A., et al. *Nursing in Society: A Historical Perspective*. 15th ed., W. B. Saunders, 1983.

Donahue, M. Patricia. *Nursing: The Finest Art*. 3rd ed., Mosby, 2011.

"Is Nursing the Right Profession for You?" *EveryNurse*, everynurse.org/blog/is-nursing-right-for-you/. Accessed 3 Sept. 2020.

Kozier, Barbara, et al. *Fundamentals of Nursing: Concepts, Process, and Practice*. 2nd ed., Pearson, 2012.

"Licensed Practical and Licensed Vocational Nurses." US Bureau of Labor Statistics, *Occupational Outlook Handbook*, 13 Apr. 2018, www.bls.gov/ooh/healthcare/licensed-practical-and-licensed-vocational-nurses.htm.

"Nursing Definitions." *International Council of Nurses*, www.icn.ch/nursing-policy/nursing-definitions. Accessed 2 Sept. 2020.

Park, Melissa, et al. "Nurse Practitioners, Certified Nurse Midwives, and Physician Assistants in Physician Offices." *Centers for Disease Control and Prevention*, 17 Aug. 2011,

Quinn, Mattie. "Should Hospitals Limit the Number of Patients Nurses Can Help?" *Governing*, 12 Sept. 2018, www.governing.com/topics/health-human-services/gov-massachusetts-ballot-nurses-patient-ratio-healthcare.html.

Reising, Virginia A. "What Is a Nurse?" *American Journal of Nursing*, vol. 119, no. 6, June 2019.

"Registered Nurses." US Bureau of Labor Statistics, *Occupational Outlook Handbook*, 13 Apr. 2018, www.bls.gov/ooh/healthcare/registered-nurses.htm.

Riley, Julia Balzer. *Communication in Nursing*. 8th ed., Elsevier, 2017.

Taylor, Carol, et al. *Fundamentals of Nursing: The Art and Science of Nursing Care*. 9th ed., Wolters Kluwer, 2018.

"What Is Nursing?" *American Nurses Association*, www.nursingworld.org/practice-policy/workforce/what-is-nursing/. Accessed 2 Sept. 2020.

ROLES ON THE HEALTHCARE TEAM

ABSTRACT

A healthcare team is a group of medical professionals who are responsible for overseeing the care of patients. Although the makeup of the healthcare team differs according to the specific setting in which they operate, most healthcare teams contain, at the minimum, a doctor and a registered nurse, although in some cases a physician assistant or nurse practitioner may replace the doctor.

MAKEUP OF HEALTHCARE TEAMS

From the smallest clinics to the largest hospitals and medical centers, a patient's care is entrusted not to a single medical professional but to a team of dedicated workers. At the minimum, this team usually consists of a physician and a registered nurse. In some cases, particularly in rural settings, the physician may be replaced by a physician assistant or nurse practitioner. In larger settings, there are many more professionals who make up the healthcare team. These may include additional specialists—either doctors or nurses—for example, a hospitalist physician, an anesthesiologist or a nurse anesthetist. They may also include physical or occupational therapists, clinical pharmacists, dietitians, social workers, office managers, or a patient transport team. A patient may not interact with all of his or her healthcare team, but each member serves an essential role in providing healthcare service.

In a hospital setting, there are a number of clearly defined roles on a patient's healthcare team that are designed to provide effective and efficient care. Chief among these professionals are the patient's attending physician. The attending physician is the chief doctor assigned to a patient and is responsible for making the decisions that affect that patient's care. The attending physician may be a hospitalist, a doctor who cares specifically for hospitalized patients but does so with a generalist's scope, or a specialist such as a cardiologist or pulmonologist. Working under the supervision of the attending physician in teaching hospitals are residents and interns, licensed physicians who are gaining practical experience in their field before practicing on their own. One or more residents often help make up a hospital healthcare team. In smaller hospitals, often in rural settings, the patient may not encounter residents and interns.

In a hospital setting, the nursing staff is usually supervised by a nurse manager, who oversees the unit's daily operations, and/or a charge nurse, who manages nursing shifts while still working in patient care.

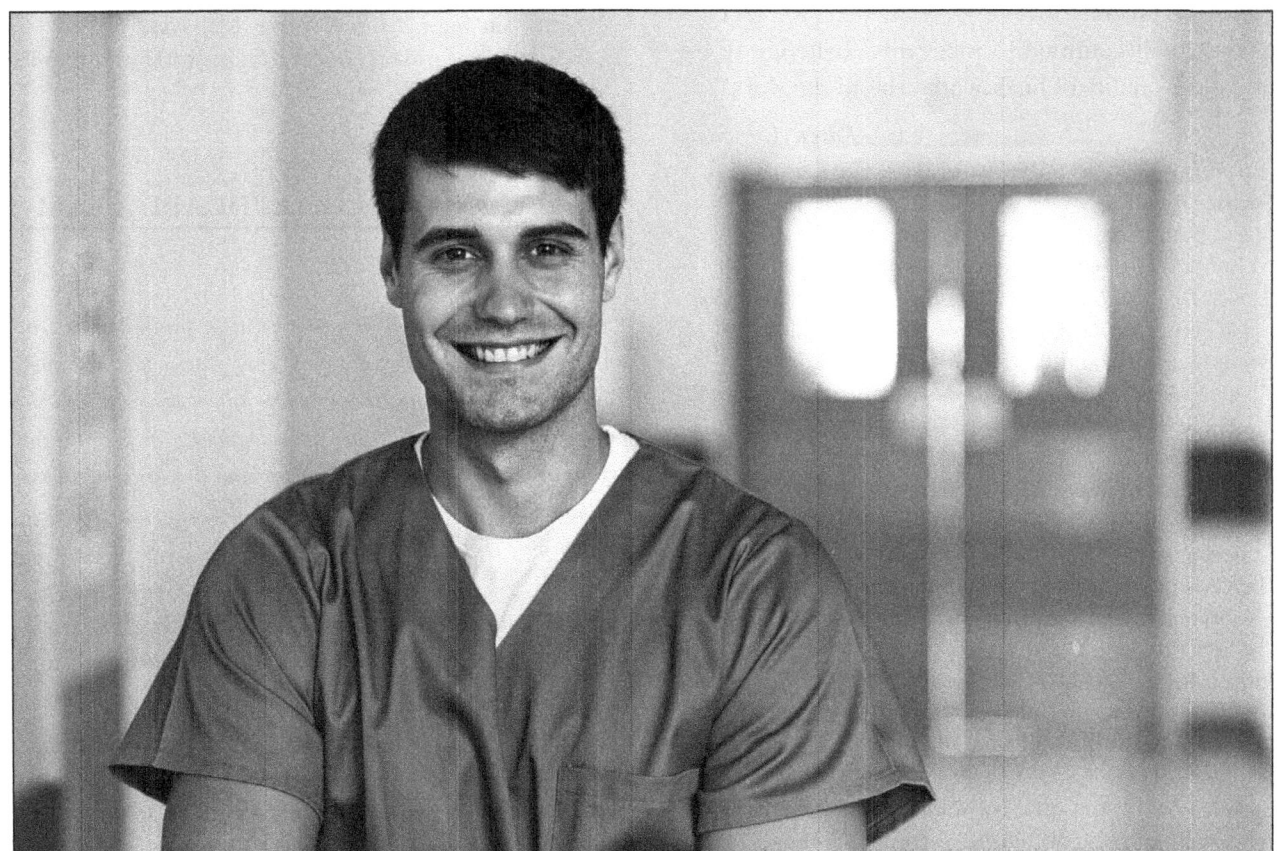

The true spirit of nursing has no gender barriers. History has seen both men and women respond to the needs of the sick. (shapecharge via iStock)

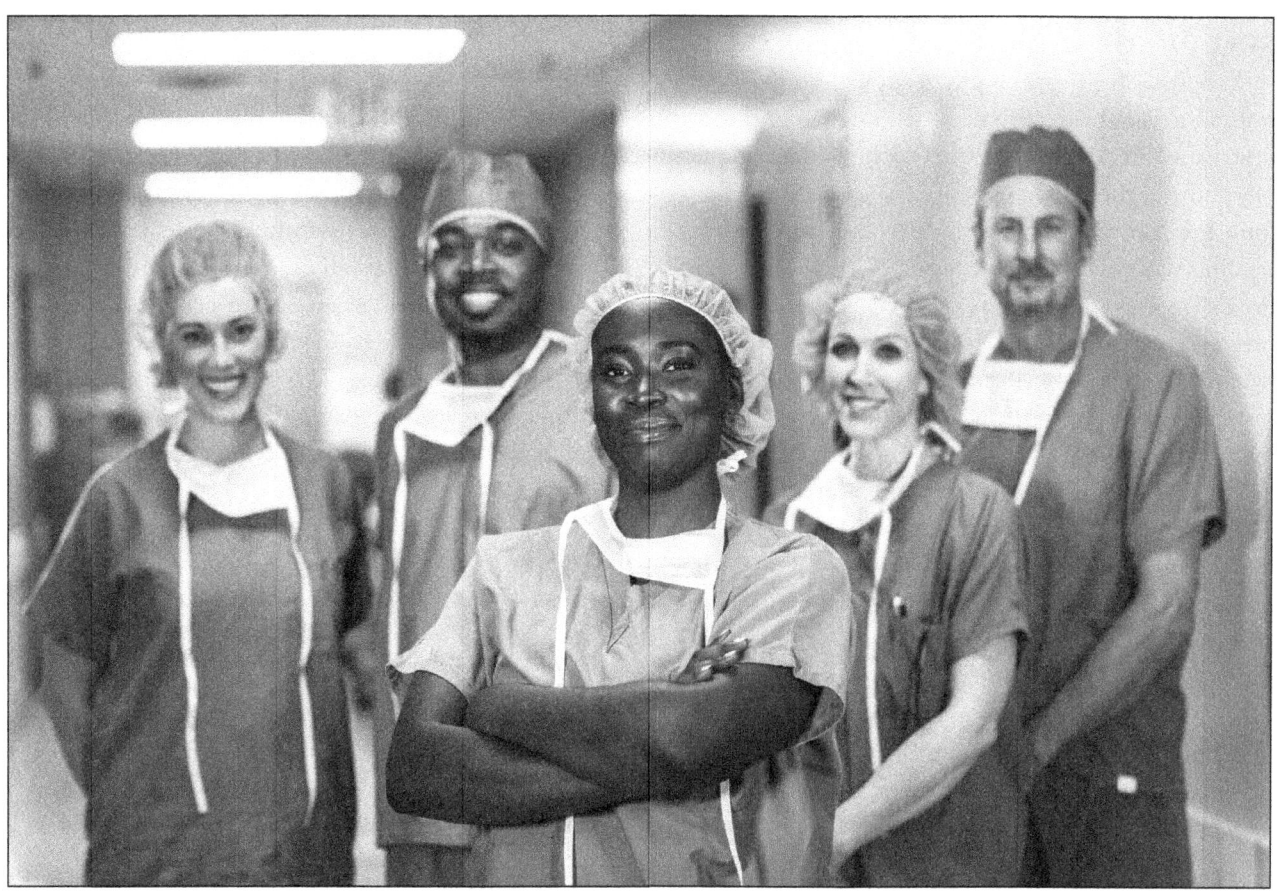
Communication and teamwork are a large part of nurses' success (kali9 via iStock)

Under these managers, work a team of nurses who provide much of the day-to-day care for patients. A patient will typically be assigned a primary nurse who is directly responsible for their care. A primary nurse will usually be a registered nurse (RN) but may also be licensed practical nurse (LPN) or licensed vocational nurse (LVN). Other nursing professionals that may be involved in a patient's care include a clinical nurse specialist (CNS), who is a master's-prepared nurse with specialized knowledge in a specific area; a nurse practitioner (NP), who may provide more direct patient care; and a certified nursing assistant (CNA).

There are also numerous other healthcare professionals that may be part of a healthcare team in a hospital setting. Among the most significant are therapists. These include physical therapists (PTs) who help patients rehabilitate the functioning of their large motor groups; occupational therapists (OTs) who help patients recover the skills needed for daily living; speech therapists; respiratory therapists; and recreation/milieu therapists. Other possible members of a patient's larger healthcare team include clinical pharmacists, dietitians, social and case management workers, Rapid Response Team (RRT) clinicians, and the patient transport team. Administrators may also be considered as part of the healthcare team. In doctor's offices, for example, office managers play an important role in providing healthcare by improving the efficiency and quality of the medical treatment the office provides and managing day-to-day operations including billing.

ROLE OF NURSES ON THE HEALTHCARE TEAM

Although in most cases a physician will play the lead role on a healthcare team, nurses often spend more time providing one-on-one care to the patient and are often the patient's first point of contact. RNs are found on almost every healthcare team and they are qualified to perform many significant medical functions. They assess patient's conditions, write nursing care plans, administer medications, provide patient treatments, help perform and analyze diagnostic tests, and help patients manage illnesses or injuries including discharge teaching. Hospitals, doctor's offices, and other institutions may also employ LPNs or LVNs, professionals who typically work under the supervision of doctors and RNs. Among the tasks that LPNs may perform are maintaining patient records, monitoring the patient's vital signs, administering some medications, assisting doctors and nurses with tests, and helping patients eat, dress, and bathe.

Advanced practice registered nurses (APRNs) are nursing professionals who possess an advanced degree, either a master's or a doctorate, and are often given the autonomy to take on a greater role on the healthcare team. For example, NPs may function as a primary or specialty care provider in place of a physician. In twenty-three states, they are given full practicing authority, although in the others they must work under the supervision, even if indirect, of a physician. Either way, they are legally allowed to examine patients, diagnose illnesses, prescribe medications, and provide treatments. Certified registered nurse anesthetists (CRNAs) administer anesthesia and provide care throughout surgical, diagnostic, or other procedures. CRNAs administer about half of the anesthesia given to patients in the United States and are the main providers of anesthesia in the military, maternity units, and in rural and underserved communities. As with nurse practitioners, CRNAs are allowed to operate independently in a number of states, currently seventeen, while in others, they are required to operate under the supervision of a physician. CNSs are another group of advanced practice nurses who are granted a good deal of autonomy within the healthcare team. They provide direct patient care in a specific area of expertise, such as pediatrics or psychiatric health, while often taking on leadership roles in a hospital or clinical setting. They may also be involved in educating staff or in performing research.

Caring for patients requires a variety of staff with expertise needed by the patient at a particular point in their illness and recovery. The healthcare team provides for the patient from diagnosis to hospitalization to home care or rehabilitation, and ultimately to recovery.

—*Andrew Schenker*

Further Reading

Bendaly, Leslie, and Nicole Bendaly. *Improving Healthcare Team Performance: The 7 Requirements for Excellence in Patient Care*. John Wiley & Sons, 2012.
"Understanding the Healthcare Team." *Creaky Joints*, creakyjoints.org/about/what-is-the-healthcare-team/. Accessed 9 Oct. 2020.
Weiss, Donna, et al. *The Interprofessional Health Care Team: Leadership and Development*. 2nd ed., Jones & Bartlett Learning, 2018.
"Who's Who on Your Hospital Team." *Patient Care Link*, patientcarelink.org/for-patients-families/whos-who-on-your-hospital-team/. Accessed 9 Oct. 2020.
"Your Health Care Team." University of Rochester Medicine, Strong Memorial Hospital, www.urmc.rochester.edu/strong-memorial/patients-families/health-care-team.aspx. Accessed 9 Oct. 2020.

NURSING CONCEPTS

ABSTRACT

There are four main concepts of nursing: person, health, environment, and nursing. Each of these concepts are defined and described by a nursing theorist.

NURSING METAPARADIGM

The nursing metaparadigm is a general presentation of the framework on which conceptual models develop. This theoretical framework focuses on the relationships between four major concepts. These concepts are person, environment, health, and nursing. Nursing theories flow from these four concepts. For example, Florence Nightingale defined the Environmental Theory as using the patient's environment to enhance recovery. Imogene King's Theory of Goal Attainment states that the nurse-patient relationship is focused on meeting goals leading to good health. Sr. Callista Roy's theory viewed the person as a set of interrelated systems with the goal of maintaining system balance in the presence of various stimuli. Ida Jean Orlando defined in her theory based on the concept of Nursing that the relationship between the nurse and the patient should be reciprocal, meaning the nurse must find out and meet the patient's immediate needs.

The nursing theorists all utilize the four major concepts in defining their theories but each brings their own nursing experience, orientation, and other factors into their definitions. The goal of the four main concepts is to provide the foundation for definitions, statements, and assumptions that make up nursing. Interrelationships between the four concepts comprise the basis for nursing and guide the development of knowledge, education, research, and practice.

PERSON

Person may be defined as the client, the patient, or the human being who receives nursing care. Person may include individuals, groups, families, and communities. The term "person" takes into consideration the whole person, not just the rationale for nursing

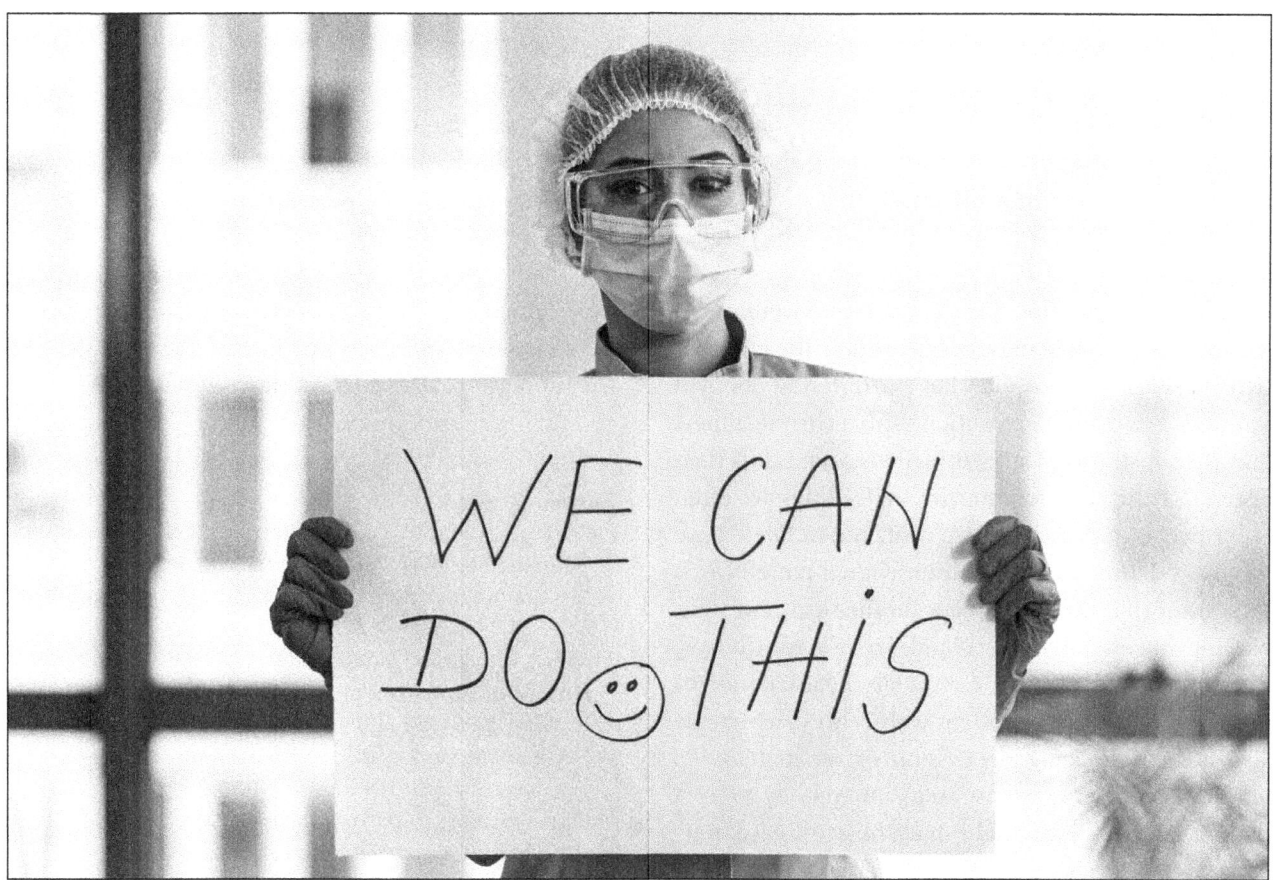

When the challenges facing healthcare workers seem overwhelming, perserverence is key (Drazen Zigic via iStock)

care. The whole person includes the psychological, physical, social, cultural, and spiritual needs of the patient in addition to the patient's medical condition.

ENVIRONMENT

The environment or situation that clients or patients operate in include both internal and external impacts. These impacts may be positive or negative such as prolonged poor health, poverty or good physical fitness. The physical environment of the patient such as home, work, and setting of healthcare is also part of this concept. Supportive families or friends or lack of support are also part of the environment of the client. The patient's environment includes access to healthcare. Patients in urban areas with high-level facilities are more likely than patient's in rural areas with limited access to care to achieve optimal outcomes. Individuals with insurance are more likely than those without to receive a different level of care. The environment is made up of a variety of factors that need to be assessed in determining the role of nursing care for the individual patient.

HEALTH

Health is better defined as the degree of wellness or the feeling of well-being experienced by the client or patient. Each patient may have a different level of wellness. For example, a patient with a chronic illness may demonstrate a degree of wellness that is less than optimal. Patients in long-term care facilities are often described as in poor health. Health and wellness have different definitions for each individual patient. It is important that the nurse focus on the health of their patients in general, not just on the reason for the hospitalization, for example. Secondary health concerns influence outcomes. A patient with heart disease may also be experiencing depression or an inability to maintain sufficient exercise to maintain body tone. A patient with cancer may also have heart disease. Recognizing all levels of health and wellness of patients and communicating with the physician is important to support this concept in nursing care.

NURSING

The nurse is responsible for nursing care of the client or patient. The actions of nursing care are focused on improving patient care, which is also the ultimate goal of nursing theories based on the four concepts. The nurse works with the client or patient to define what care will best achieve the optimal outcome for the individual. The concept of Nursing encompasses leadership, decision-making, care planning, and care delivery in meeting the patient's needs. Working within the healthcare team, communicating findings related to care, and easing suffering all flow from the fourth concept.

SUMMARY

The four main concepts of nursing on which nursing theories are based provides a strong foundation for nursing practice but the integration of these concepts into care delivery is crucial. Nursing care delivery is complex and must include all components that influence the response of the patient to the care delivered by the nurse and the healthcare team. Meeting the patient's essential needs as well as any corollary needs is the ultimate goal of nursing care.

—*Andrew Schenker*

Further Reading

Deliktas, A., O. Korukcu, R. Aydin, and K. Kabukcuoglu. "Nursing Students' Perceptions of Nursing Metaparadigms: A Phenomenological Study." *Journal of Nursing Research*, vol. 27, no. 5, Oct. 2019.

Mudd, A., R. Feo, T. Conroy, and A. Kitson. "Where and How Does Fundamental Care Fit within Seminal Nursing Theories: A Narrative Review and Synthesis of Key Nursing Concepts." *Journal of Clinical Nursing*, vol. 29, Oct. 2020, pp. 19–20, www.ncbi.nlm.nih.gov/pmc/articles/PMC7540068/.

Upson, Margo. "What Are Fundamental Nursing Concepts?" *Career Trend*, careertrend.com/

list-6196507-fundamental-nursing-concepts-html. Accessed 19 Oct. 2020.

Wayne, Gil. "Nursing Theories and Theorists." *Nurseslabs*, nurseslabs.com/nursing-theories/. Accessed 19 Oct. 2020.

Nursing Process

ABSTRACT

The nursing process, defined by nursing theorist Ida Jean Orlando in 1958, is a systematic approach to providing nursing care. It utilizes critical thinking, goal-oriented tasks, patient or client centered treatment, evidence-based practice and nursing intuition to plan quality care for a patient or client.

INTRODUCTION

The nursing process is the foundation for nursing care provided to a patient. It serves as a "roadmap" for care provided during a hospitalization, illness, or chronic condition. It is systematic, patient centered care with five steps that are considered sequential, recognizing that revisions over time may be required. The five steps are Assessment, Diagnosis, Planning, Implementation, and Evaluation. Written documentation of the nursing process is referred to as a nursing care plan. The nursing process is a core learning element of any nursing program and a care plan is written to document the plan of care derived from the steps of the nursing process. All student nurses will learn how to write a plan of care based on assigned patients during their education. The nursing process remains a crucial part of nursing throughout a nursing career. The Joint Commission, the international accrediting body for hospitals and health providers, requires a written plan of care to facilitate communication about the patient and between nurses. Often this plan of care is electronic and part of the permanent patient record and may be evaluated and added to by nurses caring for the patient. In some instances, other healthcare professionals may add to the plan of care.

ASSESSMENT

The first steps in assessment are critical thinking, observation, and data collection. The nurse must employ critical thinking to determine what is going on with the patient. When you first meet the patient after reviewing available chart data, what do you think and see that can help plan the care the patient will need going forward? Data may be objective such as vital signs, laboratory results or height, weight and blood pressure measurements or subjective such as observation of skin color, mobility and statements from the patient, family, or caregivers. Most hospitals use an electronic documentation system that may be programmed to add data into the plan of care.

DIAGNOSIS

A nursing diagnosis is formed based on knowledge gained through education and experience, observations of the patient and data gathered during the assessment. Clinical judgments guide and shape the planning and implementation of care. NANDA International, formerly known as the North American Nursing Diagnosis Association (NANDA), provides nursing diagnoses that use standardized terminology to enhance nursing practice. NANDA International's purpose is to develop, refine and promote terminology to accurately direct clinical judgments with evidence-based nursing diagnoses that direct interventions and outcomes and contribute to patient safety. Examples of nursing diagnoses include readiness for enhanced health literacy, ineffective adolescent eating dynamics, risk of metabolic imbalance syndrome, and risk for unstable blood pressure.

Abraham Maslow defined a Hierarchy of Needs based on fundamental needs of individuals and states that basic physiological needs must be met before higher needs may be achieved. Basic needs such as nutrition, elimination, breathing, and sleep are examples of basic physiological needs. Safety and security, love and belonging, self-esteem and self-actualization complete the hierarchy. Use of Maslow's Hierarchy is an important part of the nursing process.

PLANNING

Once the assessment is complete and a nursing diagnoses is formulated, the planning process begins. Planning encompasses learned knowledge, observations and data, and a nursing diagnosis that reflects the individualized needs of the patient. A problem-solving approach to patient needs based on evidence is the foundation of care planning. Evidence-based practice (EBP) comes from well-designed studies of patient care interventions, patient values, input and preferences, and the nurse's knowledge gained from education and experience.

Specific goals and desired outcomes are defined to directly influence patient care. Nursing care plans are goal and outcome directed and provide guidance to meet a patient's individual need for care. The plan of care promotes continuity of care, communication between nurses, documentation and support for reimbursement. Goals must be specific, measurable, action oriented and attainable, realistic for the patient and timely based on the time interaction between the nurse and the patient. For example, a goal for a patient post open heart surgery should not be able to run a marathon the day after discharge from the hospital. A more specific and obtainable goal might be to be able to walk fifty steps to the toilet before discharge. Planning involves writing actionable goals that are realistic and measurable.

IMPLEMENTATION

Once the plan of care has been written and actions have been listed, implementation occurs. Implementation involves providing nursing care based on the nursing care plan. Nursing interventions such as assisting the patient with walking or providing diet instruction are done to achieve the goals stated in the planning phase. Delivering nursing care based on assessment, nursing diagnoses and planning comes from basic nursing education, orientation to the job role, continuing education and in-service to enhance skills once on the job and seeking out resources to enhance the patient experience. Implementation may also include other health professionals. For example, enhancing a stroke patient's ability to communicate may also involve speech and occupational therapists. Caring for a patient is a team approach.

EVALUATION

Once nursing care is implemented, the patient response should be evaluated. Nursing interventions are designed to create a specific outcome. The evaluation process is critical to determining whether the nursing care provided achieved the desired outcome. A reassessment of the patient and an adjustment of the nursing care plan, particularly with chronically ill patients or patients moving from acute care to rehabilitative care, is indicated as needed. For example, walking fifty steps to the toilet must be achieved before discharge in order for the patient to self-care at home. If some nursing interventions are not realized, referral to a rehabilitation facility or nursing home may need to occur. This phase of the nursing care planning process is important to recognize that goals have been met or adjusted to best meet the needs of the patient.

SUMMARY

The care of the patient is dynamic and complex and requires all members of the healthcare team to work in unity to achieve desired outcomes. The nursing care plan is crucial to assuring desired outcomes. Just as the doctor leads the medical interventions for the patient, the nurse is often seen as the leader of the care team and will interact with other health professionals involved in patient care to accomplish nursing and other disciplines' goals. A comprehensive, well-constructed nursing care plan will be an excellent guide for nurses and all health professionals involved in the care of the patient.

—*Patricia Stanfill Edens*

Further Reading

"Accreditation and Certifications." *Standards*, www.jointcommission.org. Accessed 16 Sept. 2020.

"Evidence-Based Practice." *Nurse.com*, www.nurse.com/evidence-based-practice. Accessed 16 Sept. 2020.

"Free Care Plans." *RegisteredNurseRN.com*, www.registerednursern.com/free-care-plans/. Accessed 16 Sept. 2020.

Herdman, T. H., and S. Kamitsuru, editors. *Nursing Diagnoses: Definitions and Classifications 2018-2020*. (NANDA International Nursing Diagnoses.) Thieme, 2017.

"Nursing at the Joint Commission." *The Joint Commission*, www.jointcommission.org/resources/for-nurses/. Accessed 16 Sept. 2020.

Shih, C. Y., and C. Y. Huang. "The Association of Sociodemographic Factors and Needs of Haemodialysis Patients According to Maslow's Hierarchy of Needs." *Journal of Clinical Nursing*, vol. 28, nos. 1-2, pp. 270–78.

Toney-Butler, U. J., and J. M. Thayer. Nursing Process. National Institutes of Health. US National Library of Medicine. *National Center for Biotechnology Information*, www.ncbi.nlm.nih.gov/books/NBK499937/. Accessed 16 Sept. 2020.

ETHICS OF NURSING

ABSTRACT

Nurses face a host of ethical issues every day on the job. Charged with delivering the best possible health outcome for their patients, they may come under conflicting imperatives. Among the ethical issues nurses commonly face are privacy, informed consent, end-of-life, problematic workplace environments, and moral distress.

NURSING CODE OF ETHICS

Because of the sensitive nature of the work that nurses do—in which patients literally put their lives in their hands—and the complexities of the healthcare system, the profession is frequently subject to a number of moral dilemmas which the individual nurse must solve in order to provide the best possible care. These moral quandaries may arise in a number of areas in the course of a nurse's daily practice, but some of the most common might involve privacy, informed consent, end-of-life issues, difficult workplace environments, and moral distress, which is defined as a situation when a nurse knows the right thing to do but is not allowed or not able to do it. To help nurses with these difficult situations, the American Nurses Association (ANA) has developed a formal code, known officially as the Code of Ethics for Nurses with Interpretive Statements.

The idea of a nursing code of ethics dates back to 1893, when it was first suggested by Florence Nightingale. Modifying the Hippocratic Oath taken by physicians, she came up with a similar recitation that became known as the "Nightingale Pledge." Her efforts were codified in the 1950s when the ANA first developed a formal code. The code has undergone several changes since, but its core values of ethical guidance remain. Many states have incorporated the code into their individual Nurse Practice Acts.

The code is designed, according to the ANA, to offer guidance to nurses in "carrying out nursing responsibilities in a manner consistent with quality in nursing care and the ethical obligations of the profession." In service of this goal, the code identifies four main principles that should guide the ethical conduct of nurses. These principles are autonomy, the recognition of each patient's right to self-determination and decision-making; beneficence, the acting on the behalf of patient's wellness and best interests; justice, the idea that all patients be treated fairly; and nonmaleficence, the charge to do no harm. In 2015, the code was revised to include nine provisions—the "Interpretative Statements" of the title—that expand on the core principles and offer nurses additional guidance. These provisions affirm such principles as that the nurse's primary commitment is to the patient, and that the nurse is charged with collaborating with other health professionals to "protect human rights, promote health diplomacy, and reduce health disparities."

COMMON ETHICAL DILEMMAS

Although the ANA's code, along with the ethics committees in individual institutions, offer plenty of moral guidance to nurses, each professional inevitably faces ethically difficult situations that cannot be simply resolved by consulting these resources. One of the most significant moral dilemmas in the nursing profession is the question of privacy. Nurses and other medical professionals are bound by the Health Insurance Portability and Accountability Act of 1996 (HIPAA). This law created national standards that protect a patient's right to privacy. This law codifies the basic ethical issue of a patient's right not to have their information shared. Nurses and other practitioners are given access to privileged information to the patient and it is their moral duty not to unfairly disclose these details. Determining what a reasonable disclosure, though, can be a tricky issue. A health practitioner may, for example, wish to discuss the case with a patient's family or with their colleagues, against the patient's wishes.

Another ethical issue facing the nursing profession is informed consent. Informed consent is a process by which a patient is adequately informed about the treatment he or she is to receive and gives knowing permission. It is a process that is central to the principle of autonomy, one of the ANA code's four core principles. This commitment to informed consent may become complicated if a family member wishes the nurse to withhold information from a patient. This may especially be true when it comes to end-of-life decision-making. Often, a dying patient, due to cognitive difficulties or unconsciousness, is not able to make an informed decision. In these cases, the decision-making responsibility may fall to a family member. Many individuals compose advance healthcare directives, also known as living wills, to legally dictate what should be done to them if they become unable to make their own decisions. A patient may also delegate power of attorney to another individual or name a healthcare proxy. This allows the designated individual to make decisions on the patient's behalf.

Other ethical issues may involve the specific environment in which the nurse works. A nurse may notice that a colleague on their team is not competent to perform their work, or they may encounter communication difficulties or such negative behaviors as bullying. Navigating such an environment can be very difficult and nurses may not always feel comfortable addressing such behavior. Other environmental issues may include the nurse's inability to provide the proper level of care because of a staffing shortage or other institutional issue such as lack of sufficient medical equipment. In these cases, the nurse may suffer from what is known as moral distress. This results from a nurse wanting to treat a patient properly but being unable to do so.

CONCLUSION

Every nurse, at some point in their career, will encounter ethical dilemmas for which there is no clear correct answer. There are numerous resources that these nurses can draw on, from the American Nursing Association's code of ethics, to the individual ethics committees at their institution, to more experienced colleagues. Still, only with personal experience in handling ethical dilemmas that may crop up over the nurse's many years of professional practice can he or she establish a personal framework for handling these difficult, but inevitable, situations.

—*Andrew Schenker*

Further Reading

Butts, Jane B. and Karen L. Rich. *Nursing Ethics: Across the Curriculum and into Practice*. 5th ed., Jones & Bartlett Learning, 2013.

"Ethical Issues in Nursing: Explanations & Solutions." Duquesne University School of Nursing. https://onlinenursing.duq.edu/blog/ethical-issues-in-nursing/. Accessed 8 Oct. 2020.

"Health Insurance and Accountability Act of 1996 (HIPAA)." Centers for Disease Control and Prevention. https://www.cdc.gov/phlp/publications/topic/hipaa.html. Accessed 8 Oct. 2020.

"What Is the Nursing Code of Ethics?" Nurse.org, 4 Sept. 2020. https://nurse.org/education/nursing-code-of-ethics/.

Wood, Debra. "4 Common Nursing Ethics Dilemmas." Nurse Choice. https://www.nursechoice.com/traveler-resources/4-common-nursing-ethics-dilemmas/. Accessed 8 Oct. 2020.

AUTONOMY AND PHYSICIAN ORDERS

ABSTRACT

Autonomy is the ability to act based on knowledge and judgment. In nursing, autonomy is the provision of care within the full scope of practice based on professional, regulatory and organizational rules. Carrying out physician orders is implementing the physician's plan of care for the patient.

AUTONOMY IN NURSING

The Scope of Practice laws of each state legally define accepted actions within the licensure of the individual. The state legislature passes law known as the Nurse Practice Act (NPA). Currently, states each pass their own Nurse Practice Act to ensure safe, competent nursing practice and is the basis for a nursing license. While states still define their own NPA, licensure compacts are expanding to allow nurses with a registered nurse (RN) license the ability to practice in their home state and other compact states. The Nurse Licensure Compact (NLC) currently includes thirty-three states with one pending implementation. A license from a compact state allows a nurse to practice in all other NLC states but nurses are bound by the Nurse Practice Act of the state in which they are employed. If a nurse moves to a non-NLC state, an application for endorsement by the board of nursing in that non-NLC state must be completed. A license valid in that state only will be issued.

Regulatory bodies, including the State Board of Health, define rules and regulations focused on protecting the patient. In order to better meet the needs of patients, nurses must be able to practice their profession to the full extent of their education and expertise to deliver quality care to the patient and ensure optimal outcomes. Educational qualifications and work experience, organizational policies and procedures and professional expectations also define the level of autonomous practice that can occur in a healthcare setting. Nurses must make decisions for patients based on the nursing plan of care, the physician plan of care, the policies and procedures of their organization, their own education and expertise, and sound clinical judgment all within their legal scope of practice. For example, autonomous decisions made by an RN staff nurse will be significantly less than those of an advanced practice nurse such as a nurse practitioner. As education and certifications increase in scope and depth, autonomous decision making tends to expand.

There are independent nursing actions and decision making that must occur on an ongoing basis during the care of the patient while recognizing the parameters of the scope of practice and other influencing factors. For example, pain medications ordered by the physician as needed (PRN) every four to six hours for the postoperative patient require the nurse to respond to a patient request for pain medication by assessing the level of pain, determining if timing is appropriate, and giving the medication. If the patient requests pain medication too soon, the nurse decides if the physician needs to be notified or if implementing comfort measures may diminish pain until medication may be given. These are examples of autonomous actions. The fact that the physician ordered the pain medication PRN allows the nurse the autonomy to decide if medicating the patient is ap-

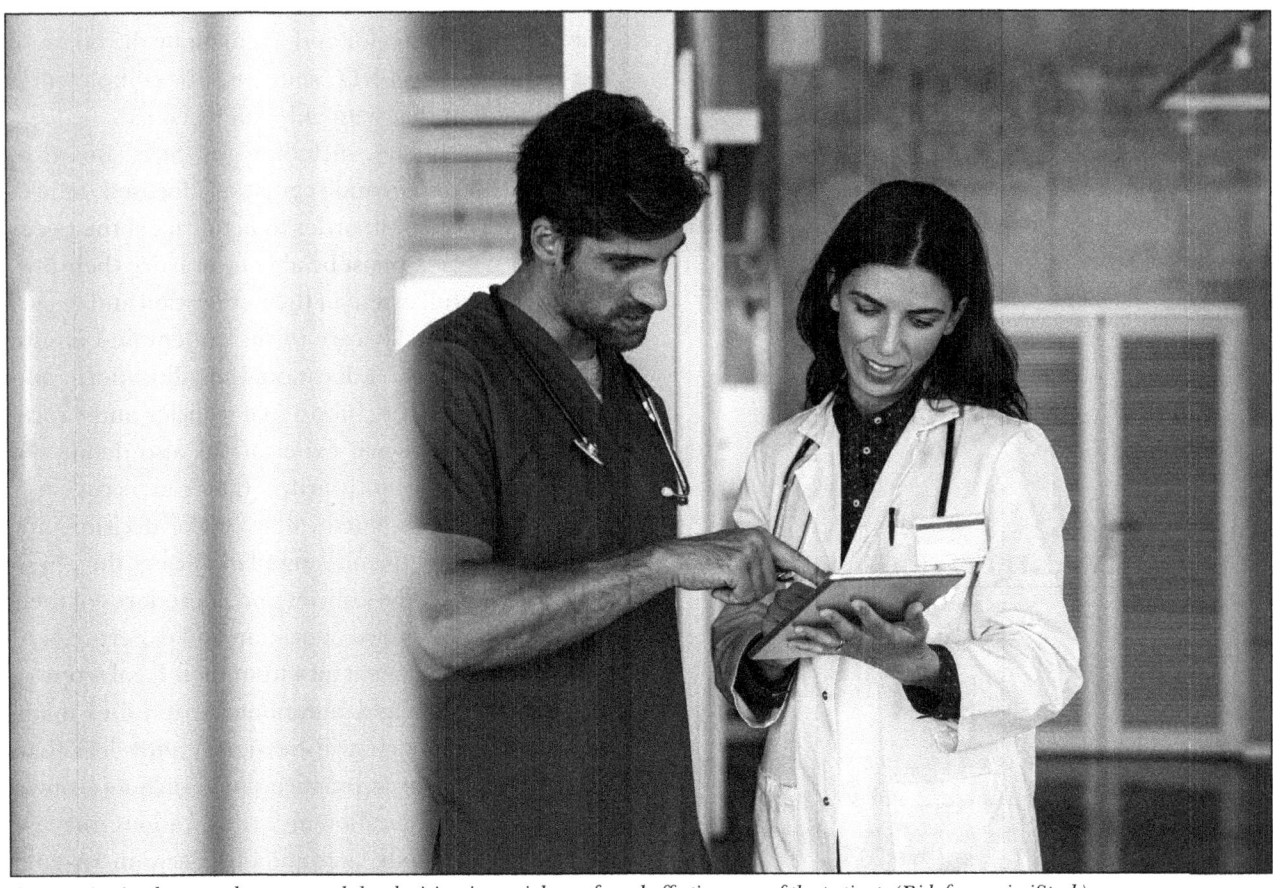
Communication between the nurse and the physician is crucial to safe and effective care of the patient. (Ridofranz via iStock)

propriate. A physician order for a medication every four hours must be honored and the nurse is charged with carrying out the order within thirty minutes either side of the hour of administration (a 4:00 p.m. dose may be given between 3:30 p.m. and 4:30 p.m.).

PHYSICIAN ORDERS

Physician orders or doctor's orders are terms used interchangeably to describe the physician's plan of care for the patient. When a patient is admitted to the hospital, for example, the physician writes admitting orders that describe the expected care of the patient during the initial period of hospitalization. Type of diet (regular, soft or cardiac), vital signs every two hours, oxygen as needed, up in chair twice daily, pain medication as needed are just a few examples of physician orders. Orders may also be written for laboratory tests, radiology tests such as computed tomography (CT) scan or magnetic resonance imaging (MRI), or cardiac catherization that the physician deems part of his or her plan of care for the patient. The nurse caring for the patient is given the responsibility to follow and implement these orders in the care of the patient. Any deviations from these orders need to be first discussed with the physician.

While nurses are expected to implement physician orders, they are also expected to challenge an order that appears incorrect. For example, a dose of pain medication or chemotherapy that seems excessively high should result in a call to the doctor. Errors do occur and the nurse is responsible for recognizing deviations from correct dosing. Pharmacists are also good resources if a medication order looks wrong. If patients are experiencing side effects such as nausea and vomiting after a dose of medication, the doctor should be notified. The dose may be held or changed or supportive care drugs may be added to minimize patient distress.

Communication between the nurse and the physician is crucial to safe and effective care of the patient. After taking a patient's blood pressure, an excessively high value should initiate a call to the physician as should any other patient status change. Following or carrying out orders does not remove the responsibility of the nurse to assess the patient and the patient's response. Just because an order has been written does not mean it should be implemented without understanding the potential patient response. Asking about allergies or previous drug or anesthesia reactions are part of nursing care. At admission, the nurse does a comprehensive nursing assessment that may uncover allergies or previous drug interactions or problems with radiology dye that may counter a physician order. The physician and nurse collaborate and coordinate to deliver safe and effective care.

IMPLICATIONS

Nursing is part of the hierarchy of patient care. The physician defines the plan of care for the patient through orders and protocols and the nurse writes the nursing care plan based on both the physician plan of care and the patient's needs. Other departments and services are also involved in the care of the patient. Strong communication between those who both plan and provide care is critical. Nurses should embrace autonomous action within the legality of their licensing, the employer's policies and procedures, their knowledge and experience and the nursing plan of care. Nurses should also understand that following the physician plan of care by implementing orders is a part of their role. Nurses should never be afraid to challenge an order in a professional manner to protect the patient.

—*Patricia Stanfill Edens*

Further Reading

"Find Your Nurse Practice Act." *National Council of State Boards of Nursing*, ncsbn.org/npa.htm. Accessed 23 Sept. 2020.

"NLC FAQs." *National Council of State Boards of Nursing*, ncsbn.org/npa.htm. Accessed 23 Sept. 2020.

Reuter C., and V. Fitzsimons. "Physician Orders." *American Journal of Nursing*, vol. 113, no. 8, 2013, journals.lww.com/ajnonline/Fulltext/2013/0800/Physician_Orders.2.aspx.

"Scope of Practice." *American Nurses Association*, www.nursingworld.org/practice-policy/scope-of-practice/. Accessed 23 Sept. 2020.

Weston, M. J. "Strategies for Enhancing Autonomy and Control over Nursing Practice." *Online Journal of Issues in Nursing*, vol. 15, no. 1, 2010, ojin.nursingworld.org/MainMenuCategories/ANAMarketplace/ANAPeriodicals/OJIN/TableofContents/Vol152010/No1Jan2010/Enhancing-Autonomy-and-Control-and-Practice.aspx.

SCOPE OF NURSING PRACTICE

ABSTRACT

Scope of nursing practice refers to the services that a nursing professional is legally permitted to perform. These practices differ by state and are regulated by each state's Nurse Practice Act (NPA).

NURSE PRACTICE ACT (NPA)

The Nurse Practice Act (NPA) is a set of guidelines developed by each state's legislature that dictates the scope of practice and professional regulations by which nurses are required to practice. Although each state's NPAs are enacted by its legislature, they are regulated by the state's Nursing Regulatory Body (NRB), also known as the Board of Nursing (BONs). NRBs were developed over 100 years ago to protect the safety and health of the public by developing standards of safe nursing care. The NRB is charged with further defining and interpreting laws surrounding the NPA. They are permitted to develop new rules and regulations that have the effect of clarifying existing laws or making them more specific, but they cannot go beyond the boundaries of the NPA as it is written. Before new laws are enacted, they are subjected to public comment periods, in which nurses and the public can submit feedback and participate in the rule-making process. All fifty states, as well as the District of Columbia and the U.S. territories, have their own NRBs. The fifty-nine NRBs in the United States are all members of the larger regulatory body, the National Council of State Boards of Nursing (NCSBN), which oversees the laws and standards practiced by each of its members.

Although each state is given leeway in writing its own NPA, the NCSBN dictates certain standards that must apply in each state. As outlined by the NCSBN, each NPA must set the following standards of practice: the authority, power, and composition of the state nursing board; the standards for educational programs; the standards and scope of nursing practice; the types and titles of licensures; the requirements for licensure; and the grounds for disciplinary action. These regulations are designed to ensure that all practitioners are prepared and competent to carry out the tasks for which they are employed. To this end, they must receive the relevant degrees or diplomas, pass the relevant certification exams, and adhere to a fixed set of practices, all of which are laid out in the NPA. All practicing nurses are bound by the NPA and are subject to disciplinary action if they violate any of its terms, even unknowingly. In 2015, in order to help nurses make informed decisions within the proper scope of practice, the NCSBN, in collaboration with the Tri-Council of Nursing, developed a uniform decision-making framework for nurses. This tool, which took the form of an activity tree, helps nurses determine whether or not they are authorized to perform a specific activity. Nurses practicing in a state are encouraged to review the NPA of their state of practice.

SCOPE OF NURSING PRACTICE BY SPECIALTY

The scope of nursing practice permitted to each practitioner differs according to their state's NPA, but it also depends largely on their official title. This title is, in turn, dictated by the nurse's level of education and certification. Registered nurses (RNs), professionals who have earned a bachelor's degree, associate's degree, or diploma in nursing and have passed the certifying exam, the NCLEX-RN (National Council Licensure Exam for Registered Nurses), are permitted to practice in a variety of settings but are limited in the tasks they can perform. In some states, nurses with higher degrees such as a Master of Science in Nursing (MSN) or a Doctor of Nursing Practice (DNP), are allowed greater autonomy and may practice skills beyond that of an RN.

Nurse practitioners (NPs), who are advanced practice registered nurses (APRNs) and hold a minimum of an MSN, are one group of nursing professionals granted this larger autonomy. Nurse practitioners work in a wide variety of healthcare settings and perform a number of important duties, that may include assessment of patient's conditions, ordering and interpreting diagnostic and laboratory tests, making diagnoses, initiating and carrying out treatment including ordering medications, counseling, and educating. They practice both autonomously and in coordination with other healthcare professionals and their degree of autonomy depends on the individual NPAs of the state in which they practice. Currently, twenty-three states, plus Guam and the Northern Mariana Islands allow NPs full practice authority. This means that they can practice without the supervision of a physician. Sixteen states, plus Puerto Rico, the U.S. Virgin Islands, and American Samoa, permit NPs reduced practice, which means that they must have a written collaborative agreement with a physician to practice. Twelve states further restrict the NPs practice by requiring them to be supervised or delegated by a physician.

Certified registered nurse anesthetists (CRNA) are another type of advanced practice nurse whose scope of practice differs by state. CRNAs are nurses who hold at the minimum a MSN and often a Doctor of Nursing Practice (DNP) degree, and who have passed the National Certification Exam (NCE) offered by the National Board of Certification and Recertification for Nurse Anesthetists (NBCRNA). CRNAs work in every setting where anesthesia is administered, including hospitals, traditional and ambulatory surgical centers, and physician's offices, and are licensed to administer both local and general anesthesia and perform other medical tasks such as placing arterial lines and administering nerve blocks. Before 2001, all nurse anesthetists in the United States were required by federal law to be supervised by a physician. In that year, the Centers for Medicare and Medicaid Services (CMS) changed the law to allow individual state governors to opt out of this requirement. Currently seventeen states, including California, Minnesota, and Wisconsin have opted out. Several other states do not have physician supervision requirements as part of their state law and are eligible to opt out at the discretion of the governor.

—*Andrew Schenker*

Further Reading
"About U.S. Nursing Regulatory Bodies." *National Council of State Boards of Nursing.* www.ncsbn.org/about-nursing-regulatory-bodies.htm. Accessed 7 Oct. 2020.
American Nurses Association. *Nursing: Scope and Standards of Practice.* 3rd ed. American Nurses Association, 2015.
"Certified Registered Nurse Anesthetists Fact Sheet." *American Association of Nurse Anesthetists (AANA).* www.aana.com/membership/become-a-crna/crna-fact-sheet. Accessed 7 Oct. 2020.
"How Is the Scope of Practice Determined for a Nurse?" *Registered Nursing.org.* www.registerednursing.org/answers/how-scope-practice-determined/. Accessed 7 Oct. 2020.
"Nursing Regulations and State Boards of Nursing." *American Nephrology Nurses Association.* www.annanurse.org/advocacy/resources-and-tools/state/nursing-regulations. Accessed 7 Oct. 2020.

Informed Consent

ABSTRACT
Informed consent occurs when the healthcare provider educates a patient about the risks, benefits and alternatives of treatment, including drugs, procedures and other interventions. It is both a legal and ethical requirement of physicians and healthcare providers in the United States to obtain informed consent as the patient has a right to control his or her body.

INTRODUCTION
Consent is the process where a patient makes a voluntary decision to enter a hospital or other setting for treatment, has specific procedures while in the hospital or setting, or to participate in other situations requiring the patient to give his or her permission before any invasive procedure is done. Informed consent is more in-depth. When a patient decides to receive a drug or treatment that may be under study in a clinical trial and subject to US Food & Drug (FDA) requirements, informed consent is required. When being admitted to the hospital, the consent forms requiring a signature are for accepted activities and procedures, are considered standard of care, are not considered research and are considered legal documents. The terms consent and informed consent are often used interchangeably.

The Joint Commission, the accrediting body for hospitals and healthcare providers, requires documentation of five elements of consent: (1) what is the procedure; (2) what are the risks and benefits of the procedure; (3) reasonable alternatives; (4) risks and benefits of alternatives; and (5) an assessment of the patient's understanding of elements 1 to 4. Some examples of required informed consent is for treatment, sharing of patient information, discussion of HIPPA laws, surgery, specific procedures, blood transfusions and anesthesia.

For clinical studies or interventions that are subject to FDA regulations, informed consent documents should meet the requirements of 21 CFR 50.25(a) and

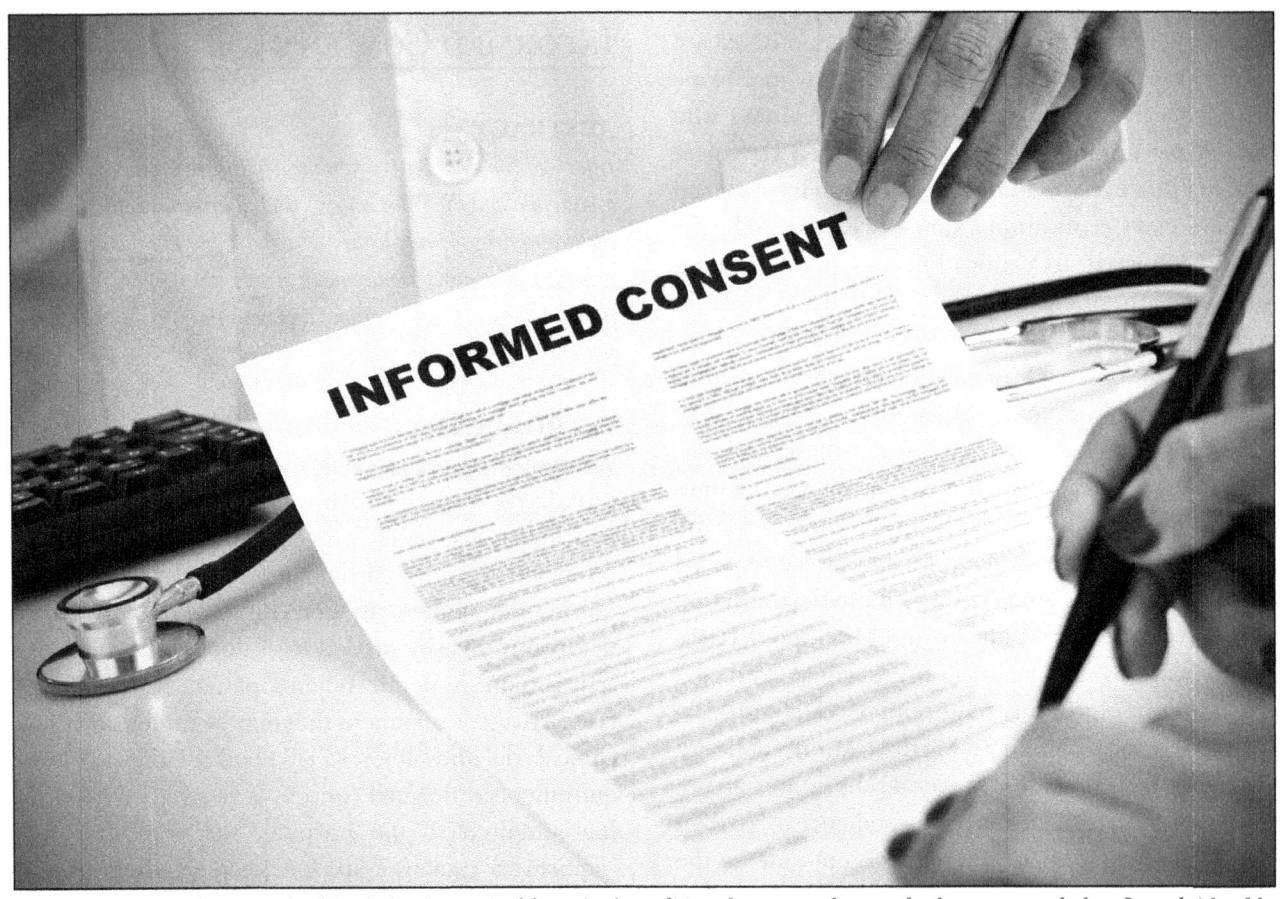

An informed consent document should include a diagnosis of the patient's condition, the name and reason for the treatment, the benefits and risks of the treatment, the benefits and risks of alternative procedures, and other information deemed necessary. (nito100 via iStock)

(b). An Institutional Review Board (IRB) has the final authority for ensuring that sufficient informed consent occurs. An IRB is an independent ethics committee, an ethical review board or a research ethics review board that has been designated to review and monitor primarily biomedical research involving humans. Its role is to protect the rights and welfare of human subjects. Using a group process, all materials are reviewed prior to presenting a consent form to the patient. IRBs generally reside in a healthcare provider setting and may review basic and clinical research and other activities as designated by the provider of the IRB.

There are three exceptions to obtaining informed consent: (1) if the patient is incapacitated; (2) in the case of a life-threatening emergency with inadequate time to gain consent; and, (3) if the patient voluntarily waives consent. If the patient has a healthcare power of attorney, others may give consent for the patient. If there is no one designated to make decisions, a designated group may intercede or, in rare cases, a court appointed legal guardian may step in to decide. Children under 17 cannot provide informed consent unless legally emancipated. Informed permission, meaning the process is explained to the child, is recommended.

In most situations, the physician, clinical investigator or provider designee is responsible for providing information, obtaining verbal agreement and negotiating a signed consent document. In some cases, the physician will provide the education of the patient and then his or her designee will obtain the actual signature.

WHAT REQUIRES INFORMED CONSENT

Any treatment or procedure with some level of perceived risk requires informed consent. Most surgeries and biopsies, blood transfusions and some blood tests, most vaccinations and anesthesia all require informed consent. In cancer care, a more extensive consent document is prepared for chemotherapy administration due to the potential life-threatening side effects. Radiation also requires a comprehensive consent document.

THE CONSENT DOCUMENT

An informed consent document should include a diagnosis of the patient's condition, the name and reason for the treatment, the benefits and risks of the treatment, the benefits and risks of alternative procedures, and other information deemed necessary. For example, a clinical research study may also outline supplemental procedures such as radiology procedures, scans, blood draws, noninvestigational drugs and any additional interventions required by the study that are not a part of standard care. The content should be written for a layperson in simple language that is easily understood. Part of the role of the IRB is to determine that consent documents are clear and understandable to the nonmedical professional.

A type of informed consent is implied consent. For example, if a patient has a fever and goes to a healthcare provider, it is implied that they are seeking care. It is less formal and does not have to be legally recorded.

SUMMARY

As a patient, you have the right to accept or refuse treatments recommended by a health professional. If you decide to seek treatment, you may be asked to give consent to the treating physician or facility. Informed consent also indicates that you have made a voluntary and educated choice to receive care. This article is a simple summary of informed consent. For more information see Further Reading that follows.

—*Patricia Stanfill Edens*

Further Reading

"A Guide to Informed Consent: Guidance for Institutional Review Boards and Clinical Investigators." *US Food & Drug Administration*, www.fda.gov/regulatory-information/search-fda-guidance-documents/guide-informed-consent. Accessed 11 Sept. 2020.

"Informed Consent: More Than Getting a Signature." *Joint Commission*, www.jointcommission.org/-/media/deprecated-unorganized/imported-assets/tjc/system-folders/joint-commission-online/quick_safety_issue_twenty-one_february_2016pdf.pdf?db=web&hash=5944307ED39088503A008A70D2C768AA. Accessed 11 Sept. 2020.

"Informed Consent-StatPearls." National Library of Medicine. National Institutes of Health. *NCBI Bookshelf*, www.ncbi.nlm.nih.gov/books/NBK430827/. Accessed 11 Sept. 2020.

Kadam, R. A. "Informed Consent Process: A Step Further Towards Making It Meaningful." *Perspectives in Clinical Research*, vol. 8, no. 3, 2017, pp. 107–12.

"What You Need to Know about Informed Consent." *Healthline*, www.healthline.com/health/informed-consent. Accessed 11 Sept. 2020.

CLINICAL RESEARCH TRIALS

ABSTRACT

Clinical research trials are observed studies of the effect of medications, treatments, activities, supplements, vitamins, and other interventions on the human body. Trials may be observational studies or clinical trials.

OVERVIEW

Clinical research trials may also be referred to as clinical trials. Nonmedical trials may be descriptive in nature and, for example, may test learning styles, methods of instruction, and evaluate situations or operational issues. Observational trials gather information by observing people in normal settings. Data may be collected through questionnaires, medical examinations and tests and may be used to define new studies for clinical trials. Clinical trials are more complex research studies in people or patients to evaluate pharmaceutical, medical or behavioral interventions with the aim of determining safety and efficacy. Clinical trials address the question: What does a particular treatment do to the human body? Trials may involve a researcher who systematically observes and collects data on the activities and behaviors of specific persons to answer a specific research question or may be used in groups of varying sizes. Trials may take place in educational settings, employment settings, healthcare settings and other sites. There are four phases of clinical trials: Phase I, Phase II, Phase III and Phase IV. The phases are designed to test a treatment, find an appropriate dosage, look for side effects and, finally, monitor safety and effectiveness in large, diverse population.

Clinical trials are developed by a wide range of researchers including doctors, sponsoring companies such as pharmaceutical or device manufacturers, and other health practitioners including nurses. All treatments that must be approved by the US Food and Drug Administration (FDA) must first undergo a clinical trial to prove that the medication or supplement is effective and safe for human use. Even for those treatments that do not require FDA approval, researchers may still use clinical trials to show patients and health consumers that a product or treatment is effective and safe. In most care sites, researchers must submit their trial to an Institutional Review Board (IRB) responsible for patient safety and informed consent oversight. Informed consent means the participant understands the risk and benefits of participating in the trial and does so freely. The IRB is responsible for reviewing all research conducted within the institution it is affiliated with, including off site offices, schools and employees conducting a study.

TRIAL DESIGN

To conduct a quality clinical trial, studies must begin with a research question and effective research design. First, the researchers must develop a specific testable question known as a hypothesis. Next, the researchers select a series of tests and questions that can accurately assess the hypothesis and provide information or data to support the study's conclusion. This is known as a study protocol.

The study protocol explains the trial's purpose, function, and methods (or the way it is to be conducted). Protocols often also include information about the reason for the study, any past research relating to the study, the number of subjects (persons) needed to perform an effective study, eligibility and exclusion criteria, details of the intervention or therapy the participants will receive, what data to gather, what demographic information about the participants to gather, steps for clinical care givers to carry out, and the study end points. If a protocol is being run by several different investigators, a single standard protocol must be used without deviation to ensure that the resulting data will be consistent and reliable. All parts of the protocol should answer the hypothesis and should try to eliminate conflicting factors that might lead to false conclusions.

Depending on the design of the study protocol, the clinical trial may be given one of two overall design labels: case-control study or double-blind study. In a case-control study, a group of persons affected by the disease being studied is compared with a group without the disease. In a double-blind study, neither the study personnel nor the study participants know who is assigned to a particular intervention. In many studies, especially in cancer, one group receives the best standard of care and one group receives the best standard of care plus a new drug or intervention. This allows the researcher to compare the groups to discover if the new drug or intervention made a difference in the outcome of the disease or activity under study.

Clinical trials are also labeled by the types of questions they are attempting to answer. The first type is a phase I trial, applied to first-ever studies of a particular treatment or product and to early studies in an overall series of clinical trials. After conclusions about the basic safety of the treatment in humans have been drawn from phase I, phase II clinical trials continue to test the safety of the drug and begin to evaluate how effective the drug is in the target population. Phase III studies compare the new treatment to the current standard treatment. This phase is particularly crucial in that it produces the primary data the FDA reviews before approving or rejecting a particular treatment. Phase IV studies take place after FDA approval and monitor and evaluate drugs or devices for effectiveness and safety in large, diverse populations of people.

Once the clinical trial is properly designed and approved by the Institutional Review Board if necessary, human volunteers can be asked to participate in the study. After all the procedures, tests, and questions are finished, the investigators analyze the data using statistical techniques and then draw a conclusion about their original hypothesis. In many cases, the conclusions establish the overall risks and benefits of any intervention.

To distribute the information learned from clinical trials to the widest audience, most investigators will present their hypotheses, procedures, results, and conclusions in oral presentations, conference posters, and journal articles. Before publication or acceptance for conference presentation, most studies undergo peer review, in which other specialists and investigators in the original author or authors' field examine the clinical trial and support or reject the accuracy and conclusions of the research. The reviewers will determine the validity of a clinical trial based on the researcher's performance in accurately testing the hypothesis. Determination of validity is based on the use of a strong set of tests and evaluations, the repeatability of the study, and the accuracy of data collection and interpretation. Studies that receive positive peer review can be published.

TRIAL IMPORTANCE

Well-designed clinical research trials are critical to practitioners and users of any new therapy, device, or intervention. Clinical trial data help consumers, patients and practitioners to determine which intervention, treatment, or device should be the most safe and effective for a particular issue. Knowing the most effective treatment and using it first can also decrease the amount of time an individual suffers from a particular health issue.

Manufacturers seeking FDA approval also require clinical trials to prove the safety and efficacy of their products. FDA approval brings an additional level of oversight to a product, and, critical to a manufacturer, also adds validation for use.

TRIAL OVERSIGHT

A clinical research trial usually has several layers of oversight to ensure that the study is designed well and that the participants will not be harmed. These layers of oversight were created to keep scientists, including medical doctors and other health practitioners, from performing unethical experiments on humans. The history of unethical research includes that conducted by the Nazis during World War II and that conducted by the US government from 1932 to 1972 with poor African American men in Tuskegee, Alabama; the men studied had syphilis but were not treated for the disease.

Institutional Review Boards (IRBs), developed in response to unethical experimentation on humans, review and monitor every clinical trial in the United States. An IRB consists of an independent committee of physicians, medical professionals, statisticians, community advocates, and others that ensure that a clinical trial is ethical and that the rights of study participants are protected. One of the main responsibilities of IRBs is to ensure that research participants are fully informed of a study's purpose, procedures, risks, benefits, and costs through a process called informed consent.

The US government also plays a role in the regulatory oversight of clinical research trials. The Department of Health and Human Service's Office for Human Research Protections (OHRP) oversees and regulates IRBs and human research in general. OHRP helps ensure the rights of persons in clinical trials by providing clarification and guidance, developing educational programs and materials, and providing advice on ethical and regulatory issues in biomedical and behavioral research. The FDA helps investigators create effective, ethical treatment studies on humans.

Many clinical trials (particularly those with more than one study site) also have data-safety-monitoring committees or boards. These independent committees are formed of experts who are familiar with the conditions and treatments under study but who are not involved in the clinical research trials themselves. The committee members review any adverse events, experimental errors, or other issues to make sure the study can continue and to ensure that investigators are performing research appropriately and effectively.

TRIAL PARTICIPATION

Clinical research trials are possible only because volunteers agree to participate in the studies. Participants often volunteer to have a more active role in their own healthcare, to gain early access to new research treatments, and to help others by contributing to medical research. The decision to join a research trial should be a reasoned one and may involve the help of friends or family members. Before participating in a clinical trial, it is critical to know the key facts about a particular trial. One should understand the trial's procedures, risks, benefits, and personal costs. These answers are provided to volunteers through the informed consent process. The main portion of informed consent occurs before a prospective volunteer agrees to join the study. Only after the conclusion of informed consent can a study subject begin his or her participation in a clinical trial.

Clinical research trials can be found through internet searches, particularly through Clinicaltrials.gov, run by the National Institutes of Health. Investigators around the world submit information to this site about ongoing research. Another option for finding clinical trials is to identify the researchers who have done past work and to contact them about recruitment for future studies.

Published research studies can be found through internet databases such as Pubmed, provided by the National Library of Medicine. Using reliable sites for finding clinical research trials is important as there are fake sites online.

—*Dawn Laney*

Further Reading

Boissel, J. P. "Planning of Clinical Trials." *Journal of Internal Medicine*, vol. 255, no. 4, 2004, pp. 427–38.

National Center for Complementary and Alternative Medicine, nccam.nih.gov. A comprehensive site of a leading US agency for scientific research on complementary and alternative medicine. Provides results and information on CAM obtained from clinical trials.

National Institute of Child Health and Human Development, www.nichd.nih.gov/health/clinicalresearch. Provides information about clinical research and the NICHD's role in this research

National Institutes of Health. *ClinicalTrials.gov*, clinicaltrials.gov.

National Library of Medicine, www.pubmed.gov.

"NIH Clinical Research Trials and You: The Basics." *National Institutes of Health*, www.nih.gov/health-information/nih-clinical-research-trials-you/basics. Accessed 24 Aug. 2020.

"What Are Clinical Trials?" National Cancer Institute. *National Institutes of Health*, www.cancer.gov/about-cancer/treatment/clinical-trials/what-are-trials. Accessed 24 Aug. 2020.

"What Are Clinical Trials and Studies?" US Department of Health and Human Services. *National Institute on Aging*, www.nia.nih.gov/health/what-are-clinical-trials-and-studies. Accessed 24 Aug. 2020.

Nursing Theory

This small but concentrated section starts by outlining the various nursing theories—the foundation of nursing—which define what nurses do and why they do it. Nursing theory has evolved from disease-centered in the mid-1800s to patient-centered theory of today. In addition to discussing the Nursing Metaparadigm, this section covers in detail Grand, Middle-Range and Practice-Level theories, comprising both abstract and evidence-based theories which is seen as the future of nursing.

Nursing Theory	31
Metaparadigm Concepts in Nursing	33
Grand Theories	35
Middle-Range Theories	37
Practice-Level Theories	39

Nursing Theory

ABSTRACT
Nursing theories are the foundations of nursing. It organizes knowledge to define what nurses do and why they do it. It provides a framework to define the discipline as separate and distinct from other health professions. Nursing theories essentially define the scope of nursing practice.

INTRODUCTION
Until the mid-1800s, nurses had little training and were not prepared to care for illnesses or injuries. Their role was to assist doctors as directed, provide comfort where possible and handle the daily needs of their patients. Many of the first nurses were involved in treating the war-wounded and learned on the job. Florence Nightingale is designated as the first nursing theorist and is seen as the driving force behind the development of formal nursing education and advocacy. In 1860, she opened the first school of nursing at St. Thomas Hospital in London. Today, nursing has its own body of knowledge that provides the foundation for the delivery of nursing care. From the mid-1800s to today, nursing theorists have participated in defining the thinking, knowledge, and beliefs that provide the foundation of nursing.

DEFINING NURSING THEORY
Nursing theory essentially defines the scope of nursing practice. The evolution of nursing theory requires a knowledge of definitions and assumptions that began with Florence Nightingale and continue to evolve today. The beliefs and values, or philosophy of nursing, define a collective group of issues accepted by the profession. The basis of nursing actions is considered theory and is used to explain, predict or describe procedures and policies. To build a foundation to support the theory of nursing, concepts and models evolved. Concepts are often described as building blocks and create an image of desired actions. Models represent the manner in which theory can be introduced into nursing practice.

The conceptual framework is a collection of ideas, statements, and concepts and may also be referred to as the conceptual model or grand theory of nursing. Process, also to mean nursing process, are organized steps that are applied to bring about a desired outcome or result. When the framework and processes are combined, a paradigm evolves to establish a shared understanding and value system that may be used to make assumptions about the reality of the world, including nursing. The most general statement of a discipline and its functions is called a metaparadigm. This evolution of nursing is focused on bringing current concepts and functions into a framework that can be applied to the person, the environment, health, and nursing.

HISTORY
The first nursing theories began in the mid-1800s and have evolved from an emphasis on educating nurses to incorporating tenants of fundamental needs of patients, scientific knowledge, nurse-client relationships, shifting from disease centered to patient-centered care, goal attainment, achieving balance in the body, and the humanistic aspects of nursing as they interrelate with scientific knowledge and nursing practice. Nursing theory began with an emphasis on nursing education led by Florence Nightingale and her Environmental Theory but has evolved to so much more. The theoretical framework of nursing theory incorporates work beginning in the 1950s from nursing leaders who recognized that nursing needed to validate itself as a profession by defining its own scientific basis for practice. (See "Nursing Theorists" section of this work for information on the most influential nursing theorists.)

THE NURSING METAPARADIGM
Nursing theory is founded on four interrelated concepts; person, environment, health, and nursing. In

each of the nursing theories that evolved through the years, each of these concepts may be identified. Persons are those who interact with nurses to receive care and may include healthy individuals, patients, families, caregivers, and communities. The environment of care is that which surrounds individuals or patients and their support system and includes both internal and external impacts. Health, also described as wellness, is the unique experience each individual experiences. Nursing includes the actions of caring for a client, their support systems and the community at large. Defining nursing remains challenging as the roles of nurses continue to evolve from the hands-on care at the bedside in the days of Florence Nightingale to a variety of sites of employment. As nursing becomes more sophisticated with increases in advanced treatments and technologies, the one thread that remains is that the ultimate goal of nursing theories is to improve the care of the individual or patient.

IMPORTANCE OF NURSING THEORY

For a theory to contribute to nursing care, it must include concepts, definitions, related statements, and assumptions that explain a situation or phenomenon and describe how these components interreact. Nursing theory has been the basis for all nursing practice over the years, from the need for nursing education to the need for humanistic, patient-centered care. Understanding its evolution will create a foundation for the individual nurse to define a personal theory of nursing care. Just as nursing has evolved from battlefield, hands-on care to advanced practice and nursing research, it also has

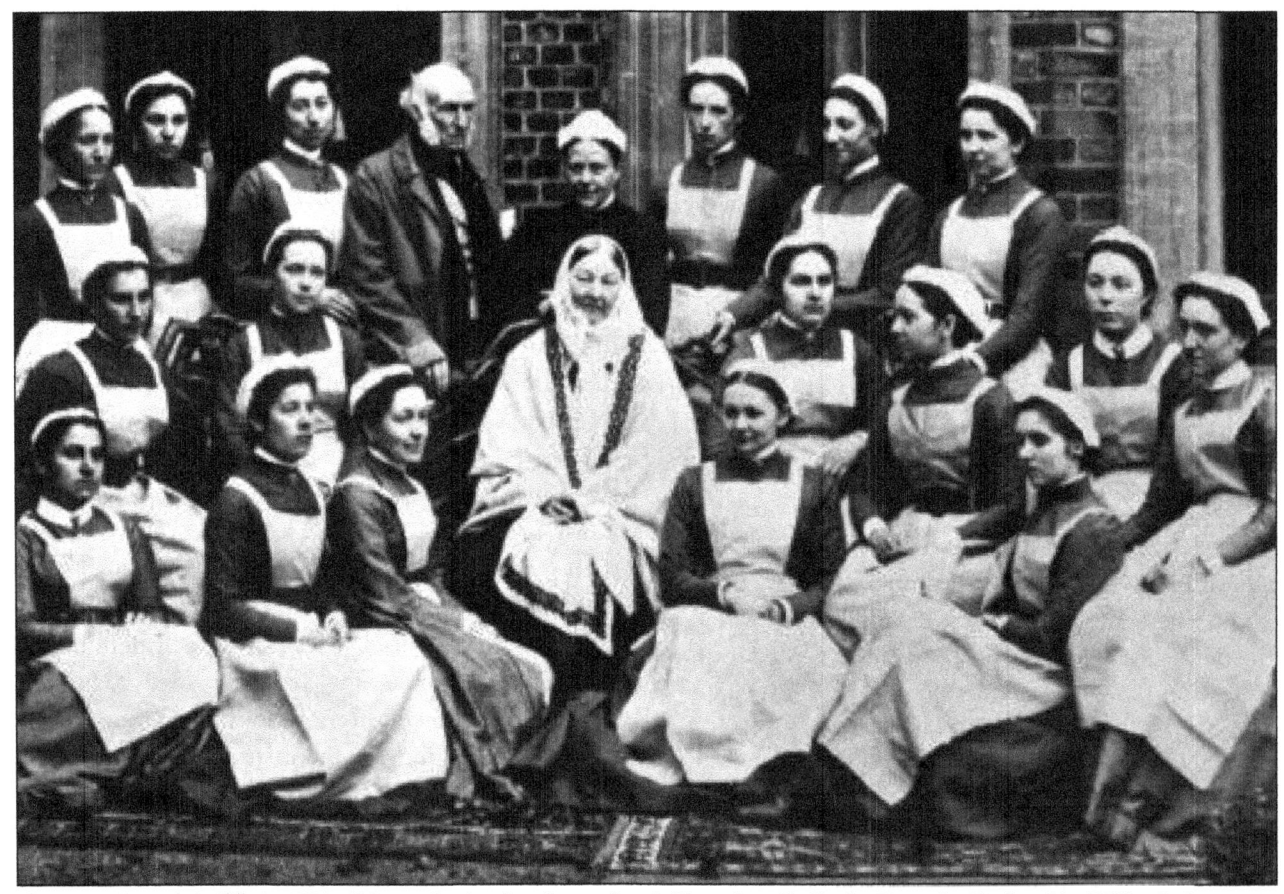

Florence Nightingale (middle) in 1886 with her graduating class of nurses from St Thomas' outside Claydon House, Buckinghamshire (Wikimedia Commons)

evolved from being recognized as only task-based to that of being recognized as an academic discipline. Theories provide a rationale for why nursing interventions are needed and provide a basis to generate further knowledge as healthcare evolves. Nursing theory focuses on the needs of both the patient and nurse to maintain a profession that guides knowledge, practice, research, and education to best deliver the optimal outcomes indicated for each patient.

OVERVIEW OF THEORIES

The goal of nursing theory is to improve nursing practice in order to positively impact the health and quality of life of individuals, patients, caregivers, and communities. Theories have allowed the recognition of nursing as an academic discipline which contributed to professional recognition of the nurse as an integral part of the healthcare team. Nursing theories begin with an understanding of the nursing metaparadigm and move to understanding the categories of grand theories, middle-range theories, and practice level theories, or abstract based theories. These theories are more foundational in nature and contribute to overall nursing practice. Goal theories focus on a specific outcome and can be descriptive or prescriptive. Theories can also be defined as needs theories, interaction theories, and outcome theories. Alligood is the most recent theorist and categorizes nursing theories into four subtypes: philosophy, conceptual models, grand nursing theories, and middle-range theories.

SUMMARY

The curriculum in all nursing education is based on a theoretical framework that most often evolved from the theories that are considered foundational in nature or those labeled abstract theories. The conceptual underpinnings of nursing are instrumental in shaping both education and practice. Additional theories come into play as the nurse graduates and moves into a variety of roles in the healthcare space. These more specific theories may relate to topics such as end of life care, mental health, postpartum depression and others more focused on a targeted field. In the future with more virtual care being employed, nursing theory and research will contribute to the advancement of care. Nursing theory provides the foundation as nurses define, redefine and challenge their scope of practice.

—*Patricia Stanfill Edens*

Further Reading
Alligood, M. R. *Nursing Theorists and their Work*. 9th ed., Elsevier eBook on Vital Source, 2018.
Colley, S. "Nursing Theory: Its Importance to Practice." *Nursing Standard*, vol. 17, no. 46, 2003, pp. 33–37.
Dallaire, C., and P. Krol. "Revisiting the Roots of Nursing Philosophy and Critical Theory: Past, Present and Future." *Nursing Philosophy*, vol. 19, no. 1, Jan. 2018.
Fronczek, A. E. "Nursing Theory in Virtual Care." *Nursing Science Quarterly*, vol. 32, no. 1, Jan. 2019, pp. 35–38.
Jairath, N. N., et al. "Theory and Theorizing in Nursing Science: Commentary from the Nursing Research Special Issue Editorial Team." *Nursing Research*, vol. 67, no. 2, Mar.-Apr. 2018, pp. 188–95.
Wayne, G. "Nursing Theories and Theorists: Your Theoretical Guide to Nursing Theories." *NursesLabs*, nurseslabs.com/nursing-theories/#what_are_nursing_theories. Accessed 14 Sept. 2020.
"What Is Nursing Theory? Key Concepts for DNPs." *Regis College*, online.regiscollege.edu/blog/what-is-nursing-theory/. Accessed 14 Sept. 2020.

METAPARADIGM CONCEPTS IN NURSING

ABSTRACT

A metaparadigm is a general statement of disciplines such as nursing and functions as a framework on which conceptual models develop. Jacqueline Fawcett's metaparadigm in nursing consists of four major components. The four nursing paradigm concepts are person, environment, health, and nursing. Fawcett's metaparadigm concepts were a framework for the development of models in the articulation of expert nursing.

INTRODUCTION

In Fawcett's metaparadigm, "Person" refers to the individual with whom the nurse interacts on a therapeutic level. These may be patients, families, or even an agency or an entire community. "Environment" refers to the internal and external factors affecting the treatment. "Health" refers to the person's well-being, including physical, psychological, emotional, and spiritual aspects. However, according to Fawcett's paradigm, what constitutes health must be defined by the patient, and nurses must allow themselves to be guided by what the person considers an acceptable level of health or standard of living. Health also includes the ability to access healthcare and other kinds of support. "Nursing" refers to the actions taken by the nurse, including applying professional knowledge, procedural and technical skills, and indirect and direct patient care. According to the American Nursing Association, nursing is the protection, promotion, and optimization of health and abilities, prevention of illness and injury, facilitation of healing, alleviation of suffering through the diagnosis and treatment of human response, and advocacy in the care of individuals, families, groups, communities, and populations. Fawcett's metaparadigm provided a framework around which nursing concepts could be organized.

BACKGROUND

Until the mid-nineteenth century, nurses had haphazard or no formal training. They might be kind but were not formally prepared to understand the nature of illness or injury.

Florence Nightingale is acknowledged as the force behind nursing education and advocacy. She was the first nursing theorist and opened the first school of nursing at St. Thomas' Hospital in London (1860). Two years later, her belief in advanced nursing education resulted in a school for midwives at Kings College. Prior to those accomplishments, she had received a total of less than four months training at two institutes, which qualified her to be superintendent of a hospital. Nightingale is best known for her work as a nurse in the Crimean War, which appears to be the first time standards of care had been set at a military hospital. She saw to it that patients were bathed and fed regularly, their psychological needs were met, and that the patients had clean dressings and clothes, as well as activities to keep them occupied. Called the "Lady with the Lamp" as she moved through the military hospital, she was a keen observer and statistician, skills that have become ingrained in the practice of nursing. Her lamp remains a symbol of nursing today.

Fawcett's metaparadigms were already evident in Nightingale's work. Nevertheless, nursing was considered a low-skilled, task-based vocation until the late twentieth century. As healthcare advanced, nursing required greater levels of professional knowledge and skill. Articulating precisely what a nurse should know and what skills a nurse must possess to be competent in the profession sparked debate within the nursing community and drove nursing education. The metaparadigm concepts provide a framework for more advanced concepts to be nurtured and developed.

IMPACT

Within nursing there is a running controversy concerning the difference between nursing theory and conceptual models. Hesook Kim, a noted nursing scholar, stated: "the functions of metaparadigms are to summarize the intellectual and social missions of a discipline and place a boundary on the subject matter of that discipline." The profession of nursing is ever changing and so are the boundaries. Technologies may be state of the art today and obsolete in five years. An intensive care unit (ICU) nurse of fifty years ago would stand in awe of computerization. Communication, a major part of person, has been facilitated by technology. Further, understanding of human behavior and physiology has changed considerably since the early days of professional nursing and continues to expand.

Concepts of person and health must be developed in order to integrate patient and family needs into care plans. For example, a patient may present with an injury or disease that needs direct care; the patient, however, is more than an injury or disease, and care requires attention to the entire patient, including alleviating discomfort, noting side effects or distress, and facilitating family participation in treatment. In some models, person may include other people who interact on behalf of the patient. In all models, caring for the physical and psychological needs of patients cannot be overstressed.

Environment, as Nightingale recognized, contributes to the continuum and quality of care. The concept of environment includes, for example, sanitary conditions—sterile equipment, a relatively germ-free facility, and keeping patients clean—as well as a culture of caring. Working (and convalescing) in a dismal physical environment is not consistent with good physical or mental health for anyone. Further, in some cases, the ability to practice nursing optimally can be impaired by the culture rather than the building structure.

As the nature of nursing education has progressed, there has been discourse on the expanding role of nurses, along with additional opportunities to engage in independent practice beyond midwifery. The medical field has seen an explosion in nurse practitioners. According to the American Association of Colleges of Nursing, there are four times as many advanced practice nurses than there are practicing physicians. Perhaps the metaparadigms will expand into the practice of medicine.

—*EBSCO CAM Review Board*

Further Reading

Alimohammadi, Nasrollah, et al. "The Nursing Metaparadigm Concept of Human Being in Islamic Thought." *Nursing Inquiry*, vol. 21, no. 2, 2014, pp. 121–29.

Alligood, Martha Raile, and Ann Marriner-Tomey. *Nursing Theorists and Their Work*. Mosby/Elsevier, 2010.

Fawcett, Jacqueline, and Susan DeSanto-Madeya. *Contemporary Nursing Knowledge: Analysis and Evaluation of Nursing Models and Theories*. 3rd ed., Davis, 2013.

Jackson, J. I. *Nursing Paradigms and Theories: A Primer*. Virginia Henderson Global Nursing e-Repository, 26 Jan. 2015, www.nursinglibrary.org/vhl/handle/10755/338888.

Jarrin, Olga F. "The Integrality of Situated Caring in Nursing and the Environment." *Advances in Nursing Science*, Winter 2012, www.ncbi.nlm.nih.gov/pmc/articles/PMC3402335/. Accessed 2 Jan. 2016.

Kim, Hesook Suzie, and Ingrid Kollak. *Nursing Theories: Conceptual & Philosophical Foundations*. Springer, 2006.

Smith, Mary Jane, and Patricia Liehr. *Middle Range Theory for Nursing*. Springer, 2013.

The National Voice for Academic Nursing. American Association of Colleges of Nursing, www.aacnnursing.org. Accessed 3 Sept. 2020.

Thompson, Cathy J. "What Is the Nursing Metaparadigm?" *Nursing Education Expert*, 3 Oct. 2017, nursingeducationexpert.com/metaparadigm/.

Thorne, Sally, et al. "Nursing's Metaparadigm Concepts: Disimpacting the Debates." *Journal of Advanced Nursing*, vol. 27, no. 6, 1998, pp. 1257–68.

"What Is Nursing?" *American Nurses Association*, www.nursingworld.org/practice-policy/workforce/what-is-nursing/. Accessed 3 Sept. 2020.

Grand Theories

ABSTRACT

Grand theory, classified as one of the three major categories of nursing theories based on abstraction, is broad and complex with abstract content that needs additional research for definition and clarification. This theory does not provide specific guidance for nursing interventions, but does provide a general framework for describing actions related to interventions.

INTRODUCTION

Nursing grand theories are formal, highly abstract, theoretical systems framing knowledge within the profession of nursing. The content of grand theories is not specific to events or patient populations, but rather they define concepts and principles applicable in a variety of situations. Grand theories are broad and address a variety of concepts that are integral to the foundations of nursing practice. These theories describe or explain situations that nurses may encounter in their scope of nursing practice. Grand theories have evolved over time and are often based on the experiences of the theorist writing the theory. For example, Florence Nightingale, considered the founder of nursing and the first nursing theorist, defined the Environmental Theory which includes the environmental factors of fresh air, clean water, efficient drainage, cleanliness, and sanitation and direct sun or light as necessary to assist the patient in recovery. Faye Glenn Abdellah developed the 21 Nursing Problems Theory, which changed the focus of nursing from disease-centered to patient-centered and was intended to guide care in hospitals. Additional theorists contributed to the development of the profession of nursing by writing grand theories that have been incorporated into the foundation and theoretical framework of nursing curriculum to this day.

EVOLUTION

In transitioning nursing care from the uneducated, hands on, trial-and-error beginnings on the battlefield to the high-tech world of nursing today, there was a need to define what constitutes the discipline of nursing. While nursing has always been perceived as a helping profession, the scientific underpinnings and complex technologies have required a more learned and academic approach to care. The argument has always been whether nursing is an art or a science. In the history of nursing, caring and comfort was the primary focus. In today's nursing, caring and comfort exist beside research, new drugs and agents, technology, equipment and a more intense care setting. Grand theories have evolved over time based on the care environment that exists and the author's own experiences in defining his or her theory on which to base nursing care.

GRAND THEORIES AND NURSING CURRICULUM

As nursing theories evolved over time, schools and colleges of nursing wrote documents that provided the foundation for curricula taught in each program. The conceptual framework, also referred to as the theoretical framework, provided the foundation on which nursing content was selected, how courses were to be ordered in the program, and how hands on learning experiences were sequenced. Interwoven in each conceptual framework was most often one or more grand theories. The conceptual framework integrates the four concepts central to the curriculum: person, environment, health and nursing. The person component incorporates concepts of learning, self, individuals, families, and communities. The environment focuses on internal and external inputs and processes that impact people. Nursing is a resource that can influence the environment of the health of a person. Health is a dynamic state of being that results from interactions between the person and the environment. Health may be influenced by nursing. Health can vary from wellness to illness and changes throughout life, including at the end of life. Nurses are influential with persons, their environment and their health. The teaching and modeling good health behaviors, the continuous care of the acutely or chronically ill patient, the provision of supportive care, educating others and conducting research to enhance the quality of care are all incorporated into the theoretical framework via nursing theories.

GRAND THEORIES AND NURSING THEORISTS

In addition to Florence Nightingale, the founder of nursing theory with her Environmental Theory, there have been multiple influential nursing theorists who have written the grand theories that shape the nursing profession. These theorists are covered in a separate section of this text. A few of the more well-recognized theorists and a short synopsis of their theories is provided here as examples. Hildegard Peplau defined the Theory of Interpersonal Relations as therapeutic interactions between an individual who is in need or sick and a nurse educated to recognize and respond to the stated or observed need. Imogene King defined the Theory of Goal Attainment that focused on the nurse's role in nurse-patient relationships designed to help the patient achieve health related goals. Virginia Henderson authored the Nursing Need Theory that emphasizes the need to increase the patient's independence and individualize care to enhance progress in the hospital. Joyce Travelbee described a Human to Human Relationship Model that stated that nursing was accomplished through human to human relationships designed to help and support in the struggles of illness. The Child Health Assessment Model was developed by Kathryn Barnard and addressed the concerns around improving the health of infants and their families. One of the most significant theorists, Ida Jean Orlando, developed the Nursing Process Theory that allows nurses to formulate an effective nursing care plan.

Each of the Grand Theories lends a significant level of support to why nurses perform in the clinical setting. The Grand Theories provide an historical frame of reference for the profession of nursing and should be recognized as shaping its evolution. In recent years, Alligood redefined the classification of nursing theories. She categorized nursing theories into four components: nursing philosophy, nursing conceptual models, nursing theories and grand theories, and middle-range nursing theories. Nursing philosophy is the most abstract of the theories and includes the works of Nightingale, Watson, Ray, and Benner. Nursing conceptual models are considered the pioneers of nursing theories and include theories that address the nursing metaparadigm. These include the works of Levine, Rogers, Roy, King, and Orem. Grand Nursing theories derive from nursing philosophies, conceptual models and other grand theories and include the works of Levine, Rogers, Orem, and King. With her new classification of nursing theories, she attempts to group theorists under a topic that reflects the purpose of their work rather than chronological and historical significance.

SUMMARY

Nursing theory, especially grand theories, will always occupy a place of historical significance in the evolution of nursing. It is important to understand how little was known of nursing care in the days of Florence Nightingale when hygiene and a good diet were considered innovative. The progress made from "handmaiden" to doctors to independent nurse is due in large part to nursing theory. While some may argue that nursing theories are old and outdated, it is imperative to see them as the foundation for a dynamic and ever evolving profession. The grand theories are abstract but foundational as they describe environment, interpersonal relationships, nursing needs and the nursing process, nurses helping patients achieve goals, and other core work that nurses do to improve patient outcome. Grand theories were integral to establishing nursing as a profession, discipline and science. Nursing theory will continue to evolve over time. While the development of new grand theories may be less, the emergence of middle-range theories focused on nursing practice will continue. This next level of theory will be both qualitative and quantitative and directly focused on the day to day provision of care. Grand theories set the future direction of both middle-range theories and practice-level theories. Understanding the history of nursing theories is crucial to understand the future of nursing practice.

—*Patricia Stanfill Edens*

Further Reading

Alligood, M. R. *Nursing Theorists and their Work*. 8th ed., Mosby Elsevier, 2014, docshare01.docshare.tips/files/29843/298436680.pdf.

———. *Nursing Theorists and their Work*. 9th ed., Elsevier eBook on Vital Source, 2018.

"Conceptual Framework." *UNC Greensboro School of Nursing*, nursing.uncg.edu/about/mission/conceptual-framework/. Accessed 14 Sept. 2020.

Higgins, P. A., and M. S. Moore. "Levels of Theoretical Thinking in Nursing." *Nursing Outlook Theory*, vol. 48, no. 4, 1 July 2000, www.nursingoutlook.org/article/S0029-6554(00)32367-3/pdf.

Mintz-Binder, R. "The Connection between Nursing Theory and Practice." *Nursing Made Incredibly Easy!*, vol. 17, no. 1, Jan.-Feb. 2019, pp. 6–9.

"Nursing Theory: Topical Overview and Research Resources for Nursing Theories." *University of Wisconsin-Milwaukee Libraries*, guides.library.uwm.edu/c.php?g+832148&p=5943165. Accessed 14 Sept. 2020.

Wayne, G. "Nursing Theories and Theorists: Your Theoretical Guide to Nursing Theories." *NursesLabs*, nurseslabs.com/nursing-theories/#what_are_nursing_theories. Accessed 14 Sept. 2020.

"What Is Nursing Theory? Key Concepts for DNPs." *Regis College*, online.regiscollege.edu/blog/what-is-nursing-theory/. Accessed 14 Sept. 2020.

MIDDLE-RANGE THEORIES

ABSTRACT

Middle-range theories are the least abstract of the nursing theories and are focused on practice applications. These theories develop evidence for nursing practice outcomes.

INTRODUCTION

Three categories classify nursing theories based on their level of abstraction: grand theories, middle-range theories, and practice-level theories. Grand theories are broad and not focused on application, but rather on developing a framework on which nursing practice can evolve. They are abstract and nonspecific in nature. Middle-range theories are the least abstract and describe how these theories apply to the practice of nursing. These theories are more targeted and limited in scope and present concepts that address a specific phenomenon. Because grand theories were difficult, if not impossible to test, scholars proposed the middle-range theory. These theories, while based on the works of the grand theorists, are defined from research, nursing practice, or from examples in other disciplines. Some of the grand theorists were actively involved in defining middle-range theories.

Much has been written in recent years about nursing practice outcomes or nursing outcomes and the need for evidence to show that the care delivered truly made a difference. These middle-range theories include nursing characteristics related to practice and nursing situations to provide theoretical evidence of applications and outcomes. The primary purpose of nursing theory is to improve practice and middle-range theories provide the framework to support this effort. As accrediting bodies, professional organizations and third-party payers require documentation of patient outcomes, the role of middle-range theories becomes more important.

Middle-range theories focus on a variety of components. The care setting and situation, the health and uniqueness of the client, the locale of practice (hospital, community, physician office), the actions of the nurse and the outcome of the intervention on the patient. The interconnectedness of theories, academics, research, and nursing care is crucial to delivering optimal quality care and enhanced patient outcomes.

MIDDLE-RANGE THEORIES

Ramona Mercer defined the theory of Maternal Role Attainment-Becoming a Mother in 1986. She stated that maternal role attainment is the period when a mother becomes bonded with her infant, learns the necessary caretaking tasks and finds pleasure and gratification in the role. Providing health teaching and interventions for both traditional and nontraditional mothers encourages a strong maternal identity and provides a better environment for the infant. Cheryl Tatano Beck defined the Postpartum Depression Theory and defines the issues surrounding the birth of a baby when joy is not experienced. This theory provides nurses with information to understand and prevent postpartum depression in their patients.

The Uncertainty in Illness Theory defined by Merle Mishel describes how patients and individuals form meaning from illness related situations. The goal of this theory is to provide a structure on which nursing interventions can be organized to promote optimal patient outcome. Pamela Reed's Self-Transcendence Theory has three basic concepts: vulnerability, self-transcendence, and well-being. Self-transcendence relates to the individual's ability to move beyond perceived boundaries. It also provides insight into the nature of humans and their circumstances.

The Theory of Illness Trajectory written by Wiener and Dodd provides a framework for nurses to better understand the uncertainty surrounding a chronic illness such as cancer. By understanding uncertainty, the nurse can better participate in the patient's trajectory of living. Uncertainty also translates to loss of control and assists nurses to work strategically to assist patients and families through the dynamics of their illness. Sorrow is a significant component of chronic health conditions for the patient, family, caregiver and the bereaved. Eakes, Burke, and Hainsworth define chronic sorrow as a normal response to loss. Good mental health is a pervasive need in the population, and especially so in the patient and family experiencing the stress of illness. Phil Barker's Tidal Model of Mental Health Recovery is widely viewed in nursing as a practical guide for psychiatric and mental health nursing. It describes relating to people in their moment of distress. The values of the Tidal model define ten commitments that define how to intervene with distressed patients such as giving the gift of time, valuing the voice, respecting the language, and developing transparency.

When comfort is enhanced, it can counteract the stressors inherent in treatments and illness. Katharine Kolbaca defined the Theory of Comfort to reflect patient comfort (relief, ease and transcendence) in physical, psychospiritual, environmental, and sociocultural contexts. As comfort needs change, the nurse must assess the situation and adjust nursing interventions. Kristen Swanson defined caring as a way of relating to someone in a nurturing manner with a personal sense of commitment to the individual. It offers a structure to bring caring to nursing practice, education, and research while providing a framework for caring and healing.

Not all patients will recover from their illnesses. End of life care is receiving an increased emphasis with the introduction of palliative care early in the disease process followed by hospice care during the dying phase. Ruland and Moore described their Peaceful End-of-Life Theory as a focus on peaceful, meaningful living in remaining time rather than on death itself. This theory reflects the complexity of caring for chronically ill and terminally ill patients.

SUMMARY

Each of these nursing theories are more in-depth than this reference can provide and further reading and exploration is always recommended. Middle-range theories, because they are applications, will continue to develop over time as the profession of nursing advances. In recent years, middle-range theories have superseded grand theories. With the advent of telehealth and telemedicine and other advances in patient care, it is likely that additional middle-range theories will be developed. Middle-range theories are recognized as a way to develop further knowledge to guide nursing practice.

—*Patricia Stanfill Edens*

Further Reading

Alligood, M. R. *Nursing Theorists and their Work*. 8th ed., Mosby Elsevier, 2014, docshare01.docshare.tips/files/29843/298436680.pdf.

———. *Nursing Theorists and their Work*. 9th ed., Elsevier eBook on Vital Source, 2018.

Wayne, G. "Nursing Theories and Theorists: Your Theoretical Guide to Nursing Theories." *NursesLabs*,

2020, nurseslabs.com/nursing-theories/#what_are_nursing_theories. Accessed 14 Sept. 2020.

"What Is Nursing Theory? Key Concepts for DNPs." *Regis College*, online.regiscollege.edu/blog/what-is-nursing-theory/. Accessed 14 Sept. 2020.

PRACTICE-LEVEL THEORIES

ABSTRACT

Practice-level theories are a type of nursing theory that focuses in a situation specific manner, is narrow in scope and directed toward a specific patient population at a specific moment in time. Nursing theory guides research and improves practice, particularly that of practice-level theories, which test specific interventions that may flow from grand or middle-level theories. Theory guided practice coupled with evidence-based data are the future of nursing.

INTRODUCTION

Grand theories and middle-range theories are interrelated with practice-level nursing theories. Practice-level theories provide a framework for nursing interventions in a specific situation and encourages expected outcomes as the result of nursing practice. This is the least abstract of the three categories of nursing theories but has a more direct effect on nursing practice. Practice-level theories may test singular components of grand and middle-range theories, creating what might be called practice-based evidence.

Nursing outcome studies measure the effectiveness of interventions to create change. Studies are often based, either accidentally or on purpose, on nursing theories. When researchers share the use of a theory to investigate a health-related phenomenon, they may build knowledge more efficiently. Theory guided research, in addition to explaining how they planned a study, aids in comparing results between and across studies. For example, a study looking at environmental impacts such as temperature of an operating room, may be labeled an outcome study but flows from the Environmental Theory of Florence Nightingale from the mid-1800s.

EXAMPLES OF PRACTICE-LEVEL THEORIES

The application of practice-level theories may not be obvious in the nursing care setting. Because these theories often flow from grand and middle-range theories, they may be seen as a quality improvement study or a research study to test an intervention in a defined setting with a defined group of patients rather than being labeled a practice-level theory. An example may also be practice-based research which defines a hypothesis and tests interventions. Specific examples might be the evidence of postpartum depression in women without partners or husbands with a defined number of participants, during a defined period, and using a defined tool to measure the evidence of postpartum depression. A corollary could be identifying postpartum depression, trying a certain approach with the subjects such as journaling feelings and frustrations, and evaluating whether it made a difference in their perceived depression. This could relate to Beck's Postpartum Depression Theory to provide evidence to understand and prevent postpartum depression.

Since the primary purpose of nursing theories is to improve practice, the understanding of grand theories and middle-range theories and their influence in developing practice-level theories, will influence the health and quality of life of patients. Theories are fundamentally important to the research process where the theory provides the framework to guide the study and validates its importance. Practice-level theories and their application connect the gap between theory and practice.

OTHER CLASSIFICATIONS

In addition to the three levels of abstract nursing theories (grand, middle-level, and practice-level), theories may also be classified based on their goals: descriptive and prescriptive. Descriptive is the first step in developing a theory and describes the phenomena associated with the potential theory. Explanatory theories describe relationships between phenomena. For example, does environment impact mental health? This incorporates two theories, the grand theory of environment proposed by Florence Nightingale and the middle-range theory of the tidal model of mental health in an attempt to describe an observed phenomenon, or a practice-level theory application. Prescriptive theories are an attempt to determine an outcome of select nursing interventions.

Some nursing theories are organized by needs-based theories, interaction theories and outcome theories. Outcome theories are an evolution from practice-level theories and describe nurses as directing care based on their knowledge of physiological and behavioral systems documenting the effect of their care.

SUMMARY

Practice-level theories are the third level of nursing theory application to practice and the least difficult to incorporate into nursing practice. It requires defining an issue, developing an approach to issue management and evaluating patient response. It is the necessary next step in determining if an intervention delivers the appropriate outcome. All nursing interventions flow from one of the three levels of abstract nursing theories. The integration of nursing theories into the curricula of nursing programs provide a learning process based on decades of grand theories, middle-range theories and practice-level theories. Practice-level theories are narrow in scope and suggest the outcomes of specific nursing interventions. They are often a test of the effectiveness of grand and middle-level theories.

—*Patricia Stanfill Edens*

Further Reading

Alligood, M. R. *Nursing Theorists and their Work*. 8th ed., Mosby Elsevier, 2014, docshare01.docsha,re.tips/files/29843/298436680.pdf.

———. *Nursing Theorists and their Work*. 9th ed., Elsevier eBook on Vital Source, 2018.

Saleh, U. S. "Theory Guided Practice in Nursing," www.pulsus.com/scholarly-articles/theory-guided-practice-in-nursing.pdf. Accessed 14 Sept. 2020.

Wayne, G. "Nursing Theories and Theorists: Your Theoretical Guide to Nursing Theories." *NursesLabs*, nurseslabs.com/nursing-theories/#what_are_nursing_theories. Accessed 14 Sept. 2020.

"What Is Nursing Theory? Key Concepts for DNPs." *Regis College*, online.regiscollege.edu/blog/what-is-nursing-theory/. Accessed 14 Sept. 2020.

NURSING THEORISTS

From Florence Nightingale, considered the first nursing theorist with her Environmental Theory in the 1850s, to Katherine Kolbaca—Theory of Comfort—and Kristen Swanson—Theory of Caring—in the 1990s, this section profiles thirteen individuals whose nursing theories are based on a variety of concepts, including patient-centered care, stress-reduction, treating a patient's inter-related systems, scientific knowledge, self-esteem, and interaction between nurse and consumer.

Florence Nightingale	45
Hildegard Peplau	47
Faye Abdellah	49
Ida Jean Orlando	51
Dorothea Orem	53
Imogene King	55
Betty Neuman	57
Callista Roy	58
Jean Watson	60
Abraham Maslow	62
Katharine Kolbaca and Kristen M. Swanson	65
Nola Pender	67

Florence Nightingale

ABSTRACT
Florence Nightingale is considered history's most famous nurse and the first nursing theorist with her Environmental Theory. Starting with caring for soldiers during the Crimean war, she went on to advocate for nursing education and advocacy. In 1860, she opened the first school of nursing at St. Thomas Hospital in London.

INFLUENCE ON NURSING

Florence Nightingale (1820–1910) was a nurse recognized for defining and shaping the modern practice of nursing. She is considered the first nursing theorist with her development of the Environmental Theory that created nursing practices to create sanitary conditions for patients receiving care. She is also considered the founder of modern nursing. Based on her work with wounded soldiers during the Crimean War, she gained the name "The Lady with the Lamp." She made her rounds on horseback carrying an oil lamp. To this day, the lamp is often used as a symbol in nursing recognition and graduation ceremonies. Born in Italy to a prominent British family, Nightingale was considered awkward in social situations. She was provided a classical education on the family's estate with an interest and expertise in mathematics. Active in philanthropy from a young age, she cared for the poor and ill in the village neighboring her home. At 17, she made the decision to dedicate her life to medical care for the sick. She made the commitment to overhaul and sanitize the appalling conditions of healthcare in England. In 1844, she enrolled in the Lutheran Hospital of Pastor Fliedner Nursing School in Kaiserwerth, Germany. She remained single throughout her life stating that Victorian women who want to go out into the world and do something could not have a marriage and children.

In addition to developing her Environmental Theory, she also wrote over 200 books, reports and papers. In 1860, she authored *Notes on Nursing* that described principles of nursing, a book still in print today with translation in multiple languages. She received money for her work from the British government and used that money to found the St. Thomas Hospital and the Nightingale Training School for Nurses. The grant for $250,000 recognized Nightingale's work. She received multiple other honors and awards during her lifetime, and was the first woman to receive the Order of Merit. She also mentored Linda Richards, America's first trained nurse. Richards returned to the United States with sufficient education and training to establish high-quality schools of nursing and was a nursing pioneer in both the United States and Japan. During the American Civil War, the

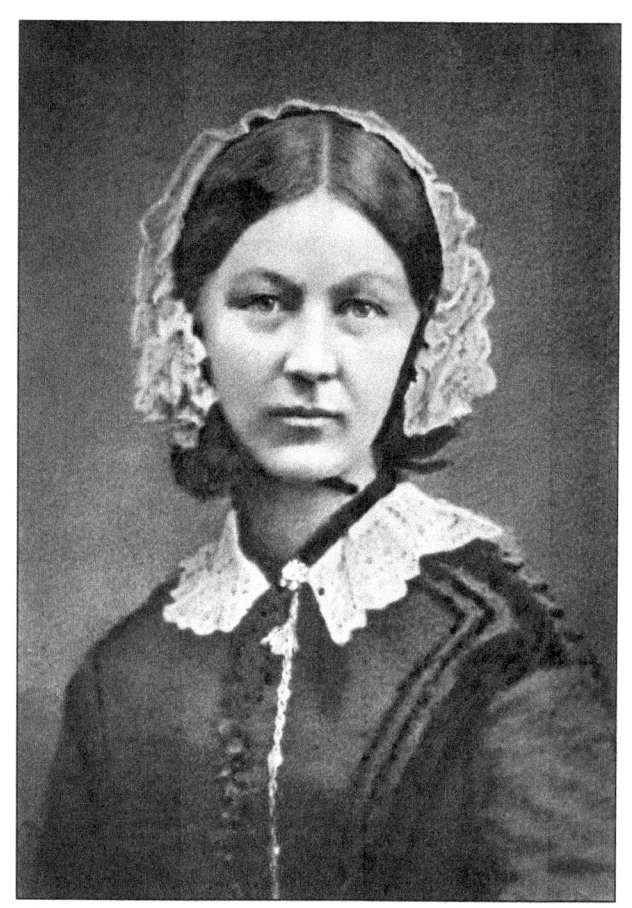

Florence Nightingale, c. 1860 (Wikimedia Commons)

Union government asked her advice in organizing field medical hospitals.

Florence Nightingale was also one of the first to recognize that data collection and statistics could influence care. William Farr, a noted government statistician and her mentor, helped her gather data from military hospitals. She was able to confirm that more than seven times as many soldiers died from disease than from combat. She also showed that deaths dropped dramatically when hospitals were clean and sanitary. These findings clearly supported that improved sanitation decreased death rates. In 1858, she was the first woman named as a Fellow in the Royal Statistical Society.

ENVIRONMENTAL THEORY
Florence Nightingale based her Environmental Theory on her work in the Crimean War. She defined the theory as "the act of utilizing the environment of the patient to assist him in his recovery." The goal for nurses is to ensure that the environment of care settings are appropriate to encourage the return to health. She theorized that external factors of the patient's environment and surroundings affect life, biologic, and physiological processes, and ongoing development. The five environmental factors theorized to impact recovery are: (1) fresh air, (2) pure water, (3) efficient drainage, (4) cleanliness, and sanitation, and, (5) direct sunlight or light.

She wrote an 830-page report entitled *Notes on Matters Affecting the Health, Efficiency and Hospital Administration of the British Army*, analyzing her experiences and proposing reforms for military hospitals operating under poor conditions. The book led to the development of the Royal Commission for the Health of the Army in 1857.

The Environmental Theory of Florence Nightingale has direct application today in hospitals and other healthcare settings. Maintaining a clean environment for the patient is essential. Isolation of patients with infections contributes to a decreased spread of disease. Many hospitals have laminar flow rooms, a type of air handling system using high energy particulate air (HEPA) filters, with the focus on cleaning the air in a patient or operating room. Phototherapy, a treatment with a special light is often used to treat newborn jaundice. Many of these nursing actions are based in Environmental Theory. Exposure to hazardous substances in the hospital setting are managed to decrease the risk of negative impacts. Safety is a part of environmental theory as patients are protected from exposures to hazardous factors.

SUMMARY
While Florence Nightingale is recognized historically as a leader in nursing and the author of a theory still recognized as necessary today, she does have some detractors. Some nurses in the British public service union, UNISON, feel she promoted a hierarchical approach to nursing, opposed higher education and wanted nurses to remain chaste and obedient. In general, Nightingale is recognized as a leader in the development of the profession and for her promotion of a safe and secure environment of care even as advances in nursing education move far beyond her basic education tenants.

The profession of nursing today is in debt to Florence Nightingale. She advocated for the role of education for individuals in formal schools of nursing. As other theorists defined their theories of nursing, the foundation Nightingale provided is still quite evident. Hygiene, fresh water, and air are important parts of life whether in the hospital or in the community. Current events such as lead-contaminated water in a community, lack of fresh water in parts of the world, and pollution and fires contaminating the air all have negative health impacts. Florence Nightingale provided a strong foundation for nursing education and for a safe and protective environment to impact healthcare.

Her life was quite interesting. An investor recently bought her family estate and is restoring it to what it would have been during her life. There are museums in her honor and she is recognized in nursing as having set the principles and priorities for nursing education. Nightingale's lamp is an internationally recognized symbol that represents her transforming work, compassion, and goodwill. The pinning ceremony at graduation, when the new nurse receives the pin representing her school, is often accompanied by the lighting of replicas of Florence Nightingale's lamp. Florence Nightingale truly founded nursing education and nursing theory and her impacts are still felt today.

—*Patricia Stanfill Edens*

Further Reading

Gonzalo A. "Florence Nightingale: Environmental Theory." *Nurseslabs*, Updated Aug. 2019, nurseslabs.com/florence-nightingales-environmental-theory/.

Hammer J. "Thou Shalt Not Underestimate Florence Nightingale." *Smithsonian*, vol. 50, no. 10, Mar. 2020, pp. 24–33, 78–79.

Wayne, G. "Nursing Theories and Theorists: Your Theoretical Guide to Nursing Theories." *NursesLabs*, nurseslabs.com/nursing-theories/#what_are_nursing_theories. Accessed 14 Sept. 2020.

"What Is Nursing Theory? Key Concepts for DNPs." *Regis College*, online.regiscollege.edu/blog/what-is-nursing-theory/. Accessed 14 Sept. 2020.

Zborowsky, T. "The Legacy of Florence Nightingale's Environmental Theory: Nursing Research Focusing on the Impact of Healthcare Environments." *HERD: Health Environments Research & Design Journal*, vol. 7, no. 4, pp. 19–24.

HILDEGARD PEPLAU

ABSTRACT

Nursing theorists are responsible in great part, for the evolution of nursing. By dedicating her professional career to nursing and nursing theories, Hildegard Peplau made a major impact on the development of these fields, especially psychiatric nursing. She was particularly influential in promoting reforms in mental health nursing and in increasing understanding of interpersonal relations between nurses and their patients.

BACKGROUND

Hildegard Peplau was born on September 1, 1909, in Reading, Pennsylvania, into a German American family as one of six children. Even as a young child, she was a keen observer of human behavior. At the age of nine, a major flu epidemic raged across the world, striking down between 30 and 50 million people worldwide and killing approximately 675,000 Americans. The pandemic had a major impact on Peplau, and she determined that she wanted to become a nurse. She was trained in her home state of Pennsylvania at the Pottstown Hospital School of Nursing, completing her nursing degree in 1931. Nursing was still a relatively young field at the time, and professional aspects of the field were still being developed.

From 1932 to 1936, Peplau worked as a private duty and general staff nurse in both Pennsylvania and New York. In 1936, she accepted a position as head nurse at the College Health Services department of Bennington College in Vermont. During the school year, she continued to pursue her education, studying with Erich Fromm, the internationally acclaimed German American psychologist, and training in the field of nursing psychiatry at Chestnut Lodge with Frieda Fromm-Reichmann, a German American psychotherapist, and Harry Stack Sullivan, a noted American Freudian. By the time she left Bennington College in 1942, she had become executive officer of the Health Services department.

American nurses were recruited for military services after the Japanese attacked Pearl Harbor on December 7, 1941. Peplau joined the Army Nurse Corps and was ordered to report for duty with neuropsychiatric units within the United States and in England between 1943 and 1945. Following the end of World War II, she began studying for advanced degrees at Columbia University's Teachers College. While obtaining both a master's degree and a doctorate, she taught nursing classes. Between 1948 and 1953, she also served as director of the school's psychiatric nursing program and worked as a psychoanalyst at the William Alanson White Institute in New York.

Peplau became a mother in 1945 when her daughter Letitia Anne (Tish) was born. She chose not to marry the child's father, Donald McIntosh. Illegitimacy and single motherhood were not accepted social practices at the time, and Peplau agreed to let her brother adopt Tish. It was not until 1984 that she openly acknowledged her daughter and moved to Sherman Oaks, California, where her daughter served as a social psychology professor at the University of California. She died in 1999.

ESTABLISHING THE THEORY OF INTERPERSONAL RELATIONS

As her career developed, Peplau helped to define the field of psychiatric nursing in the United States. She had become one of the most respected names in the field by the early 1950s and was the first professor to teach graduate classes for psychiatric nurses at Columbia University. Between 1956 and 1974, she taught at Rutgers University, where she trained clinical specialists in psychiatric nursing with funding from the National Institute of Mental Health. Her work at Rutgers led to a greater understanding of the complexities of the field and to the development of new theories based on that understanding. Using data collected through clinical interviews, Peplau became an expert at bridging the gap between theory and practice.

Throughout the 1950s and 1960s, Peplau spent summers giving workshops at mental hospitals in both the United States and overseas. These classes dealt with topics such as individual, family, and group therapy, interpersonal communication, and interviewing techniques. She also traveled widely, speaking and lecturing on topics relevant to nursing in general and to psychiatric nursing in particular. She stressed the need for greater professionalism within nursing and emphasized the need for advanced degrees for nurses while continuing to produce a growing body of research.

The work for which Peplau is best known is *The Theory of Interpersonal Relations* (1952), which clearly reflects the influence of noted names in the field, such as Sullivan and American psychologist Percival Symonds, and advocated that psychiatric nursing move away from the custodial method and toward more therapeutic care. She developed four components to explain her significant nursing theory of interpersonal relations, suggesting that the person component refers to a natural inclination to attempt to meet individual needs by reducing anxiety, the environment component is composed of external forces dictated by culture, the health component reflects personality development, and the nursing component involves community-wide cooperation. Within this nursing model, she examined the phases of orientation, identification, exploitation, and resolution. As interpersonal relationships develop, she argued that the role of nurse in relation to the patient sequences from stranger to resource provider to teacher to counselor to surrogate to active leader and, finally, to technical expert.

Peplau served as president of the American Nurses Association from 1970 to 1972 and as second vice president from 1972 to 1974. Though she retired from her position at Rutgers in the mid-1970s, she continued to teach periodically. Throughout her career, she served as visiting professor at universities in the United States, Africa, Latin America, and Europe. She also further advanced the field of psychiatric nursing by serving on a number of advisory committees, working with the World Health Organization and the International Council of Nursing, among others.

IMPACT

Peplau's greatest impact was on the development of the understanding of interpersonal relationships between nurse and patient. As a pioneer in the field, she brought greater insight into how this relationship functions, helping to redefine the relationship as a dynamic process and eradicating earlier beliefs that nurses were intended to function solely as channels for transmitting information from physicians to patients. In 1996, she was declared a Living Legend by the American Academy of Nursing.

—*Elizabeth Rholetter Purdy*

Further Reading

Alligood, Martha Raile. *Nursing Theorists and Their Work*. Elsevier, 2014.

Callaway, Barbara J. *Hildegard Peplau: Psychiatric Nurse of the Century*. Springer, 2002.

D'Antonio, Patricia, et al. "The Future in the Past: Hildegard Peplau and Interpersonal Relations in Nursing." *Nursing Inquiry*, vol. 21, no. 4, 2014, pp. 311–17.

Masters, Kathleen. *Nursing Theories: A Framework for Professional Practice*. 2nd ed., Jones, 2015.

Smith, Marlaine C., and Marilyn E. Parker, editors. *Nursing Theories and Nursing Practices*. 4th ed., Davis, 2015.

Stuart, Gail Wiscarz. *Principles and Practice of Psychiatric Nursing*. 10th ed., Elsevier, 2013.

Winship, Gary, et al. "Collective Biography and the Legacy of Hildegard Peplau, Annie Altschul, and Eileen Skellern: The Origins of Mental Health Nursing and Its Relevance to the Current Crisis in Psychiatry." *Journal of Research in Nursing*, vol. 14, no. 6, 2009, pp. 505–17.

Faye Abdellah

ABSTRACT

Nursing theorists are responsible in great part, for the evolution of nursing. In a public health career that spanned more than seven decades, Faye Abdellah changed the traditional conception of the role of the nurse by moving the focus away from understanding illness and administering medical protocols and toward responding to patients as people with a complex of emotional and psychological needs.

BACKGROUND

Faye Glenn Abdellah was born in New York City on March 13, 1919, the daughter of first generation immigrants: her father was Algerian, her mother Scottish. Concerned over raising children in a large city, Abdellah's parents moved the family to New Jersey, near the small town of Neptune City, just south of Asbury Park, along the Atlantic coast.

A precocious child with a gift for helping neighbors, Abdellah would later recount how she decided to pursue nursing on the afternoon of May 6, 1937. She was eighteen years old, and she and her brother had driven to Lakehurst Airfield to watch the arrival of the massive German zeppelin the *Hindenburg*. When the aircraft exploded and crashed just above the mooring mast, Abdellah was among the first to get to the wounded, many with deep burns, who were strewn about the airfield. She felt helpless. When emergency

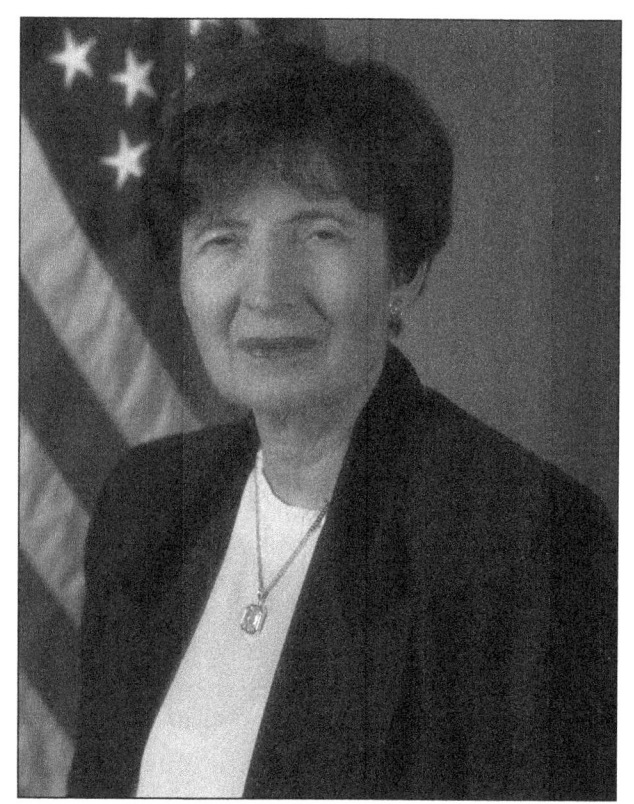

Faye Abdellah (Wikimedia Commons)

responders arrived, Abdellah watched the care and confidence of their work, and she knew then she would pursue nursing.

She completed her nursing certificate at the nursing school at Fitkin Memorial Hospital (now part of the Jersey Shore Medical Center). Although such certification was all nurses were required to have, Abdellah felt that the school's program of study, which stressed basic protocols nurses would apply across the board to all patients, was too limited. Nurses, she believed, needed to be more grounded in cutting-edge research and more in tune with individual patient needs.

Abdellah retired from USU in 2002, after more than fifty years of working for the government. She was living in Maryland at that time. She died in 2017.

NURSING CAREER
Abdellah continued her studies at Columbia University, completing a BA in nursing and then expanding her expertise by completing post graduate work in both psychology and education. During this time, she worked as a nurse in a private school. After completing her doctoral work, she was determined to reshape the role of the nursing profession.

Her first teaching post was with the prestigious Yale University School of Nursing. Reviewing the textbooks available for nursing instruction, Abdellah became frustrated; the protocols did little to encourage hands-on care and treated nurses like robots completing rounds. Nurses were not expected to think or to approach a patient as an individual. Nursing programs did little to prepare nurses to actually work with patients. Within a year of her appointment, she gathered her colleagues and students outside Yale's nursing building and dramatically burned a stack of the required textbooks—although she would have to pay for the books later, she recalled that the moment set her free.

Over the next decade, Abdellah, by gathering massive amounts of data from practicing nurses, created what she called the Twenty-one Problems. For Abdellah, elements of a patient's recovery were best approached as problems that nurses were there to address. The protocol listed critical elements of patient care divided into three broad areas: physical needs (such as providing medicines, charting tests, ensuring adequate nutrition and hydration, and securing a stable and restful environment); emotional needs (such as listening to patient worries, addressing patient anxiety, and communicating clearly and regularly and honestly with the patient), and sociological needs (such as interacting and communicating with the patient's family and friends and taking into account a patient's background as part of recovery and treatment).

In 1949, Abdellah left private hospital work and joined the Commissioned Corps of the United States Public Health Service (USPHS), a uniformed branch of the federal government. After a stint overseas during the Korean War, Abdellah dedicated forty years to creating innovative templates for nursing. Her most notable creations include the Progressive Patient Care Protocol, which developed three stages for nursing care (Intensive Care, Immediate Care, and Home Care, the last introducing the revolutionary concept that nurses need to be involved in developing a patient's self-care and regimens for recovery after a hospital stay) and the PACE standards (Patient Assessment of Care Evaluation), which asked patients themselves to respond to the effectiveness of nursing care.

In 1974, she became the first nurse commissioned as a two-star rear admiral. In 1981, she was named deputy surgeon general, the first time a nurse had been so honored. Over the next eight years she worked tirelessly to promote public health awareness, most notably about acquired immunodeficiency syndrome (AIDS) and drug addiction (part of First Lady Nancy Reagan's "Just Say No" initiative). In addition, she began to work in gerontological care, particularly in the areas of hospice care and treatment of Alzheimer's disease.

After her retirement from the USPHS in 1989, Abdellah undertook a global campaign to raise awareness of the changing role of nurses. In 1994, she was the recipient of the inaugural American Academy of Nursing's Lifetime Achievement Award, often called the Nobel Prize of nursing. She was named to the Nursing Hall of Fame in 1999 and to the National Women's Hall of Fame in 2000. She also cofounded the Graduate School of Nursing at the Uniformed Services University (USU) and served as its first dean.

IMPACT

Faye Abdellah is widely regarded as one of the most significant figures in nursing in the twentieth century. By introducing the ideas that nursing care needed to be grounded in researched data and that nurses cared for people, not patients, Abdellah created revolutionary templates for virtually all areas of hospital nursing care. As a teacher, as a researcher, and as a charismatic speaker, she pioneered nursing protocols that introduced the cornerstone concept that a nurse creates the therapeutic environment in which a patient can best cope with illness.

—*Joseph Dewey*

Further Reading

Alligood, Martha Raile. *Nursing Theorists and Their Work.* Elsevier, 2014.
"Faye Glenn Abdellah." *National Women's Hall of Fame*, n.d. Accessed 19 Aug. 2016.
Johnson, Betty, and Pamela Webber. *An Introduction to Theory and Reasoning in Nursing.* 4th ed., LWW, 2013.
McEwen, Melanie. *Theoretical Basis for Nursing.* 4th ed., LWW: 2014.
Meleis, Afaf Ibrahim. *Theoretical Nursing: Development and Progress.* 5th ed., LWW, 2011.
Reed, Pamela. *Perspectives on Nursing Theory.* 6th ed., LWW, 2011.
Wayne, Gil. "Faye G. Abdellah's 21 Nursing Problems Theory." *Nurseslabs*, 29 Sept. 2014.

IDA JEAN ORLANDO

ABSTRACT

Nursing theorists are responsible in great part, for the evolution of nursing. Ida Jean Orlando set the standard for effective nursing practices with her theories on the nursing process in the 1960s and 1970s. She spent many years observing thousands of nurse-patient relationships to formulate more successful nursing systems. Orlando's methods found extensive support within the medical community and are still used in modern nursing education.

BACKGROUND

Ida Jean Orlando was born on August 12, 1926, in New York. Her parents were Italian immigrants, and she grew up during the Great Depression (1929–1939). Orlando began her nursing education at the New York Medical College School of Nursing, earning her nursing diploma in 1947. She then earned a bachelor's degree in public health nursing in 1951 from St. John's University. Orlando continued her education at Columbia University Teachers College, receiving her master's degree in mental health consultation in 1954. Throughout her years of higher education, Orlando held an array of jobs in the nursing field in areas including obstetrics, medicine, and emergency room nursing. After earning her master's, she took a job as a teacher at the Yale School of Nursing in Connecticut.

During the eight years she spent at Yale, she also worked as a research associate and principal investigator for a federal project entitled Integrations of Mental Health Concepts in a Basic Curriculum. The project called for Orlando to collect data from observing students' interaction with patients and members of educational and healthcare teams. She reported her findings in her first book, *The Dynamic Nurse-Patient Relationship: Function, Process, and Principles* (1961). The book established what became known as Orlando's nursing process theory.

Orlando married Robert Pelletier in 1961. She died in 2007 at the age of 81.

LIFE'S WORK

Orlando's nursing practice and research-based theory blends nursing practices, psychiatric mental health nursing, and nursing education. The theory is based on a mutual nurse-patient relationship that acknowledges how the actions of one affect the other. Orlando stressed the importance of patient participation during nurse questioning. She also outlined a detailed strategy to ensure the most accurate calculations resulted from a nurse's inquiry.

Orlando's nursing process theory can be broken down into three concepts: patient behavior, nurse reaction, and nurse action. In terms of patient behavior, nurses must take into account the patient's verbal and nonverbal behavior when assessing a situation. A nurse's capacity to understand a patient's ability to communicate what is wrong is critical to an effective resolution of the issue. The nurse's reactions and actions are designed around this understanding. A nurse's reaction marks the beginning of the nursing process and consists of a series of steps that lead to an action. First, the nurse observes the patient's behavior and shares his or her thoughts and feelings about the observations with the patient. The patient will either confirm or deny the point of view, at which point the nurse must weigh his or her personal opinion with the patient's input. This focus on mindfulness is meant to ensure the best possible reaction to a situation and produce professional, deliberative action rather than automatic, impulsive action. Nurse actions must be dictated by patient need and not by medical orders. According to Orlando, professional nursing actions are designed to correctly identify the best way to help a patient independent from the input of physicians and other healthcare providers. Such actions must take into account how the interaction between patient and nurse can affect each other's perceptions, thoughts, and feelings. Correct action can then be verified as effective or ineffective immediately after being implemented.

Orlando spent the next decade honing her theory, which quickly gained popularity within the medical community. The National Institute of Mental Health provided Orlando with funding to develop improved educational methods that would teach nurses how to improve their interpersonal skills when dealing with patients. Orlando later worked as a clinical nurse for the McLean Hospital in Belmont, Massachusetts, where she took advantage of her surroundings to further her studies in nursing practice. She studied the interactions nurses had with patients, hospital staff members, and other nurses. Her observations convinced her that the hospital was in need of a nursing education program. She later established an educational program and nursing service department for McLean, which utilized her nursing practice theory in its daily functions.

The program at McLean helped Orlando conceive her next book, *The Discipline and Teaching of Nursing Process* (1972). The book redefined parts of her original theory. Her writings continued to stress the importance of the nurse-patient relationship. Orlando served on the board of Harvard Community Health Plan in Boston, Massachusetts, throughout the 1970s and 1980s. She also began teaching at Boston University School of Nursing in 1981. Orlando held various administrative positions at the Metropolitan State Hospital in Waltham, Massachusetts, in the late 1980s before being named assistant director of the hospital's Nursing for Education and Research.

Orlando's *The Dynamic Nurse-Patient Relationship: Function, Process, and Principles* was reprinted in 1990 and was eventually translated into five languages. Orlando retired in 1992. She was honored with a Living Legends in Nursing award by the Massachusetts chapter of the American Nurses Association in 2006. She passed away on November 28, 2007.

IMPACT

Orlando's work was the first known theory related to the nursing process. Her nursing theory continues to be widely used within the nursing education community and her texts remain a critical part of nursing process strategy around the world. Orlando is responsible for bringing more awareness to the significance of the nurse-patient relationship. Many scholars believe this focus has brought greater success and discipline to the healthcare community.

—*Cait Caffrey*

Further Reading

Alligood, Martha Raile. *Nursing Theorists and Their Work*. Elsevier, 2014.

Butts, Janie B., and Karen L. Rich. *Philosophies and Theories for Advanced Nursing Practice*. Jones & Bartlett Learning, 2015.

Fawcett, Jacqueline, and Susan DeSanto-Madeya. *Contemporary Nursing Knowledge: Analysis and Evaluation of Nursing Models and Theories*. F.A. Davis Company, 2013.

Meleis, Afaf Ibrahim. *Theoretical Nursing: Development and Progress*. Wolters Kluwer, 2012.

Sitzman, Kathleen, and Lisa Wright Eichelberger. *Understanding the Work of Nurse Theorists*. Jones & Bartlett Learning, 2015.

Smith, Marlaine C., and Marilyn E. Parker. *Nursing Theories and Nursing Practice*. F.A. Davis Company, 2013.

Dorothea Orem

ABSTRACT

Nursing theorists are responsible in great part, for the evolution of nursing. Dorothea Orem developed the self-care deficit nursing theory, sometimes known simply as the self-care theory or the Orem Model of nursing, which redefined the role of nurses in healthcare by suggesting that when a formerly healthy person becomes a patient, nurses should address deficiencies in that patient's ability to take care of themselves and their own health.

BACKGROUND

Born on July 15, 1914, Dorothea Elizabeth Orem was raised in Baltimore, Maryland, in a comfortably middle-class environment. Her father worked in construction and her mother was a homemaker. The example of her mother tirelessly devoting her time and energy to maintaining the household and taking care of Orem and her older sister influenced Orem's perception of the role of a nurse. Before she graduated from high school, she knew her life would be dedicated to the service of others. Although she briefly considered becoming a nun or a teacher, she opted rather to pursue nursing.

She earned her nursing certification from the Providence Hospital School of Nursing in Washington, DC. At the time, such certification was considered ample education for an occupation that was perceived to be largely an administrator of doctors' protocols. Orem was not content with that; after working for a brief stint as a nurse at St. John's Hospital (now Saints Medical Center) in Lowell, Massachusetts, she decided to continue her education at the Catholic University of America in Washington, where she earned a BS in nursing education in 1939, followed by an MS in nursing education in 1945.

DEVELOPING NURSING EDUCATION

After working as a nurse for several years, Orem came to believe that the value of nursing began in the classroom, and she decided to devote herself to working with nursing students. In addition, she began to gather data on nurses and their function in hospital operations, original research at a time when little attention was paid to the role of nurses. She became the director of the Providence Hospital School of Nursing in Detroit, Michigan. She also taught there, working in biological sciences and nursing from 1945 to 1948. She then returned to Catholic University and taught there for more than a decade, serving for a time as the dean of the university's school of nursing. Determined to develop teaching curricula that matched

53

what she had observed as a practicing nurse, Orem worked as a nursing curriculum consultant for more than a decade, working with hospitals and nursing schools across the country.

By the 1970s, Orem was convinced that nurses had a critical role to play in patient treatment, a role that had yet to be clearly defined in the literature of the field. Orem was convinced that patients needed to be treated as people—individuals with medical histories, certainly, but also with families and friends, all of whom played a role in the treatment and recovery from illness. She published her landmark book, *Nursing: Concepts of Practice*, in 1971. The success of this book established Orem among the leading nursing theorists in America. Because of its flexibility, her theory has been used mostly for rehabilitation and primary care. The theory is based on the idea that patients wish to care for themselves and that they are more likely to recover if encouraged to do so.

Orem theorized that a person, by nature, desires self-reliance, to be empowered to control and direct their own life. Illness, of course, challenges that assumption. For Orem, nursing actually begins with the person maintaining a lifestyle that encourages health and well-being, taking care to provide themselves with adequate sustenance, for instance, to pursue generally healthy activities, and to maintain a safe lifestyle that balances social interaction and necessary solitude and that avoids self-destructive habits such as smoking and excessive eating. In addition, the individual needs to stay informed about potential symptoms, monitor their own health, take prescribed medications, and modify their lifestyle to adjust to any long-term medical conditions.

When catastrophic illness or accidents occur to disrupt that self-reliance, the person becomes a patient and suddenly faces a deficiency in their ability to care for themselves. That can be traumatic—and that is where the nurse comes in, to address that self-care deficit. The nurse's goal then is to restore the patient's independence and self-reliance through dedicated care, communication, and careful and methodical regimens designed specifically to assist that individual in their recovery of self-reliance. That is a process of necessary interaction—the nurse is part of the patient's return to independence. That process necessarily involves, for Orem, the nurse using all the resources of the patient's life: family, friends, even religious beliefs.

For Orem, the nurse's role is divided into three basic stages: first, the nurse assesses the patient's condition, and that assessment changes day to day under their care and must be informed by regular communication from the attending physicians and with the patient; second, the nurse diagnoses the patient's specific responses to treatments and medications—everything from biological reactions to medications and treatments to overall psychological reactions, such as emotions and mood; and third, the nurse implements protocols and regimens that are tailored for that patient. In each stage, the nurse is dedicated to restoring the patient's ability to care for themselves. For Orem, illness is itself an interruption of a healthy life—and the nurse's job is to return the patient to the status of a person.

IMPACT

Orem tirelessly promoted her humanistic theory of nursing in numerous journal publications, in the classroom, and on the lecture circuit. Because the theory seemed self-evident, some criticized Orem for simplifying the recovery and treatment process and for assuming that people would maintain a healthy lifestyle when such a lifestyle was, in fact, quite demanding. But Orem staunchly defended her theory well into her seventies. She became an inspiration for nurses who saw nursing as compassionate and involved with patients as people. Orem retired to Georgia's affluent Skidaway Island near Savannah and died there at the age of ninety-two in 2007.

—Joseph Dewey

Further Reading

Alligood, Martha Raile. *Nursing Theorists and Their Work.* Elsevier, 2014.

Clarke, Pamela N., et al. "The Impact of Dorothea Orem's Life and Work: An Interview with Orem Scholars." *Nursing Science Quarterly*, vol. 22, no. 1, 2009, pp. 41–46.

"Dorothea Orem Collection." *Alan Mason Chesney Medical Archives*. Johns Hopkins Medical Inst., n.d. Accessed 28 Aug. 2016.

Fawcett, Jacqueline. "The Nurse Theorists: 21st Century Updates—Dorothea E. Orem." *Nursing Science Quarterly*, vol. 14, no. 1, 2001, pp. 34–38.

Orem, Dorothea E. "Views of Human Beings Specific to Nursing." *Nursing Science Quarterly*, vol. 10, no. 1, 1997, pp. 26–31.

Pearson, Alan. "Dead Poets, Nursing Theorists and Contemporary Nursing Practice." *International Journal of Nursing Practice*, vol. 14, no. 1, 2008, pp. 1–2.

Renpenning, Kathie McLaughlin, and Susan G. Taylor. *Self-Care Theory in Nursing: Selected Papers of Dorothea Orem.* Springer, 2003.

Wayne, Gil. "Dorothea E. Orem." *Nurselabs*, 11 Aug. 2014.

IMOGENE KING

ABSTRACT

Nursing theorists are responsible in great part, for the evolution of nursing. Imogene King revolutionized the clinical practice of nursing by creating innovative conceptual models to define the relationship between a nurse and a patient. King's models emphasize patient-environment and patient-nurse interactions, as well as goal-setting.

BACKGROUND

Imogene Martina King was born in 1923 in the small Iowa town of West Point, a crossroads town in the southeastern corner of the state. King was precocious child who early on felt restless within the tight confines of rural life. By the time she was a teenager, she had decided she would be a teacher. But money was tight—King was one of three sisters. When an uncle, the town's only practicing doctor, offered to pay her tuition if she went to nursing school, King accepted his offer.

Raised Catholic, King enrolled at the St. John's School of Nursing in St. Louis. It was affiliated with the St. Louis University School of Nursing and run by the Sisters of Mercy, an order long devoted to patient care. Although at the time certification was all that was required for nurses (King completed hers in 1945), King went on to earn a bachelor's degree in nursing at St. Louis University in 1948. King began hands-on nursing in 1945, accepting a position as clinical instructor in medical-surgical nursing at St. John's. But she was frustrated by the nursing curriculum which, at the time, regarded nurses as appendages of doctors, providing care at the instruction of the attending physician. King felt that nurses were far more crucial, and their role far more complex.

LIFE'S WORK

From 1952 to 1958, King served as an instructor and as assistant director of nursing at St. John's School of Nursing. During that time, King began to gather firsthand data on the actual work nurses performed. After she completed her doctoral work in education at Teachers College, Columbia University, King accepted a teaching position at Chicago's Loyola University in 1961. In 1966 she worked as assistant chief in the nursing division's research grants department at the Bureau of Health, Manpower, and Welfare. She then left to direct the nursing program at The Ohio State University from 1968 to 1972, before returning to Loyola as a professor in the university's graduate nursing program.

In the late 1960s, King first promulgated what became known as the Theory of Goal Attainment, a landmark conceptual model of nursing. A patient, King argued, was a person in constant interaction with themselves and with their environment. A nurse, far from simply administering service at the direction of a physician, was involved in promoting, maintaining, restoring, and sustaining good health in a patient who day to day, really hour to hour, changed. In fact, a nurse could be seen only in relation to the patient, an ongoing dyad that had to be open to change as the care protocol developed. A patient could best be seen as a complex system of interrelated levels: a personal level (how the patient sees and evaluates themselves, their health, and their body); the interpersonal relationship (how the patient responds to and interacts with the nurse as primary caregiver); and the larger social system (how the patient interacts with family and friends). Each system needed to be factored in to how the nurse would best approach the ultimate goal of restoring the patient to health.

To achieve that goal, King proposed a five-step model: nurses (1) assess the patient, the patient's background and attitude; (2) diagnose the patient's medical record, examine the monitored signs and understand the specific health issue(s) by drawing on experience as well as their skills and expertise; (3) create a clear plan for achieving a return to health, a doable and realistic plan with a specific time schedule; (4) implement that plan in carefully measured steps with the patient's cooperation; and (5) most importantly, evaluate the plan even as it is being executed, and continue to adjust and improve its efficiency as needed. If the nurse was not in tune with the patient, stress would be generated and the goal of good health could not be attained. King argued there must be open communication with the patient—the lack of such openness only created anxiety.

King's model—first published in 1968, further developed in *Toward a Theory of Nursing* (1971), and formally named in 1997—became a template for nursing care even as King herself tirelessly promoted the concept of transactional nursing in conference forums and in professional publications. She relocated in 1980 to St. Petersburg, Florida, accepting a professorship at the University of South Florida. Even when she retired from teaching as professor emeritus in 1990, she maintained an international presence in the nursing community as a consultant for curriculum development in nursing schools around the world.

King was widely recognized for her contributions to nursing theory and practice. Her honors include an honorary doctorate from Loyola in 1989, the American Nurses Association's Jessie Scott Award in 1996, and a gold medallion from the governor of Florida for advancing the nursing profession in 1997. In 2004 she was inducted in the American Nurses Hall of Fame; in 2005, she was given the Living Legend Award by the Academy of American Nursing. She died on December 24, 2007, two days after suffering a stroke.

IMPACT

King merged nursing theory with nursing experience. Her principle, that a nurse interacted with a patient by both communicating and listening, was a radical concept when it first appeared. By interacting with the patient, a nurse maintained clear and specific goals and initiated clear and specific steps toward each goal. Goal setting became a way for nurses to direct a patient's recovery. King was a teacher by nature—her greatest achievement, she told audiences, was not her writing but rather the impact she had on each new generation of nurses in her classroom and the impact they would have, in turn, on their patients.

—*Joseph Dewey*

Further Reading

Alligood, Martha Raile. *Nursing Theorists and Their Work*. 8th ed., Mosby, 2013.

Evans, Christina L. Sieloff. *Imogene King: A Conceptual Framework for Nursing*. Sage, 1991.

Frey, Maureen A., and Christina L. Sieloff, editors. *Advancing King's Systems Framework and Theory of Nursing*. Sage, 1995.

Sitzman, Kathleen, and Lisa Wright Eichelberger. *Understanding the Work of Nurse Theorists: A Creative Beginning*. Jones, 2015.

Smith, Marlaine C., and Marilyn E. Parker. *Nursing Theories and Nursing Practice*. 4th ed., Davis, 2015.

Betty Neuman

ABSTRACT
Betty Neuman is a nurse who developed the influential Neuman systems model, which is a holistic treatment model designed to be adaptable for use in a wide variety of health-related concerns.

BACKGROUND
Betty Neuman was born Betty Maxine Reynolds on September 11, 1924, on her parents' farm in Lowell, Ohio. She had an older brother, Adrian, and a younger brother, Larry. Her father died of kidney disease when she was eleven years old. When she was in junior high school, her mother moved with her and Larry to nearby Marietta, Ohio, leaving Adrian to manage the farm.

Neuman graduated from high school in 1942 and began working at the Air Force Technical Base (now Wright-Patterson Air Force Base) just outside Dayton, Ohio, as an aircraft instrument technician. In fall 1944, the year after the US Cadet Nurse Corps was established, she joined the cadet nurse training program in Akron, Ohio. Neuman trained at the Peoples Hospital in Akron (now Akron General Medical Center) and received her nursing diploma in 1947.

Neuman's first marriage, to physician Richard Neuman, lasted from 1954 until 1963. The couple had a daughter, Nancy, born in 1959. In the 1970s Neuman married her second husband, Kree Dicklich, and they settled in Watertown, Ohio. Dicklich passed away in 1995.

NURSING CAREER
After graduating from the Peoples Hospital School of Nursing in 1947, Neuman moved to Los Angeles, California. She began working in the communicable diseases department of Los Angeles County General Hospital, starting as a staff nurse and working her way up to head nurse. After some time, she decided to continue her nursing education, entering the University of California, Los Angeles (UCLA) School of Nursing in 1956 and earning her bachelor of science in nursing (BSN) degree the following year.

Neuman returned to UCLA in 1964 for graduate studies and completed her master's degree in mental health and public health consultation in 1966. Her master's thesis examined the relationship between individuals' personality patterns and suicide attempts. She was subsequently appointed chair and faculty member of the same program in which she had studied. While there, she designed a teaching model to train nurses in community mental health, laying the foundations for what would eventually become the highly influential Neuman systems model.

In 1970, Neuman was certified as a marriage, family, and child counselor in the state of California. (She would later be certified as a marriage and family counselor by the American Association for Marriage and Family Therapy.) Around the same time, she adapted the teaching model she had previously developed to make it more broadly applicable to nursing in general. After testing the adapted model in her graduate community mental health courses, she presented the results in an article titled "A Model for Teaching Total Person Approach to Patient Problems," coauthored by Rae Jeanne Young and published in the peer-reviewed journal *Nursing Research* in 1972. A refined version of the model was published in the first edition of Joan P. Riehl and Callista Roy's *Conceptual Models for Nursing Practice* (1974) under the title "The Betty Neuman Health-Care Systems Model."

The Neuman systems model takes a comprehensive, flexible, and holistic approach to nursing. It is based on general systems theory, viewing patients or clients as open systems that respond to both internal and external stressors. The model starts from the basic assumption that each "client system" is unique, comprising a number of different influences and characteristics all contained within a basic structure that is surrounded by a "normal line of defense" and a "flexible line of defense." The basic structure consists of the client's own unique energy resources, specifically the genetic, environmental, physical, and psychological traits that are geared toward the client's survival. These energy resources are linked to the client's defenses against stressors. Each possible stressor differs in its potential to disrupt a client's lines of defense, and each client is unique in their responses to these disruptions.

Neuman returned to Ohio in 1973 to care for her ailing mother. While there, she used a clergy counseling grant to teach and fund field supervision for both lay and clergy counselors at Washington County Mental Health Services. She also worked as a mental health consultant for West Virginia's Department of Mental Health. Throughout the 1970s, as Neuman continued to work as a lecturer, consultant, and occasional counselor, the Neuman systems model grew in popularity and was increasingly adopted by nursing schools. After 1978, when the model was officially implemented for the first time, Neuman began to work more closely with those schools in a consultant capacity.

The first edition of *The Neuman Systems Model: Application to Nursing Education and Practice* was published in 1982. Neuman then returned to school once more, completing her doctorate in clinical psychology at Los Angeles's Pacific Western University in 1985.

The Neuman systems model went global in 1986, when Neumann College (now Neumann University) in Aston, Pennsylvania, sponsored the first International Neuman Systems Model Symposium; the event was subsequently repeated every other year, with the fifteenth international symposium being held in Philadelphia, Pennsylvania, in June 2015.

Neuman has received a number of honors for her work over the years, including two honorary doctorates, one from Neumann College in 1992 and the other from Michigan's Grand Valley State University in 1998. In 1993 she was made an honorary fellow of the American Academy of Nursing.

IMPACT
The Neuman systems model has been massively influential in nursing education, particularly mental health nursing. It is widely used by nursing schools, postgraduate programs, and healthcare organizations around the world, especially in the Netherlands, where it was first introduced in the early 1990s. A biennial international symposium about the model has been held regularly in the United States since 1986, and the first European symposium was held in Belgium in 2012. The fifth edition of *The Neuman Systems Model* was published in 2010.

—*Patrick G. Cooper*

Further Reading
Brook, Marian. "Betty Neuman." *American Nursing: A Biographical Dictionary*, edited by Vern L. Bullough and Lilli Sentz, vol. 3, Springer Publishing, 2000, pp. 218–21.
Gonzalo, A. *Betty Neuman: Neuman Systems Model*, nurseslabs.com/betty-neuman-systems-model-nursing-theory/. Accessed 24 Aug. 2020.
Lawson, Theresa G. "Betty Neuman: Systems Model." *Nursing Theorists and Their Work*, edited by Martha Raile Alligood, 8th ed., Mosby, 2014, pp. 281–302.
Masters, Kathleen. *Nursing Theories: A Framework for Professional Practice*. 2nd ed., Jones & Bartlett Learning, 2015.
Neuman, Betty, and Jacqueline Fawcett, editors. *The Neuman Systems Model*. 5th ed., Pearson, 2011.
Neuman Systems Model. Neuman Systems Model Trustees Group, www.neumansystemsmodel.org/index.html. Accessed 4 Oct. 2016.
Ostroff, Donna, preparer. "Betty M. Neuman Papers." Updated by Gail E. Farr. *University of Pennsylvania Finding Aids*, U of Pennsylvania, Jan. 2013, hdl.library.upenn.edu/1017/d/ead/upenn_bates_MC160. Accessed 4 Oct. 2016.

CALLISTA ROY

ABSTRACT
Nursing theorists are responsible in great part, for the evolution of nursing. A researcher into the relationship between nurse and patient, Callista Roy pioneered a landmark para-

digm, now called the Roy Adaptation Model, that redefined the role of the nurse in treatment protocols.

BACKGROUND

Callista Lorraine Roy was born in 1939 on the feast day of Saint Callistus I, a slave who rose to become pope, and for whom she was named. Her parents were devout Catholics; her mother, a nurse in a city hospital in Los Angeles, raised Roy to appreciate the importance of selfless service and the need for compassion. Roy often accompanied her mother to the hospital, and, at age fourteen, Roy volunteered to work in the hospital's kitchen; within a year, however, she was working with patients as a nurse's aide. She loved the interaction with patients and knew early on she would become a nurse.

A precocious student and avid reader, Roy matriculated at nearby Mount St. Mary's College (now University), an all-women's Catholic liberal arts college that stressed the importance of community service. By the time she graduated in 1963 with a bachelor's degree in nursing, she had undergone a significant religious experience and had determined she would become a nun as well, joining the Sisters of St. Joseph of Carondelet, whose members had pioneered healthcare services for more than a century, staffing hospitals, rest homes, and orphanages. Completing a master's in pediatric nursing at University of California, Los Angeles (UCLA) in 1966, Roy decided to expand her expertise by pursuing first a master's and then a doctorate (1975) in sociology, also at UCLA. She was certain that sociology, with its emphasis on how the individual is defined by interaction with larger communities, was crucial to understanding the nature of how patients cope with illness, the core mission of a nurse.

After completing her doctoral work, Roy taught at Mount Saint Mary's and the University of Portland until 1983, and was then a postdoctoral fellow at the University of California, San Francisco. Since 1987, she has been a professor and resident nurse theorist at the Boston College School of Nursing.

ESTABLISHING THE ROY ADAPTATION MODEL

At the time Roy began her nursing studies, there existed no conceptual model to define the actual role of a nurse; nurses were largely seen as adjuncts to physicians. Roy's groundbreaking work in nursing theory began in 1964 when a professor in her graduate classes, Dorothy E. Johnson, challenged her students to come up with an actual model that would reflect the day-to-day responsibilities of a nurse.

Over the next decade, Roy developed a revolutionary conceptual model that would become known as the Roy Adaptation Model, first published in 1976. Roy began with two fundamental assumptions: first, health and illness were part of the same continuum, a patient did not "get" sick; second, nurses did not treat a patient, nurses treated a person, a complicated cooperative system of parts, physical, mental, emotional, and spiritual, and that in adapting to the reality of illness each patient drew on all four levels. Roy concluded then that a nurse, to be both effective and compassionate, needed to design a response program to each individual patient that in turn recognized these different levels of adaptation, or response, systems that worked in cooperation with the others. Under this system, patients were seen as more complex than nursing theory to that time had advanced; their treatment demanded that the nurse recognize the vital role of the patient's self-concept as well as their perception of their family, friends, and ultimately God.

In short, Roy was instrumental in advancing the human factor in nursing. Roy theorized that the appropriate goal of a nurse was to assist the patient in adapting to the onset of illness and its continuing impact. In gathering data on patient care across more than three decades, Roy showed that patients responded positively to encouragement, clear direction, honesty, and interpersonal communication, and demonstrated a remarkable capacity to change, adapting to the reality of illness. The nurse provided day-to-day, direct and clear stimuli.

Roy's model, as it evolved across four decades of research, came to endorse six levels of response that collectively provided patients integrated care. First, the nurse observes patient behavior, creating a patient profile grounded in measureable data; second, the nurse observes stimuli, or protocols, that clearly had no evident impact on the patient's health status—that is, the nurse observes (and rejects) what does not work for the patient; third, the nurse, in close communication with the attending physicians, creates a patient profile that diagnoses why such protocols proved ineffective; fourth, the nurse sets reasonable, achievable goals for charting the patient's adaptation to the illness; fifth, the nurse executes the actual interventions, beginning to apply the selected protocols as a way to direct the patient's adaptation program; and sixth, the nurse must continually evaluate the efficacy of the designated protocols—what is working and what is not—as a way to enhance and encourage short- and long-term recovery.

IMPACT

Roy's theoretical premise—that a patient is a complex individual who responds to the challenge of illness on multiple levels—has become a working assumption in contemporary nursing practice. Her model has been applied to a variety of nursing fields, from pediatric care to hospice work, as well as both short-term care and long-term rehabilitation protocols. In short, Roy redefined the concept of the nursing profession. She continues her research in the dynamics of coping with illness, as well as lecturing, helping universities around the world develop nursing school curricula, and teaching graduate courses in nursing theory. Her tireless efforts to promote a concept of compassionate care have made her one of the most recognized scholars in her field, and in 2007 the American Academy of Nursing named her a Living Legend, the organization's highest honor.

—*Joseph Dewey*

Further Reading

Akinsanya, Justus A. *The Roy Adaptation Model in Action*. Macmillan, 1994.
Alligood, Martha Raile. *Nursing Theorists and Their Work*. 8th ed., Mosby, 2013.
Alligood, Martha Raile, and Ann Marriner-Tomey. *Nursing Theory: Utilization and Application*. 5th ed., Mosby, 2013.
Frederickson, Keville. "Callista Roy's Adaptation Model." *Nursing Science Quarterly*, vol. 24, no. 4, 2011, pp. 301–3.
Sitzman, Kathleen, and Lisa Wright Eichelberger. *Understanding the Work of Nursing Theorists: A Creative Beginning*. 3rd ed., Jones, 2017.
"Sr. Callista Roy, PhD, RN, FAAN." Trustees of Boston College. *Boston College William F. Connell School of Nursing*, 20 July 2016.
Vera, Matt. "Sister Callista L. Roy." *Nurselabs*, 18 Aug. 2014.

JEAN WATSON

ABSTRACT

Nursing theorists are responsible in great part, for the evolution of nursing. Jean Watson is a nursing theorist whose theory of human caring is taught in nursing schools throughout the world. The theory emphasizes the importance of the transpersonal caring relationship in nurse-patient encounters and the need for the nurse's authentic presence.

BACKGROUND

Jean Watson was born Margaret Jean Harman in Welch, West Virginia, in 1940. The youngest of eight children, Watson was a devoted student with plans to go to college to major in literature, in an era when only about a third of women who graduated high school went to college and a quarter of women overall did not even finish high school. When her father died of a heart attack, her plans shifted and she decided to pursue a career in nursing. She enrolled in the Lewis

Gale School of Nursing in Roanoke, Virginia, but although she completed her registered nurse (RN) training and earned her diploma in 1961, she was disappointed that the environment was not more academic.

After graduating, Watson relocated to Colorado, where she was able to continue her education at the University of Colorado Boulder. She earned a bachelor of science in nursing in 1964, a master's degree in psychiatric and mental health nursing from the University of Colorado Medical Center in Denver in 1966, and a doctorate in educational psychology and counseling from the University of Colorado Boulder in 1973.

Watson credits her husband Douglas Watson, who died in 1998, with supporting her while she pursued her education, as well as encouraging her in her career. Watson has two daughters and five grandchildren. In 1997, an accident resulted in Watson losing her sight in her left eye.

THEORY OF HUMAN CARING

Watson began developing her theory of human caring in 1975, shortly after completing her doctoral work, and it continues to be the foundation of her theoretical work. The recurring theme in her work is the relationship between caring and curing, something she draws attention to with her term "carative factors," coined to evoke the medical term "curative factor." Watson's theory of human caring stresses the importance of human contact in the healing process and of the quality of that human contact—the transpersonal caring relationship, as Watson calls it. It is the nurse's responsibility to be authentically present and loving in order to create this relationship and create the opportunity for "caring occasions"—when the nurse and patient can learn from one another by sharing personal experiences.

The ten carative factors Watson defined were later redefined as "caritas processes," from one of the Latin words for love (from which both "care" and "charity" are derived). The list includes being authentically present, cultivating the nurse's own spirituality, supporting the patient's expressions of both positive and negative emotions, and "being open to miracles." As with this latter phrase, Watson's theoretical work often stresses the spiritual and transcendent, not simply the moral and pragmatic, reflecting her commitment to a model of health as encompassing the body, mind, and soul, and the importance of self-conception and self-esteem in that model. In part, this aligns with her view that while curative practices are geared toward curing conditions, carative practices must include preparing both nurse and patient for the possibility of a compassionate death.

Love, respect, and human dignity are at the core of Watson's caring theory. Whereas "bedside manner" is sometimes spoken of as an adjunct to a doctor's skill set, Watson positions the nurse-patient relationship as essential to nursing theory and the practice of nursing. That extends, too, to relationships with patients' families, who naturally are emotionally and spiritually invested in their loved ones' care, and Watson focuses on the importance of one-to-one connections even when the nurse is addressing multiple people, rather than assuming the mannerisms and tone of a lecturer or meeting leader.

Watson has received numerous awards recognizing her contributions to nursing, the healthcare field, and theory, including nine honorary doctoral degrees, and she is a distinguished professor of nursing and chair in caring science at the University of Colorado Health Sciences Center. She has previously served as the university's dean of nursing and as the president of the National League for Nursing. In 2008, she founded the nonprofit Watson Caring Science Institute. In 2013, the American Academy of Nursing declared her a Living Legend, its highest honor.

IMPACT

Watson is one of the nursing theorists instrumental in getting nursing recognized as a discipline grounded in theory and backed by evidence, a feat commemorated by the many honors bestowed upon her by the field. The theory of caring as she developed it promoted the idea of nursing as a field both scientific and humanistic and emphasized the importance of human contact, transpersonal relationships, and emotional connections in the healing process. Nursing that follows this theory demonstrates respect for the patient and upholds human dignity.

Watson continues to develop the theory of human caring throughout her career, and numerous hospitals, clinics, and nursing schools implement or teach her carative factors (also known as caritas processes, caring practices, and caritas literacy).

—Bill Kte'pi

Further Reading
Alligood, Martha Raile. *Nursing Theorists and Their Work.* Elsevier, 2014.
Butts, Janie B., and Karen I. Rich. *Philosophies and Theories for Advanced Nursing Practice.* Jones, 2014.
Fitzpatrick, Joyce J., and Geraldine McCarthy. *Theories Guiding Nursing Research and Practice.* Springer, 2014.
Potter, Patricia A., Anne Griffin Perry, and Patricia Stockert. *Fundamentals of Nursing.* Mosby, 2016.
Purnell, Larry. *Transcultural Health Care: A Culturally Competent Approach.* Davis, 2013.
Sitzman, Kathleen, and Jean Watson. *Caring Science, Mindful Practice: Implementing Watson's Human Caring Theory.* Springer, 2013.
Smith, Marlaine, and Marilyn E. Parker. *Nursing Theories and Nursing Practice.* Davis, 2015.
Watson, Jean. *Human Caring Science: A Theory of Nursing.* Jones, 2012.
Watson, Jean. *Nursing: The Philosophy and Science of Caring.* UP of Colorado, 2008.

Abraham Maslow

ABSTRACT
Abraham Maslow's theory Hierarchy of Needs describes five levels of needs that must be met in order to have both physical and emotional health. His theory provides a base of Basic Physiological Needs and Safety and Security Needs that are the basis for the implementation of nursing care and nursing interventions. These both lay the foundation on which other needs are realized in the pursuit of physical and emotional health.

INTRODUCTION
Abraham Maslow (1908–1970) was an American psychologist and philosopher recognized for his self-actualization theory of psychology, an integration of the self. Considered a motivational theory, the hierarchy remains popular and well-accepted, but some critics question the validity that meeting levels of needs helps the individual to realize full potential. Maslow argued that not having needs met can lead to illness or psychiatric illness and not having safety needs met can lead to posttraumatic stress. While not a nursing theorist by the truest definition, Maslow and his Hierarchy of Needs became an integral part of nursing care. Nurses routinely learn about Maslow's levels of needs that must be achieved in order to realize self-actualization, or achieving one's full potential with the ability to recognize the view of others. Nurses use his theory to set patient care priorities beginning with meeting the patient's Basic Physiological Needs and the need for Safety and Security.

Maslow's Hierarchy of Needs has five levels arranged in a pyramid:
- *Basic Physiological Needs.* These are needs that must be met in order for the individual to survive. Nutrition (water and food), elimination, a clear airway, breathing (oxygen), circulation including pulse, blood pressure, sufficient sleep, sex, shelter, and exercise are examples of Basic Physiological Needs.
- *Safety and Security.* Individuals must feel safe and secure. In the hospital setting, Injury prevention (call lights, side rails, hand hygiene, isolation, fall precautions, suicide precautions, for example), a climate of trust and therapeutic relationships, pa-

tient education for modifiable risk factors such as stroke prevention, healthy heart and patient privacy are examples of Safety and Security Needs.
- *Love and Belonging.* Individuals have the need for supportive relationships, help with defining methods to avoid social isolation, learning how to employ active listening skills and using therapeutic communication, and sexual intimacy which all support Love and Belonging.
- *Self-Esteem.* Individuals desire to have sufficient self-esteem to recognize their place in their work environment or even as they face illnesses. Beginning with acceptance in the workforce and community, defining personal achievements, having a sense of control, and accepting one's physical appearance or body contribute to self-esteem.
- *Self-Actualization.* Self-actualization is defined by reaching one's maximum potential. Prospering in an empowering environment, recognizing the point of view of others, and experiencing spiritual growth may all indicate self-actualization.

Maslow's levels are not sequential. Individuals may not have all basic needs met but may still have high self-esteem. Individuals flow between levels and up and down the pyramid based on their situation and challenges.

Nurses in the hospital setting generally focus on the patient's basic physiological needs and the need for safety and security. Nurses also focus on their place in the hierarchy as they provide care for patients. For example, nurses are expected to provide active listening and therapeutic communication in dealing with patients. Nurses need to feel accepted in the workforce and need to feel a level of personal achievement in their role. A self-actualized nurse recognizes the point of view of others, is empowered by the environment and reaches personal maximum potential. Maslow believed that people will seek self-actualization requiring lower level needs to be met before moving up his levels. Because Maslow's hierarchy is not static, individuals may move up and down this pyramid between the various levels at different points in life.

MASLOW'S HIERARCHY AND ITS APPLICATION TO NURSING

As part of the nursing care process and the nursing care planning process, nurses must assess the needs of patients in their care. Nurses in a clinical setting will be involved in providing for the Basic Physiological Needs of patients, including nutrition. While the physician orders the diet for the patient and the clinical dietician ensures the nutritional quality of the provided food, the nurse must ensure that the patient eats and takes in sufficient fluids during the admission to the hospital. Carefully monitoring intake of foods and monitoring output (elimination) is part of attending to the physiological needs of the patient. Maintaining an open airway for the patient and monitoring oxygen levels is also critical. Taking blood pressure measurements as ordered, monitoring sleep cycles and providing opportunities for appropriate exercise such as walking to the toilet or in the hall are just a few of the activities involved in meeting the basic physiological needs of the patient.

Safety is the second step in Maslow's pyramid. With a focus on precautions in the hospital to protect the patient, the needs of the patient can be met in a safe and secure manner. For example, having a call light available to ask for help in using the toilet, using bedrails to prevent falls out of bed, posting notes for fall risk or allergies on the door to the patient's room and others will help ensure the safety and security of the patient.

The remaining three steps in Maslow's pyramid may not be accomplished during a short hospitalization but in patients with repeat admissions for a chronic illness, opportunities may present to provide comfort and support for patients and caregivers (love and belonging) and to enhance a patient's self-esteem. For example, when cancer patients lose their hair, they need to experience a sense of love regardless of physical appearance (Level 3, Love and Belonging) and need to be coached to accept their physical appearance (Level 4, Self-Esteem). While nurses may not see patients in a fully self-actualized manner, recognizing that nursing interventions throughout the hospitalization or repeated hospitalizations may assist the patient in ultimately achieving one's full potential.

Patients will move up and down the pyramid over time. Some needs will be more prevalent, for example, after a surgical procedure, while hospitalization for a psychiatric issue may move the patient to a different level of the hierarchy.

MASLOW'S HIERARCHY AND THE NURSING PROFESSIONAL

In most nursing management courses, Abraham Maslow's Hierarchy of Needs Model is used to explain the challenges of understanding, developing and motivating employees in the dynamic healthcare industry. Constant change, reorganization, mergers and increasing technology can threaten the nurse attempting to navigate the care of patients. A nursing career is challenging and stressful. Maslow's hierarchy applies as easily to the professional nurse as it does to the patient. Recognizing workplace concerns such as the need for security and manageable stress,

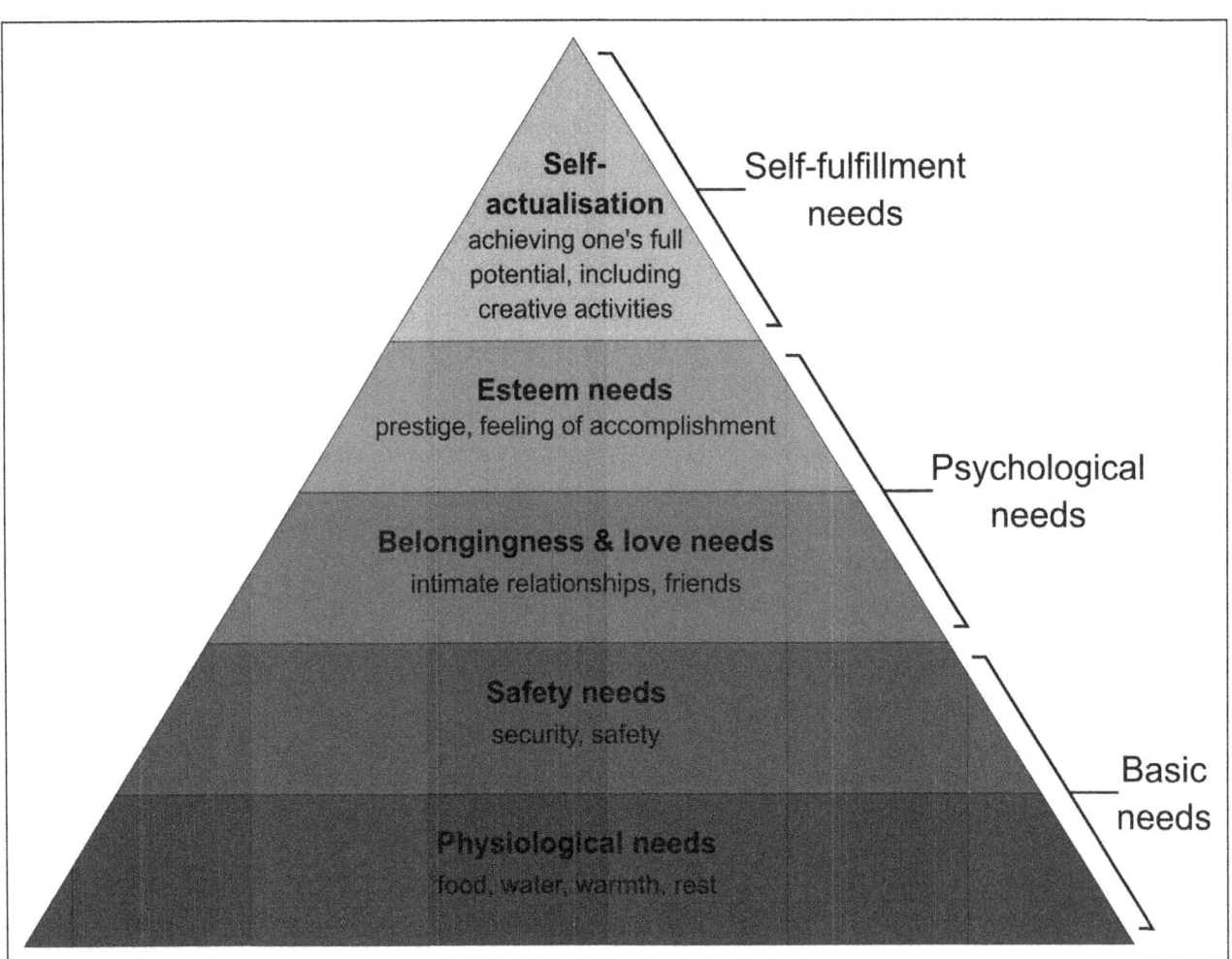

Maslow's Hierarchy of Needs (Wikimedia Commons)

social belonging in the nursing unit, new opportunities for learning, and recognition enhancing self-esteem will support the growth toward self-actualization of the employee. As employees become self-actualized, the care of the patient will be enhanced. The employee needs to feel needed, secure in his or her role, and most importantly feel appreciated.

SUMMARY

Maslow's Hierarchy of Needs is one of the most robust theories in supporting both nurses and the patients under their care. Understanding where the patient is on the hierarchy pyramid will help the nurse focus on the specific needs of the patient. It is also important that the nurse understands how the Hierarchy of Needs can impact personal needs for self-actualization. The more an individual studies Maslow's Hierarchy, the greater the realization that basic human needs must be met before self can become more balanced and productive.

—*Patricia Stanfill Edens*

Further Reading

Benson, S. G., and S. P. Dundis. "Understanding and Motivating Health Care Employees: Integrating Maslow's Hierarchy of Needs, Training and Technology." *Journal of Nursing Management*, vol. 11, no. 5, 2003, pp. 315–20.

Freitas, F. A., and L. J. Leonard. "Maslow's Hierarchy of Needs and Student Academic Success." *Teaching and Learning in Nursing*, vol. 6, 2011, pp. 9–13, files.transtutors.com/cdn/uploadassignments/1551711-1-maslow-theory.pdf.

Jennifer K. "How to Apply Maslow's Hierarchy of Needs to Nursing." Updated 18 Jan. 2018, www.theclassroom.com/how-7727994-apply-maslows-hierarchy-needs-nursing.html.

McLeod S. "Maslow's Hierarchy of Needs." *Simply Psychology*, updated 20 Mar. 2020, www.simplypsychology.org/maslow.html.

Toney-Butler, U. J., and J. M. Thayer. "Nursing Process." US National Library of Medicine. National Center for Biotechnology Information. *National Institutes of Health*, updated 10 July 2020, www.ncbi.nlm.nih.gov/books/NBK499937/.

Vertino, K. A. "Effective Interpersonal Communication: A Practical Guide to Improve Your Life." *Online Journal of Nursing*, vol. 19, no. 3, 30 Sept. 2014, p. 1.

Winter T. "Maslow's Hierarchy: Separating Fact from Fiction." *Association for Talent Development*, www.td.org/insights/maslows-hierarchy-separating-fact-from-fiction. Accessed 16 Sept. 2020.

KATHARINE KOLBACA AND KRISTEN M. SWANSON

ABSTRACT

Katharine Kolcaba defined the Theory of Comfort as an antidote to stress in the healthcare setting. She felt that when comfort is enhanced, patients and families grow stronger. Kristen M. Swanson defined the Theory of Care as a nurturing way of relating to others. In viewing these theorists together, a patient's comfort and an informed caring for others are interrelated.

KATHARINE KOLBACA

Katharine Kolbaca's Theory of Comfort was developed in the 1990s and is considered a middle-range theory. A middle-range theory presents concepts that address a specific phenomenon in nursing. Most middle-range theories flow from a grand theory that is too broad to fully measure. Middle-range theories evolve from research, nursing practice and other disciplines. Her theory evolved when she conducted a concept analysis of comfort from the literature of nursing, medicine, psychology, and others. She defined three forms of comfort: (1) relief, (2) ease, and (3) transcendence. These three comforts exist in four contexts: (1) physical, (2) psychospiritual, (3) environmental, and, (4) sociocultural.

Using the three forms of comfort and the four contexts of comfort, Kolbaca described a method to assess, measure and evaluate patient comfort. She feels comfort is a part of holistic nursing. For example, a patient receiving pain medication is receiving relief comfort. Ease is when a patient feels a sense of peace after interventions such as the visit from a counselor or chaplain. Transcendence is when a patient is able to achieve comfort despite the challenges of the disease or situation of care.

The Theory of Comfort includes patients, individuals, families or communities in need of care. The environment may be manipulated to provide comfort measures to relieve patients' pain and discomfort. While healthcare providers may have little control over some facets of healthcare for the patient, identified healthcare needs may be managed to deliver comfort measures and evaluate responses. Assessment of comfort can be subjective, such as asking patients to describe their level of comfort, or objective, observing healing of surgical incisions or sleep patterns.

KRISTEN M. SWANSON

Swanson's Theory of Caring was developed in 1991 and is also considered a middle-range theory. She outlines five caring processes: (1) knowing, (2) being with, (3) doing for, (4) enabling and, (5) belief. In later iterations, the theory is also described as caring capacity, concerns and commitments, conditions, caring actions, and consequences. Her theory derived from nursing research and provides a description of the relationships between the caring process and patient well-being. The theory posits that nurses who exhibit that they care about their patients is as important as the actual care provided. While clinical activities such as administering medications and treatments directly impact care outcomes, delivering these activities in a caring manner is equally important.

Dr. Swanson defines caring as a nurturing way to relate to others. It describes a need to feel the individual has value and also that the nurse has a personnel sense of commitment and caring to the patient and family. Nurturing is a set of interrelated processes. Maintaining belief begins with a fundamental belief that patients can get through events and challenges. Knowing encourages understanding the patient's condition and reality. A bond of empathy develops during the knowing phase of the Theory of Caring. Being-with describes the nurse-patient relationship as being emotionally present, assuring the patient of the nurse's readiness to be in the patient's reality, and giving time. Doing-for is the function of nurses to assist the individual in activities that contribute to health and recovery. Enabling is the facilitation of the patient's progress through unfamiliar events and transitions. Enabling fosters self-healing.

The application of the Theory of Caring by Dr. Swanson in her research focuses primarily on pregnancy issues in dealing with miscarriage and the healing needed by patients and families. The goal of the theory is to assist nurses to deliver care that promotes dignity, respect, and empowerment.

SUMMARY

The Theory of Comfort states that comfort is an important outcome for the delivery of patient care. The Theory of Caring states that nurses care by establishing meaningful, healing relationships with patients and families. In viewing Kolbaca's theory and Swanson's theory, it makes sense to consider nursing as providing and enhancing comfort and care to patients and families. Nursing requires humanitarian behaviors of compassion, reflection, concern, commitment and communication. A focus on others, respect for individual dignity and worth and being present are all a part of both Kolbaca's Theory of Comfort and Swanson's Theory of Caring. Ultimately the welfare of the patient and family is supported by both comfort and caring, two essential theories of nursing.

—*Patricia Stanfill Edens*

Further Reading

Alligood, M. R. *Nursing Theorists and their Work*. 9th ed., Elsevier eBook on Vital Source, 2018.

Colley, S. "Nursing Theory: Its Importance to Practice." *Nursing Standard*, vol. 17, no. 46, 2003, pp. 33–37.

Dallaire, C., and P. Krol. " Revisiting the Roots of Nursing Philosophy and Critical Theory: Past, Present and Future." *Nursing Philosophy*, vol. 19, no. 1, 2018.

Jairath, N. N., et al. "Theory and Theorizing in Nursing Science: Commentary form the Nursing Research Special Issue Editorial Team." *Nursing Research*, vol. 67, no. 2, Mar./Apr. 2018, pp. 188–95.

"Kolcaba's Theory of Comfort." *Nursing Theory*, www.nursing-theory.org/theories-and-models/kolbaca-theory-of-comfort.php. Accessed 19 Sept. 2020.

"Kristen Swanson Theory of Caring and Healing." *Psych-Mental Health NP*, pmhealthnp.com/kristen-swanson-theory-of-caring-and-healing/. Accessed 19 Sept. 2020.

McKelvey, M. M. "Finding Meaning through Kristen Swanson's Caring Behaviors: A Cornerstone of Healing for Nursing Education." *Creative Nursing*, vol. 24, no. 1, connect.springerpub.com/content/sgrcn/24/1/6?implicit-login=true. Accessed 19 Sept. 2020.

Tonges, M., and J. Ray. "Translating Caring Theory into Practice." *Journal of Nursing Administration*, vol. 41, no. 9, pp. 374–81, prd-medweb-cdn.s3.amazonaws.com/documents/evidencebasedpractice/files/KS_Translating%20Caring%20Theory.pdf. Accessed 19 Sept. 2020.

Wayne, G. "Nursing Theories and Theorists: Your Theoretical Guide to Nursing Theories." *NursesLabs*, nurseslabs.com/nursing-theories/#what_are_nursing_theories. Accessed 14 Sept. 2020.

Nola Pender

ABSTRACT

Nola Pender is a nurse educator and theorist who developed the Health Promotion Model in 1982. The model focuses on preventive health, rather than the treatment of illnesses.

BACKGROUND

Nola Pender was born on August 16, 1941, in Lansing, Michigan. In 1962 she earned her registered nursing (RN) degree from the School of Nursing at West Suburban Hospital in Oak Park, Illinois. She then studied at Michigan State University, earning a bachelor's degree in nursing in 1964 and a master's degree in human growth and development in 1965. In 1969 she earned two PhDs, in psychology and education, from Northwestern University.

NURSING CAREER

Pender began her nursing career while completing her bachelor's degree. From 1962 to 1964 she worked as a head nurse in the medical-surgical unit at Ingham Medical Hospital in Lansing, Michigan. She then began working as an instructor at Mercy School of Nursing, in Lansing.

After a year at the Mercy School of Nursing, she moved to Grand Forks, North Dakota, and worked as an instructor in the College of Nursing at the University of North Dakota from 1965 to 1967. She moved to Illinois in the late 1960s, and began a twenty-one-year career with Northern Illinois University (NIU) in DeKalb, Illinois. Starting as an assistant professor in the School of Nursing in 1969, she was promoted to associate professor after one year and then to professor in 1976. In 1984 she became the director of the Health Promotion Research Program at NIU's Social Science Research Institute.

Pender simultaneously worked in several other positions. From 1979 to 1990 she was an adjunct professor at Rush University's College of Nursing in Chicago. She also was a coordinator for the DeKalb County Health Department's Relaxation and Biofeedback Program.

Early in her career at NIU, Pender began developing a nursing theory. Concerned that patients typically first received treatment after they had acquired an illness, she believed preventative measures could reduce illnesses and promote healthier lifestyles. While this belief was not unique, prevalent preventive health theories of the time, such as the Health Belief Model, used negative motivations to frighten individuals into adopting more healthy behaviors. Pender's theory, the Health Promotion Model (HPM), uses a positive approach to encourage a healthy lifestyle and behaviors that promote health. In 1975 she published an article, "A Conceptual Model for Preventive Health Behavior" in *Nursing Outlook*. Pender's theory became an integral part of many nursing students' educations. It was first published in her textbook *Health Promotion in Nursing Practice* (1982). Pender has revised the model twice since its original publication.

The Health Promotion Model is based on five key concepts and the interrelationships between them: the person, the environment, nursing, health, and illness. Its goal is to encourage health professionals, especially nurses, to work with individuals to create the best conditions to foster optimal health.

In 1990 Pender joined the School of Nursing at the University of Michigan, Ann Arbor. From 1990 to 1994 she was a professor and director of the Center for Nursing Research. She then became the associate dean of academic affairs and research. From 1998 to 2001, she was professor and associate dean of research. She was named a professor emerita in 2001.

Pender has conducted extensive research throughout her career. She has been the principal investigator, director, or chair for research studies on a diverse array of health topics, including relaxation and biofeedback, corporate fitness programs, and exercise. Throughout her career, Pender has shown a particular interest in adolescents and counseling them to adopt physically active lifestyles. In 2005 the Midwest Research Society awarded Pender a Lifetime Achievement Award in recognition of her contributions to nursing research.

Pender has also maintained a prolific speaking career, presenting at professional meetings such as conferences, workshops, and universities both nationally and internationally. She has also served as a consultant to health departments, schools of nursing, and federal institutes such as the National Institute of Aging, and has taught seminars and consulted with universities in Asia and the Caribbean.

An active member of the nursing and research communities, Pender has been involved with many national associations and organizations. She was a founding member and president of the Midwest Nursing Research Society and the president of the American Academy of Nursing.

In 2004, Pender became a distinguished professor at the School of Nursing at Loyola University, Chicago.

IMPACT

Pender's theory has been widely accepted and is one of several nursing theories that is taught to nurses during their training and during continuing education. Her textbook *Health Promotion in Nursing Practice* has been in print for over thirty years, with the seventh edition (with coauthors Carolyn Murdaugh and Mary Ann Parsons) published in 2015. She consults nationally and internationally on health promotion and research after retirement and is a Professor Emerita at the University of Michigan.

—*Barb Lightner*

Further Reading

Murdaugh C. L., M. A. Parsons, and N. J. M. Pender. *Health Promotion in Nursing Practice*. 8th ed., Pearson. 2019.

"Nola J. Pender." *School of Nursing, University of Michigan*. Regents of the University of Michigan. Accessed 29 Aug. 2016.

"Nola Pender." *WhyIWantToBeANurse.org*. WhyIWantToBeANurse.org. Accessed 29 Aug. 2016.

Pender, Nola J. *Health Promotion Model (HPM): Frequent Questions and Answers*. U of Michigan, Deep Blue, 2011.

Peterson, Sandra J., and Timothy S. Bredow, editors. *Middle Range Theories: Application to Nursing Research*. 4th ed., Wolters, 2017.

Petiprin, Alice. "Nola Pender—Nursing Theorist." *Nursing Theory*. Alice Petiprin, Nursing-Theory.org, 2016. Accessed 29 Aug. 2016.

Becoming a Nurse

This robust section includes fourteen essays—from Selecting the Right Program and Finding the Right College to Models of Nursing Care—designed to identify the steps necessary to not only become a nurse but to understand the different options available in becoming a successful nurse in a way that matches expectations with the reality of the profession. Practical issues like taking entrance exams, writing a cover letter, interviewing, career testing, professional organizations—it's all here.

Selecting the Right Program and Finding the Right College	71
Learning Styles and Study Skills	75
Cover Letter and Resume Writing	80
Interviewing	83
Career and Personnel Testing	87
College and Nursing Entrance Examinations	92
Succeeding at Work	95
Nursing Certifications and Degrees: Licensed Practical Nurse and Registered Nurse	102
Advanced Practice Nurses	104
Licensure and Certification	107
Professional Nursing Organizations and Certification	109
Magnet Recognition Program in Nursing	111
Nurse-Patient Ratio	113
Models of Nursing Care	115

Selecting the Right Program and Finding the Right College

ABSTRACT

Choosing a college that is right for you may be the first important decision you make as a young adult. When considering a nursing career, there are multiple levels of entry. Deciding if you want to be a licensed practical nurse or a registered nurse, a staff nurse or nurse manager, an educator or an advanced practice nurse will all help determine your choice of college. Confirm your interest in attending that particular college and ask about any possible scholarships or grants that may be available to you. Paying for college is an important part of program selection.

INTRODUCTION

Finding the college that is right for you is usually the first big decision you make as an adult. It is a decision that needs to be well thought out, as you will be spending the next few years of your life at the college you choose.

There are multiple options for becoming a nurse based on job description and level of schooling. For example, a licensed practical nurse (LPN) or licensed vocational nurse (LVN) is usually educated in a vocational school or school of applied health and requires approximately one year and an estimated 46 credits to graduate. The practical or vocational nurse graduate must pass a state administered nursing examination called the NCLEX-PN. The sites of practice and activities of an LPN are less than that of an RN and depending on site of practice is usually supervised by an RN or other licensed medical professional. An associate degree in nursing is usually a two-year commitment followed by passing state licensure to become an RN. You may need to be admitted to the college or university first and complete required prerequisite courses before applying to the nursing school. A bachelor level nursing program requires four to five years and is more rigorous and extensive than both the LPN and Associate level programs.

Most college guidebooks will suggest applying to seven or eight schools, divided into three groups. Group one is your "safe schools," or colleges you know you will get into based on admissions criteria. Group two are termed "fit schools," and are colleges you have a very good chance of being admitted to. Group three are your "reach schools," which are more selective schools that you may get into. Decide first if you can commit to a registered nurse career track or if the shorter, quicker LPN route is preferable. LPNs are more limited in job hiring and make less money than RNs but it is a quicker and somewhat easier route to becoming a nurse. Look also at the rate of acceptance into the nursing program for each of your selected schools. Admission into a nursing program is often highly competitive requiring both excellent grades and appropriate level courses while also demonstrating desirable character and common sense. For example, be cautious in your use of social media as more and more colleges are reviewing your online presence.

In thinking about colleges or universities you would like to attend, the following criteria is important to consider:

Location. If you plan to live on campus, do you prefer an urban, rural, or suburban environment? Although you will be spending most of your time at classes inside the campus, it is also important to think about how everyday life may be outside campus. If you choose a school in an urban area, you may have to quickly get used to subway schedules and crowds. However, in urban areas, there are usually lots of museums, libraries, and historical sites, in other words a lot to do and see outside of campus. Because nursing requires work in a clinical setting as part of the curriculum, an urban setting may offer a greater variety of hospital and healthcare experiences and major medical centers that may be important to later employment opportunities. In a rural area, there may be little access to public transportation, and more farmland than anything. If you crave quiet and easy access to the natural world, a school in a

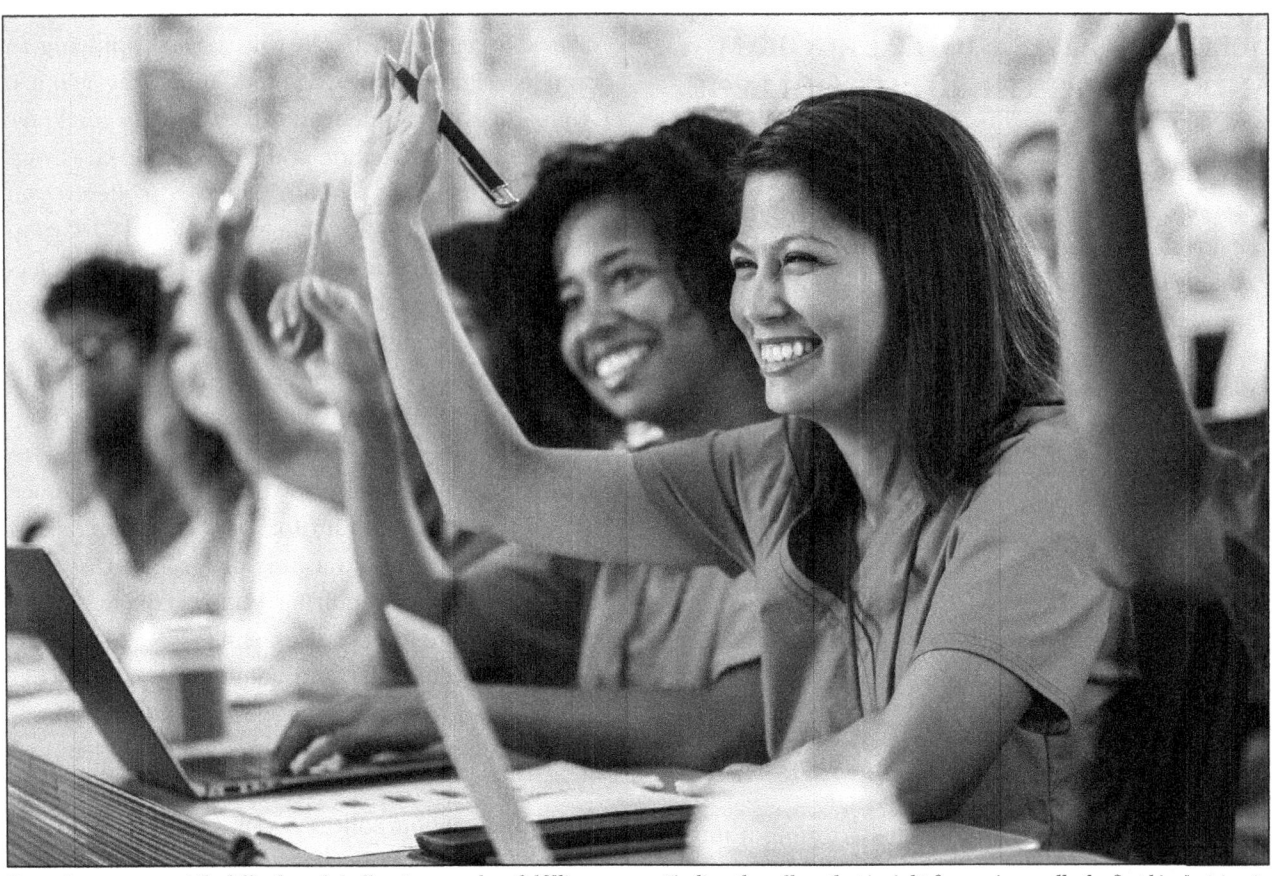

Becoming a nurse, while difficult and challenging, can be a fulfilling career. Finding the college that is right for you is usually the first big decision in the process. (SDI Productions via iStock)

rural area may be the way to go. In a rural setting, access to medical centers may be limited requiring relocating for clinical locations.

If you plan on commuting, how far is your commute? Are you commuting by car, bus, or subway? Commuting is a great way to save money on room and board if the school of your choice is close to your home. Many colleges and universities are known as "commuter schools," because they have a high number of commuter students as compared to students who live on campus. Commuter schools may not have as many on campus activities as schools with more on campus residents. You also will need to be able to travel to either local or more distant clinical settings for a portion of your nursing curriculum. Reliable transportation is important.

Large University or Small College? Larger universities tend to have a higher student to professor class ratio than smaller colleges. In your freshman year at a large university, many of your classes may be held in lecture halls, where you will be one of a hundred or more students. Classes in large universities get smaller as you begin to concentrate on your nursing major. The great advantage to going to a large university is that the professors there are usually at the top of their fields. Their knowledge and experience are incredible, and usually they have published extensively. Larger universities may have access to large medical centers for clinical rotations as part of the nursing curriculum.

At small colleges, student to professor class ratio is small. This means you will get more individualized attention from your professors, and more meaningful in-class interactions with your fellow classmates. It may also be easier in a small college to "break into" extracurricular activities or athletic teams. Campus life may be cozier, and class cohorts tighter.

Regardless of the university or college selected, be sure that the nursing school is accredited. Some states will not allow licensure if a school is not accredited. Be sure that the state licensing board pass rate is high. Look at how long the nursing program has been in existence. While new programs may admit more students, the learning curve for the college may be difficult making the program less than desirable. Talk to recent graduates and ask if they would recommend their school.

Private or Public? The great advantage to going to a public college is cost. Many public colleges are funded by state governments, and so in state residents pay significantly less in tuition and fees. This means that a majority of students at the public college will be students from your state or local area. Private contributions, alumni donations, and tuition fees fund private colleges or universities. Although private colleges tend to be costlier than public colleges, students tend to get access to greater resources and more individualized service. Because class size at private colleges tends to be smaller than class sizes at public colleges, faculty at private colleges are more likely to know you personally and be supportive of your goals and dreams.

Whatever college you choose, it is important to remember that the college or university has to be right for you. Although it is tempting to apply to and attend the same schools your high school friends are going to, what is a good fit for them may or may not be a good fit for you. Visit the colleges you are interested in and get a real sense of how the campus works. Attend a sample class in the nursing program at the college or university with the instructor's permission. Visit the school's financial aid office and tell them of your interest in the college. College is a wonderful opportunity to expand your horizons, meet new people, and become immersed in your chosen field. When you love the college you choose, academic success usually follows.

PAYING FOR COLLEGE

After you have been admitted to the college or university of your choice, the next step is to explore how you will pay for your education. How you choose to fund your education is an important financial decision, and may possibly be one of the first financial decisions that you make for yourself. One of the first things you should do after you send out your applications to colleges is to fill out the Free Application for Federal Student Aid (FASFA) found at fafsa.ed.gov.

Once you are admitted to a college or university, that college's financial aid office will send you a financial aid package based on the data submitted via your FASFA, outlining the scholarships, grants, loans, and work study opportunities you may be eligible for. No matter what colleges and universities say, this package is negotiable to a point. If you or your families' financial situation has changed since applying, do let the financial aid office know.

It is important that all avenues be explored in finding money to pay for a vocational school or college. Start investigating potential tuition sources early in high school as competition is high the closer you get to graduation. In addition to organizations, local, state, and federal assistance, the armed services offer tuition assistance through Reserve Officers' Training Corps (ROTC) on many college campuses. If you have an interest in serving in the military after graduation, this may be worth investigating.

SCHOLARSHIPS AND GRANTS

Scholarships and grants are wonderful because they are funds you do not have to pay back. Community organizations, religious organizations, and music, art, and athletic groups are great resources for scholarship money, especially if you or a family member has been involved in the organization for a significant amount of time. Many organizations such as the Rotary Club or Exchange Club may offer scholarship money. If you are active in a church, ask if any members have sponsored nursing students in school. Search online as there are many opportunities specific to a group of people.

Scholarships are generally available from states, schools, and organizations. Many states have lottery scholarship money that is provided to high school graduates with a certain grade point average. Some states have free tuition for community college and vocational schools. Scholarships generally do not have to be paid back unless the applicant does not finish the commitment for receiving money. Grants are awards that you don't have to pay back such as the Federal Pell Grant. A list of nursing scholarships may be found at www.nurse.org. The US Department of Labor also has a free scholarship search site that can be found at www.careeronestop.org/findtraining/pay/scholarships.aspx.

FEDERAL WORK STUDY AND WORKING OFF CAMPUS

Many times, work opportunities are available on campus via the Federal Work Study program. The payment per hour is equal to or more than minimum wage, and the college or university that employs you and the federal government splits the cost of paying you. Federal work-study opportunities may include working in the library or cafeteria on campus, working within department offices, or tutoring. There may also be off campus jobs available outside the college or university, at local malls, stores, coffee shops, or garden centers. If you do choose to work and go to college, make sure your work does not interfere with your academics or extracurricular activities. Ten to fifteen hours per week working on or off campus is the maximum suggested for first-year college students.

STUDENT LOANS

Many students do need to take loans to cover the cost of their education. Generally, taking out federal loans, instead of private loans, is the suggested route. Federal student loans tend to have lower interest rates and greater options for repayment as compared to private student loans. There are three major types of Federal Student Loans offered by the US Department of Education. Subsidized loans are offered to undergraduates who need them. When you take out a subsidized loan, the US Department of Education pays interest on those loans while you are in school at least half time, as well as paying the interest six months after graduation and/or during periods of deferment. Taking out an Unsubsidized Federal loan means that you are responsible for paying the interest through the lifetime of the loan. If your parents would like to help pay for your education, but cannot immediately cover the cost of tuition, a PLUS loan, is an option. PLUS loans are loans that may be offered to professional degree students as well as parents of dependent undergraduates. These loans are also covered by the US Department of Education. Parents do need good credit to qualify for these loans.

If you do take out loans to pay for the cost of school, it is important to remember that you are responsible for paying those loans back after graduation. The Department of Education does offer income based and pay as you earn repayment programs. It is essential that after graduation you keep in contact with your loan servicer, so you can choose the repayment program that is right for you.

There have been issues related to particularly private colleges not delivering on promises so investigate your school of choice carefully before signing loan documents.

SUMMARY

It is important to determine what level of education you seek in nursing, select a college or university that provides the best education at a price you can afford, and be committed to completing the program especially if loans are needed to afford school. Becoming a nurse is an academic challenge as well as a challenge to caring for patients in the hospital or clinic during the education process. Becoming a nurse, while difficult and challenging, can be fulfilling though the course of a career.

—*Gina Riley and Patricia Stanfill Edens*

Further Reading

"Career Onestop." US Department of Labor. Scholarship search, www.careeronestop.org/FindTraining/Pay/scholarships.aspx. Accessed 27 Aug. 2020. This website, sponsored by the US Department of Labor, focuses on helping individuals find the job or career that is right for them. Within the website, the scholarship search tool has over 7,000 legitimate graduate, undergraduate, and professional scholarship opportunities to explore.

"Choosing a Nursing Degree? Here's What You Need to Know." *Nurse.com*, www.nurse.com/blog/2017/11/30/choosing-a-nursing-degree-heres-what-you-need-to-know/. Accessed 27 Aug. 2020.

"Finding Colleges That Fit." *The College Board*, parents.collegeboard.org/planning-for-college/applications-and-admission/finding-colleges-that-fit. Accessed 1 Sept. 2020.

"Federal Student Aid: An Office of the US Department of Education." FASFA: Free Application for Federal Student Aid, 2020, fafsa.ed.gov/. The Office of Federal Student Aid provides scholarships, grants, loans, and work study opportunities for undergraduate and graduate students attending school in the United States. To apply for student aid, all college and university students, or prospective students, should fill out the Free Application for Federal Student Aid (FASFA).

"Nursing Scholarships." *Nurse.org*, nurse.org/scholarships/. Accessed 27 Aug. 2020. A comprehensive list of available nursing specific scholarships.

"Pell Grant: Federal Student Aid." US Department of Education, studentaid.gov/understand-aid/types/grants/pell. Accessed 27 Aug. 2020.

Learning Styles and Study Skills

ABSTRACT

There are both passive and active learners. The participation of passive learners is limited and attempts to encourage interaction and serious commitment are less than stimulating. Other learners embrace every word, volunteer, participate, manipulate the learning environment to their advantage, and practice skills that enhance success and positive consequences for their behaviors. They characterize active learners. In other words, active learners apply the ideas, concepts, and learning objectives presented in class. Individuals can learn and practice skills that increase their chances for academic success and renewed confidence in their abilities.

INTRODUCTION

You notice that all your best friend needs to do is to practice listening to the teacher—she remembers everything! You know you are smart, but simply taking notes while she lectures from the textbook is not working for you. You feel lost in the maze of words and wish the teacher would slow down. Your instructor turns away from the audience and makes little eye contact. The tone of her voice never changes and she does not offer visual examples, graphics, or maps. You feel bored and doodle on your notebook pages. The time passes slowly, and you can't wait for the end of class.

You change classes and for some magical reason everything starts to fall in place. Your teacher uses PowerPoint, hand-outs, and often writes key words and concepts on the board. She makes eye contact with the audience, pauses for questions, and offers vivid illustrations to explain the content. Her presentations are bold, colorful, and reinforcing. You particularly benefit from the charts and graphics that support the course outline. It's easy to focus on the learning content because it's especially appealing to the eye. However, there's no real social interaction between members of the class.

Learning styles differ between students and teaching styles differ between teachers and classes. Having a favorite class or teacher, while making learning easier, limits success if less enjoyable classes lead you to do poorly. In a nursing program, all classes are important, and a very defined curriculum is the norm. You can't drop a class if you don't like the teacher or content. The first step in defining your personal learning style is to list those things that work for you. Hearing the content, visualizing the content, using handouts, class size, working in groups, and taking extensive notes are all examples of defining what works for you. Ask questions, read and follow instructions, and visualize success. Set a reasonable goal for the next text or assignment and do whatever is necessary to reach it. In other words, I can see myself earning an "A" grade and I'm going to do everything possible to achieve it. This is going to require some action on your part.

When it comes time to study alone, what time is best? How do I minimize distractions? Do I need quiet or soft background music or TV? Do I have a designated place to study with good lighting? Can I put my cell phone on silence or put it out of reach? Take study breaks, walk around, and refresh yourself. Then go back for another learning burst. If you need help, ask for it. One very important habit is to begin assignments early so you don't have to rush.

Visualize your personal presentation. Remember, you represent yourself when you hand in an assignment, project, examination, make a speech, or participate in a group activity. Did you rush, wait until the last moment, hand it in late or not at all? So, how do you look? Is how you visualize your personal assignment matching the result?

Defining your learning style, learning study skills, and developing techniques to do well in classes where the teacher's teaching style does not best fit your learning style are the keys to success. The study of nursing is challenging. Core courses taught in the classroom setting must be applied to the hands-on practice of skills. Understanding the theoretical basis for nursing care is ongoing. The knowledge learned in a nursing curriculum must be retained for classes that follow as all content builds on previous nursing. For example, a pharmacology class is used in every other class in the curriculum as new drugs are introduced in the treatment of increasingly complex diseases.

BECOMING AN ACTIVE LEARNER

It takes time to adjust to your new skills as you journey down the road to becoming an active learner. Your positive behavior changes and fresh academic success may cause others to wonder what's going on. They will have to adjust. Perhaps you are not hanging out with them as much, your grades are improving, and you are feeling better about yourself. That's not a bad trade. It's working for you. Keep going!

You incorporate all your senses when you become an active learner. Get to know and understand the words in your textbook by actually looking at the pages. The SQ3R Learning System can help:

- SURVEY the chapter assignment. It should only take about fifteen minutes. Look at all the titles, headings, vocabulary, bold and italicized words, illustrations, captions, etc. You become familiar with the content and have a mental hook about the sequence of information prior to the teacher's presentation.
- FORMULATE QUESTIONS: Review all the bold headings and words. What questions would you ask? In other words, play school, and you're the teacher. Use who, what, where or when to help you formulate your questions.
- READ the sections in your textbook that answer the questions you formulated.
- RECITE your questions and answers. Manipulate the information by putting it into your own words. Express your answers in different ways. You soon begin to understand and not simply memorize the material.
- REVIEW your questions and answers again and again in preparation for the test. Focus on the questions that you get wrong and check-off those you consistently get right. It's a waste of time to focus on what you already know even though it is easier, and you may feel comfortable answering the question correctly.

Sometimes reading your textbook might seem boring. Active reading can help because you engage with the words and simulate your mind to receive and retain new concepts. Some students learn best from listening only, auditory learners, and they are rare. Many students learn best by seeing, visual learners. The majority typically benefit from seeing, hearing, and doing. When learners apply multiple senses at the same time, retention increases. Application of newly acquired knowledge is beneficial. Group problem-solving, case studies, and student-to-student active learning strategies that incorporate multiple senses have positive results. There are many opportunities to learn from each other.

MANAGING LEARNING AND STUDYING

Teaching styles differ from class to class. Learning styles are different. The one constant is this equation is study skills. Individuals have different learning styles or preferences. In other words, they thrive in some environments better than others.

When a teacher incorporates all of your senses and facilitates group interaction that enhances the chance for discussion, retention, and the application of concepts most students learn better. It allows the individual to be an active learner in a classroom and allows better implementation or manipulation of the concepts being taught. Individuals who like the idea of actually doing the work and who find the social

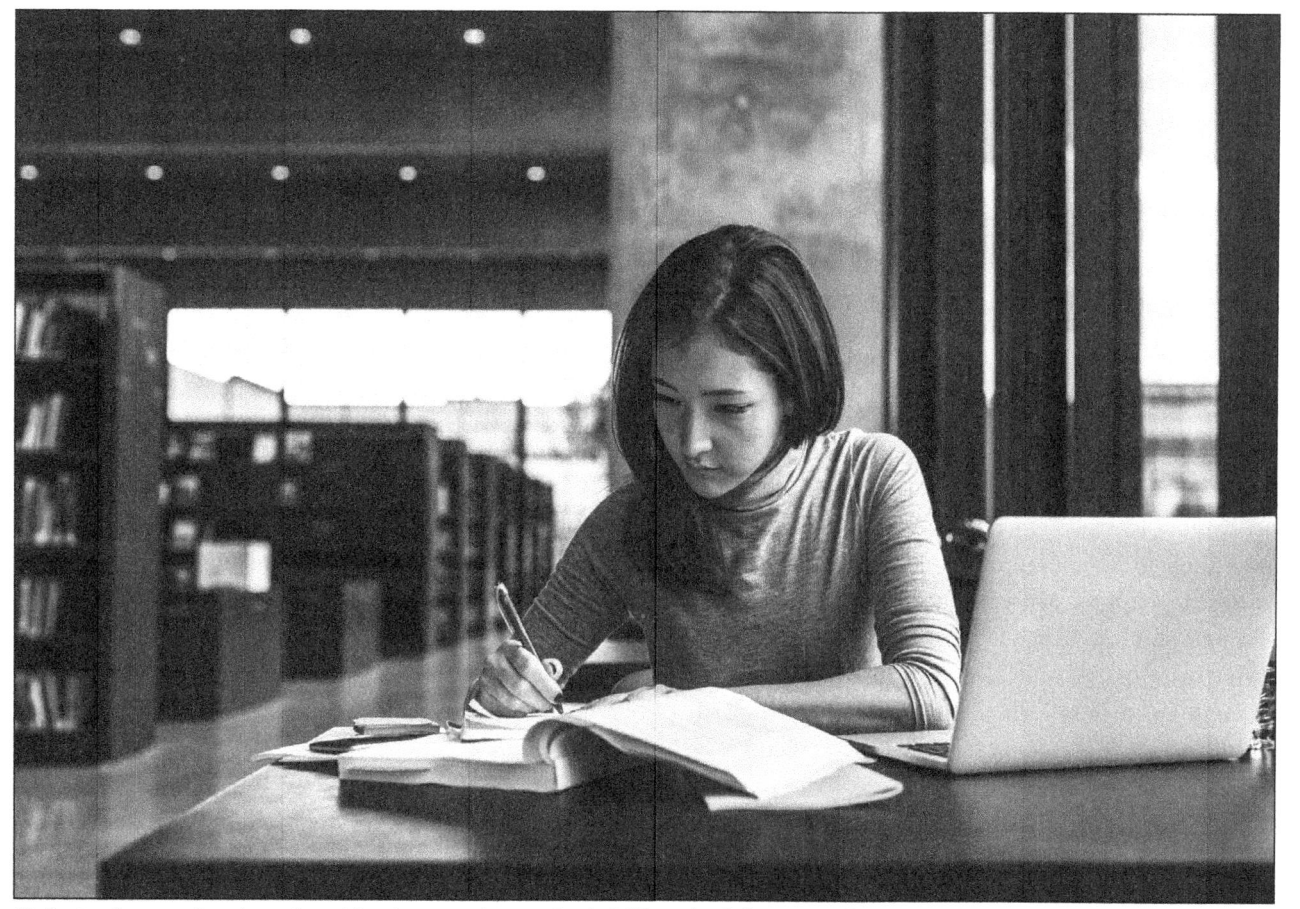

Understanding your learning style and how best to study to retain vital, life-saving information allows you to ultimately provide the best care for your patients. (Jacob Ammentorp Lund via iStock)

interaction of exchanging ideas to come to logical conclusions in a safe, nonjudgmental, environment stimulating.

The teacher who simply lectures appears the least effective in stimulating learner interest and participation. However, auditory learners are satisfied with the learning environment and earn positive grades. Others may feel safe because they do not have to participate in active learning exercise. They simply sit, take notes, and listen.

Solitary learners prefer to learn without interacting with others. Study groups would not be an option they would endorse. Online learning is something they might consider. Therefore, classroom environments that encourage group interaction, discussion, and presentation requirements could prove intimidating. However, learning to mingle with others and force yourself to face your fears may prove beneficial to your development. You can't always choose what kind of environment you will be in and getting along with others is an essential developmental task.

Individuals benefit by understanding what learning environment works best. In addition, identifying learning style or preferences will help determine the best way to study. Think about your individual learning style for a moment. What could you do to help achieve improved success because you acknowledge differences in learning styles?

Auditory learners enjoy listening to instructors and read their study notes out loud. They like to talk things out. Visual learners create mental images to remember and have the need to write in the margins of their textbooks. Tactile learners like to touch and move things around. They enjoy labs where they can handle actual objects—not simply look at pictures.

Orient your study skills to managing the teaching styles of the teachers in your classes that correlate with your learning style. At the beginning of the class, ask how testing will be handled. Do tests come primarily from the lecture, the textbook, handouts, or a combination of all three? Most teachers state at the beginning of the course how testing is handled, or it may be covered in the syllabus for the course.

While taking notes is important, be sure you listen as you write. Ask for copies of slides or presented materials. Most teachers will share if you explain you study better visually. Consider starting a study group for more difficult courses. Reading others' notes may point out topics you missed. Read the text and supplement your class notes with content or page numbers. Read your notes daily and fill in missing content when it is fresh. Each day go back to the beginning and read all your notes including the most current. Reading notes daily and reading the assigned text more than once will make studying for the test easier! Do not try to cram the night before a test. Remember, nursing school class content will be needed during your entire career. It is not good enough to pass a course; you must apply the knowledge gained to your patients.

The Cornell note taking system steps developed by Dr. Walter Pauk is one system that may help you become a better note taker. Divide your notebook paper into sections. It's easy to simply fold your paper along the margin, leave space on the right side.

Step 1: Record your lecture notes in the appropriate space on notebook pages.

Step 2: Use the Review and Self-Test area, the space you've left on the right side, to insert key words, concepts, and formulate your own practice test questions that reflect content in the notes. Review your notes frequently and as soon as possible after class lectures. Constant review aids retention and prevents last minute crash study sessions.

Step 3: Briefly summarize your notes at the bottom of the page.

Step 4: See if you can answer the questions you generated while reviewing your notes. Also, attempt to define the terms you listed. Make an effort to search for understanding. Your goal is to answer questions presented in different test formats and require you to use your critical thinking skills.

There are numerous study skill activities that have the potential to enhance your ability to achieve academic success. Active learners experiment to find what works best for them. Some prefer to study with others, while others find that technique distracting. Active learners often use index cards as a tool to manipulate facts and concepts. They constantly shuffle their self-made cards that have questions on the front and answers on the back. Publishers often give students access to websites that enhance their textbook reading/learning experience. The links offer practice tests, flashcards, chapter outlines and summaries, important terms, outside resources, and an abundance of related supplementary learning aids.

There is no substitute for repetition and practice. Some subjects have clearly defined instructional requirements that demand offering the content in a specific format. Flexibility is a necessity in all learning environments, and you must review prior learning to preserve it. For every learning curve there is a forgetting curve. Regardless of your study method, remember learning requires work.

SUMMARY

Acknowledging your learning style(s) or preference(s) is your strength. Orient your study skills with the goal of retaining information to either augment or compensate for the teaching style of your professors. Understanding your learning style and how best to study to retain vital, life-saving information allows you to ultimately provide the best care for your patients. How you approach your learning journey is important. Unlike other chosen professions, nursing can make the difference in life and death for others. You cannot learn just for grades; you learn for the life of others.

—*Jane Piland-Baker, Thomas E. Baker, and Patricia Stanfill Edens*

Further Reading

Barnier, C. *The Big What Now Book of Learning Styles: A Fresh and Demystifying Approach*. Emerald Books, 2009. This book delivers a fresh and demystifying approach to learning styles.

Brown, P. C. *Make It Stick*. Harvard UP, 2014. This book offers techniques for becoming more productive learners. In addition, it cautions against counterproductive study habits.

Burger, E., and M. Starbird. *The 5 Elements of Effective Thinking*. Princeton UP, 2012. The book presents practical and inspiring techniques for learners to become more successful through better thinking strategies.

Fuller, C. *Talkers, Watchers, and Doers: Unlocking Your Child's Unique Learning Style*. Piñon Press, 2004. By understanding your child's basic learning style and intelligence gifts, you can craft and tailor a learning environment to their needs. These practical suggestions will change the way you approach your child's education. No matter how your child learns, you can help him or her learn better and more efficiently.

Goldberg, D., and J. Zwiebel. *The Organized Student: Teaching Children the Skills for Success in School and Beyond*. Simon & Schuster, 2005. The book presents hands-on strategies for teaching disorganized children how to organize for success. In addition, it offers special tips for children with attention deficit disorder/attention deficit/hyperactivity disorder (ADD/ADHD) and learning disorders.

Guare, R., and P. Dawson. *Smart but Scattered Teens: The "Executive Skills" Program for Helping Teens Reach Their Potential*. Guilford Press, 2013. Detailed examples demonstrate how to teach your teenager the skills needed for success. Clever strategies help address creative resistance to making necessary changes.

Pritchard, A. *Ways of Learning: Learning Theories and Learning Styles in the Classroom*. Routledge, 2013. Provides an understanding of the ways in which learning takes place. Teachers can implement suggestions in their planning and teaching.

Siegel, D., and T. Bryson. *The Whole-Brain Child: 12 Revolutionary Strategies to Nurture Your Child's Developing Mind*. Delacorte Press, 2011. Helps parents teach children about how their brain works, giving young children the self-understanding that can lead them to make better choices that ultimately lead to meaningful and joyful lives.

"Study Skills for Students." *Education Corner: Education that Matters*, www.educationcorner.com/study-skills.html. Accessed 30 Aug. 2010.

Waitley, D. *Psychology of Success: A Positive Approach to Lifelong Learning.* Irwin, 1990.

Waitley, D. *The Psychology of Winning.* Berkley Books, 1984. Best-selling author and speaker, Denis Waitley has painted word pictures of optimism, core values, motivation and resiliency that have become indelible and legendary in their positive impact on society. His works are easily understood and offer positive applications to living a meaningful and successful life.

COVER LETTER AND RESUME WRITING

ABSTRACT

Cover letter and resume writing are critical skills that are sometimes neglected in formal curriculum. As a result, these documents are often misconceived as documents of "objective accomplishments," not unlike a transcript. Cover letter and resume writing are presented as much more effective when approached as a crafted argument of fit as determined by the desired school or employer, and that each application should be tailored to the specifications of the objective.

INTRODUCTION

Despite being required for almost all employment and increasingly as a part of the school admission process, resume and cover letter writing is seldom taught in standard curriculum. Often resume and cover letters are born out of necessity, cobbled together in response to an application deadline for school or work and subsequently recycled for all future applications. Often, applications land in the rejection pile due to issues on the resume or cover letter that would have been easy fixes.

The most common misconception of resume and cover letter writing is that these are objective documents of accomplishments, not unlike a transcript. However, what counts as an "accomplishment" is often based on what the applicant is proud of, or what his or her peers have deemed remarkable. This would work if not for the problem that accomplishments valued by the applicant may not be similarly valued by a school, college or employer. For example, while winning the regional science fair in physics may be a source of pride for an applicant, it may be less valuable for a job that relies heavily on people skills.

In truth, a resume with a cover letter is more like a persuasive argument than a transcript. These documents should convince the application committee or employer that the applicant is the best fit for the position by presenting a collection of supporting evidence. Consider this analogy: If you were buying a birthday cake for someone you want to impress, the smart strategy would be to figure out what flavors and texture they like, and use that information to pick the best cake. Since people have widely varying tastes, the optimal cake will differ based on the individual's preferences. This philosophy leads to a focus on determining the reason for the cover letter and resume and the artful crafting of an argument for admission or employment in resume and cover letter form.

FIRST RULE OF WRITING: KNOW YOURSELF AND YOUR AUDIENCE

As with all good writing, the first step is to understand yourself, what you desire to achieve and who your audience is, and how they will be reading your writing. In this case, the audience is usually a school admissions office seeking the best fit for the school or nursing program or an employer looking to hire someone to do something specific. Note that the three variables of interest here are (1) why you desire admission to a particular school or want a particular job;(2) the person who will review your cover letter and resume, and (3) the requisite skills available for learning or for the job.

Understanding why you are interested in pursuing a nursing role is critical to success. Many times, a decision to be a nurse is based on a family member's illness. Talking to the high school guidance counselor, volunteering at a hospital or clinic, following a registered nurse as part of a career day, and talking with nurses you or your family may know all help define why you want to become a nurse. Some positions in nursing such as a licensed practical nurse (LPN) may be available after one year of education right out of high school at a local vocational school. An associate degree in nursing is usually a two-year commitment in a community college and allows the student to sit for the Registered Nurse Boards after graduation. Bachelor's degrees and advanced nursing degrees require additional education, from four to five years for a Bachelor's in Nursing and additional years for advanced practice.

So how do you secure this information? The easiest place to look is in the admission or course catalogue or in the job description. Being admitted into a nursing program or school is increasingly difficult as individuals realize there are many options for nursing employment, the salary ranges are generous and flexibility in location and schedule is attractive. Competition is stiff for applicants as accrediting bodies such as the National League for Nursing set stringent requirements for faculty to student ratios and curriculum and all states require a licensure examination, often referred to as Nursing Boards, at the end of the program. Schools with low pass rates may be put on probation or accreditation may be lost. Students who do not pass Boards may not work as a licensed or registered nurse unless a successful pass is achieved and may even require going back to repeat courses. Employment requires a current nursing license gained by passing the licensure exam and all employers will verify licensure with the State Board of Nursing before offering a position. To be successful, applicants for limited school positions must stand out. Applications to multiple schools is often the norm to get one acceptance. Also, don't send a cover letter or resume to School B that shows School A's name! Take the time to proofread your application.

After graduation and licensure, applying for a job will require a new cover letter and resume tailored to the position desired. Information about what the employer is seeking in the way of skills and experience is most often found in the job description or the posting of a job on an online career site. Finding information about the employer is available on their internet site or by talking to people who work in the facility. Often, career centers in the school or college will assist in the search for a position after graduation. Be sure that your cover letter and resume are specific to the job you are applying for in the facility. For example, if you are applying for multiple jobs, don't use the resume that says you want a job working with children when you are applying for an adult critical care unit position. Tailor your cover letter and resume to the job you want. You may need to apply for multiple positions to get the one that matches your interest and the employer's needs. Once employed, there is always flexibility to move within an organization.

WRITING THE RESUME CONTENT

Once you have identified the attributes and skills that are consistent with the school requirements for admission or those that best fit the position, the rest should follow logically. Each piece of information on your resume and cover letter should be strategically selected based on the relevant attributes and skills. The simplest method is to showcase experiences that demonstrate the specific skills or attributes desired by the school or employer. For example, you may write about your experiences on student council to showcase leadership skills, or volunteering at a hospital to illustrate compassion and commitment to nursing. Keep in mind that life experiences are rarely unidimensional, which means that different aspects of the same experience can be highlighted to demonstrate various skills and attributes. For instance, you may focus on your successful campaign for student council to illustrate interpersonal skills in connecting with a larger student body, or write about the care you helped provide for a sick family member.

Armed with the strategic collection of evidence that correlates with the admission requirements or job description, the final step is to write a document with precision and impact. Decisions in writing (including wording, organization, and formatting) should be guided by who your audience is and how they will be reading your writing. In most cases, your audience will be the admission committee of a college or nursing program or employers. Gaining admission and obtaining employment are competitive processes. Resumes may be searched by a computer so be sure format is straightforward and words in the document are targeted to the desired outcome. Proofread, reread, and proofread again and ask others to read your resume! Spelling and grammatical errors may be enough for your resume to be tossed in the trash. Most admission committees or employers who encounter a sloppily drafted application or resume assume that translates into how the individual will conduct themselves in class or work.

A few final tips for writing the content of the resume. With limited time, the challenge is to present yourself as an ideal fit for the school or position in as few words as possible. The document must be easy to read (i.e., clean font, clear sections, no cuteness like hearts or smiley faces), and present compelling evidence about your fit with the organization. Here are some general guidelines specific for resumes:

Be concise. For example, I organized a health promotion fair at my high school.

Use action verbs. These are verbs that succinctly communicate skills and attributes. For example, instead of "Served on Yearbook Committee," you may write "Collaborated with peers to publish and distribute a 200-page yearbook" to illustrate interpersonal skills, and organizational skills in managing large tasks.

Follow the general structure. Most resumes follow a standard format. A school may provide an idea of what they are looking for in a resume or you may find examples of college application resumes online. Employers will likely expect to see specific information in specific places and templates are available for professional resumes. Most resumes begin with your name, followed by contact information, an objectives section, your education, selected honors/awards, your (strategically selected) experiences, and any other relevant skills.

Visual presentation matters. Just like how your attire in an interview communicates specific attributes, visual presentation on a résumé can be leveraged to your advantage. Efficient use of space can demonstrate organizational skills. Attention to detail and clearly presented content are important. While many applications are online, if a paper cover letter and resume are requested use white paper and be sure all contact information is accurate.

THE COVER LETTER

A common error of cover letter writing is duplication of the resume, except in prose form. The cover letter is your opportunity to communicate the larger context in which the evidence on your resume fits. The letter should clearly state why you are writing such as applying for admission to the college of nursing or applying for a staff nurse position. Your cover letter may state that your desire to help others and learn new skills along with an ability for critical thinking under pressure, coupled with brief examples, is your goal. This is then followed by the resume that might include leadership roles in team sports, volunteering in disaster relief efforts or at a local hospital, and/or medals won in academic competitions. The cover letter explicitly communicates why you should be admitted or hired, but also allows you to guide the reader through the contents on your resume. Finally, your cover letter should also be concise and easy to read.

—*Patricia Stanfill Edens and Philip Cheng*

Further Reading

Brizee, A., N. Jarrett, N., and K. Schmaling. "What Is an Action Verb?" *Owl Purdue*, 2 Apr. 2010, owl.english.purdue.edu/owl/resource/543/01/. This article reviews what an "action verb" is and how it should be used. A link is also included for a list of action verbs categorized by skill sets.

Brizee, A., and A. Olson. "What Is a Cover Letter?" *Owl Purdue*, 14 Dec. 2011, owl.english.purdue.edu/owl/resource/549/01/. This article reviews what a cover letter is and contains further links such as video instructions and sample documents.

"The Do's and Do Not's of Getting Accepted into Nursing School." *Registered Nursing*, www.registerednursing.org/dos-donts-nursing-school-acceptance/. Accessed 27 Aug. 2020.

Giang, V., and M. Stanger. "How to Write the Perfect Resume." *Business Insider*, 29 Nov. 2012, www.businessinsider.com/how-to-write-the-perfect-resume-2012-11?op=1. This article reviews the general principles of writing an effective resume, and also provides mechanical details regarding the formatting of a resume (e.g., where to put your name, how to make use of space, etc.)

"How to Write a High School Resume for College Applications." *The Princeton Review*, www.princetonreview.com/college-advice/high-school-resume. Accessed 27 Aug. 2010.

INTERVIEWING

ABSTRACT

Interviewing is one of the most popularly adopted methods to select and recruit committed nursing students and productive employees. Interviewee competences are critical to obtaining admission to the desired nursing school and to get attractive job offers after graduation, the first step to success in the workplace. Adolescents face a developmental task to construe their identity, a part of which is career identity. One meaningful path is to get working experience through volunteer activities or employment. In modern society, adolescence is probably the first time in life for a youngster to go through a formal interviewing process to be hired for a job or admitted to the school of choice.

INTRODUCTION

This article focuses on interviewee skills, and not interviewer skills, because realistically, the majority of the adolescents will be interviewees.

According to the late psychologist Erik Erikson, adolescents' developmental task is to construe identity ("who you are"). In this process, career becomes a salient part to adolescence as they start to participate in the labor force. If work is balanced well with school, employment can be beneficial to adolescent development. The longitudinal data from the Youth Development Study of high school students showed benefits of employment to the "steady workers" (less than twenty hours per week most of the time) and "occasional workers" (less than twenty hours per week in a few months only), giving them a sense of accomplishment. Supported by work experience they were strong at achieving educational goals, accumulating savings and bettering their time management skills. Another group, identified as "the most invested workers" (more than twenty hours per week most of the time), also benefited. Employment gave them an opportunity to practice agency and helped them move faster into their self-selected career path to achieve a full-employee identity. In addition, obtaining job-related training, receiving mentoring, and enjoying advancements in the workplace were positively associated with the adolescents' self-efficacy. Negative effects like work stress tended to be short-lived, and more noticeably, might actually have fostered psychological resilience and expanded stress management skills. Students who work during school also have a more robust resume when the time comes to seek admission to their college of choice.

INTERVIEWING BASICS

Interviewing information is applicable to work and other types of interviewing for different purposes, for example, for admission to colleges/graduate programs or for scholarships.

For the sake of reliability (consistency) and validity (job-related qualifications), interviews are most likely to be structured, that is, a predetermined set of designed interview questions will be asked to all of the student or job candidates in the same way by all interviewers and there is a standardized scoring key to evaluate each candidate's performance, although the level of structure may vary.

Adolescents should be prepared for all three phases in an interview: the preinterview phase, the actual interviewing phase, and the postinterview phase. A face-to-face interview may have only one interviewer or a panel of interviewers. Interviews may be conducted in an alternative medium: a phone interview or a video interview.

TYPICAL INTERVIEW QUESTIONS

Interview questions are designed to assess the candidate's personality, knowledge and skills, quality of thinking, ability to handle difficult situations, values and ethics, motivation, career goals, etc. Michael G. Aamodt, an American industrial and organizational psychology professor at Radford University, has listed six types of interview questions:

Clarifier questions—to clarify information in the application files. Work-history and volunteer activity questions belong to this group. Be prepared to answer questions such as "Why are you applying for this school, scholarship or job?" "Why do you want to leave your current job?" or "Why did you chose this school?" Your answers should highlight your career interest, motivation for career development, and realistic necessities such as location and school commitment. You should avoid mistakes like criticizing former employers/coworkers, complaining about previous jobs, or emphasizing benefits.

Disqualifier questions—to disqualify a candidate if he/she cannot satisfy the specific requirements of the school, scholarship or job. In the case of school, the academic record or test results will be discussed, and most schools require minimum levels of competency.

In rare instances a strong academic record might make up for poor standardized test scores. The interviewer may ask if the candidate tests poorly and why the school should give the candidate another chance. A more specific example, if the job requires the candidate to work on night shifts, a candidate who answers "no" to "Are you able to work on night shifts?" is disqualified for this job.

Skill-level determiners—to tap the candidate's job-relevant skills. Applicants for admission to a school may be asked questions about study skills, computer skills and using software. Brainteasers may be included in an interview for competitive jobs that require logical reasoning and creative thinking.

Past-focused questions (behavioral questions)—to get information about the candidate's previous behavior. For example, "Share with me an example of how you reacted to negative feedback from your teacher or boss."

Future-focused questions (situational questions)—to get information about the candidate's probable behavior in the future. For example, "Imagine that you are a nurse in a hospital and a family member becomes impatient with a long wait for a test. How would you handle this situation?"

Organization fit questions—to find out if the candidate will fit into the culture of the school, nursing program, company or work unit. For example, the candidate may be asked to tell the interviewer about his/her preference for team-based work or independent work. Some schools use case studies with study groups or team projects while others ask students to work on their own.

THE PREINTERVIEW PHASE

Caldwell and Burger have reported the power of social preparation and background preparation in predicting interview success (getting subsequent interviews or job offers). Social preparation is to utilize social resources (teachers, school counselors, parents, friends, someone currently enrolled in the college or working in the company, and people in similar jobs) for advice and information about the school or company. Background preparation is to research the college or company to determine if you think it is a fit for you. Study the website. Find brochures, news and business reports in the college or career center, public libraries, and business publications. Read the information carefully. Get educated about factors that impact your choice.

Preparation is not just for gathering information to answer the interviewer's questions but also is for you to prepare questions for the interviewer. You may ask questions about the specific programs or job (e.g., academics, nursing licensure pass rate, responsibilities, authority), growth opportunities (e.g., training, promotion), or peers, faculty or management (e.g., culture of the nursing program or work unit, immediate supervisor). Prioritize your questions. Caution: Do not ask any question about the information readily available. Otherwise, you are telling the interviewer that you have not done your homework. Remember, your questions are not just questions; they are part of the interviewing because they tell something about you—your conscientiousness, intelligence, personality, and career interests and goals.

Preparation should include practice. Practice your role as a job interviewee. Get feedback and improve. Role play again. Familiarity helps reduce anxiety and nervousness. Practice improves speech fluency. Pay attention to your articulation, volume, tone, rhythm, and stress. Get rid of "um," "like," "and," or "you know." Keep good eye contact with "the interviewer." Emphasize with proper gestures without excessive hand movements. The body should be relaxed but alert.

Get familiar with the interview location and how to get there. Consider a drive to locate the interview site before the day of the interview. On the interview day, give yourself plenty of time to arrive at the interview site ten to fifteen minutes earlier than the scheduled interview time. Build in time for traffic or other unexpected delays. Never be late for an interview. Dress appropriately. Look clean. Smile. Be professional and friendly to all the people you meet once you set your feet on the site of the interview (you never know who that person is and what role that person plays). If possible, decline coffee (you may spill it and look clumsy and messy). Keep mentally alert and focused. Organize all of the materials you will need during the interview neatly and get into the interview room with confidence.

If it is a phone/video interview, find a quiet location without any distraction or interference. Check the device, volume, clarity of the visual images, and all of the connections. Have a back-up plan in case technology fails. Familiarize yourself with how to operate the machine(s).

THE INTERVIEWING PHASE

The interviewer will start interviewing with a brief welcoming introduction. Give a warm greeting with a firm handshake. Practice your handshake. Respond to "small talk" naturally. Take your seat with a comfortable position without casualness. The interviewer then proceeds to give you some information, including explaining the interviewing process. Listen attentively. Make some mental notes as the information may be usable later when you answer or ask questions. You may ask if you can take notes which often indicates you are serious about the interview. Have a portfolio with pen ready.

After this information giving phase comes the time for you to answer the interviewer's questions. Listen carefully to get an accurate understanding of each question. If you are not sure about what is being asked, politely ask for clarification. Provide focused answers in specific and personalized language that goes straight to the point (demonstrating your clear way of thinking). Speak up and speak clearly with good eye contact. Do not ramble or use vague/general expressions (indicator of a cloudy mind or lack of knowledge). Cite specific examples to vividly illustrate the key points. Avoid reciting a memorized answer. Interact with the interviewer and monitor your approach. When it is your turn to ask questions, select a few questions that can show your independent thoughts, values, and goals. You may also develop questions based upon what the interviewer has been saying on the spot. When the interview approaches conclusion, you may inquire about the timeline for the decision making and also, encourage the interviewer to contact your references. Leave a good impression that you are interested and enthusiastic. Remember to thank the interviewer.

If this is a phone interview without visual imaging, be aware that you are deprived of nonverbal and paralinguistic cues (e.g., facial expressions, eye contact). Your articulation and speech features become even more important here than in a face-to-face interview. It is advisable to dress up so that you won't get too relaxed and lose your alertness.

Here is a last note specific to adolescents. While it is important to effectively deliver your job-relevant qualifications, it is equally, if not more, important to convince the interviewer that you have great potential. Show your career interest and goals, motivation and enthusiasm, modesty and willingness to learn and improve, and courage to welcome challenges.

THE POSTINTERVIEW PHASE

Remember to do follow-up work after an interview in a timely manner. Send a thank-you note right after the interview. Be patient and wait. After a week or two, you may send a letter or make a call to the contact person reinforcing your continued interest, and provide new supportive documents, if any. But do not be a stalker. After two such inquiries without a reply, it is a sign for you to move on.

Reflect critically upon your interview experience. Find strengths to keep and weaknesses to improve. You may even contact the interviewer for constructive feedback.

CONCLUSION

In the time leading up to sitting for college or job interviews, be sure you become well-rounded as a young adult (e.g., schoolwork, sports, volunteering, strong academic performance), which will contribute to a successful interview performance. Identify your strengths and weaknesses. For example, if you know you don't test well or have test anxiety, consider taking a test taking course as entrance examinations are important. Have you participated in health profession clubs or volunteer activities that show commitment to pursuing nursing? Well-rounded adolescents are highly likely to get interview opportunities. They will be able to do conscientious preparation and perform well in the actual interviews. Getting into a school of nursing is highly competitive. Academic performance is only one factor considered in the admission process. All of these skills will also translate into the career setting.

—*Ling-Yi Zhou*

Further Reading

"33 Common Nursing School Interview Questions." *Indeed.com*, www.indeed.com/career-advice/interviewing/nursing-school-interview-questions. Accessed 28 Aug. 2020.

Aamodt, M. G. *Industrial/Organizational Psychology: An Applied Approach.* 8th ed., Cengage Learning, 2016. A segment of chapter 4 describes types of employment interviews and interview questions, as well as how to conduct interviews.

Caldwell, D. F., and J. M. Burger. "Personality Characteristics of Job Applicants and Success in Screening Interviews." *Personnel Psychology*, vol. 51, 1998, pp. 119–136. The paper reports the mediating functions of personality traits of conscientiousness, extraversion, and openness to experience in the associations of social preparation and background preparation to interview success.

Huffcutt, A. I., C. H. Van Iddekinge, and P. L. Roth. "Understanding Applicant Behavior in Employment Interviews: A Theoretical Model of Interviewee Performance." *Human Resource Management Review*, vol. 21, 2011, pp. 353–367, doi:10.1016/j.hrmr.2011.05.003.

The authors present a theoretical model composed of multiple factors in interviewer-interviewee dynamics and ideas for future research.

Mortimer, J. T. *The Benefits and Risks of Adolescent Employment* (PMCID: PMC2936460), www.ncbi.nlm.nih.bov/PMC2936460/. This document reviewed the longitudinal Youth Development Study and identified four types of high school students who participated in employment.

CAREER AND PERSONNEL TESTING

ABSTRACT

The popularity of career and personnel testing reflects the trend toward the utilization of interest surveys, ability and aptitude tests, and personality tests for the systematic development of personal careers.

INTRODUCTION

Psychologists have developed numerous testing devices for assessing human capabilities. The groups of tests that have been used most frequently for career and personnel purposes have been those measuring interests, abilities and aptitudes, personality, and values.

Inventories that survey interest patterns are useful in providing indications of the areas in which individuals might work. Research by psychologist Edward K. Strong Jr. has shown that people in the same line of work also tend to have similar hobbies, like the same types of books and magazines, and prefer the same types of entertainment.

Psychological research by John L. Holland concluded that most occupations can be grouped into six vocational themes reflecting certain employment preferences: "realistic," favoring technical and outdoor activities such as mechanical, agricultural, and nature jobs; "investigative," interested in the natural sciences, medicine, and the process of investigation; "artistic," favoring self-expression and dramatics such as the musical, literary, and graphic art occupations; "social," reflecting an interest in helping others, as in teaching and social service; "enterprising," interested in persuasion and political power, as in management, sales, politics, and other areas of leadership; and "conventional," including enjoyment of procedures and organization such as office practices, clerical, and quantitative interest areas.

Tests that measure ability include intelligence tests, achievement tests, and aptitude tests. Intelligence tests purport to measure objectively a person's potential to learn, independent of prior learning experiences. Attempting such objective measurement is a highly complex task; whether it can truly be achieved is open to debate. The very concept of "intelligence," in fact, has been controversial from its inception. The most highly developed tests of individual intelligence include updated versions of the Stanford-Binet test, a scale originally developed in 1916, and the Wechsler Adult Intelligence Scale, originally developed in 1939.

Achievement tests are designed to measure how much a person has learned of specific material to which he or she has been previously exposed. Aptitude tests measure a personal ability or quality (such as musical or mechanical aptitude) to predict some future performance. For example, the military would like to be able to predict the likelihood that a given candidate for pilot training will successfully complete the complicated and expensive course of training. Flying a plane requires good physical coordination and a good sense of mechanical matters, among other things. Therefore, candidates for flight training are given a battery of aptitude tests, which include tests of mechanical aptitude and eye-hand coordination, to estimate later performance in flight training. People who score poorly on such aptitude tests tend to fail pilot training.

Psychologists recognize that it is important to understand a person's interests and abilities—and personality tendencies—if a thorough appraisal of career potentials is to be made. Personality tests, also often known as personality rating scales, measure dispositions, traits, or tendencies to behave in a typical manner. Personality tests are described as either objective (a structured test) or subjective (a projective personality test). Objective tests are structured by providing a statement and then requiring two or more alternative responses, such as in true-or-false questions in the Woodworth Personal Data Sheet. In contrast, projective personality tests ask open-ended questions or provide ambiguous stimuli that require spontaneous responses (as in the Rorschach inkblot test). The two types of personality test reveal different information about the respondent.

The development of objective personality tests was greatly improved when studies showed that personality tests did not have to rely completely on face validity, or the apparent accuracy of each test question. Through empirical research, the accuracy of a question can be tied to the likelihood of a question being associated with certain behavior. Consequently, it does not matter whether a person answers the question "I am not aggressive" as either "true" or "false." What does matter is whether that question is accurately associated with aggressive or nonaggressive behavior for a significant number of people who answer it in a particular way. This approach is referred to as criterion keying: The items in a test are accurately associated with certain types of behavior regardless of the face validity of each question.

Beginning with Gordon Allport's study of values, psychologists have recognized that personal values affect individual career choices. Allport found six general values that are important to most individuals: theoretical, economic, aesthetic, social, political, and religious. Occupational values represent a grouping of needs, just as abilities represent a grouping of work skills. René Dawis and Lloyd Lofquist found that there are six occupational values: achievement, comfort, status, altruism, safety, and autonomy.

TESTING IN PRACTICE

For people to enter careers that will be satisfactory for them, it is desirable to make an effort to match their personal interests with the day-to-day activities of the careers they will eventually choose. Interest inventories are one method of helping people make career choices that compare their interest patterns with the activities of persons in the occupation they hope to enter.

The Strong Vocational Interest Blank (SVIB) was developed by Strong. It matches the interests of a person to the interests and values of a criterion group of employed people who were happy in the careers they have chosen. This procedure is an example of criterion keying. Strong revised the SVIB in 1966, using 399 items to relate to fifty-four occupations for men and a separate form for thirty-two occupations for women. The reliability of this test to measure interests is quite good, and validity studies indicate that the SVIB is effective in predicting job satisfaction.

The Strong-Campbell Interest Inventory (SCII) was developed by psychologist D. T. Campbell as a revision of the SVIB. In this test, items from the men's and women's forms were merged into a single scale, reducing the likelihood of gender bias, a complaint made about the SVIB. Campbell developed a theoretical explanation of why certain types of people like working in certain fields; he based it on Holland's theory of vocational choice. Holland postulated that interests are an expression of personality and that people can be classified into one or more of six categories according to their interests and personality. Campbell concluded that the six personality factors in Holland's theory were quite similar to the patterns of interest that had emerged from many years of research on the SVIB. Therefore, Holland's theory became incorporated into the SCII. The SCII places individuals into one of the six Holland categories, or groupings of occupations, with each group represented by a national sample.

The Kuder Occupational Interest Survey (KOIS) was first developed in 1939. This survey also examines the similarity between the respondent's interests and the interests of people employed in different occupations. It can provide direction in the selection of a college major. Studies on the predictive validity of the KOIS indicate that about half of a selected group of adults who had been given an early version of the inventory when they were in high school were working in fields that the inventory suggested they enter. The continuing development of this measure suggests that it may be quite useful for guidance decisions for high school and college students.

The Self-Directed Search (SDS) was developed by Holland as a means of matching the interests and abilities of individuals with occupations that have the same characteristics. Holland uses a typology that groups occupations in the categories of realistic, investigative, artistic, social, enterprising, and conventional. There are three forms of the SDS: Form E is designed for use with middle-school students or older individuals with limited reading ability; Form R is for use with high school students, college students, or adults; and Form CP is designed for use with college students and adults. The test is also available in other languages, such as Spanish.

Several ability and aptitude tests have been used in making decisions concerning employment, placement, and promotion. The Wonderlic Personnel Test (WPT), later renamed the Wonderlic Cognitive Ability Test, was based on the Otis Self-Administering Tests of Mental Ability. The Wonderlic Cognitive Ability Test is a quick test of mental ability in adults. Normative data are available for more than fifty thousand adults between twenty and seventy-five years of age. The Revised Minnesota Paper Form Board Test (RMPFBT) is a revision of a study in the measurement of mechanical ability. The RMPFBT is a twenty-minute speed test consisting of two-dimensional (2D) diagrams cut into separate parts. The test seems to measure those aspects of mechanical ability requiring the capacity to visualize and manipulate objects in space. It appears to be related to general intelligence.

The US Department of Labor developed an instrument to measure abilities known as the General Aptitude Test Battery (GATB). The GATB measures nine specific abilities: general learning, verbal ability, numerical ability, spatial ability, form perception, clerical perception, eye-hand coordination, finger dexterity, and manual dexterity. Another ability test that was developed by the US government is the Armed Services Vocational Aptitude Battery (ASVAB). The ASVAB is used by the Department of Defense to assist individuals in identifying occupations that match their personal characteristics.

Personality tests were developed in an effort to gain greater understanding about how an individual is likely to behave. As tests have been improved, specific traits and characteristics have been associated with career development, such as leadership propensities or control of impulses. Several personality tests have been used in career and personality development. The Minnesota Multiphasic Personality Inventory II Restructured Form (MMPI-2-RF) is the 2008 version of a scale developed in 1943 by S. R. Hathaway and J. C. McKinley. The test was designed to distinguish normal from abnormal behavior. It was derived from a pool of one thousand items selected from a wide variety of sources. The California Psychological Inventory (CPI) was developed by Harrison Gough in 1957 and was revised in 1987. The test is regarded as a good measure for assessing normal individuals for interpersonal effectiveness and internal controls.

The Sixteen Personality Factor Questionnaire (16PF) was developed by Raymond Cattell in 1949 and was revised in 1993. Considerable effort has been expended to provide a psychometrically sound instrument to measure personality, and it remains an exemplary illustration of the factor-analytic approach to measuring personality traits. The Personality Research Form (PRF) was developed by Douglas Jackson in 1967. It was based on Henry A. Murray's theory of needs. The PRF includes two validity scales and twenty multidimensional scales of personality traits. It has been favorably reviewed for its psychometric rigor and is useful in relating personality tendencies to strengths and weaknesses in working within a corporate or employment setting.

Tests to measure occupational values include the Minnesota Importance Questionnaire (MIQ), developed by David Weiss, René Dawis, and Lloyd Lofquist, and the Values Scale (VS), developed by Doris Nevill and Donald Super. The MIQ compares individual needs with reinforcers found in occupations. The VS measures work values that are commonly sought by workers, such as personal development and achievement. The values in the test are also cross-referenced with the occupational groups found in Holland's typology.

An alternative to paper-and-pen tests is the use of computerized career guidance systems, which may consist of specialized software or web-based programs. The common elements of these systems include the use of an assessment instrument, the provision of an individualized detailed occupational profile, and instructions on how to use the information in career planning.

FUNCTIONS OF TESTING

These instruments are examples of tests that are frequently used for career and personnel assessment. The range of psychological assessment procedures includes not only standardized ability tests, interest surveys, personality inventories and projective instruments, and diagnostic and evaluative devices but also performance tests, biographical data forms, scored application blanks, interviews, experience requirement summaries, appraisals of job performance, and estimates of advancement potential. All these devices are used, and they are explicitly intended to aid employers who make hiring decisions to choose, select, develop, evaluate, and promote personnel. Donald N. Bersoff notes that the critical element in the use of any psychological test for career and employment purposes is that employers must use psychometrically sound and job-relevant selection devices. Such tests must be scientifically reliable (appropriate, meaningful, or useful for the inferences drawn from them) and valid (measuring what they claim to measure).

Each of the test procedures previously described would be used for different purposes. Ability tests can be used to determine whether a person has the potential ability to learn a certain job or specific skills. Ability tests are used for positions that do not have a minimum educational prerequisite (such as high school, college, or professional degree). They are also used to select already employed individuals for challenging new work assignments and for promotion to a more demanding employment level. The United States Supreme Court has held that the appropriate use of "professionally developed ability tests" is an acceptable employment practice; however, the employer must demonstrate a relationship between the relevance of the selection test procedure and job qualification. This requirement is to ensure that the ability test provides a fair basis for selection and is nondiscriminatory. The goal of Title VII of the Civil Rights Act of 1964 was to eliminate discrimination in employment based on race, color, religion, sex, or national origin in all of its forms. The use of a selection procedure or test must meet this standard.

Interest inventories have been developed to identify a relationship between the activities a person enjoys and the activities of a certain occupation. For example, a salesperson should enjoy meeting people and persuading others to accept his or her viewpoint. An interest inventory can validly link a person's preferences and interests with associated social activities and can thereby identify sales potential. Interest inventories are frequently given when an employer seeks more information that could lead to a good match between a prospective employee and a job's requirements. Interest inventories typically survey a person's interests in leisure or sports activities, types of friends, school subjects, and preferred reading material.

Personality, or behavior traits, can be identified by test inventories and related to requisite employment activities. Once again, these personality dimensions must be demonstrated to be job-related and must be assessed reliably from a performance appraisal of the specific position to be filled. For example, behavior traits such as "drive" or "dependability" could be validated for use in promoting individuals to supervisory bank teller positions if demonstrated to be job-related and assessed reliably from a performance appraisal.

The use of psychological tests has grown immensely since the mid-twentieth century. Increased public awareness, the proliferation of different tests, and the use of computer technology with tests indicate that continually improving career and personnel tests will emerge. Yet these developments should proceed only if testing can be conducted while protecting the human rights of consumers—including their right not to be tested and their right to know test scores and how test-based decisions will affect their lives. Psychological testing must also be nondiscriminatory and must protect the person's right to privacy. Psychologists are ethically and legally bound to maintain the confidentiality of their clients.

Making a selection among the many published psychological tests is a skill requiring experienced psychologists. In personnel selection, the psychologist must determine if the use of a psychological test will improve the selection process above what is referred to as the base rate, or the probability of an individual succeeding at a job without any selection procedure. Consequently, the use of a test must be based on its contributing something beyond chance alone. This requirement necessitates that a test be reasonably valid and reliable, in that it consistently tests what it was designed to test. Consequently, the use of a test is only justified when it can contribute to the greater likelihood of a successful decision than would be expected by existing base rates.

Existing theories of career selection have related career choices to personal preferences, developmental stages, and the type of relationship a person has had with his or her family during childhood. More extensive research will continue to assess other relationships between one's psychological makeup and successful career selection. This positive beginning should eventually result in more innovative, more objective, and more valid psychological tests that will greatly enhance future career and personnel selection.

—*Robert A. Hock; updated by Debra S. Preston*

Further Reading

American Psychological Association. "Ethical Principles of Psychologists." *American Psychologist*, vol. 36, 1981, pp. 633–38.

Bersoff, Donald N., Laurel P. Malson, and Donald B. Verrilli. "In the Supreme Court of the United States: Clara Watson v. Fort Worth Bank and Trust." *American Psychologist*, vol. 43, 1988, pp. 1019–28.

Buros Institute of Mental Measurement. *The Fourteenth Mental Measurements Yearbook*. U of Nebraska P, 2001.

Campbell, Donald Thomas. *Manual for the Strong-Campbell Interest Inventory*. Stanford UP, 2001.

Capuzzi, David, and Mark D. Stauffer, editors. *Career Counseling: Foundations, Perspectives, and Applications*. Routledge, 2012.

Committee to Develop Standards for Educational and Psychological Testing. *Standards for Educational and Psychological Testing*. American Psychological Association, 1999.

Darley, John M., Samuel Glucksberg, and Ronald A. Kinchia. *Psychology*. 5th ed., Prentice-Hall, 1991.

Holland, John L. *Manual for the Self-Directed Search*. Consulting Psychologists, 1985.

Kapes, Jerome T., Marjorie Moran Mastie, and Edwin A. Whitfeld. *A Counselor's Guide to Career Assessment Instruments*. National Career Development Association, 2008.

Koppes, Laura L., editor. *Historical Perspectives in Industrial and Organizational Psychology*. Psychology, 2014.

"Policy, Data, Oversight: Assessment & Selection." *Office of Personnel Management*, www.opm.gov/policy-data-oversight/assessment-and-selection/other-assessment-methods/job-knowledge-tests/. Accessed 24 Aug. 2020.

Swanson, Jane L., and Nadya A. Fouad. *Career Theory and Practice: Learning through Case Studies*. Sage, 2010.

Zunker, Vernon. *Using Assessment Results for Career Development*. Brooks, 2006.

COLLEGE AND NURSING ENTRANCE EXAMINATIONS

ABSTRACT
College entrance examinations have been used since the 1920s in the United States to assist college administrators in making admissions decisions. The two most widely used exams are the American College Test (ACT) and the Scholastic Aptitude Test (SAT). A separate nursing school entrance examination may be required before admission to a nursing program or college of nursing.

INTRODUCTION
College entrance examinations (exams) are standardized tests designed to predict student grades in the first year of college. Because research has shown that students' scores on these assessments are related to their grade point averages as college freshmen, many US colleges and universities use these scores as a source of information for selection and admissions decisions. In addition, college entrance exam scores are used for decisions about financial aid, scholarships, and placement into remedial course work.

Nursing schools may also require an entrance exam to measure aptitude for the profession. The exams rate abilities such as comprehension, critical thinking, communication, and knowledge of the core subjects that may have been a component of the courses required before taking the exam. There are a variety of exams that may be required depending on the type of program and level of degree. Often both a college entrance examination and a test specific to nursing may be required. Some nursing programs require admission first to the college and successful completion of pre-requisite courses before sitting for the nursing examination.

The most used college entrance exams in the United States are the SAT Reasoning Test and the ACT. In 2012, about 1.6 million high school students completed the ACT, and 1.6 million completed the SAT. ACT test takers are largely residents of the Midwest and the South, while SAT test takers tend to be residents of the Northeast and West, although most institutions will accept scores from either assessment. The most used nursing specific exams are the NLN PAX, NET, Kaplan Admissions Test, PSB Aptitude for Practical Nursing Exam, PSB Registered Nursing School Aptitude Exam, TEAS, and HESI A2.

THE SAT
Before the development of the SAT Reasoning Test, information used to make college admissions decisions varied widely. Many elite institutions selected the children of alumni or graduates from highly ranked preparatory schools for admission. Some colleges did have entrance exams; however, these differed from college to college, so students interested in multiple institutions had to take multiple exams. The aim of the SAT as designed by its developers, the College Entrance Examination Board (later the College Board), was to provide a standardized way to assess students' aptitude for college-level work, regardless of previous education or family lineage and, consequently, to select students for admittance on the basis of their own merits.

The SAT Reasoning Test, developed in the 1920s and originally called the Scholastic Aptitude Test, has evolved over the years. It was originally designed to measure aptitude, or an individual's innate ability to perform well in school. The SAT is a three-hour test—three hours and fifty-minutes when including the essay—with three sections: critical reading (formerly verbal), mathematics, and writing. Both the critical reading and mathematics sections consist of multiple-choice and fill-in-the-blank questions. In the critical reading section, students complete sentences, read, and assess written passages, and in the math section, they apply mathematical concepts and interpret data. The writing section is made up of an essay-writing portion which was made optional in 2014 and multiple-choice questions requiring students to recognize writing errors and improve sentences and paragraphs. Scores on each section of the SAT range from 200 to 800. The average score varies slightly from year to year, but is relatively stable at approximately 500 on each of the sections with a standard deviation of about 100.

THE ACT
In the 1950s, E. F. Lindquist developed the American College Test (later known as the ACT) and founded the testing and measurement company ACT, Inc., in Iowa City, Iowa. Lindquist believed that although tests of aptitude such as the SAT measured an individual's innate ability, such tests failed to recognize achievement, or what individuals had done with their ability. The ACT, therefore, was designed to measure what students had learned in core college-preparatory curriculum areas. ACT regularly conducts a survey of high school and college faculty to ensure that the assessment stays consistent with high school curricula.

The ACT is a two-hour, fifty-five-minute test. The writing section of the ACT is optional and takes an additional thirty minutes to complete. Besides writing, the ACT has four sections—English, mathematics, reading, and science—consisting entirely of multiple-choice questions. The English test measures knowledge of punctuation, grammar, sentence structure, organization, and style. Mathematics measures algebra, geometry, and trigonometry skills. Reading measures skills in reading college-level material, and the science section measures scientific reasoning skills, assuming that students have completed three years of science, including biology. The optional writing test is a single thirty-minute essay.

Scores on each of the four ACT scales range from 1 to 36. A composite score, which is the mean, or average, of the scores on all four scales, is also provided on a range from 1 to 36. The mean score varies slightly from year to year but remains relatively stable at approximately 20 on each of the scales and the composite, with a standard deviation of about 5. Scores on the writing section range from 2 to 12 and are reported in combination with the English subscale on a scale of 1 to 36.

Although the ACT is used for college admissions decisions, it is also designed to provide feedback to teachers and students on academic areas of strength and areas for development. Students can use ACT subscale scores to plan what courses to take and where to focus their studies to improve their achievement and, consequently, their level of preparation for college. In addition, teachers and high school administrators can use ACT scores to evaluate the effectiveness of their teaching and of the curriculum. Because the ACT is linked to high school course content, several states have also mandated its use as a high school exit exam.

NLN PAX
One of the most frequently used nursing entrance exams administered by the National League for Nursing (NLN), it measures verbal ability and understanding of math and science. This exam is most often used for individuals who desire to enter certificate, associate, or bachelor's degree programs in nursing. The test allows up to three hours to answer three sections of multiple-choice questions: 80 verbal, 54 math and 80 science. Acceptable scores are determined by each school. In rare exceptions, schools may overlook a low score if high school and college pre-requisite course grades indicate an ability to do the work required in nursing school. The NLN Study Guide is an excellent way to prepare for the test, offering 1,000 practice test items and suggestions about taking standardized tests.

NET

The Nursing Entrance Test (NET) is primarily used for those entering a Licensed Practical Nurse (LPN) or Registered Nurse (RN) program. It is designed to cover basic high school level knowledge related to reading and math, decision making skills, learning styles and other factors. There are 60 math, 33 reading, 44 learning style, 17 social decisions, 49 stressful situations, and 30 exam-taking questions over 2 1/2 hours. A study guide is available.

KAPLAN ADMISSIONS TEST

Both LPN and RN potential students may be asked to take the Kaplan Admissions Test to determine performance and gaps in reading, math, science, writing and critical thinking. In two hours, 45 minutes, the test taker is asked to complete four sections of multiple-choice questions: 22 reading, 28 math, 21 writing, and 20 science. Acceptable scores vary by school but a score of approximately 70 percent is the usual pass rate.

PSB APTITUDE FOR PRACTICAL NURSING EXAM

A Licensed Practical Nurse (LPN) provide more basic nursing care and work under the license of a Registered Nurse or Physician in most cases. Jobs are primarily in hospitals, nursing homes, long-term care facilities and office settings. The test measures vocabulary, math, analytical reasoning, spelling, natural science, judgment on practical nursing situations, and the Vocational Adjustment Index in a 2 1/2-hour test with 225 multiple-choice questions. Both sample questions and a study guide are available at www.psbtests.com.

OTHER NURSING ENTRANCE EXAMINATIONS

The most used nursing specific exams are the NLN PAX, NET, Kaplan Admissions Test, and PSB Aptitude for Practical Nursing Exam. Other exams may be more generic and designed for a variety of healthcare professionals. The Test of Academic Skills (TEAS) is broader in knowledge tested and predicts a student's preparedness to enter the field of healthcare. The HESI A2 includes a personality profile and learning style inventory. Each school or college has their own set of requirements and aspiring nurses are encouraged to obtain a copy of requirements, use targeted study guides, take practice exams if offered, and realize that exams are only one part of the admission process.

THE ROLE OF ENTRANCE EXAMINATIONS

The SAT, ACT, and all nursing entrance examinations have both advantages and limitations. Critics suggest that college entrance exams measure only one determinant of success in college and ignore other influential variables. For example, the motivation to perform well, feelings of connection to the college, and study skills have all been shown to predict college performance and are marginally related, if at all, to performance on the SAT and ACT. The nursing entrance exams test for more targeted factors relating to potential success in the field of nursing. No standardized test can fully measure the ability of an individual to succeed in a nursing program. Multiple factors should be considered by those evaluating applicants and applicants should be realistic about their abilities to be successful in an academically and often physically challenging field.

—*Patricia Stanfill Edens and Christina Hamme Peterson*

Further Reading

Adams, Caralee. "College Board Begins Redesign of SAT Exam." *Education Week*, 6 Mar. 2013, p. 4.

Barton, P. E., and R. J. Coley. "Windows on Achievement and Inequality." *Policy Information Report*, PIC-WINDOWS. Educational Testing Service, 2008.

"Health Careers Aptitude Tests." *Psychological Service Bureau*, www.psbtests.com.

"Kaplan Nursing School Admissions Test." *Kaplan Nursing*, www.kaptest.com. Accessed 27 Aug. 2020.

Lewin, Tamar. "A New SAT Aims to Realign with Schoolwork." *New York Times*, 6 Mar. 2014, p. A1.

Mattern, K., W. Camara, and J. L. Kobrin. *SAT Writing: An Overview of Research and Psychometrics to Date. College Board Research Report no. RN-32*. The College Board, 2007.

"NLN PAX." *National League for Nursing*, www.nln.org. Accessed 27 Aug. 2020.

"Nursing Entrance Exams: What You Can Expect." *All Nursing Schools*, www.allnursingschools.com/how-to-get-into-nursing-school/entrance-exams/. Accessed 27 Aug. 2020.

Sackett, P. R., M. J. Borneman, and B. S. Connelly. "High-Stakes Testing in Higher Education and Employment: Appraising the Evidence for Validity and Fairness." *American Psychologist*, vol. 63, no. 4, May/June 2008, pp. 215–27.

"Solutions for College and Career Readiness." ACT, www.act.org. Accessed 27 Aug. 2020.

"The SAT." *College Board*, www.collegeboard.org. Accessed 27 Aug. 2020.

SUCCEEDING AT WORK

ABSTRACT

The adolescent years generally provide the first experience in the more formal work environment. Jobs such as grass cutting and babysitting may occur before taking a job such as food service, retail, or lifeguarding. Jobs and work environments can seem alien because of the norms and expectations employee's face. Understanding how organizations work and what it takes to "fit" in will encourage success as adolescents' transition through college and ultimately into their chosen career.

INTRODUCTION

During adolescence, many people begin working at their first job. For some, this first work experience may be a revelation due to the expectations for performance, the complexity of demands, and the diversity of social interactions. Working adolescents often must adjust to the lack of direct adult supervision at work and the need to work independently and autonomously. This article examines critical aspects of work and employee behavior that adolescents should be aware of as they begin working. The emphasis is on what it takes to be successful—the do's and don'ts. The discussion examines: finding the right personal work "fit," work expectations, building good relationships with supervisors and coworkers, communicating effectively at work, and the necessity for continuous growth and learning. Successful mastery of this information will lead to success in a career role such as nursing.

PERSON-ENVIRONMENT FIT

The key to work success is finding the right job and organizational fit. This is also true when selecting a college or nursing program. Many students must work part time to make ends meet while in school. As the Greek aphorism admonishes, "Know thyself." This involves self-discovery. Adolescents seeking work should get to know themselves first by identifying their personal interests, personality characteristics, values, skills, knowledge, and abilities. What tasks do they like to do? What skills do they have? Are they detailed oriented? Are they sociable and gregarious? Can they manage both school and work? Adolescence is a time of exploration and discovery focused on uncovering areas of competence and the things they care about.

Jobs vary in terms of requirements, duties, tasks, and activities. Person-job fit focuses on matching the person's characteristics with the jobs. Prospective employees should figure out what knowledge, skills, abilities, and other (KSAO's) job characteristics (e.g., personality, attitudes, values) are required to succeed at a particular job. For example, how much interaction does the job require with people? O*Net Online, a database sponsored by the US Department of Labor, describes the tasks, KSAO's, work activities, work context, interests, values, educational requirements, and credentials for a wide range of occupations.

Person-organization fit emphasizes the fit between the individual and the organization's culture. An organization's dominant culture can be thought of as its personality. Culture reflects shared employee assumptions, values, and norms. Shared assumptions are common underlying beliefs about human nature and the way the organization should operate. Often these are revealed in decisions and choices made by employees. Values of the organization reflect what is important and prioritized at the organization. Norms reflect how employees should and should not behave. Corporate artifacts represent physical manifestations of these shared assumptions, values, and norms. Common cultural artifacts include stories about the founder, the company logo, its branding, its ceremonies (e.g., an award recognition ceremony), the style of its office furniture, and the organization's public image. For example, corporate slogans spell out priorities and responsibilities, such as Google's slogan "Don't be evil." Similarly, Starbucks' purchase of only fair-trade coffee beans represents the value it places on sustainability.

Organizations design their employment systems to recruit and hire employees who will fit their culture. In 2013, Cubiks conducted an international survey that found 82 percent of respondents felt that cultural fit was important in their hiring decisions and 59 percent said they rejected a candidate because of lack of cultural fit.

Benjamin Schneider developed the Attraction, Selection, Attrition (ASA) model to describe how organizations promote fit by attracting, selecting and retaining key employees. In terms of attraction, individuals are drawn to apply for jobs at organizations that have appealing cultures. Organizations, likewise, attempt to attract and to recruit workers who share their values. From the pool of applicants, organizations select candidates who are perceived to match their culture. Attrition happens when employees, who do not fit, either quit or are fired.

Adolescents should be encouraged to examine each of these three areas: getting to know themselves, understanding the KSAO's required of jobs, and exploring how organizational cultures vary. Exposure to a wide range of careers and learning experiences will help them explore their opportunities and help them find the right fit.

WORK EXPECTATIONS

Once adolescents are hired, they need to recognize what they are expected to do. Each organization is in business for a specific purpose. The individual should pay attention to the types of products their organization makes or the services it provides. Organizations pay their employees for productivity, and not simply for showing up and socializing with their coworkers and customers.

An essential source of information about work expectations is the individual's supervisor. New employees should be encouraged to talk to their supervisor to find out what tasks should be done and when these should be done. Many organizations provide new employees with training and other activities to help them transition into their new roles within the organization. These activities are called onboarding and are designed to help socialize new employees. They can involve meetings, videos, mobile apps, or computer programs. New employees should take advantage of these to learn the ropes and get to know what is expected. Most organizations will also have some type of performance evaluation. The supervisor conducts these evaluations once or twice a year. The performance evaluation rating form is a good source of information about what represents effective performance and what it takes to succeed. Whenever you receive a formal performance evaluation, ask for a copy for your files. New employees should ask their supervisors for a blank copy of the form.

There are some work expectations that apply to almost all jobs. These are considered the "ropes" all employees should know and are summarized below. Many of these will show up on the performance evaluation.

"ROPES TO KNOW"

Know the Schedule and Show Up When Scheduled to Work. Employees must keep track of their work shifts and show up ready to work. Missing a shift means that your work group will be short staffed. Others will have to scramble to complete the work for the missing employee. If an employee would like a certain shift off, he/she should follow the prescribed process for requesting the time off. Some supervisors will be reluctant to change a schedule once it is posted. Also, employees must keep in mind that supervisors must staff all shifts. Requesting Saturday off every week may be seen as an unreasonable demand.

Miss Work Only for Legitimate Reasons. If an employee must miss work; he/she should let the boss know as soon as possible, so that the boss might schedule another worker. In general, you must have a legitimate reason for missing work (e.g., being ill, a death in the family, an emergency). The employee may need to bring a doctor's note or other appropriate documentation for an absence to be excused. A note from a parent is usually not considered proper documentation.

Be on Time. Being punctual and dependable reflects on the individual's work ethic. When employees are late, either their work goes undone or a coworker or boss must cover for them.

Observe and Learn from Your Coworkers. You can learn a lot about what is expected from watching your experienced coworkers. Bandura's Social Learning Theory suggests that by modeling (imitating) desired behaviors and avoiding undesired ones, individuals will learn to be effective, high performers.

Take Pride in Work. Employees should strive to do the work as accurately and quickly as possible. They should take pride in their tasks and outcomes. Workers represent their organization. Often, they are the face of the organization that the public sees. An organizations' image, reputation and profitability rests on the quality of its employees' work.

Time Management. Employees should identify tasks that need to be done and do the ones that have the highest priority first. Employees should avoid spending a lot of time on something that is not important or not a central job task. They should also recognize what is work and what is not. Personal phone calls, web browsing, social media (e.g., Facebook, Instagram), and responding to personal texts or emails are not productive. Employees may find time for these activities during their scheduled breaks, but these activities should not distract them from their main duties. Using time effectively allows employees to focus on providing the best service or making the highest quality products possible.

Seek Feedback from Supervisor. New employees should ask for feedback from their supervisors to assess how well they are doing on the job. What is being done right? What needs to be changed? What is missing? By seeking feedback, the individual indicates that they are willing to learn and improve.

GOING ABOVE AND BEYOND WORK EXPECTATIONS

In addition to meeting work expectations, many organizations reward "organizational citizenship behaviors" (OCBs). These behaviors reflect performance that goes above and beyond the call of duty, such as: filling in for others when needed; working extra hours; helping a coworker when your tasks are done; taking on additional responsibilities; helping a customer, when it is not directly related to your job; and helping your supervisor accomplish last minute tasks. Employees who engage in OCBs typically get higher performance ratings and are more satisfied with their jobs.

BUILDING RELATIONSHIPS WITH THE BOSS AND COWORKERS

All new employees should focus attention on building high quality relationships with their bosses and coworkers. High quality relationships increase effectiveness and employee well-being for five fundamental reasons: (1) developing friendships, (2) building cohesiveness, (3) social support, (4) making connections, and (5) networking.

When you must work closely with a group of people, developing friendships makes it more enjoyable and fun. Coworkers who become friends create a more satisfying work environment. They eat lunch together and may go out together after work. Friends develop mutual trust and cultivate a sense of camaraderie. Your coworkers become people with whom you can share your successes and commiserate with over your failures.

Cohesion refers to the positive atmosphere created by working with people you like, respect, and trust. Employees spend a lot of time with their coworkers. Some of that time will be spent on challenging tasks, under pressure. Cohesion makes it easier to work together. When employees receive help and encouragement from their coworkers, they are more likely to chip in and help out, take necessary risks, and pull together to get the work done.

Coworkers, because they spend time in the same work environment, understand the challenges and difficulties and can buffer a person's experience of stress. This social support can help workers deal with crises and difficult work situations by improving their ability to cope with these situations and reducing their stress.

Connections employees make through building work relationships provide them access to the information network. Being connected allows employees to access knowledge about how to get their tasks done and overcome obstacles. Coworkers can also be source of good advice about how to handle difficult situations.

Building a network of connections may increase an employee's opportunities and increase his/her influence (e.g., being able to get things done, swaying decision makers). Part of building a network is developing relationships with mentors. Mentors are more experienced, higher-ranking individuals, who can provide guidance, counsel, and serve as role models. Making connections and networking will open doors and lead to opportunities. Employees who are liked and trusted are the ones who will get an opportunity at the more challenging work assignments, client referrals, and promotion opportunities.

DEVELOPING A GOOD RELATIONSHIP WITH YOUR BOSS

Inexperienced employees often view their boss as someone who tells them what to do and when to do it. They do not realize that their role is to help their boss meet his/her goals. According to the Leader-Member Exchange (LMX) theory, bosses place employees into one of two groups. Bosses have limited resources they can expend on their employees. These resources include time and effort. Bosses must accomplish their objectives through influence and because of this, they strategically invest their scarce resources where they think there will be the highest payoff. One group (the in-group) has high quality relationships with the boss, while the other (the out-group) has low quality relationships. In high quality LMX relationships, employees spend more time with the boss, receive more information, and earn more trust and respect. These workers are more likely to get difficult and challenging assignments because the boss depends on them to work hard and produce quality work. Individuals in the low quality LMX relationships get little attention from the boss and typically get assigned more mundane repetitive tasks. High LMX employees get higher performance reviews, better raises, more recognition, and more promotion opportunities than those in low LMX relationships. For new employees, it is important to realize that leaders make these decisions quickly, typically within the first week. These early decisions influence work-related judgments six months, a year, and even two years later.

BUILDING RELATIONSHIPS WITH COWORKERS

Developing warm and friendly relationships with your coworkers have many benefits. New employees should socialize with their coworkers. They should seek opportunities to eat lunch together, share a joke, and connect personally. There are, however, some risks to keep in mind:

Avoid Excessive Socializing. It is good to make friends, but coworkers have to get their tasks done, too.

Avoid Unnecessary Conflict. Picking your battles wisely is a good rule. If task conflict arises, keep the conversation focused on the task and avoid criticizing the person.

Avoid Gossip. Gossiping is seen as immature and unprofessional. Gossip can damage collegiality and ruin friendships. You want to keep an upbeat and positive attitude and don't want to be dragged into another coworker's conflict or jeopardize your reputation as a trustworthy individual.

Be Discreet. Social media posts are not private. Posting nasty comments on Facebook or another social media site about your boss or coworkers is likely to get back to them. Human Resource Departments routinely look at social media posts.

Intimate Relationships with Coworkers Can Be Tricky. Dating someone you work with may be prohibited by policy in your company. There is no way to keep a dating relationship perfectly secret and may lead to one or both parties being disciplined, reassigned or even terminated. If not prohibited, dating a coworker may still be awkward and may strain your relationships with other coworkers. Others may perceive that coworkers who date will give each other special treatment and may resent the favoritism. Also, relationship conflict can spill over to the workplace. Consider how you would feel having to face your ex after you break up?

COMMUNICATION

Work success and building high quality relationships with coworkers and your supervisor, depend on effective communication. Communication involves both the transmission of information by a speaker and the interpretation of that information by the receiver. The receiver must decode the message and take meaning from it. Social perception plays an important role in how the receiver interprets what is being communicated. These interpretations are based not just on what is said, but how it is said. Here are some tips for getting your message across without being misunderstood.

WHAT YOU SAY

First and foremost, the language used must be appropriate for the workplace. When discussing work-related issues, be informed. Sound, rational arguments are more persuasive than relying on hearsay or another person's opinion. Employees should avoid using curse words and too much texting jargon (e.g., LOL). Communication should stay work focused and employees should avoid sharing too much personal information. Weekend escapades might be fun to relay to your coworkers, but they may cast you in an unprofessional light. When discussing your work with others, be sure to maintain privacy, especially about information the organization feels is proprietary. The healthcare environment has strict rules about confidentiality. Under no circumstances should patient information be shared with others or online.

Because your boss will be very busy, you should make the most of the limited time you have to communicate. If you are asked to present in a meeting, be prepared. If you have a chance encounter with your boss, you should have a brief message ready that describes your recent successes. This is sometimes referred to as a one-minute elevator speech. You should be able to convey important information to your boss in the short time it takes to ride the elevator.

It is important to acknowledge the assistance of others. Thank you notes and emails are appropriate to recognize the help others have provided you.

COMMUNICATION IS MORE THAN WHAT YOU SAY

The way you communicate has a big impact on how others react to what you are saying. You should speak with confidence. Avoid using filler words like "uh," "like," and "you know". Speak clearly and address your intended audience directly. You want to avoid being seen as a mumbler.

Modulating your voice and finding the right volume for the situation is important. If you speak too softly, you may not be heard. On the other hand, you do not want to speak too loudly (e.g., the voice level you would use on a basketball court). Avoid putting an upward inflection (i.e., up-talking) at the end of a sentence. This makes the statement sound like a question and the speaker appear uncertain. Women tend to do this more than men. Up-talking can damage both your credibility and influence.

While speaking in a group or meeting, sharing the airspace is essential. You must not dominate the conversation and hog the airtime. On the other hand, you want to make your point and have a voice in the discussion. Pay attention to turn taking and avoid rudely interrupting, but speak up when you have a good idea or major concern.

NONVERBALS

Nonverbal signals are an important part of the message that you are sending. Eye rolls, head nods, and gestures all contribute to how receivers interpret a message. There are seven key nonverbal behaviors that you want to manage to communicate effectively.

Facial Expressions. Facial expressions provide a lot of information about a person's emotional state and reactions. A look of disgust (a curled lip and narrowed eyebrows) can tell a speaker that you are repulsed by what they are saying. Smiling indicates a positive attitude and that the listener is receptive to the information being communicated.

Eye Contact. Eye contact establishes a connection with the listener. During interviews, when individuals established eye contact with interviewers, they received higher ratings and were more likely to be hired for the job.

Posture. An open and receptive posture creates a positive and warm interpersonal interaction. An open posture is one where the person's arms are open and vulnerable parts of the body are exposed. Open postures invite warm, friendly communication. On the other hand, in a closed posture the person folds his/her arms across the chest or crosses his/her legs. A person adopting a closed posture is seen as setting up obstacles to communication. Posture can also provide information about an individual's energy level. Sitting slumped in a seat or slouching when walking is typically interpreted as low energy and a lack of enthusiasm.

Gestures and Touching. Many people speak using their hands and movements of other parts of their bodies (e.g., raising your shoulders to indicate that you do not know an answer). Gestures can convey a great deal of information quickly. A head nod indicates that you understand what a person is telling you. At work, individuals should refrain from using controversial gestures. If working in an international environment, you should be aware that some common US gestures might be considered offensive. Typically, in the United States, you can indicate "okay" by connecting your thumb and finger to form an "O." In some cultures, this would be considered a vulgar, sexual reference.

Adapters are gestures that are not meant to communicate your message but give off subtle clues about what you are feeling and how you are reacting. Examples of adapters include fidgeting, adjusting your hair or clothes, and toe tapping. These can be interpreted as boredom, nervousness, and discomfort.

Light noninvasive touches are viewed as warm and caring. Wait staff that simply touched a customer's hand when returning money, earned larger tips. Handshakes and high fives are examples of noninvasive touching. But being too touchy feely, unwanted hugging, and sexual overtures, will be received negatively and may even result in sexual harassment charges.

Physical Space. When interacting with others, there is typically an acceptable amount of physical space that we like to maintain between ourselves and other people. Encroaching on someone's personal space (close talking) can be viewed as threatening and uncomfortable. Keep in mind that people from different cultures may have different default personal distances. People from the United States like more space than individuals from more crowded countries like India.

Appearance and Dress. Dressing appropriately (e.g., always dressing neatly and cleanly) signals your professionalism. Adolescents should look the part for the clientele they serve and the type of organization they represent. For example, flip-flops are not acceptable when working in a bank, but are essential when working as a lifeguard. "Sexually charged" clothing should be avoided. If you are interested in getting promoted, one recommendation is to dress for the job you want, not the job you have.

Jewelry, tattoos, and piercings are also part of your appearance. An organization may have a specific "dress code" or set of policies that dictate how employees should look on the job. For example, if you are working at a resort that serves a conservative religious group, they may be offended by body piercings. You may be asked by your employer to remove your tongue ring. Organizational policies may even discuss the appropriate length and style of hair and whether or not facial hair (beards and mustaches) is acceptable. Challenging a dress code is never wise. Many states have an "at will" policy that means the employer can terminate an employee for any reason, including noncompliance with the dress code. Ask about the dress code during the interview and be prepared to walk away if you cannot live by the employer's rules. Some exceptions may be made, but this should be established at employment. A private company has the right to make its own rules.

Fragrance. Believe it or not fragrance, bad breath and body odor can be emotionally charged workplace issues. Working near someone who gives off an offensive odor can be unpleasant and cause friction among coworkers. Some of the people you encounter at work may also be very sensitive to smell, while some may even be allergic to perfumes and scents in soap, skin lotion, or shampoo. Some workplaces have been declared scent-free zones. Your goal is to smell clean and fresh by bathing regularly and using deodorant or antiperspirant. A light fragrance might work but be careful not to use too much cologne or perfume. Most healthcare settings discourage fragrances, scented body lotions and other smells that may be unpleasant to patients.

GROWTH AND CONTINUOUS LEARNING

Learning does not end when adolescents finish school. It continues throughout their lives. In school, adolescents should be encouraged to develop work habits that can benefit them in future endeavors. Learning how to learn is important. This includes developing critical thinking skills, learning how to apply knowledge, and knowing how to search for and use information to make sound decisions. Growth is also about being flexible and adaptable. Workplaces are dynamic which means they are constantly changing. Taking change in stride and avoiding resistance to change can be useful skills. Adolescents should not be afraid to try new things and be innovative. Facing failure and learning from the experience are keys to ultimate success at work.

CONCLUSION

Work will take up a large part of an employee's life. Selecting the right job or career will lead to a much happier life. Adolescents should develop good work habits that will serve them throughout their careers. They should find work that they like to do and that they find meaningful and fulfilling. A good foundation begins with learning work expectations and building good relationships with their coworkers and supervisors. Succeeding at work requires developing both verbal and nonverbal communication skills. Adolescents must strive for excellence and recognize that learning is a lifelong endeavor.

—*Maryalice Citera*

Further Reading

Freedman, E. *Work 101: Learning the Ropes of The Workplace without Hanging Yourself.* Delta Trade Paperbacks, 2007. This book is written for people who are starting their first job and describes common workplace norms, rules of etiquette, and business know-how. It contains insights, tips, and practical advice for succeeding on the job.

"Managing Employee Dress and Appearance." *Society for Human Resource Management*, www.shrm.org/resourcesandtools/tools-and-samples/toolkits/pages/employeedressandappearance.aspx. Accessed 31 Aug. 2020.

O*NET Online. online.onetcenter.org, 2015. This website sponsored by the US Department of Labor provides detailed job descriptions for career exploration and job seekers. This database can be searched by job title and by occupation. It details the knowledge skills, abilities, and other characteristics required for particular jobs, the future outlook in terms of hiring potential, the typical salary range, as well as other key information.

Riordan, C. M. "We All Need Friends at Work." *Harvard Business Review*, 3 July 2013, hbr.org/2013/07/we-all-need-friends-at-work. This describes the benefits of developing warm and friendly relationships with coworkers.

Ritti, R. R., and S. Levy. *The Ropes to Skip and The Ropes to Know: Studies in Organizational Theory and Behavior.* 8th ed., Wiley, 2009. Using a case study approach, this book highlights some of the key pitfalls that new employees make.

Nursing Certifications and Degrees: Licensed Practical Nurse and Registered Nurse

ABSTRACT

A number of different certifications and degrees are available to people who wish to enter the nursing profession. Among the most common are the Licensed Practical Nurse (LPN) certification, which allows the nurse to assist physicians and registered nurses in taking care of basic duties in hospitals, nursing homes, and related settings. Those who wish to become a registered nurse (RN) typically pursue an ADN (associate's degree in nursing), a BSN (bachelor of science in nursing) degree, or a diploma.

LICENSED PRACTICAL NURSE (LPN)

A licensed practice nurse (LPN) is a nurse who works under the supervision of doctors and registered nurses. A licensed practical nurse performs a variety of duties in a hospital or nursing home setting including maintaining patient records, monitoring the patient's vital signs, administering medication, assisting doctors and nurses with tests, and helping patients eat, dress, and bathe. LPNs may be the first people that the family members of the patient interact with and LPNs are occasionally tasked with explaining procedures and care programs to the family. For LPNs, good communication skills and a good beside manner are essential. Over a third of all LPNs work in nursing homes and residential care facilities, with the other most common settings including hospitals, doctor's offices, and positions as home healthcare workers.

The licensed practical nurse may also supervise certified nursing assistants (CNAs), although this is often done by registered nurses (RNs). CNAs are the healthcare professionals tasked with providing entry-level care to patients. They perform some of the same tasks as LPNs such as taking vital signs, cleaning rooms, and helping patients with daily activities. Unlike LPNs, they are not likely to administer medications but may record vital signs, food and fluids taken in by the patient, and urine and bowel outputs. CNAs generally are required to complete a training program which can take as little as 4 weeks. For those who wish to become licensed practical nurses, there are direct CNA-to-LPN programs.

To become a licensed practical nurse, a candidate must complete an LPN program. (In Texas and California, the title licensed vocational nurse (LVN) is used instead, although the job is virtually identical.) LPN/LVN programs are usually offered at community colleges and vocational schools. Each program is accredited through the Accreditation Commission for Education in Nursing (ACEN). The majority of LPN/LVN programs last about twelve to eighteen months, although some may be as short as seven months and some may last up to two years. Coursework that candidates usually complete may include nursing fundamentals, nutrition, mathematics, leadership principles, pharmacology, and general anatomy.

After the candidate completes the certification program, he or she must then apply for a nursing license. Obtaining this license is contingent on passing an exam known as the National Council Licensure Examination (NCLEX), which is administered through the National Council of State Boards of Nursing. The test covers four principles categories: Safe, Effective Care Environment; Health Promotion and Maintenance; Physiological Integrity; and Psychosocial Integrity. Once licensed as an LPN, they are typically expected to earn continuing educational credits every few years to maintain their license. LPNs may also have the option of earning additional certifications in order to specialize in specific areas of nursing. Employment settings may offer or require additional education that allows LPNs to take on additional tasks such as medication administration and wound and dressing care.

REGISTERED NURSE (RN)
Unlike the more limited role of LPNs, the role of the RNs is more comprehensive. Depending on the site of care and nursing care model, registered nurses may provide direct patient care, such as in hospitals with a primary care model or in a nursing home where supervision of LPNs and CNAs is provided and tasks such as medication administration are the norm. Sixty percent of RNs work in hospitals, with other sites of care such as ambulatory healthcare services, nursing and residential care facilities, educational services, physician offices and government services making up the difference. The duties of a RN may vary with the type of environment in which they work, but among the more common tasks performed by RNs are: assessing patients' conditions, planning nursing care and writing nursing care plans, administering medications, providing patient treatments, helping perform and analyze diagnostic tests, and helping patients manage illnesses or injuries. Registered nurses may also be assigned nurse manager roles and supervise other nurses.

There are three ways to become a registered nurse: an associate's degree, a bachelor's degree, and a diploma. Both diploma and associate's programs take about two years to complete and are considered entry-level degrees. The primary difference between the two is that the associate's degree in nursing (ADN) is a college degree, while the diploma is not typical offered in an academic setting, but generally in a hospital setting or a vocational or technical school. Although diploma programs are known for being hands on, ADN programs also offer a high degree of clinical training in addition to classroom instruction. Because the ADN is an academic degree, students typically take a wide variety of courses including offerings in the humanities, history, math, and communications in addition to nursing classes. Transitioning to a bachelor's degree is less difficult with an associate degree.

The bachelor of science in nursing degree, by contrast, is a full four to five-year academic program. Graduates of BSN programs are eligible to apply for more jobs than those with a diploma or associate's degree, including many of the more well-compensated positions. In addition, people with a BSN degree have greater opportunity for specialization and promotion to supervisory or management roles. The BSN program generally consists of a two year curriculum of general education and prerequisite courses followed by two years of nursing coursework and clinical training. The curriculum for all programs in the United States is set by the American Association of Colleges and Nursing.

Regardless of which degree or diploma a candidate has pursued, he or she is required to take the National Council Licensure Exam for Registered Nurses (NCLEX-RN) in order to practice. Some states allow the graduates of nursing programs to work under a temporary permit while they wait to take the test. Those who do not pass the exam on their first chance must wait forty-five days before taking it again.

Registered nurses who earned an associate's degree or a diploma can go back to school to earn a BSN through a special RN-to-BSN program so that they do not need to start from scratch. RNs looking for further advancement can pursue a master's or doctoral program in nursing. Professionals in other fields who already hold a bachelor's degree but wish to transition to nursing may qualify for an accelerated nursing program.

SUMMARY

Making the decision to become a nurse requires thought and preparation. Being admitted to a nursing program requires determining the resources available to pay for the program, the length of time available to complete the program, and the ultimate career goal of the individual. Regardless of the nursing program selected, be sure that the program is accredited and that the cost of the program is reasonable. Scholarships and grants are available to assist in paying for nursing programs and should be explored with the program or school of choice.

—*Andrew Schenker*

Further Reading

Gutkind, Lee, editor. *I Wasn't Strong Like This When I Started Out: True Stories of Becoming a Nurse*. In Fact Books, 2013.

"How to Become an RN: Begin Here." *NursingLicensure.org*, www.nursinglicensure.org/articles/how-to-become-an-rn.html. Accessed 21 Sept. 2020.

Kleinfield, Sonny. *Becoming a Nurse*. Simon & Schuster, 2020.

"Licensed Practical Nursing: Education Requirements, Career Paths, & Job Outlook." *All Nursing Schools*, www.allnursingschools.com/licensed-practical-nurse/. Accessed 21 Sept. 2020.

"Registered Nurses" US Bureau of Labor Statistics, *Occupational Outlook Handbook*, www.bls.gov/ooh/healthcare/registered-nurses.htm. Accessed 21 Sept. 2020.

Advanced Practice Nurses

ABSTRACT

Advanced practice nurses (APNs), also called advanced practice registered nurses (APRN), are registered nurses with postgraduate education in nursing, either a master of science in nursing (MSN) or a doctorate. APNs typically fall into four categories: clinical nurse specialists (CNSs), nurse anesthetists, nurse midwives, and nurse practitioners (NPs). The scope of practice laws in each state may dictate duties that APNs can provide.

DIFFERENT TYPES OF ADVANCED PRACTICE NURSES

Nurses with advanced degrees in their field typically pursue one of four different specializations in the field, although there are numerous other positions available.

A CNS is a professional who provides direct patient care in a specific area of expertise, such as pediatrics or psychiatric health. They may work with a specific population or specialize in a specific disease or subspecialty. They often take on leadership roles in a hospital or clinical setting and may be involved in educating staff or in performing research.

A certified registered nurse anesthetist (CRNA) is a nurse who administers anesthesia and provides care throughout surgical, diagnostic, or other procedures. CRNAs administer about half of the anesthesia given to patients in the United States and are the main providers of anesthesia in the military, maternity wards, and in rural and underserved communities. Nurse anesthetists also provide pain management as well as some emergency services.

A nurse midwife is a professional who provides a wide range of health services for women, especially during and after pregnancy. Among the services performed by a nurse midwife are delivering babies, providing surgical assistance to physicians during cesarean (C-section) births, performing gynecological exams, and offering family planning services and prenatal care. In some cases, nurse midwives may serve as a woman's primary maternity care provider.

NPs function as both primary and specialty care providers. They are considered mid-level practitioners and are trained in basic disease prevention and coordination of care. In some states they have full practicing authority, while in others they must work under the supervision of a physician. Either way, they are legally allowed to examine patients, diagnose illnesses, prescribe medications, and provide treatments. NPs generally work with a specific population of people in areas such as geriatric health, pediatric health, or psychiatric and mental health.

The type of APN designation defines practice authority in conjunction with state laws. The Scope of Practice describes what a healthcare practitioner is permitted to do based on the terms of their professional license and certification. For example, in twenty states NPs have full practice authority and do not have to work under a physician supervisor. CRNAs may work without supervision in some states. Certified Nurse-Midwives (CNMs) practice in consultation and collaboration with licensed physicians in most states. Less than ten states allow CNSs the authority to practice without a supervising physician. Each state defines in their Scope of Practice law the authority to practice autonomously and should be referenced for additional information.

EDUCATIONAL AND LICENSURE REQUIREMENTS

While the specific requirements for APNs differ by specialty, all APNs are required to obtain a master's degree as the minimum requirement. Typically, this master's takes the form of a master of science in nursing (MSN) degree. After obtaining this degree, nurses can enter the field directly or go on to earn a doctorate. Candidates for the MSN degree usually already work as registered nurses and their path to obtaining their master's differs based on whether they hold an associate's degree, a bachelor's degree, or a diploma in nursing. For example, if they hold an associate's degree, they may apply for an ADN-MSN bridge program. Students that are not nurses but who earned a bachelor's degree in a related health science field may also be eligible for an MSN.

The MSN degree can vary in length from one year to several years depending on the program. Typically, students take generalized coursework such as advanced health assessment, advanced pharmacology, and nursing research, as well as coursework in the specific area in which they want to specialize. These specializations determine the student's subsequent career path and include nurse midwife, nurse anesthetist, neonatal nurse practitioner, family nurse practitioner, clinical nurse specialist, and psychiatric nurse practitioner, among others.

After completing the MSN, students must complete a number of additional requirements in order to practice as an APRN. Although the requirements may differ by state, most APRNs are required to pass a national certification exam in addition to successfully completing the NCLEX-RN exam to become a registered nurse. The certification for APN or APRN is not to be confused with certifications by professional organizations open to all registered nurses regardless of education level, such as the Oncology Certified Nurse (ONCC) or Certified Pediatric Nurse (CPN), that validate experience and knowledge measured by a test to obtain a nationally recognized credential. Currently there are five organizations that provide national certification to nurse practitioners, with two of these also providing certification to CNSs. The certification exams are different depending on the candidate's specialty. Nurse anesthetists take the National Certification Exam (NCE) through the National Board of Certification and Recertification for Nurse Anesthetists (NBCRNA) and are referred to as CRNAs. Nurse midwives take the CNM exam through the American Midwife Certification Board. Nurse practitioners have several options for certification exams including those offered through the American Academy of Nurse Practitioners Certification Board (AANPCB), the American Nurses Credentialing Center (ANCC), the American Association of Critical Care Nurses (AACN), the National Certification Corporation (NCC), and the Pediatric Nursing Certification Board (PNCB).

Some advanced practice nurses may choose to pursue a doctorate; either a doctor of nursing practice (DNP) or a PhD. Nurses who wish to gain advanced practice knowledge or who wish to take on leadership roles may elect to pursue this course. In addition to advanced practice nurses, graduates of these programs may work in nurse management, organizational leadership, health policy, or health informatics systems. In 2004, the member schools of the American Association of Colleges of Nursing (AACN) voted to endorse the *Position Statement on the Practice Doctorate of Nursing*, which called for the minimum educational requirement for advanced nursing to be moved from master's to doctorate-level by 2015. Although this has not yet happened, it may in the future as professional organizations such as the American Association of Nurse Anesthetists and the National Association of Clinical Nurse Specialists have echoed the AACN's call in recent years.

Both the doctor of nursing practice and the PhD in nursing are terminal degrees and are generally completed in three to five years. They differ in their focus, with the PhD designed for those who wish to pursue research or an academic career, while the DNP is designed for those interested in direct patient care. The DNP builds on the MSN degree and offers students a chance to pursue either a leadership or administration focus or to study one of the specialties of advanced practice nursing, such as nurse midwife, nurse anesthetist, clinical nurse specialist, family nurse practitioner, or neonatal nurse practitioner. DNP programs are designed to prepare students in eight key competencies, including organizational and systems leadership, healthcare policy, and evidence-based practice. All DNP students are also required to fulfill 1,000 clinical practice hours. For doctorate students studying to be a nurse anesthetist, the degree they earn is sometimes known as a doctor of anesthesia practice (DNAP) rather than a DNP.

—*Andrew Schenker*

Further Reading

DeNisco, Susan M. *Advanced Practice Nursing: Essential Knowledge for the Profession.* 4th ed., Jones & Bartlett Learning, 2019.

Dunphy, Lynne M., et al. *Primary Care: Art and Science of Advanced Practice Nursing–An Interprofessional Approach.* 5th ed., F. A. Davis Company, 2019.

"FAQ: What Are the Different APRN Certification Options for NPs, CNSs, CNMs and CRNAs?" *Online FNP Programs*, www.onlinefnpprograms.com/faqs/aprn-certification-organizations/. Accessed 23 Sept. 2020.

LeVeck, Danielle. "Doctorate of Nursing Practice (DNP)–What Is a DNP and Is It Worth It?" *Nurse.org*, 11 Sept. 2020, nurse.org/articles/how-to-get-a-dnp-is-it-worth-it/.

"Nurse Anesthetists, Nurse Midwives, and Nurse Practitioners: Occupational Outlook," *US Bureau of Labor Statistics*, www.bls.gov/ooh/healthcare/nurse-anesthetists-nurse-midwives-and-nurse-practitioners.htm.

Licensure and Certification

ABSTRACT

Licensure and certification are two very important components of becoming a professional nurse. Licensure defines what nurses can do and gives them authority under the law to perform as a nurse. There are different licenses based on the knowledge that nurses complete in their program. Certification, on the other hand, is the validation that a nurse has knowledge, skills and abilities to perform in a specialized area of nursing and has met the requirements of an accrediting body. Many times, having a certification in nursing meets the requirements for nurses to renew their licensure. It also provides an opportunity to advance their practice and add additional responsibilities for what they can do.

LICENSURE

All nurses need a license in order to get a job and practice nursing. Since licensure is a requirement for the practice of nursing, there are several different types of licensure that apply to the different types of nurses and what they do. The levels of nurse licensure are vocational or practical nurse (LVN/LPN), registered nurse (RN), and advanced practice nurses (APNs). Safe, competent nursing practice is provided in the law as written in the state nurse practice act (NPA) and the state rules/regulations. NPAs can vary from state to state, but include standards and scope of nursing practice, requirements for licensure, and grounds for disciplinary action. Every nurse is responsible for reading the nurse practice act in the state where they are licensed in order to follow the rules. Nursing licensure is only available to those nurses who have completed a nursing program and taken and passed the National Council Licensure Examination (NCLEX). Multiple steps must be completed before a nurse can become licensed and safely enter the profession. These steps typically include graduating from a recognized nursing program, meeting the specific requirements of the state board of nursing, and passing the National Council of State Boards of Nursing (NCSBN) National Council Licensure Examination-Registered Nurse (NCLEX-RN exam) for RNs or LPN/LVNs.

CERTIFICATION

Nursing certification is a formal but usually voluntary process for individuals that hold an RN or advanced practice license. It can be mandatory in certain types of employment or job roles, such as chemotherapy administration, or encouraged by employers who recognize the additional validation of skills as desirable. It recognizes a nurse's knowledge, skills, and abilities in a defined area of clinical practice. Certification allows nurses to show commitment to exceptional patient safety and follow, as well as practice, current nursing care in their field of work. The purpose of being certified in nursing allows nurses to be recognized by their fellow nurses and employers, continue their education of current nursing practice in their work, perhaps increase their salary and also provide greater opportunities for job promotion. All certifications follow rules of an accrediting body which is recognized by the professional organization of nursing practice for certification. The most common accrediting body for nursing certification is the American Nurses Credentialing Center which is part of the American Nurses Association. Certification requires many of the same steps that Licensure requires.

COMPONENTS OF LICENSURE

Upon graduation from an approved nursing school in the state in which you will practice, you will be required to take the nursing licensure exam. To take the exam you will need to complete an application for licensure/registration in the state where you reside.

This includes a fee and requires proof of citizenship, permanent residency address, official school transcripts and in most states, a criminal background check. Once submitted, you will be notified to sit for the NCLEX exam. You must present this notice in order to schedule an appointment to sit for the exam. Your identification used for the licensure application and information you submit for making the appointment for the exam must match exactly. You will have a ninety-day window to schedule your exam. After the exam you will be notified in about six weeks by your state board of licensure of your results.

All state boards of nursing licensure (which are legal bodies in the state legislature) belong to the National Council on State Boards of Nursing (NCSBN). NCSBN is responsible for all nursing regulatory standards and to make sure safe and qualified nursing care is provided by licensed nurses. Another group that is part of this organization is the Nursing Licensure Compact Commission. They developed the state legislation for nurses to practice in multiple states. Each state can pass legislation called the Nurse Licensure Compact (NLC). It is important to know whether your state is an NLC state as it will allow an RN or LPN/LVN to practice across state lines without having to obtain another license in other states. The NLC requires nurses to adhere to the nurse practice act and rules of the state in which they reside under their compact license. If a nurse moves to another state and establishes residency, they must apply for licensure in that state whether or not it is a "Compact state." Not all states are part of the NLC so it is important to find out if your license is in a compact state.

Nursing license renewal is every two years. The license renewal process includes requirements and may vary in each state. Most, but not all states, require continuing education hours be completed over the course of the renewal period and also proof of practice/employment in nursing. Questions regarding any criminal or disciplinary activity must also be answered in addition to questions regarding allegations of unprofessional conduct, incompetent practice, unethical practice or criminal convictions. A renewal fee is also charged.

COMPONENTS OF CERTIFICATION

Just as in licensure, many of the components to achieve certification are similar. Nursing certification is regulated by the professional association in that type of nursing practice or specialty. Many specialty nurse associations exist such as for the operating room, critical care nurses, oncology, or emergency nurses. The largest professional nursing association, the American Nurses Association, uses the American Nurses Credentialing Center (ANCC) for nursing certifications. Whatever the regulatory body that does certification for the area of nursing for which you apply, several components are identical.

All nursing certification processes include rules you have to meet in order to apply for certification. Typical requirements include current practice for a number of hours/years in the area of certification, have an active RN license, work as an RN full time for at least two years, and complete continuing education in the area of the specialty (i.e., thirty continuing education hours over three years, as an example). More advanced certifications may also require an advanced degree in that area of specialty—such as nurse practitioners or nursing administrators. Certification fees must be paid prior to taking the exam.

Certification exams are developed by a Content Expert Panel (CEP) CEPs identify the required test questions which consists of about 200 questions and takes three to four hours to complete. Results are processed within a period of four weeks. You will receive an official letter regarding your certification that includes your renewal period. You are awarded additional credentials such as RN-C to use in your signature.

Your certification start date is the date you successfully completed the exam and most certifications last five years before renewal is required. Renewing your certification requires documentation of continuing education nursing hours over the five-year period and can include various professional development and practice activities. Certification renewal may also permit you to apply it to continued nursing licensure, reimbursement, and potential employer recognition. Certification renewal is required for continued use of your credentials.

SUMMARY

Nursing Licensure is a requirement to enter and practice nursing as a profession. Nursing certification is a recognition and can be voluntary or mandatory to demonstrate special skills, knowledge and practices of nursing in a unique area. Both of these processes demonstrate the unique practices that the nursing profession brings to healthcare and the public. Regulatory processes are an important part of the nursing profession that makes sure the public receives a standard of care by an individual that is meeting state license requirements. The nursing profession requirements of licensure and certification provide those same safeguards as are done across the professions of medicine, dentistry, and even the police professionals.

—Carol Beehler

Further Reading
LICENSURE
Betts, Joe. "2020 NCLEX Fact Sheet NCLEX Statistics." NCLEX Examinations.
"NCSBN Welcomes You to the Nursing Profession." *New Nurse Booklet*, National Council of State Boards of Nursing, 2018, www.ncsbn.org/New_Nurse-Booklet-Web.pdf.
"What You Need to Know about Nursing Licensure and Boards of Nursing." National Council of State Boards of Nursing, 2011, www.ncsbn.org/licensure.htm.
CERTIFICATION
ANCC Certification General Testing and Renewal Handbook. American Nurses Credentialing Center, April 2017.

"Certification and Career Progression." CCI (The Competency and Credentialing Institute), 2019, www.cc-institute.org/why-certify/.
Van Wicklin, Sharon Ann. "What Is the Perceived Value of Certification Among Registered Nurses? A Systematic Review," Alpha Iota & Xi Alpha, Perioperative Consultant, Competency and Credentialing Institute, June 2020.

PROFESSIONAL NURSING ORGANIZATIONS AND CERTIFICATION

ABSTRACT
Numerous professional organizations exist for the purpose of advancing the profession of nursing. Perhaps the most venerable of these institutions in the United States is the American Nurses Association (ANA) which was founded in 1896. Many of these professional organizations also offer certification to nurses in their specific fields including the ANA which does so through its subsidiary organization the American Nurses Credentialing Center (ANCC).

THE AMERICAN NURSES ASSOCIATION (ANA)
The American Nurses Association, a professional organization that represents registered nurses in the United States, was founded in 1896 as the Nurses Associated Alumnae and adopted its current name in 1911. Their stated mission is to "lead the profession to shape the future of nursing and healthcare." The ANA is involved in many aspects of the nursing profession, including establishing standards of nursing practice, credentialing nurses, promoting the rights of nurses in the workplace, and advancing the economic claims of nursing. The organization is run by the ANA Membership Assembly, which is the organization's official governing and voting body. The Membership Assembly works closely with the nine-member Board of Directors which is responsible for fulfilling the ANA's corporate and fiduciary duties and setting and monitoring the organization's strate-

gic direction. The Board includes Ernest J. Grant who is currently the ANA's president. In addition, the ANA's leadership group consists of three standing committees and a Leadership Council, which is the organization's advisory board.

The ANA operates 54 constituent member associations throughout the United States and also has three subsidiary organizations. The subsidiary organizations include the American Academy of Nursing (AAN), which generates and spreads nursing knowledge in order to contribute to public health policy and practice, the American Nurses Foundation, the organization's nonprofit philanthropic and charitable arm, and the American Nurses Credentialing Center (ANCC). Founded in 1991, the ANCC is the largest certification body for advanced practice nurses in the United States, although it offers certification to registered nurses as well. Even before the founding of the ANCC, though, the ANA had been certifying nurses for close to two decades. In 1973, the ANA first announced its national certification program and the next year, the first certificates were awarded.

Today, the ANCC provides four basic services: their accreditation program which certifies nursing continuing education organizations, their Magnet recognition program, which recognizes nursing organizations that consistently meet standards of excellence, their Pathway to Excellence program, which recognizes "a healthcare organization's commitment to creating a positive practice environment that empowers and engages staff," and its certification program. This certification program provides the opportunity for nurses to become credentialed in an area of specialization. Certification is based on competency-based examinations designed to test the candidate's entry-level clinical knowledge and skills in the area in question. Once candidates pass the test and earn their credentials, the certification usually remains valid for five years. Certifications are currently offered in eighteen different areas, which are subdivided into nurse practitioner certifications, clinical nurse specialist certifications, and specialty certifications. The ANCC also offers a certificate in National Healthcare Disaster Certification (NHDP-BC) which is considered an interprofessional certification. The cost to take an exam begins at $395, although this is reduced to $295.00 for ANA members.

OTHER ORGANIZATIONS

Although the ANA is the principal nursing organization in the United States, several other organizations represent nurses as well, both domestically within the United States and internationally. The principal international organization is the International Council of Nurses (ICN), a federation of more than 130 national nurses' organizations which was founded in 1899 and today is headquartered in Geneva, Switzerland. The ICN's stated mission is "to represent nursing worldwide, advance the nursing profession, promote the wellbeing of nurses, and advocate for health in all policies." The National League for Nursing (NLN), founded in 1893, is the oldest nursing organization in the United States and is focused on nursing education and faculty development, nursing research grants, and public policy initiatives. The National Student Nurses Association (NSNA) offers resources for students who are preparing for their initial nursing licensure.

Most professional organizations for nurses offer a specialty certification that recognizes experience and knowledge in a particular field of nursing. Through submitting documentation of education and experience and taking a certification test, nurses may be recognized for their expertise in a chosen specialty. Any registered nurse meeting eligibility requirements defined by the organization, regardless of education level, may apply for recognition through certification. For example, the Oncology Nursing Society offers a nationally accredited, oncology-specific certification designated ONCC. The American Association of Critical-Care Nurses offers a CCRN certification that validates knowledge of adult, pediatric and neonatal care for critically or acutely ill patients.

Additionally, other nursing specialties have their own organizations as well as their own certification boards. For example, nurse practitioners are represented by the American Association of Nurse Practitioners (AANP) which was formed in 2013 via a merger of two older organizations, the American Academy of Nurse Practitioners and the American College of Nurse Practitioners. The organization, which advocates for nurse practitioners on the local, state, and federal levels, has over 100,000 members. Nurse practitioners can earn their certification either though the ANCC or through the American Academy of Nurse Practitioners Certification Board (AAPCB), an independent, nonprofit certifying body established in the early 1990s. The ANCC offers four different certifications for nurse practitioners, while the AAPCB offers three.

Nurse anesthetists in the United States are represented by the American Association of Nurse Anesthetists (AANA), an organization that was founded in 1931 and has over 53,000 members. Nurse anesthetists are certified through the National Board of Certification and Recertification for Nurse Anesthetists (NBCRNA). Nurse midwives are represented by the American College of Nurse-Midwives (ACNM) and are credentialed through the American Midwifery Certification Board (ACMB). The National Association of Clinical Nurse Specialists (NACNS) is the only organization in the United States representing clinical nurse specialists. Certification for clinical nurse specialists is offered through the ANCC.

In order to become licensed, all registered nurses are required to take the National Council Licensure Examination (NCLEX-RN). This exam is administered through the National Council of State Boards of Nursing.

—*Andrew Schenker*

Further Reading

American Nurses Association (ANA), www.nursingworld.org/ana/.

American Nurses Credentialing Center (ANCC), www.nursingworld.org/ancc/.

"Complete List of Common Nursing Certifications." *Nurse.org*, 8 July 2017, nurse.org/articles/nursing-certifications-credentials-list/.

"Nurse Anesthetists, Nurse Midwives, and Nurse Practitioners." US Bureau of Labor Statistics. *Occupational Outlook Handbook*, www.bls.gov/ooh/healthcare/nurse-anesthetists-nurse-midwives-and-nurse-practitioners.htm.

MAGNET RECOGNITION PROGRAM IN NURSING

ABSTRACT

The Magnet Recognition Program is an initiative run by the American Nurses Credentialing Center (ANCC) that is intended to compare and promote healthcare organizations with strong nursing staffs. To qualify as part of the program, a designation called "Magnet Status," healthcare organizations are required to demonstrate their compliance with a preestablished set of criteria. Magnet Status healthcare organizations, which may include hospitals, clinics, and other healthcare facilities, are characterized by their ability to attract and retain nurses deemed to be among the best in their profession. This program is one of the barometers used by U.S. News & World Report *to rank hospitals in its annual survey of the American medical system.*

OVERVIEW

The ANCC is a subsidiary of the American Nurses Association (ANA), a nonprofit professional organization dedicated to addressing workplace issues in nursing. The Magnet Recognition Program was initially begun in 1981 as part of a research project initiated by the American Academy of Nursing (AAN), a branch of the ANA, to determine how hospitals identified and prioritized nurses deemed to be particularly good at their jobs. To examine why these top nurses stayed at particular healthcare facilities, the task force created a set of parameters to identify the best hospital nursing staffs. Of the 155 hospitals originally considered, only forty-six met the standards of these criteria. From there, the group then sought to identify the shared characteristics of these institutions and use them to promote better healthcare on a national basis.

The group ultimately identified a set of fourteen common traits. Researchers found that these healthcare institutions shared elevated levels of reported job satisfaction by nurses, low staff turnover, good workplace conflict mediation, strong nurse-oriented research programs, and high rates of positive patient outcomes. The research also showed that such institutions had noticeably better care for patients than those that did not have these characteristics. Because of this work, the ANA established the Magnet Hospital Recognition Program for Excellence in Nursing Service as a forerunner to the Magnet Recognition Program, and named the University of Washington Medical Center in Seattle as the first designee of this elevated status in 1994. Over time, the program has broadened to include long-term care facilities and other healthcare institutions.

The staffs of healthcare institutions have been shown to have higher rates of job satisfaction and pride in their workplace after transitioning to Magnet Status. This often translates to even better patient care on a long-term basis. However, research has also indicated that at some facilities, once the institution has attained the elevated prestige that comes with Magnet Status, less effort is made to maintain or improve conditions by the administration. In other words, strong effort is often made to gain the prestige of Magnet Status, but these facilities may then see a reversion to prior standards having earned this heightened level of recognition. Nonetheless, many nursing groups and healthcare researchers acknowledge that the program has tremendous potential value to improve the working conditions of nurses and enable better overall healthcare in the United States and abroad.

As of December, 2019, 505 US hospitals had achieved magnet status. Magnet status can also be achieved by international facilities outside the United States. The full list is available at the American Nurses Credentialing Center website.

—*Eric Bullard*

Further Reading

Aiken, Linda. "The Magnet Nursing Services Recognition Program: A Comparison of Two Groups of Magnet Hospitals." *American Journal of Nursing*, vol. 100, no. 3, 2000, pp. 26–36.

ANCC Magnet Recognition Program.(r) *American Nursing Credentialing Center*, www.nursingworld.org/organizational-programs/magnet/. Access 3 Sept. 2020.

Bulla, Sally A., and Elaine M. Scherer. "What Does 'Magnet' Have to Do with Research?" *Real Stories of Nursing Research: The Quest for Magnet Recognition*, edited by M. Maureen Kirkpatrick McLaughlin and Sally A. Bulla, Jones and Bartlett Publishers, 2010, pp. 9–13.

"Find a Magnet Hospital." *American Nurses Credentialing Center*, www.nursingworld.org/organizational-programs/magnet/find-a-magnet-organization/. Accessed 3 Sept. 2020.

Kutney-Lee, Ann, et al. "Changes in Patient and Nurse Outcomes Associated with Magnet Hospital Recognition." *Medical Care*, vol. 53, no. 6, 2015, pp. 550–57.

"Magnet Recognition Program: Areas for Improvement." *The Truth about Nursing*, www.truthaboutnursing.org/faq/magnet.html#gsc.tab=0. Accessed 3 Sept. 2020.

McHugh, Matthew D., et al. "Lower Mortality in Magnet Hospitals." *Medical Care*, vol. 51, no. 5, 2013, pp. 382–88.

Ponte, Patricia Reid. "Structure, Process, and Empirical Outcomes—The Magnet Journey of Continuous Improvement." *Journal of Nursing Administration*, vol. 43, no. 6, 2013, pp. 309–10.

Westendorf, Jennifer J. "Magnet Recognition Program." *Plastic Surgery Nursing*, vol. 27, no. 2, 2007, pp. 102–4.

Nurse-Patient Ratio

ABSTRACT

Nurse-patient ratio refers to a fixed number of patients a nurse provides care for at one time. The ratio is dependent upon numerous factors and differs according to the severity of patients. Understaffed hospitals present risks to both nurses and patients. In the United States, no federal law exists to mandate minimum nurse-patient staffing ratios at hospitals. As of 2020, California is the only state that has enacted nurse-patient ratio legislation for all hospital care units.

OVERVIEW

Nurses care for several patients with varying needs at one time. They must be able to juggle multiple patients and tasks, while still giving the best care they can. Having too many patients to look after can hinder a nurse's ability to do his or her job and can endanger patients. Mandated nurse-patient ratios can help ease the burden on nurses and provide patients with better care.

Hospital administrators argue that nurse staffing requirements set by law would financially burden many hospitals, especially rural ones. Nursing union leaders argue that laws are needed to protect nurses from being overworked. Too many patients per nurse puts too much strain on the nurses themselves and could lead to mistakes that could endanger patients.

Because no federal legislation exists, the debate continues over what appropriate staffing should be. States have proposed federal and individual bills that would set differing staffing ratios. For example, a pe-

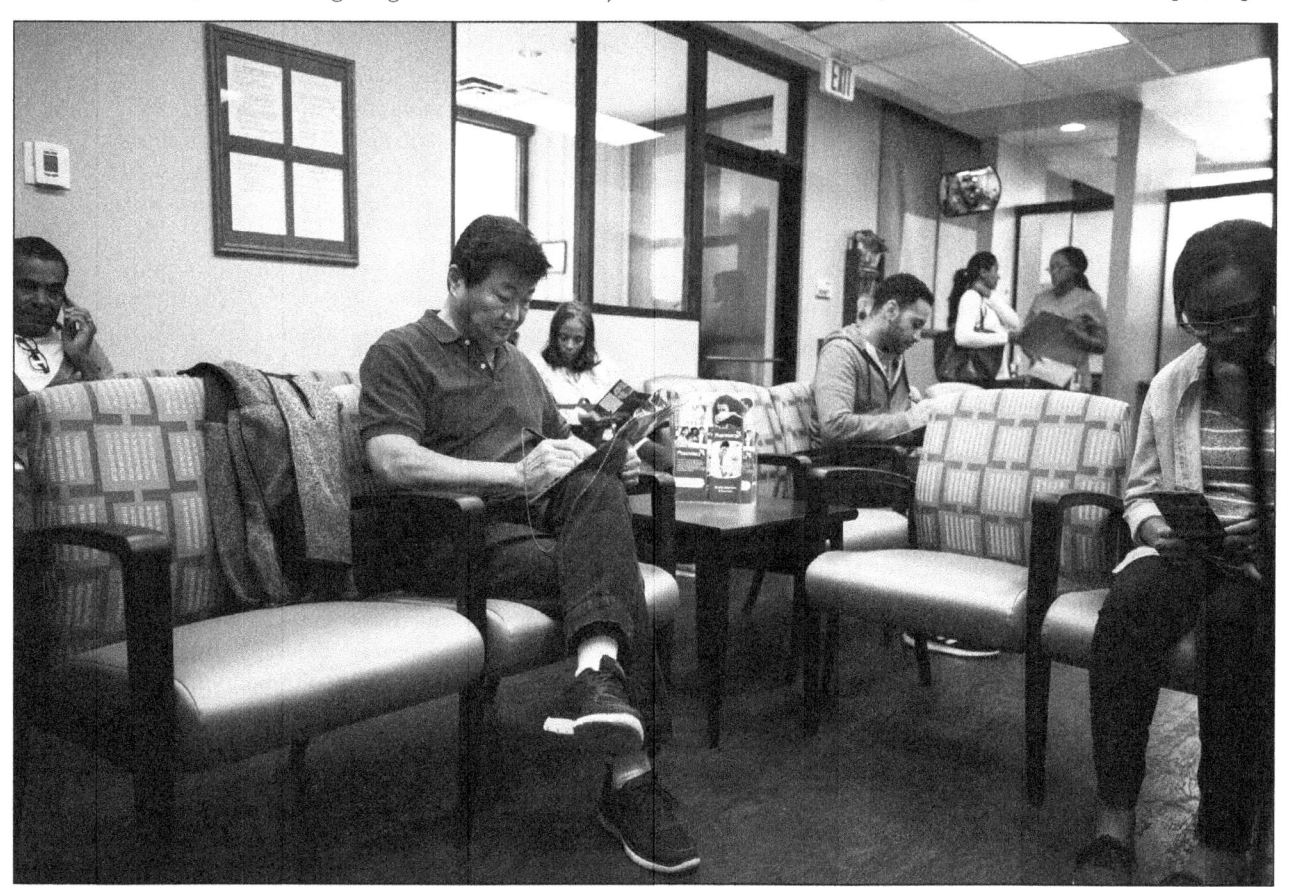

Above, a nurse attends to one of many patients waiting in a busy medical office (SDI Productions via iStock)

diatric nurse would be required to care for no more than four patients at a time, while an intensive care nurse would only care for one or two patients at once. If these bills become law, hospitals would be required to maintain these ratios unless the hospital has an emergency such as a multiple-vehicle crash or an outbreak of a contagious disease.

In 1999, California passed a law that required all hospitals to implement nurse-patient ratios. It took effect in 2004. Hospitals must adhere to staffing ratios at all times, except in the event of healthcare emergencies. For example, oncology nurses cannot exceed caring for more than five patients at one time. While the law has eased the workload for nurses, it does have its shortcomings. For instance, staffing must be covered at all times. When a nurse takes a break, he or she must have a replacement. This has made scheduling more challenging for hospital officials.

In the years that followed, many hospital officials and nursing unions looked to California's law for guidance when they were in the process of designing nursing-patient ratio legislation. Many states proposed staffing ratios for nurses, but only one other state, Massachusetts, had passed legislation. The Massachusetts law passed in 2014 and was implemented for academic hospital ICUs in 2016 and for community hospitals and neonatal ICUs in 2017. It mandates that nurses working on ICUs and burn units may only be assigned up to two patients, and only one patient if the patient's care requires it. A study published by Beth Israel Deaconess Medical Center in 2018 found that the state's law did not have much impact on the number of nurses on the job or on patient outcomes, mortality, or complications. The Massachusetts Nurses Association filed the Patient Safety Act, a 2018 state ballot question to decide whether the state should set nurse-to-patient ratios for all hospital units, with ratios set depending on the type of unit. The initiative is endorsed by the Committee to Ensure Safe Patient Care, comprising a broad coalition of elected officials, healthcare organizations, nurses' associations, community groups, Democratic town committees, and labor councils and unions. The Coalition to Protect Patient Safety, whose members include the Massachusetts Health & Hospital Association, the Organization of Nurse Leaders, Massachusetts Council of Community Hospitals, and Conference of Boston Teaching Hospitals, formed in December 2017 to oppose the initiative.

Several states have passed laws requiring hospitals to appoint committees to oversee and create staffing plans appropriate for each unit. These plans must be flexible and account for numerous factors, including the severity of the patients needing care; experience level of nurses; layout of the hospital; and availability of resources.

—*Angela Harmon*

Further Reading

"Coalition Launched to Oppose Nurse Staffing Ballot Question." *Massachusetts Health & Hospital Association*, 11 Dec. 2017, www.mhalink.org/MHA/MyMHA/Communications/MondayReportItems/Content/2017/12-11/Items/Coalition-Launched-to-Oppose-Nurse-Staffing-Ballot.aspx.

Lampert, Lynda. "Nurses Storm the U.S. Capitol to Demand Safe Staffing Ratios." *Daily Nurse*, 2 June 2016, dailynurse.com/nurses-storm-u-s-capitol-demand-safe-staffing-ratios/.

Law, Anica C., et al. "Patient Outcomes after the Introduction of Statewide ICU Nurse Staffing Regulations." *Critical Care Medicine*, vol. 46, no. 10, Oct. 2018, pp. 1563–69, doi:10.1097/CCM.0000000000003286, pubmed.ncbi.nlm.nih.gov/30179886/.

Manjlovich, Milisa. "Seeking Staffing Solutions." *American Nurse Today*, vol. 4, no. 3, Mar. 2009, www.myamericannurse.com/seeking-staffing-solutions/.

"Nurse Staffing Advocacy." *American Nurses Association*, www.nursingworld.org/practice-policy/nurse-staffing/nurse-staffing-advocacy/. Accessed 3 Sept. 2020.

"Nurse Unions Continue to Push for Nurse-Patient Ratio Legislation." *Littler*, 20 Feb. 2014, www.littler.com/publication-press/publication/nurse-unions-continue-push-nurse-patient-ratio-legislation.

"Nurses Association Pushes for Federal, State Nurse-to-Patient Ratio Laws." *AHC Media*, 1 July 2015, www.reliasmedia.com/articles/135642-nurses-association-pushes-for-federal-state-nurse-to-patient-ratio-laws.

Pecci, Alexandra Wilson. "Nurse-Patient Ratio Law in MA Raises Cost, Quality Concerns." *HealthLeaders Media*, 23 June 2015, www.healthleadersmedia.com/nursing/nurse-patient-ratio-law-ma-raises-cost-quality-concerns.

"Safe-Staffing Ratios: Benefiting Nurses and Patients." *Department for Professional Employees, AFL-CIO*, www.dpeaflcio.org/factsheets/safe-staffing-critical-for-patients-and-nurses. Accessed 3 Sept. 2020.

Schultz, David. "Nurses Fighting State by State for Minimum Staffing Laws." *Kaiser Health News*, khn.org/news/nurse-staffing-laws/. Accessed 3 Sept. 2020.

Models of Nursing Care

ABSTRACT

Nursing care can be provided using a variety of organizational methods. Among the most significant models of nursing care are functional nursing, team nursing, modular nursing, primary nursing, and total patient care. The model that an organization or healthcare provider uses varies from institution to institution and according to the specific needs of each patient.

FUNCTIONAL NURSING

One of the earliest models of nursing care to develop in the United States is functional nursing. Functional nursing arose during the Great Depression when there was a shortage of available nurses, a shortage that continued into World War II. Because of this lack of nurses, many hospitals had to rely on less skilled personnel. In order to adjust to this lack of all-around expertise, hospitals began assigning nurses and nursing assistants specific functions rather than training them in the full range of activities nurses had previously performed. In this way, it was easier to train less skilled practitioners.

Functional nursing is a task-oriented model that values efficiency as its primary objective. Generally, in this model, each nurse or nursing assistant is given one or two responsibilities and is not required to learn the tasks performed by the rest of the nursing staff. The head nurse is charged with assigning the individual duties. Although this model has numerous advantages—in addition to more efficiently employing less-knowledgeable professionals, it allows staff members to acquire their skills more quickly and is more efficient and cost-effective than other models—it also has its drawbacks. Among the negative features of the model are that it leads to an impersonal relationship between nurses and patients and limits the job growth of each individual nurse.

TEAM NURSING AND MODULAR NURSING

The team nursing model was developed in the 1950s as a response to the criticisms being leveled at functional nursing. Under a grant from the W. K. Kellogg Corporation, Eleanor Lambertson at Columbia University's Teachers College in New York developed her new model as a way of making functional nursing more patient-centric. In team nursing, a group of four to six people work together to care for a group of assigned patients. This team usually consists of a team leader or head nurse who is an RN (registered nurse) and several other nursing professionals, often LPNs (licensed practical nurses), CNAs (certified nursing assistants), or nurse's aides. Unlike in functional nursing where caregivers are only concerned about their individual tasks, team nursing focuses on providing comprehensive nursing care with all team members, regardless of their specific duties, involved in care provision.

This team-oriented approach is carried out through various means of communication which ensure that all team members are involved in directing and carrying out the patient's care. Chief among these modes of communication is the team conference, with each team member reporting on his or her patients and where plans for continued care are discussed as a group. All nursing professionals are able to have a stake in the care of the patient and the system is able to combine the efficiency of functional nursing with a more patient-centric approach when employing a team conference. Some disadvantages of team nursing are the amount of time that is necessary for coordinating the team members and the instability of care that may result from team members being moved around to work with other patients.

Modular nursing is a variation of team nursing that focuses on the patient's geographic location in order to allocate nursing assignments. In this model, the patient unit is divided into several different modules (also known as pods or districts) and each team is assigned to a different module. As in team nursing, each team has an RN as the team leader who is responsible for supervising both patient care and their own team members. Generally, in modular nursing, the teams are smaller than in team nursing and are consistently assigned to the same location, leading to greater continuity of care than in team nursing.

PRIMARY NURSING AND TOTAL PATIENT CARE

Primary nursing was developed by nurses working in an acute medical care ward at the University of Minnesota Medical Center in 1969. Reacting to the chaotic arrangement of their unit, these nurses, led by a woman named Marie Manthey, created a model in which nurses would play a more central role in determining the care the patient would receive. This model helped flatten the hierarchy in hospitals, granting nurses greater autonomy, and streamlining the process of nursing supervision.

Primary nursing, as it is practiced today, involves the designation of a single nurse as the primary caregiver of a patient during his or her stay at the hospital. This primary nurse, who is always a RN, typically leads a small team that may be composed of LPN or nursing assistants. In addition to greater autonomy for the primary nurse, this model allows for more direct and holistic patient care and the development of a strong relationship between the primary nurse and the patient. It is not a particularly cost-effective model as it often requires the hiring of more RNs. It also places a high degree of responsibility on the primary nurse which may be demanding for many professionals.

Total patient care is an even more patient-centric approach than primary nursing. In this model, a variant on primary nursing, an RN proves one-on-one care to a single patient or a group of patients over the course of his or her shift. This approach allows the nurse to allot the most care to a single patient but it is also the most financially burdensome model, as it requires a large team of nurses in order to properly carry out.

SUMMARY

Regardless of the model of nursing, the nursing process and its related written nursing care plan (NCP) are an integral part of patient care. For example, team conferences may not be held daily so communication of the plan of care come from the NCP. While team conferences may not be held daily, change of shift reports are done daily at shift change. If additions or deletions are needed in the NCP between team conferences, the change of shift report is the place the NCP may be updated. With patients staying fewer days in the hospital, the nursing plan of care assumes an even more important role in communication.

—*Andrew Schenker*

Further Reading

Dunphy, Lynne M. et al. *Primary Care: Art and Science of Advanced Practice Nursing–An Interprofessional Approach*. 5th ed., F. A. Davis Company, 2019.

Michaels, Davida. "Nursing Care Models: Historical Review." *American Nursing History*, 22 Feb. 2020, www.americannursinghistory.org/models-nursing-care.

Pointer, Emma "What Is Team Nursing?" *Trusted Health*, 3 Mar. 2020, www.trustedhealth.com/blog/what-is-team-nursing.

"Understanding the Primary Nursing Care Model." *HealthStream*, 29 Aug. 2019, www.healthstream.com/resources/blog/blog/2019/08/29/understanding-the-primary-nursing-care-model.

SKILLS NEEDED IN NURSING

Indeed, some skills are obvious to succeed at nursing. This section discusses more general skills, like leadership, time management, interpersonal communication, writing skills, technical skills, community service, public speaking and networking. These collection of skills will no doubt help you in many chosen professions, and these essays will make it clear why having these skills will help you not only further your nursing career, but become a better nurse.

Leadership	119
Leadership Skills	121
Volunteering and Community Service	124
Time Management	127
Communicating Effectively: Interpersonal Communication, Skills, and Technology	131
Writing Skills	140
Public Speaking	142
Networking	146

LEADERSHIP

ABSTRACT
Leadership is comprised of basic human traits that any individual can embrace and develop. Understanding the basic components of leadership and then implementing the areas in your own unique and individualized manner is an essential aspect of being a great leader. Everyone is different and therefore leadership traits work in ways that reflect a person's uniqueness and individuality.

INTRODUCTION
The traditional concept of leadership evokes images of individuals in positions of authority; an established hierarchy with defined roles and responsibilities. However, is there more to leadership than a title and position? Surely "leadership" does not simply happen once you reach a particular position. What is the real substance that lies behind leadership that allows an individual to be looked upon as a leader? This article explores the characteristics and actions instrumental to the act of leading.

A commonly accepted definition of leadership is "the action of leading a group of people." What does this actually mean though? If you were told to go and "lead a group of people," what would that actually mean? There are countless ways people could interpret the aforementioned task. Instead of attempting to create one standard definition of leadership we instead focus in detail on the individual aspects that feature in good leadership. The features have been grouped into four overarching categories: moral traits, people-oriented traits, task-oriented traits, and improvement-focused traits. It is important to understand that while key leadership characteristics can be individually identified, in practice they frequently intertwine with one another.

MORAL TRAITS
An important aspect for leadership relates to the person's overall integrity. Some people have a talent for speaking in a persuasive and enticing manner but their end objectives are not well intentioned. While they may appear to be leaders due to their charisma and ability to get others to listen to them, these types of individuals are not honest and therefore lack an essential aspect of genuine leadership: being trustworthy. Real leaders do not hide their motives nor do they operate under false pretenses.

The question then arises, how do leaders gain other's trust? Trust grows over time as a leader's words and actions translate into reality. Therefore, it is highly important for leaders to be open and honest in what they say and what they actually do. While strong leaders genuinely do have other's best interests in mind it is equally important for leaders to not make promises that cannot be kept, even if the promises are well-intentioned. In essence, real leaders while they strive to create high quality outcomes also genuinely care about those working for them and treat people with respect.

PEOPLE-FOCUSED TRAITS
Similar to the moral-focused traits, this area shares the underlying principle of caring about others. However, it also highlights the need for leaders to understand how each individual's personality and abilities impact their work. Being aware of peoples' work styles along with the areas they excel and struggle in, is a first important step. Great leaders take it a step farther and tailor their leadership approach based on the individual characteristics of the person. For example, if one person thrives when working independently and creatively while another person performs best when given specific guidelines and deadlines, a strong leader knows how to tailor tasks to match each individual's preferred working style.

Additionally, great leaders have a positive energy that motivates people and also builds others' self-confidence. While some people use the fear tactic to get results, real leaders do not resort to scaring others. They lead by cultivating a supportive environment that focuses on utilizing people's strengths, building upon their areas of weakness, and igniting their motivation and passions.

TASK-ORIENTED TRAITS

The ability to have a vision and break that end goal down into smaller, objective, and more manageable steps is an important quality for leadership. Attention to detail and an ability to organize is important. Often people have grand plans but fail to make their target goal because the road needed to reach the end result is too ambiguous or difficult. A strong leader is able to see the larger and the smaller picture at the same time and successfully implement a strategic plan to reach both goals. Good leaders commit to their plans without being inflexible and rigid and are always open to ways to enhance the process. Often times the wide range of options can overwhelm an individual; strong leaders are knowledgeable about the pros and cons of the different routes but are able to make a decisive decision and be accountable for their choice. Sometimes when a "leader" makes a decision the person does everything in their power to make that option work. The ability to see when a plan is not working and admit to the fact is not a sign of weakness but rather one of great strength. Strong leaders maintain composure in difficult situations and modify plans in a rational versus panic-like state; the emphasis is placed on how to reach the goal and what steps need to be taken in order to get closer to the desired outcome.

IMPROVEMENT-FOCUSED TRAITS

Another essential component of leadership is one's ability to both give and receive feedback. Knowing how to provide helpful feedback is highly important. Some people are hesitant to give constructive feedback and only focus on peoples' strengths, while other individuals tend to focus on the negatives. Leaders understand the importance of equally focusing on both the positive attributes of others while also highlighting their areas for improvement. At the same time, true leaders also ask others for feedback on their own performance (e.g., the leader's strengths and areas to improve), and moreover actually make modifications based on the suggestions received. Strong self-reflection and self-awareness skills coupled with a genuine openness to feedback from others makes people respect, trust and want to listen to the leader's instructions or advice.

In addition to inviting and embracing feedback from individuals that work for the leader, another important aspect related to strong leadership rests in the leader's proactive approach to seeking counsel and advice from people both within and outside the group or agency. Soliciting suggestions from others generates additional ideas; having a wide range of options allows the leader to consider more techniques and strategies to implement. Another key factor within this improvement-focused traits domain is the leader's ability to communicate clearly and effectively. When instructions are not clearly outlined it increases the likelihood of mistakes being made. Confusion regarding the task at hand not only causes the workers to feel frustrated but it also reduces the efficiency of the overall work. Therefore, it is important that leaders are able to provide clear instructions when allocating tasks to individuals and provide people with both positive and constructive feedback.

ANYONE CAN BE A LEADER

The aforementioned are characteristics that can be championed by anybody. The characteristics are not reserved for only certain people, or people in certain positions. By displaying the above qualities every individual can be deemed a leader in some capacity. True leadership is the recognition that people bestow upon you; simply telling people what to do does not make one a leader. A position of power does not make one a leader. Unless individuals truly view and relate to the "leader" as their leader, there is no leadership, simply a person with a title. Every company has a chief executive officer (CEO), not every company has a leader. All teams have a captain, not every team has a leader.

Everybody has his or her own style. People tend to associate the concept of a leader with someone who is extroverted and exudes self-confidence. Leaders can be, but by no means "have" to be confident, charismatic individuals. The range of personality types of well-known and admired leaders ranges greatly. The real key to being a true leader is to embody the positive leadership elements that are attainable to people across all personality types.

—*Stefan Leonte and Kimberly Glazier*

Further Reading

Ashkenas, R. "Seven Mistakes Leaders Make in Setting Goals." *Forbes*, 2015, www.forbes.com/sites/ronashkenas/2012/07/09/seven-mistakes-leaders-make-in-setting-goals/.

Folkman, J. "The Best Gift Leaders Can Give: Honest Feedback." *Forbes*, 2013, www.forbes.com/sites/joefolkman/2013/12/19/the-best-gift-leaders-can-give-honest-feedback/.

Fries. K. "8 Essential Qualities that Define Great Leadership." *Forbes*, www.forbes.com/sites/kimberlyfries/2018/02/08-essential-qualities-that-define-great-leadership/#5ad70be73b63. Accessed 24 Aug. 2020.

Horsager, D. "You Can't Be a Great Leader Without Trust. Here's How to Build It." *Forbes*, 2012, www.forbes.com/sites/forbesleadershipforum/2012/10/24/you-cant-be-a-great-leader-without-trust-heres-how-you-build-it/.

"Leadership." *Psychology Today*, www.psychologytoday.com/us/basics/leadership. Accessed 24 Aug. 2020.

Silverstein, R. "Good People Make Good Leaders." *Entrepreneur*, 2010, www.entrepreneur.com/article/206832.

LEADERSHIP SKILLS

ABSTRACT

Some individuals start to groom their leadership skills early in life in anticipation of future success. They have some sense of where they are going and how they are going to get there. However, it's difficult to visualize yourself in a leadership position when you spend much of your time surrounded by adults who dictate the rules and hold you accountable for completing homework assignments, chores, and practice sessions, etc.

Adolescence is an excellent time to begin training to be a leader. Leadership skills unfold in and outside the classroom, on the playing field, and any other place where you encounter others in your daily life. You can easily identify those who stand out, take the lead, initiate, motivate, and encourage others. Those individuals are the ones who are beginning to demonstrate essential leadership qualities before society labels their "can do" behaviors. Leaders are not born; they are made.

INTRODUCTION

Leaders can communicate effectively, are able to observe and learn, are honest and demonstrate integrity, can build relationships and innovate rather than copy. The ability to learn and react is a core leadership skill. Leadership skills endorse peer feedback; you *listen* and *relate* to the concerns of others. Friends seek your advice because you appear to understand their plight and are willing to listen. They trust you. It's an awesome responsibility because adolescence can be a very confusing time in someone's life. You are experiencing many of the same emotions and are in the midst of your own emotional storm. This is an excellent time to start applying your emotional intelligence.

A leader is not bossy, but rather inclusive of the ideas of the group being led. Coaching peers requires time, energy, communication skills, and accurate feedback. Leaders demonstrate a good balance of individual and social competencies. Maintaining those qualities requires persistent and consistent efforts. It's easy to be distracted by all the sideshows in life—some are especially appealing. The road to becoming a person is jam-packed with emotional traffic, seductive images, noise, conflict, and enticements that make good decision-making and problem-solving strenuous exercises in character, self-control, and endurance. Positive leadership requires individuals to step outside the norm. The "going rate" is just not good enough. Your actions inspire others to dream more, learn more, reach higher, and exceed their grasp. In doing so, you reap the benefits of seeing others as well as yourself achieve success. It's a team approach to learning, a win/win situation, and the best possible outcome.

BEHAVIORS OF LEADERS

Leadership skills require role modeling behaviors that earn admiration from teachers, friends, and family. Participants experience less conflict because they obey the rules, are pleasant, and respect authority. In addition, they have courage. This does not mean they are fearless. It means that in spite of being afraid, they face adversity and difficult challenges. Leaders demonstrate confidence—you are not inclined to make comparisons or put others down—you help them up.

Positive leaders have a vision. They are not satisfied with the ordinary. These people look ahead and see possibilities that may improve the present condition and that of the future. In addition, they are enthusiastic in their pursuit of new ideas that benefit everyone. There is no room for one-upmanship because everyone is working toward the same goal. The classroom climate can become a motivating factor when ideas are allowed to flourish and students respect differing opinions. Student leaders encourage a mutually shared experience that stays in balance during change or uncertainty.

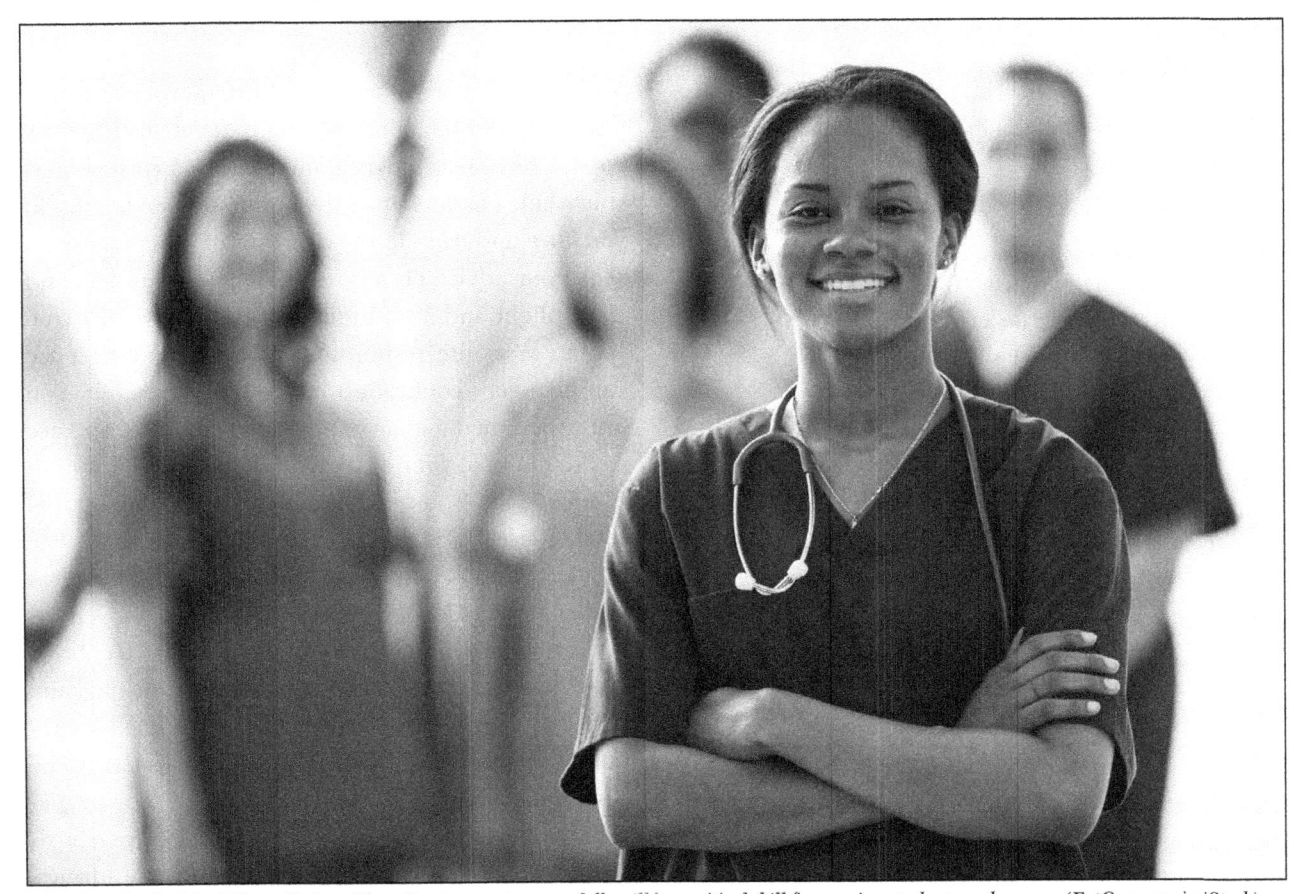

Identifying leadership skills and being able to direct a group successfully will be a critical skill for nursing students and nurses. (FatCamera via iStock)

Leadership skills require students to persevere even during difficult times. Losses, defeats, and mistakes are all learning lessons. Leaders have the strength and tenacity to see it through. They don't quit because some task or performance is boring, inconvenient, or seems too tough. Strength doesn't surface from knowing what we can achieve—it comes from overcoming obstacles that once lead us to believe we couldn't—resiliency.

Leaders are willing to take calculated risks. They understand that sometimes things do not work to their advantage and the result is—lesson learned. Information gleaned from failed attempts is noted and stored for later use. We build confidence while learning what works and doesn't work. Positive leaders are fast learners and refrain from making the same mistakes. They constantly evaluate decisions to determine the best possible approach to solving problems.

SELF-DISCIPLINE AND HONESTY

Leadership skills require self-discipline. That means you take responsibility for your behavior even when you are angry. In addition, there are numerous ways to demonstrate self-discipline that include: respecting authority, arriving on time, presenting a neat appearance, being prepared, completing tasks, being cooperative, refraining from temper outbursts, refraining from gossiping, managing emotions. Leadership skills require you to listen fully to others, without trying to figure out what you're going to say next.

Leadership skills require you to be honest with yourself and others. It's difficult to earn respect when trust is an issue. Trust is an essential ingredient to successful leadership. Without trust, there are no followers—therefore leadership is not possible. Fear tactics may work in the short run, but over time, people will drift away and find a better way. *Remember, even the nicest people have their limits.*

ADDITIONAL SKILLS

You need a sense of humor. There will be days when a good laugh is the best leadership style. Don't take yourself too seriously. Also, try to see the lighter side of a situation. *Classroom drama kings and queen do not a fun place make.* Attention-seeking devices abound everywhere. Positive leaders learn early that drama cannot exist in a void—it needs participants and observers.

It's nice to have friends but beware of cliques. Cliques are different from groups. Groups welcome everyone and there is a free exchange of ideas. Group members can move about several groups at the same time without consequences. However, in cliques, members exclude others, gossip, and make fun of those who are not in the clique. In addition, prior group members may act differently when they join a clique and any change in their behavior is likely negative.

Leadership skills are at their worst in cliques. They determine who is "in" and who is "out." Leaders often tell members how they must dress, act, and who they can talk to. They may be mean or victimize others to maintain their power position. You may become a target if you demonstrate you have no interest in following their rules or seem threatening because you have positive leadership skills and are strong in your convictions—that's a good thing and it takes courage!

HOW BEHAVIOR IMPACTS OTHERS

Adolescence is a time when many young people are often focused on how the world impacts their lives. Once you understand your emotions, step outside yourself and evaluate how your behaviors affect others—that's the beginning of building leadership skills. You are using emotional intelligence skills that help you achieve better relationships and ultimately become better leaders.

Your life-long journey to improve leadership skills takes work and dedication—a desire to reach your peak leadership performance and future leadership destination. What are your strengths and weaknesses?

What can you do to change your behaviors? Can you identify good leaders in your circle of friends or school? What teachers demonstrate leadership? What society and world leaders do you admire? How would you model, or integrate, observed leadership skills into your life?

Begin the process of evaluating your behaviors and how they impact others. The application of positive leadership skills enhances the learning environment and makes a contribution. It also makes life easier for everyone around you, including yourself. Your ability to make and keep friends is enhanced and your relationships with family and teachers benefit. Although conflict is weaved in the fabric of life, you will experience less and handle resolution more efficiently.

LEADERSHIP ROLES

Leadership can take many roles. Class officer, president of a club, leading a volunteer group or leading a study group are all examples of leadership roles. Students helping other students can offer extra benefits. A classroom of learners who unite together in the learning process is a wonderful thing. Nursing school often involves groups of students working together to achieve a common goal. Identifying leadership skills and being able to direct a group successfully will be a critical skill for nursing students and nurses. Sometimes the true test of a leader is to encourage the group to define the agenda and shape the responses to achieve the goal. Being a leader is different than being a boss.

—*Jane Piland-Baker and Thomas E. Baker*

Further Reading

"5 Leadership Skills Found in Managers." Villanova University. Updated 6 May 2009, www.villanovau.com/resources/leadership/5-leadership-skills-found-in-managers/.

"The Core Leadership Skills You Need in Every Role." *Center for Creative Leadership*, www.ccl.org/articles/leading-effectively-articles/fundamental-4-core-leadership-skills-for-every-career-stage. Accessed 30 Aug. 2020.

Covey, S. *The 6 Most Important Decisions You'll Ever Make: A Guide for Teens*. Fireside, 2006. This book shows teens how to make smart choices about the six most crucial choices they'll face during these turbulent years.

Covey, S. *The 7 Habits of Highly Effective Teens: The Ultimate Teenage Success Guide*. Miniature ed. Running Press, 2002. Based on his father's bestselling book, *The 7 Habits of Highly Effective People*, Sean Covey applies the same principles to teens, using a vivacious, entertaining style.

MacGregor, M. *Teambuilding with Teens: Activities for Leadership, Decision Making & Group Success*. Free Spirit Publishing, 2008. The 36 activities in this book make learning about leadership a hands-on, active experience. Young people are encouraged to recognize each other's strengths, become better listeners, communicate clearly, identify their values, build trust, set goals, and more.

VOLUNTEERING AND COMMUNITY SERVICE

ABSTRACT

The positive effects of volunteering on teenagers include physical, mental, social, and vocational benefits attributed to volunteer work. There are many ways of becoming involved in local organizations or independent service work. Most college admissions offices and many employers look for volunteering and community service on a resume.

INTRODUCTION

The *Merriam-Webster Dictionary* defines volunteering as, "offering to do something without being forced to or without getting paid to do it." This action acts in combination with the act of community service, which is defined by Google as "voluntary work intended to help people in a particular area." Since the time of colonization, Americans have been initiating, working towards, and establishing nonprofit and community service geared organizations. It is proven that participation in community service projects and volunteering both locally and abroad as a teenager can have lifelong positive benefits on both mental and physical health. Enforcing positive action and habits starting from a young age can lead to a healthy, happy, and productive life in the future. The seeds of a lifelong dedication to service, expansion of viewpoints, and collaboration among others are instilled within teen volunteers through their work.

There are many resources and possibilities for involvement both within local programs and beyond. National nonprofit organizations, local service groups, or independently established movements are all potential outlets for teenage volunteering. Many individuals throughout history have advocated for the positive aspects of reaching out and assisting others including Audrey Hepburn. In a famous quotation she stated, "As you grow older, you will discover that you have two hands, one for helping yourself and the other for helping others." By instilling volunteer habits in a teenager, this understanding and call to take action to enact change will come even sooner. There has been a documented increase in the amount of teen volunteers over the years. The following outlines the key reasons to volunteer and its positive benefits. Assistance on getting involved and helpful volunteering tips are also located below.

BENEFITS OF VOLUNTEERING

The benefits of volunteering are endless especially for teenagers. Getting involved within their community, learning life skills, and understanding their role and capacity to enact change can all positively enrich a teen's life. Volunteering and committing to an organization, event, or activity will teach time management, productivity, and responsibility. A study at the University of Pennsylvania by a Wharton professor, Cassie Mogliner, for the *Harvard Business Review* found that those who volunteer their time feel a balance and find they have more time. Skills that promote organization, dedication, work ethic, and perseverance are all attributed to the work of volunteers and prove very beneficial to the character development of a teenager. There is a particular development of social responsibility linked to a broadened global perspective and understanding of the value of education and everyday resources. A new sense of humility and gratitude can be forged in the service of others. Multiculturalism and understanding of the shared identity and need of all people around the world can be directly grasped through hands-on volunteering. College applications and resumes can be enforced with the skills, connections, and abilities developed through involvement with a community service organization. A study conducted in 2012 at the University of Michigan for the publication, *Monitoring the Future*, found that 40 percent of high school seniors who planned to finish college were already active volunteers.

Volunteering allows a teen to develop new skills and pursue areas of potential interest. By honing in on skills and attributes beginning as a young adult, a teen can be prepared to enter future academic and vocational endeavors. Interests exemplified through work done as a teen can lead to a lifelong calling and discovery of a particular passion. Winston Churchill stated, "We make a living by what we get, we make a life by what we give." By establishing new connections and bonds with likeminded individuals, a great support system is created for a teen. Sharing in a common cause and contributing towards its success directly enforces critical thinking skills. Social skills are developed through shared activity and striving for a common goal. Volunteering allows an active participation and application of academic knowledge and skills towards everyday problems and their solutions. While students are given factual information and written knowledge in a classroom setting, community service allows this knowledge to be applied and strengthened. Participation in volunteer work has shown a decrease in a teenager's likelihood of participating in illegal and harmful activities.

Volunteering promotes overall well-being, both mentally and physically. A report published by the Corporation for National and Community Service found that "those who volunteer have lower mortality rates, greater functional ability and lower rates of depression" going forward in life. Active movement and interaction with peers and mentors develop a teen into a well-rounded and high-functioning adult. Interaction and hands-on volunteer work grants teens a global perspective and better understanding of society and the world around them. Volunteering promotes self-confidence, fulfillment, and happiness. There is a great reward and sense of satisfaction derived from helping others. As a teen, finding a personal role in society can sometimes be challenging. By directly doing something to benefit someone or something else, a teen will gain a sense of pride, value, and identity. No matter how young, all people have the ability to make a positive difference in the world. Studies have proven an actual "happiness effect" linked to volunteer and community service work. In a report published by Harvard Health Publications, the London School of Economics found that there was a direct positive correlation in the relationship between the frequency of volunteering and an inclination to be happy. There was a 16 percent rise in happiness levels for those who volunteered weekly.

VOLUNTEER IDEAS AND OPPORTUNITIES
There are many outlets for volunteer work spanning a variety of interests. Whether dealing with the environment, healthcare, hunger and poverty relief, animal welfare, community development and infrastructure, human rights, or politics, there are both local and national organizations in need of teen volunteers. Teens can volunteer in both large and small-scale settings. As Mother Teresa stated, "Do small things with great love." Any contribution that can be made proves influential no matter how big or small. Assisting with everyday tasks at home is an easy way to perform an act of community service. Visiting and talking to elderly family members or mentoring and tutoring young relatives, are each positive contributions made without the sole intention of personal gain. Within a hometown or community, local soup kitchens and community centers can provide positions assisting with outreach programs and volunteer events. Nationally, nonprofit organizations, such as, the American Cancer Society, Special Olympics, and Habitat for Humanity provide youth leadership and volunteer programs within their campaigns, events, and advocacy. Many hospitals and health systems encourage volunteers who might be interested in a career in healthcare. High school clubs provide a platform for student-led and hands-on work. Many organizations provide the ability to form local chapters and branches making it easy for teens to form their own movement. For those interested in even more service-based immersion, community service programs exist abroad allowing students to travel and assist others around the world. The organization, Do Something, outlines a variety of ways in which teenagers can get involved in a variety of volunteer ideas and opportunities. By keeping one's perspective and options open, an array of resources and chances for worthwhile service can be found.

TIPS FOR OPTIMIZING THE VOLUNTEER EXPERIENCE
There are a few tips to ensure that volunteer work as a teenager is worthwhile. The first is to remember safety and always follow sanitation, health codes, and protective measures. Being open to new experiences, people, and activities can broaden a teen's perspective and lead to a lifelong path. By incorporating passions, interests, and hobbies the best match in a community service program can be discovered. It is important to ask questions and fully understand your role, commitment, and participation. Never overstep your bounds. Knowing what to expect by asking questions and doing research prior to serving will allow the most comfort and transitional ease. As a teen, it is easy to become discouraged or feel insignificant. It is key to remember that anyone has the ability to change the world with the right work ethic and dedication. Setting a personal goal and timeline will allow a sense

of achievement and fulfillment while eliminating the daunting and overwhelming stresses of taking on a large task all at once. Finally, it is vital to the entire experience to approach volunteering as a positive and fun activity. Volunteering can also help you decide a career path going forward. In participating in new experiences, helping others, meeting new people, and finding one's identity and passions, a teen can have a truly enjoyable and rewarding experience in volunteering and community service!

—*Christina Maher*

Further Reading

DoSomething.org. America's largest organization for youth volunteering opportunities. This organization provides an online resource for teenagers looking for effective and feasible volunteer and community service opportunities. There are many resources spanning a variety of opportunities and subject matters allowing students to have easy access to community service and inspiration to enact change.

Grubisich, Kelsi, "The Relationship Between Participation in Community Service and Students Academic Success." Masters Theses 2620, 2017, thekeep.eiu.edu/cgi/viewcontent.cgi?article=3621&context=theses. Accessed 31 Aug. 2020.

Mogilner, C. "You'll Feel Less Rushed If You Give Time Away." *Harvard Business Review*, 1 Sept. 2012. This article discusses the positive benefits of volunteering. In this study, the positive correlation between committing time to service work and personal freedom, organization, and enjoyment is proven.

"Simple Changes, Big Rewards: A Practical, Easy Guide for Healthy, Happy Living." *Harvard Health*, n.d., www.health.harvard.edu/special-health-reports/simple-changes-big-rewards-a-practical-easy-guide-for-healthy-happy-living. In this article, researchers for Harvard Health identified actual positive physical and mental benefits and an inclination towards happiness associated with volunteering and community service.

"Volunteering." *Child Trends Databank*, 2014, www.childtrends.org/?indicators=volunteering; www.childtrends.org/?indicators=volunteering#sthash.BaxYKMHw.dpuf. This article outlines specific positive trends related to student's academic and vocational plans in relation to service work. Through the presentation of graphics and statistics the correlation found through study is clearly outlined.

Time Management

ABSTRACT

The key to time management lies within the understanding of how the brain perceives the construct of time. Several theories abound, trying to explain the science to managing time and to increasing awareness of how to effectively accomplish tasks within an allotted time frame. Understanding both the science of time management and its antonym, procrastination, have proven to be very effective in using time appropriately and effectively with physical and mental benefits. Because of the difficulty of nursing programs, managing time between study, perhaps work and recreation is critical.

INTRODUCTION

Adolescence is an important developmental stage when youngsters start to spend more time outside of the home and to explore and experiment with different roles. They try to achieve autonomy by taking on more responsibilities. Among many decisions that adolescents need to make is deciding when to do what and how long they should spend on an activity. Most adolescents are making the transition from being present-oriented to future-oriented. Engaged in an amazing array of activities including school, homework, employment, sports, extracurricular/club activities, outside-school training programs (e.g., dancing, music), traveling, socializing with friends, dating, leisure, and entertainment, in addition to personal care and housework, adolescents have to manage time in one way or another. How to use time effectively and keep one's life productive and happy is one of many critical skills for adolescents to learn.

Sense of time is intricately related to cognitive development and cognitive functioning. For example, intentional planning is practically impossible for very young children who haven't got the time concept yet or people who have lost track of time due to various mental disorders. In order to manage time well, adolescents need to develop a good sense of time through participatory learning and thinking.

Scientists have trouble finding an exact definition for the term "time management," but the most widely agreed upon understanding of it is the planning and execution of activities. It is therefore a twofold concept—it involves both the preparation and the actual doing of the idea. Though it may appear counterintuitive, it is vital to dedicate some time to the organization of ideas and seeing to the completion of the tasks. And oddly enough, it is that time spent planning that is so essential to proper time management; without it, a person would be blindly acting out assignments. A plethora of literary sources agree that with proper time assessment a person can feel more in control of their time, more content with academic or professional careers, and most of all less stressed. Additionally, individuals who exercise time management report high productivity and numerous benefits from extra free time. Many researchers and theorists have explored what happens to a person psychologically and biologically when planning a course of action. Moreover, for many to fully comprehend time organization, it is easier to compare it with its complete opposite—procrastination, the act of delaying tasks and "putting off" assignments to very last-minute.

THE SCIENCE TO MANAGING TIME
The conventional way of managing time includes assessing needs and setting goals, planning-prioritizing goals/tasks to construct a hierarchy, determining strategies/tactics to complete the tasks, allocating time (scheduling), and carrying it out with monitoring and making adjustments as necessary.

Many see the perception of time as the key to understanding time management. One major theory in this field of study is the Planning Fallacy. Pioneered by researchers Roger Buehler, Dale Griffin, and Michael Ross, it is the concept that a person underestimates how long a task will require of them, particularly if he or she spends a large amount of planning time foreseeing a pleasant outcome without accounting for possible obstacles. Professor Douglas Hofstadter's law states that no matter how much planning goes into an activity, every task takes longer than anticipated. Alternatively, other studies turn to past experiences with similar circumstances rather than looking to at the future; they find that previous experience provides both a realistic result as well as a fairly accurate gauge for how long the activity will take. The University of Belgium conducted a study in which they found that the more details imagined on a future project, the more imminent and critical it feels.

Perhaps the reason time management may be so difficult to achieve for some is because of the nature of the brain. According to Dr. Timothy A. Pychyl, the limbic system (the portion of the brain primarily concerned with instinct and emotion) uses its reflexes to avoid activities that cause distress. In other words, it is an unconscious coping mechanism to evade tasks considered unpleasant. In the same study, Pychyl found that the prefrontal cortex may be both a newer and weaker portion of the brain. Because this portion of the brain is where the response to problems originates, it requires active thought and energy to generate a solution. However, particularly if the problem at hand is unpleasant, the limbic system reacts and creates a drive to ignore the task. But when an individual carves out the proper time to plan before acting, a surge of dopamine is released in the brain, producing a euphoric feeling of accomplishment.

UNDERSTANDING TIME MANAGEMENT IN COMPARISON TO PROCRASTINATION
Perhaps the key to understanding how to properly manage time is to understand what happens when time is improperly managed through procrastination. A coping mechanism for avoiding displeasing tasks, it leads to higher stress levels than if the task was com-

pleted sooner. Again, the limbic system's response to unpleasant situations tends to push people to not accomplish the assignment, leaving less time to accomplish it as well as a variety of physical symptoms associated with heightened anxiety—nausea, headache, weakness of limbs, etc. The two main types of procrastination are linked to behavior and decisions respectively. In one form of procrastination, a person self-sabotages to avoid action; in the other, a person avoids conflict and decisions. Both involve a multitude of psychological factors, including negative self-image, anxiety, high stress, and more.

Having proper time management boosts productivity, reduces stress, and the release of neurotransmitters such as dopamine creates a happy feeling that further boosts productivity. The process of collecting oneself and allotting time to finish a job is surprisingly more effective than going into a plan without the proper planning it requires, even leading to successes both short-term (such as good test grades or commendation on work presentations) and long-term (such as graduating with honors or receiving a promotion).

STRATEGIES TO ACCOMPLISH PROPER TIME MANAGEMENT

Mastering effective time management skills may seem daunting, but with a few basic skills, it can prove to be quite easy. Maintain a routine using a planner or daily "to-do" list. Use of one of these makes managing time easier, helping to establish continued, long-term success. The following tips are helpful to proper time management.

Prioritize goals and tasks. The following factors should be considered (a chart or a table will be helpful):
- The purposes and importance of each task relative to your short-term and long-term goals
- The deadline for each task
- The difficulty level of each task relative *to you*— How familiar are you with the task? If you encountered a similar task in the past, what was your performance? What did you learn from that experience? If the task is novel to you, what do you need to learn? How long will that take?
- Resources needed to complete each task—What resources do you need (information, money, instruments, social contacts)? How to locate them? How long will all this take?

Construct a time table/schedule.
- Generate a make-to-do list, with a deadline assigned to each task (schedule)—be practical and realistic. Build in some flexibility and have a back-up plan.
- Use smaller time units (hours/days) instead of larger units (weeks, months, years) when scheduling the tasks, especially when the tasks are related to long-term, future goals. Research has suggested that smaller time-unit frames (fine-tuned time metrics) help people connect their current self to a desired future self and prompts them to take action.
- Pool some tasks together so that you can multitask *safely* and *efficiently*. For example, taking a shower or having a ride in a car and mentally reviewing the key concepts for a test or outlining a paper is a good combination; but driving while eating or talking to a friend on a phone is a bad one and should be avoided.
- Develop a task matrix that includes easy, simple, familiar tasks and challenging, complex, novel ones—completion of an easy task gives you a break and a sense of accomplishment. In a similar fashion, make the schedule balanced with work, leisure, and rest, which in the long run will keep you psychologically sound and satisfied with your life.
- Break a challenging, lengthy task into smaller steps to make it more manageable. Give each step a deadline. Finishing each step not only makes a challenging task more hopeful but also satisfies

the basic psychological need for completion. Furthermore, it facilitates monitoring and adjusting.

Cultivate time-management attitudes and behaviors.
- Respect for and commit to the schedule. This not only helps you make steady progress toward the goal but also helps you avoid causing inconveniences to other people. Understand that your life is linked to other lives. There is a chain effect in teamwork; your task may be a step in a larger task or a necessary part to your peers' work. This is true when dealing with seemingly individual, independent work. For instance, not turning in an assignment to your teacher incurs disruption in the teacher's schedule—she won't be able to know your mastery level, finish the current learning unit and plan for the next unit accordingly.
- Be responsible and accountable. Manage your time well and complete all your tasks in a timely manner. Procrastinating or social loafing (being a free rider in group work) is irresponsible, showing a lack of respect for others and a poor work ethic.
- Start work early. Do not procrastinate. Life is full of surprises. Changes and unexpected things do occur. Waiting until the last minute does not give you any leeway to respond to the unexpected. It increases the risks of missing the deadline and compromising the work's quality. Procrastination usually leads to cramming, burning night oil, disrupting daily routines, all of which can result in stress and poor personal care (e.g., eating junk foods and lack of sleep). The stress-related toll on your body and mind may cause interpersonal conflicts, too. In contrast, starting work early has multifaceted benefits. You will have time to think and rethink, discuss the project with others, conduct further research, and revise and refine the work. Quality work will contribute to your own success and that of your social or work unit. This energizes a positive, healthy developmental cycle and is good for your well-being.
- Be flexible. Monitor your work progress and adjust your time allocation accordingly. An early start gives you flexibility for adaptation but procrastination leaves you no time to adjust.
- Instill the belief that the willpower needed for self-control and self-regulation is of great importance. In order to stick to the schedule to get the job done, it is necessary for adolescents to resist temptations, delay immediate gratifications, and sacrifice some personal desires. People holding the limited-willpower view think that fighting with temptations depletes ego energy, and they tend to display more problematic behaviors, including procrastination. In contrast, people holding the nonlimited-willpower view, that is, exercising willpower will be "self-generating," exhibit better self-regulating behaviors when they have many tasks to handle.
- Concentrate while working. Get rid of temptations and other distractors in your study and work environments. Undivided attention can save your cognitive energy. A quiet and comfortable environment can keep you cool (imagine how unpleasant noise and uncomfortable room temperature can irritate you). For serious cognitive work, multitasking is not recommended.

Another one of the most important time management skills is sleeping. An exhausted brain cannot think as quickly or with as much clarity as a well-rested brain can. Proper rest is also physiologically important; with sleep being such a vital life process disrupting it could lead to health complications as well. Shorter breaks should be used to refocus energy on the matter at hand, and longer weekend breaks and vacations should be used to retain long-term productivity. Proper nourishment is just as important for keeping the mind alert and attentive.

IMPLICATIONS FOR NURSING

Having knowledge and insight into the concept of time management through the concepts of time itself and procrastination have proven to be quite beneficial. Because nursing programs require both academic and clinical education, managing the time element of a difficult curriculum is critical. Being able to organize time appropriately allows commitments to study, perhaps work and recreation without shortchanging any life element. With an understanding of the various theories associated with the construct of time as well as comprehension of its polar opposite procrastination, one can take this knowledge and go forth with strategies to succeed in the nursing program.

The complexities of nursing require an ability to manage time. In all roles, multitasking, delegation and the ability to handle pressure are requisite skills. Planning the care delivery process for the working shift requires the ability to assess needs, prioritize activities and deliver care. Medications may be on a tight administration schedule. Blood pressure monitoring after surgery may be every fifteen minutes for two hours and then every hour after that initial period. Factor in that nurses may care for more than one patient and time management takes on an even greater need.

—*Courtney Brogle and Ling-Yi Zhou*

Further Reading

Booth, F. "30 Time Management Tips for a Work-Life Balance." *Forbes*, 28 Aug. 2014, http://www.forbes.com/sites/francesbooth/2014/08/28/30-time-management-tips. This article provides helpful tips to live a life with effective time management skills.

Herbet L. "How Your Brain Perceives Time (and How to Use It to Your Advantage)." *Lifehacker*, http://lifehacker.com/how-your-brain-perceives-time-and-how-to-use-it-to-you-511184192. This article evaluates the theories many researchers hold on the perception people have of time and how they manage their time.

Job, V., G. M. Walton, K. Bernecker, and C. S. Dweck. "Implicit Theories about Willpower Predict Self-Regulation and Grades in Everyday Life." *Journal of Personality and Social Psychology*, vol. 108, no. 4, pp. 637-47, doi:10.1037/pspp0000014. Reports a longitudinal study on how university students' limited or nonlimited view of willpower affected self-regulation behaviors.

Letham, S. "The Procrastination Problem." *Success Consciousness*, n.d., www.successconsciousness.com/guest_articles/procrastination.htm. This article examines the study of procrastination. Using scientific studies, it attempts to fully explain different concepts associated with procrastination and poor time management.

Lewis, N. A., and D. Oyserman. "When Does the Future Begin? Time Metrics Matter, Connecting Present and Future Selves." *Psychological Science* (OnlineFirst), 2015, doi:10.1177/0956797615572231, pss.sagepub.com/content/early/2015/04/23/0956797615572231.full.pdf+html. Reports how time metrics affected people's connection of future and current selves, which mediated their action even the perceived importance of future events was unchanged.

Spencer, A. "The Science Behind Procrastination." *Real Simple*, n.d., www.realsimple.com/work-life/life-strategies/time-management/procrastination. This article delves further into the ideas of Dr. Pychyl and the effect of the brain's structure on time management

COMMUNICATING EFFECTIVELY: INTERPERSONAL COMMUNICATION, SKILLS, AND TECHNOLOGY

ABSTRACT

Interpersonal communication is the process of sending and receiving messages. Interpersonal communication is effective when the message is received as the sender intended. Communication is an essential component of safe and effective nursing care. This can involve written communication, nonverbal communication, or face-to-face communication, but in today's world, interpersonal skills do not just relate to in-person interactions. Strong interpersonal skills now also relate to an individual's ability to effectively communicate with people through technology-based settings such as emails, texts, telehealth applications, and social media sites. While there are some similarities regarding how interpersonal skills present within face-to-face versus remote settings there are also important differences. Building one's interpersonal skills within the technology-medium is essential in today's era, which embraces technology-based methods for communication.

INTRODUCTION

Perhaps the most important critical skill to master is effective communication because it helps others to understand you, increases your understanding of others, increases others' positive feelings toward you, and decreases conflict.

Communication is the process of sending and receiving messages. Communication is effective when the message is received as the sender intended. This process can involve written communication, nonverbal communication, or interpersonal communication utilizing a variety of methods.

WRITTEN COMMUNICATION

Letters, papers, books, magazines, scripts, notes, texting, and social media all use written communication to convey a message. To be effective, written communication requires more than just jotting down a few words. It requires constructing the message to appeal to a particular audience and proofreading to catch any phrases that might cause a misunderstanding as

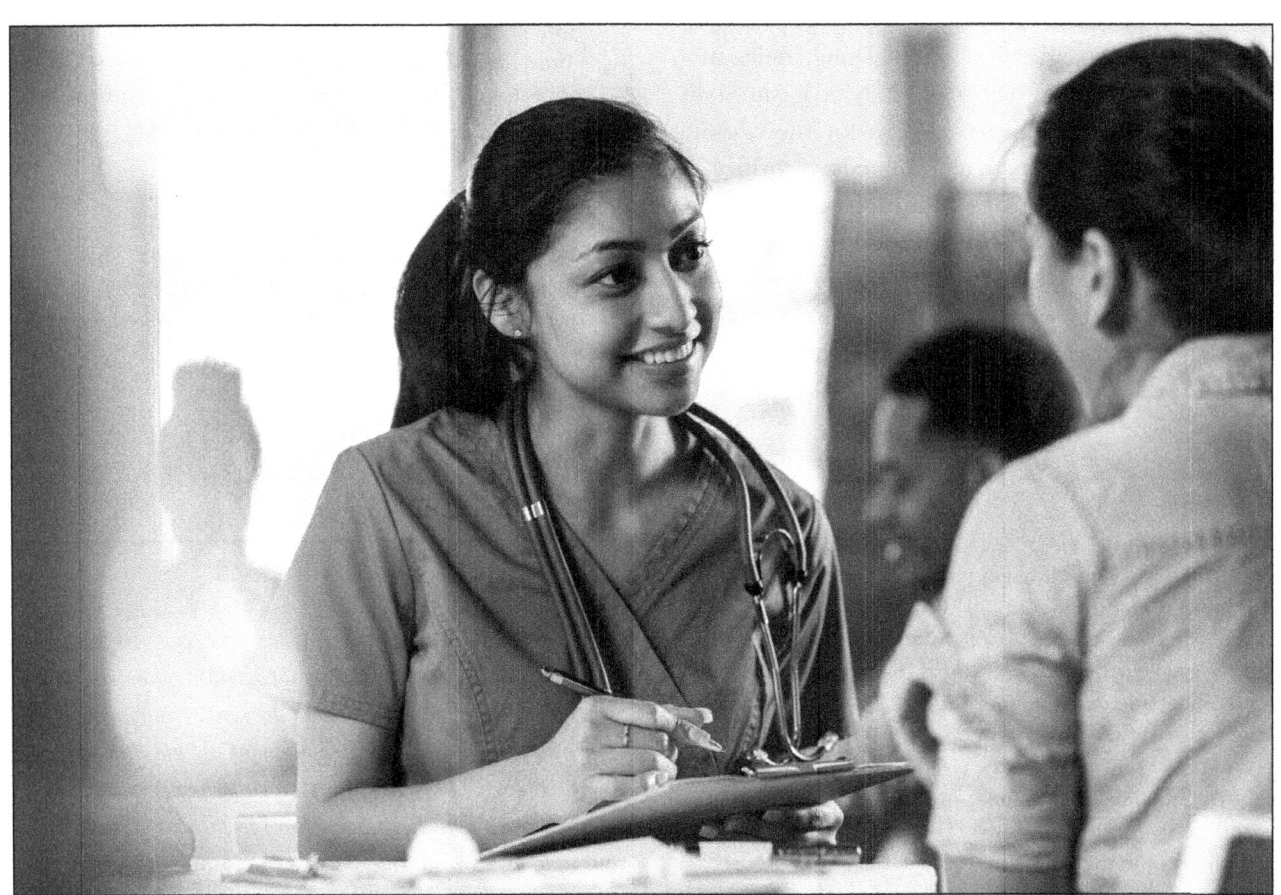

Signs that you are paying attention to the other person include: adopting an open posture, leaning forward, and making eye contact. (SDI Productions via iStock)

well as grammatical errors. In nursing, documentation online or in a paper chart is critical to communicate patient status to members of the healthcare team.

NONVERBAL COMMUNICATION

"It's not what you say, it's how you say it" describes the importance of nonverbal communication. According to Albert Mehrabian, only 7 percent of a message is conveyed through words. Thirty-eight percent is conveyed through vocal paralanguage (intonation, pitch, regional accent, hesitations). This paralanguage reveals our gender, age, geographic background, level of education, emotional state, attitudes, and our relationship with the person spoken to. Other nonverbal elements such as facial expression, gestures, physical appearance, posture, and proxemic behavior, comprise 55 percent of the message conveyed. Judgments are made based on these physical nonverbal elements and some of them are cultural or out of one's conscious control. Misunderstanding can then arise. Suspending judgment, not assuming anything based on a person's cultural group membership, and asking the other person their interpretation of their nonverbal communication helps dispel misunderstandings.

An important message that is sent through nonverbal behavior is whether you are paying full attention to the other person. If you sit facing that person with an open posture, slightly leaning forward, and making good eye contact, that person will know you are interested in what they are saying. Attending to the other person with these nonverbal cues also will cause the other person to like you more since everyone wants to feel listened to. Besides showing you are paying attention to the other person, smile. A smile goes a long way in establishing a good relationship. And, when one smiles, the other person usually smiles back, making you feel less nervous. As the saying goes, "smile and the whole world smiles with you." In nursing, assessment of both verbal and nonverbal cues is integral to knowing the status of the patient.

FACE-TO-FACE COMMUNICATION

Face-to-face communication involves at least two people in a meaningful exchange. The sender intends to affect the response of a particular person or persons. The message may be received in the way it was intended or it may get distorted. So, the sender needs to monitor how the message is sent and then how it was received by asking for feedback. In this way, any confusion or misunderstanding can be reduced.

SENDING MESSAGES EFFECTIVELY

Although saying what is on one's mind seems effortless, it really takes a great deal of skill to send a message so that the receiver does not become defensive and then distort the sender's message. For example, people who are straightforward with the messages they send, avoid the distortions that can occur when a person just hints at what they have in mind or they tell a third person, hoping the message will get to the intended recipient indirectly.

Owning one's messages by using "I" instead of "you" reduces the receiver's defensiveness. Notice the difference when you hear "I am concerned that you are spending too much time with her" instead of "You are spending too much time with her". Another skill involved in sending effective messages is being complete and specific as well as separating fact from opinion. A specific and complete statement is, "When you look away from me, I feel you are being insincere" as opposed to the vague and opinionated statement, "Nobody likes people who don't look at people."

One way of diminishing the natural tendency of the receiver to engage in mindreading, that is reading more into the message than what was sent, is for the sender to ask for feedback. The sender can ask, "Can you let me know your understanding of what we just talked about?" Or, "What is your reaction to what I just said?"

ROADBLOCKS TO INTERPERSONAL COMMUNICATION

Often, the sender does not stop to think how the message is going to be received before sending it. You, as the sender, may be in a rush to say what is on your mind. Or you may be thinking about what you want to say rather than closely paying attention to what the other person is saying before formulating a response. As Stephen R. Covey said, "Most people do not listen with the intent to understand; they listen with the intent to reply. They are either speaking or preparing to speak. We all want to be heard—that is why we speak. But most of the time we are so busy speaking that we don't listen. We don't listen to the other person. We don't even listen to ourselves."

For effective communication to occur, you must monitor yourself for at least the following three roadblocks that intensify interpersonal problems rather than alleviate them.

The first roadblock is judging, as in "You're just jealous" or "That's really wrong." The second roadblock is avoiding the other's concerns, as in "That happened to me too and it was awful" or "Don't worry, things will work out fine." The third roadblock is sending solutions, as in "You ought to do this...," or "Go make friends with someone else," or "If you do that, you'll be sorry."

You can prevent these roadblocks from occurring by pausing instead of giving a quick reaction to what the other person said. Before giving a reply or even initiating a conversation, it is important to listen to yourself. Notice any thoughts you are having or any strong emotional response that is arising. Instead of just impulsively expressing these thoughts, stop and ask yourself, "Am I saying this for my benefit rather than for having a good relationship with the other person?"

Listening closely and actively to what the other person is saying affects interpersonal communication even more than how a message is sent. When employers were asked to describe the communication skill they considered most important, listening was the number one response. Yet the average worker listens at only a 25 percent efficiency level.

Research also shows that immediately after a ten-minute presentation, a normal listener can recall only 50 percent of the information presented. After 48 hours, the recall level drops to 25 percent. This dismal state extends to students listening to a lecture or to patients listening to self-care procedures or discharge teaching. Active listening is important for both presenter and listener and asking for feedback to determine that the listener is hearing the presenter say is critical.

Poor listening not only causes a decrease in academic performance or patient outcomes, but it can lead to interpersonal conflict as well as frustration and a breakdown in communication. Yet, most people do not develop the ability to listen actively.

One of the reasons people do not make the effort to develop listening skills is they think they have more to gain by speaking than by listening. One big advantage of speaking is that it seems to give the speaker a chance to control others' thoughts and actions. Telling the other person what they should do is easier than first listening to what they want to do. Engaging the patient rather than telling the patient will result in better outcomes.

Another apparent advantage of speaking is the chance it provides to gain the admiration, respect, or liking of others. Tell jokes, and everyone will think, "there's a fun person". Offer advice, and they'll be grateful for the help. Make them impressed with your wisdom by pontificating. As you can quickly imagine, none of these strategies really work. Thus, there is a false assumption that the way to win friends and influence people is to talk rather than listen.

Finally, talking gives a person the chance to release energy in a way that listening can't. When you are frustrated, the chance to talk about your problems can often help you feel better. In the same way, you can often lessen your anger by letting it out verbally. And, sharing your excitement with others by talking about it helps when you feel as if you will burst if you keep it inside.

Although it's true that talking does have some advantages, it's important to realize that listening can pay dividends, too. Being a good listener is one good way to help others with their problems—and what better way is there to gain their appreciation? As for controlling others, it may be true that it's hard to be persuasive while you are listening, but your willingness to hear others out will often encourage them to think about your ideas in return. Like defensiveness, listening is often reciprocal: People get what they give.

Sometimes, even if a person wants to listen well, they're hampered by a lack of skill. A common but mistaken belief is that listening is like breathing, an activity that people do well naturally. "After all," the common belief goes, "I've been listening since I was a child. I don't need to study the subject in high school or college." The truth is that listening is a skill much like speaking: Virtually everybody does it, though few people do it well.

In today's rushed society, there are several reasons people don't listen well. The first reason is message overload. The amount of communications received through verbal and digital forms every day makes carefully attending to everything impossible. Almost half the time people are awake they are listening to verbal messages from teachers, coworkers, friends, family, salespeople, and total strangers, not to mention radio, television, and digital media. Research has shown people spend an average of five hours or more a day listening to people talk, 4 hours 28 minutes watching television and 5 hours 46 minutes with digital media. It looks like there is very little time spent in silence.

Another reason people don't always listen carefully is that they're often wrapped up in personal concerns that are of more immediate importance to them than the messages others are sending. It's hard to pay attention to someone else when you are anticipating an upcoming test or thinking about the wonderful time you had last night with good friends. A nurse must always put the patient first and set aside personal issues in order to focus on patient needs.

RECEIVING MESSAGES EFFECTIVELY

All of us are guilty of forming snap judgments, evaluating others before hearing them out. We also often listen to only what we want to hear. This tendency is greatest when the speaker's ideas conflict with our own. To really listen to another person is to set aside all of your distractions, expectations, judgments, anxieties, and self-concerns. Take a slow deep breath and open your ears, eyes, and heart to give center stage to the other person.

By focusing on the other person, you are putting him/her at ease and creating an atmosphere of trust. You may think it is important to talk about yourself to create a good impression, but just the opposite is true. Everyone wants to be listened to, so by attending to the other person instead of nervously talking about yourself, you are creating the best impression. To be listened to and acknowledged as heard is the greatest gift we can give or receive.

HOW TO SHOW YOU ARE LISTENING

As was mentioned in the section on nonverbal communication, show you are paying attention to the other person by adopting an open posture, leaning forward, and making eye contact. Then listen so closely to the other person that you can state back, in your own words, the essence of what you heard that person say. This is called paraphrasing. If your paraphrase is accurate, the person will, in some way, verbally or nonverbally, confirm its accuracy and usefulness.

Suppose a classmate tells you, "It's just a rough time for me—trying to work and keep up with school assignments. I keep telling myself it will slow down someday." You first ask yourself, "What has this person told me?" (That it's hard to keep up with everything he has to do.) Next you ask yourself, "What is the content of this message—what person, object, idea, or situation is the person discussing?" (Trying to keep up with work and school.) Finally you give a response, in your own words, such as, "It sounds like you're having a tough time balancing all your commitments" or "There are a lot of demands on your time right now."

When we paraphrase the listener relinquishes the leadership role, and "follows" the other person through the conversation. Sometimes, too, paraphrasing feels artificial when we first practice it. But, with added practice, paraphrasing sounds more natural.

To show you are listening at an even deeper level, use empathy. Empathy is the ability to identify with another person's experience. Empathy literally means "to feel in"—to stand in another's shoes, to get inside his/her feelings. It is listening so closely to another person that you can feel what he/she is feeling. And then it is the communication of this empathic understanding that creates trust, closeness, safety, and growth in relationships.

Empathy has been demonstrated to be one of the most important qualities for healthy relationships and for an individual's psychological health. Since the 1950s, empathy has been theorized to be essential for an individual's healthy development and has been identified as one of the most important skills parents need to develop psychologically healthy children. Empathy is essential for successfully resolving conflicts between individuals, between opposing groups of people, and even between nations.

GIVING FEEDBACK

Feedback gives clients an understanding of how others may view them. It is a reflective mirror, like empathy is, but it concentrates on the performance or behavior of the client whereas empathy deals with the statements the client makes.

Written and oral feedback is used in performance evaluations in families, education, sports, and healthcare. It is a primary strategy in documenting that patient teaching is being heard by the patient and is being internalized. The intent is to create behavior change and effective learning. Yet, in all of these settings, feedback is often given in a way that damages the relationship or the receiver. Damage occurs when the feedback concentrates on traits rather than behavior. Instead, feedback that is based on specific, observable behaviors leads to increased learning, fewer opportunities for misunderstandings, and gives clear criteria for what is and is not acceptable performance. Feedback does not give conclusions about the "goodness" or "badness" of behavior; it simply describes the behavior that is observed. When giving feedback based on behavior, think, "Who did what, when, and how?"

Feedback is effective when it is given:

- After asking the receiver's permission
- As promptly as possible after the observed behavior
- In a nonjudgmental way. For example, say, "When you look away from me, I feel you are not hearing the health information teaching you need to go home," as opposed to "Nobody likes people who don't look at people." Or, say, "I saw you relax and heard your joy as you went through that exercise," as opposed to, "You did that exercise very well."
- About the individual's strengths as well as his or her weaknesses.
- By being checked-out with the receiver to see how your feedback was received. Ask, "How do you react to that?" to begin a discussion between the two of you that doesn't end until both of you feel the feedback was accurately received and determine how useful it was. Asking if you feel comfortable with the information communicated can also be as simple as asking the person to repeat what they heard or do a return demonstration of the skill taught.

HANDLING CONFRONTATION

Confrontation can occur when you are trying to make a request or refuse a request. Assertive responding is an important way of getting your point across without increasing the other person's anxiety and creating a defensive reaction. The first step is to learn to make "I" statements instead of "you" statements. Here are some typical "you" statements that show aggression or passivity instead of appropriate assertion.

"Don't ever do that again."

Stop blaming the other person and, instead, tell the other person what you want. To change these statements into "I" statements use the following formula to tell the person how you feel and what you want.

"I feel...when you...and I want...."

The "I feel" part of the statement stops the other person from becoming defensive because it focuses on you rather than the other person and the other person is able to hear you better. The "when you" part of the statement is a pure description of what is bothering you about the other person's behavior.

Before you make an assertive statement, though, you must make an empathic statement. When you are asserting your position, you want the other person to accurately hear what you have to say. The other person won't hear you accurately if he/she is anxious and defensive. So, to prevent the other person from getting defensive or to disarm an already defensive person, make an empathic reflection. Then, state your assertion.

For example, if your friend criticizes you with, "You're not a good listener. Every time I try to talk with you, you act like you are just waiting for me to shut up so you can talk." You would first make an empathic reflection such as, "You feel I don't really listen to what you have to say...that I'm just waiting for you to finish so I can say what I want to say."

Then you can make an assertive statement about your own feelings such as, "Sometimes I have a difficult time trying to figure out what the main point is when you are giving me a long story about something. I would like you to be a little less wordy."

INTERPERSONAL SKILLS AND TECHNOLOGY

Interpersonal communication is a set of skills that require practice but, once these skills become your usual way of communicating, you will find your relationships to be more successful and satisfying. As technology increases within healthcare, interpersonal skills must evolve to meet the challenge. One issue with communication and technology is patient privacy if health-related messages are being transmitted. It is also imperative to protect patient privacy as required by the Health Insurance Portability and Accountability Act (HIPAA) developed in 1996. A primary component of the law is to require the healthcare industry to become more efficient in the use of electronic media for transmission of certain patient data. The government also developed privacy and security rules to protect health data.

The meaning of interpersonal skills has greatly expanded over the past couple of decades. Prior to the emergence of the internet and cellular phones, interpersonal skills were basically limited to in-person interactions. However, the abilities, advancement, and pervasiveness of today's technology have changed the way society as a whole interacts and communicates. While face-to-face communication remains an integral part of life, technology-based communication such as texting, emailing, and social networking (e.g., Facebook, Twitter, Instagram) has become a standard part of day-to-day communication. The emergence of telemedicine and telehealth, the use of electronic information and telecommunications technologies to support long-distance clinical care, includes videoconferencing, the internet, store and forward imaging, streaming media, and land and wireless communication. Due to the high prevalence of email, text, and social media forums as a standard way of communication, the aim of this article is to highlight both how interpersonal skills present within technology-based communication mediums and why having strong interpersonal skills related to one's email, texting, and social media use are so important.

EMAILING AND TEXTING

Since its inception, the use of emailing as a form of communication has exponentially increased. Reports from 2012 show that 144.8 billion emails are sent worldwide every day and the email rates are projected to increase to 206.6 billion emails per day in 2017. Email is the most widely used facility of the internet.

Similarly, texting is also a relatively recent medium tracing its entry into popular usage in the 1990's. The popularity of texting grew on the back of the massive technology boom in the personal mobile phone industry. The convenience and appeal of communicating by text was, and continues to be, immense; people can send messages instantly from anywhere. The convenience of text is so strong that it is the preferred form of communication for many people, particularly amongst younger individuals.

Since emailing and texting are common avenues for both professional and social interactions, the importance of having strong interpersonal skills in these areas is essential. However, when communicating via email or text valuable interpersonal information that is inherent to in-person communication is absent; the missing components relate to eye contact, body language, and rate of speech. Therefore, the remaining key interpersonal skills associated with email and text are the following: (1) Tone of voice intended by the writer, (2) Tone of voice interpreted by the receiver, (3) Intended meaning of the words typed, and (4) Interpretation of the meaning of the words typed.

TONE OF VOICE

Tone of voice relates to the emotion or attitude of how one's words are being conveyed. Some descriptors for tones of voice include but are not limited to: happy, angry, optimistic, negative, rude, empathic, frustrated, or sarcastic. The tone of voice adds significant meaning to the words being stated, but if misunderstood can be highly problematic since misunderstanding the tone of a message creates an entirely new meaning. Furthermore, interpreting the tone of voice from written words compared to an in-person verbal exchange increases the likelihood of the tone of voice being misjudged. Emails and texts do not allow one the privilege of assessing the speaker's nonverbal behaviors for cues on how to read their tone of voice. As recipients of an email or text all we have to go by are the words and punctuation contained in the written message.

Without being able to *hear* the actual tone it is challenging to properly identify how the person sending the message intended it to come across. This highlights why it is so important for the person writing the email or text to relay their tone clearly. The tools available to control tone include punctuation, sentence length, and word choice. The extra time you spend ensuring that your punctuation reflects your intended tone and that you have carefully chosen the words to convey your message properly, the stronger your interpersonal skills will become.

MEANING OF WORDS

Word choice serves two functions in written communication; firstly, it directly provides the meaning understood by recipients, secondly, it indirectly contributes to the tone of the message. When we write an email or text to somebody, we are seeking to communicate a message to the individual; our ultimate goal is for the individual to understand the message. It is crucial to remember that when interacting with people this way, particular attention needs to be given to the words used. The words people read directly impact their understanding of and reaction to the message. Making assumptions that the reader will know what is meant by the message is dangerous. Always be sure you are communicating your message clearly.

Use specifics like names rather than he or she, complete date, time and locations of meetings and other facts that are being communicated. By including more detail in the message through a different choice of words the friend is able to communicate their position much more clearly. Choosing your words carefully as the sender of a message reduces the onus of the reader to try and decipher what you mean based on the limited cues inherent in written communication.

SOCIAL MEDIA

The advent of social media has heralded unparalleled interaction and connection between individuals. Its reach across the globe and sharing based platform allows for communication to occur between people who have never even met before. While there are many benefits and significant positives to social media, users need to be aware of how they use social media so as to avoid the pitfalls presented by the numerous platforms

Similar to emails and texts, social media is primarily a written based medium, whether that is text only or also pictures. As such it is subject to the same limitations; eye contact, body language, and rate of speech is removed. Users of social media therefore need to be vigilant to ensure they create their messages carefully to be understood as intended. However, unlike email and texts, the sharing nature of social media presents some unique areas to take into consideration around interpersonal skills. The two biggest areas to be aware of are people sharing posts and information residing on the internet permanently. Patient privacy and the HIPAA regulations are important in nursing and the healthcare industry. Most employers have a significant set of policies and procedures related to patient and patient data protection that must be followed.

SHARING POSTS

The ability for information to be disseminated through social media so quickly is built on the function of it being able to be shared by users. A post can be shared between many, many people who spread it extremely quickly, in the extreme making it viral. It is very difficult for the original poster to have any control over their post in this circumstance. The inability to control such rapid dissemination demands that users be vigilant about their posts, particularly as it exposes individuals to miscommunication that can lead to unfavorable outcomes. In some cases, this can be harmless, however, it can have real life consequences.

An additional feature of the sharing aspect that is important to understand revolves around the fact that people are able to post and share anything they want. That includes information about you! This creates a fusion between events in the real world and the cyberworld; think of social media as a giant scrapbook where everybody has control over what is included in the scrapbook. The demands placed on interpersonal skills are huge!

Information Residing Permanently on the Internet

If you say something you regret in-person more often than not the situation is short lived. For example, you may be temporarily embarrassed, or you may have angered somebody but you are usually able to smooth it out shortly afterwards. However, information that finds itself into social media has a much more permanent nature. Even for posts that you originate, you only have very limited control. The availability of this information presents a unique interpersonal frontier: people formulate opinions, pass judgment, and make decisions based on something online. It is not uncommon for both prospective and current employers trawling through social media accounts to get information about individuals. Due to the very real consequences related to social media activity it is important to keep in mind the same key concepts when expressing yourself via Facebook as you do when writing an email or text.

SUMMARY

Communicating effectively is a life skill that will benefit the individual regardless of career choice. In nursing, effective communication can be the difference in life and death. The ability to communicate with people directly or without actually being in their presence is amazing and has many positive implications. It is important however to realize how speaking to someone face-to-face versus via technology requires a different interpersonal skill set. As the use of telemedicine and telehealth increases, it will allow both a combination of effective communication and the ability to observe the patient during the visit process. Without being able to see the other person, read their body language, or hear their tone of voice the words used to convey a message whether by email, text, or a social media page are extremely important. Understanding the basic principles that are the foundation for both effective communication and effective technology-based communication is essential to actively building these interpersonal skills and has immense value in today's technology dominant society.

—*Patricia Stanfill Edens, Beverly B. Palmer, Stefan Leonte, and Kimberly Glazier*

Further Reading

Barclay, J. "Text Messaging: Does It Destroy Relationships?" *Snowdrift*, 2013, www.snowcollegenews.com/text-messaging-does-it-destroy-relationships/. This article discusses that while texting has benefits, the ease and frequency in which people's texts are misinterpreted can lead to significant negative outcomes. The author focuses on how texts have led to many break-ups, specifically among college students.

Bolton, R. *People Skills: How to Assert Yourself, Listen to Others, and Resolve Conflicts*. Simon and Schuster, 1986. This paperback book was published a while ago, but it is still available, and it contains additional information and specific examples of the skills mentioned in this article.

Demangone, A. "That's Not What I Meant!—Technology and Miscommunication." *National Association of Federal Credit Unions*, 2014, www.cuinsight.com/thats-not-what-i-meant-technology-and-miscommunication.html. This article focuses on how easily technology-based communication can be misinterpreted. It highlights the importance that the person writing the message take time when composing the email to increase the likelihood that the intended and received message are the same.

Ferrazzi, K. "How to Avoid Virtual Miscommunication." *Harvard Business Review*, 2013, hbr.org/2013/04/how-to-avoid-virtual-miscommun/. This article discusses how simple things can be misinterpreted when communication occurs remotely versus in-person. The author outlines six techniques to help increase the accuracy and effectiveness of technology-based communication.

"Health Information Privacy." HHS.gov, www.hhs.gov/hipaa/index.html. Accessed 27 Aug. 2020.

"What Is Telehealth? How Is Telehealth Different from Telemedicine?" *HealthIT.gov*, www.healthit.gov/faq/what-telehealth-how-telehealth-different-telemedicine. Accessed 27 Aug. 2020.

Winerman, L. "E-mails and Egos." *American Psychological Association*, www.apa.org/monitor/feb06/egos.aspx, 2006. This article discusses how the message intended in an email is often quite different than the actual message received. The inability to accurately convey one's tone of voice when writing an email is a key component that causes the discrepancy between the intended and received message. The authors discuss how people need to learn to see how others may perceive their message.

Wood, J. F. *Interpersonal Communication: Everyday Encounters*. Cengage Publishing, 2016. This book can be obtained online and it expands the information in this article by including ways to deal with many of the communication issues of today's relationships.

WRITING SKILLS

ABSTRACT

Writing is one of the most essential skills that anyone should develop not only as an employment skill, but as part of a rewarding, educated life. Today we live in a world that is rich in access to information. As always, command of basic skills (such as spelling and grammar) remains important, but in addition, writers must learn how to explore vast amounts of information, then choose and organize what is relevant to a specified task.

INTRODUCTION

The ability to organize one's thoughts in written form is an essential skill in most professional employment, including in sometimes surprising places. The desk sergeant in a police precinct house, for example, appreciates a police officer who can spell, compose cogent sentences, and communicate relevant information in an accurate and comprehensive manner. Taking phone messages that can be read and understood, writing a school paper, or sending thank you letters after interviews are all reasons for developing good writing skills. In nursing programs, writing care plans and papers is expected. Once school is complete, communicating information takes on an even greater role.

Today's informational landscape, with its constant barrage of information, contains its own dangers, and requires a degree of focus and purpose. In any given profession, the same basic skills may be applied, but adapted to different traditional formats. For example, nurses write on patient charts and enter information into electronic health records, news reporters write stories, social workers must keep case notes, and lawyers file briefs, but all require a knowledge of correct spelling and grammar and an ability to craft a message.

WRITING IN A WORLD OF TMI (TOO MUCH INFORMATION)

When given an assignment to write, define the subject as precisely as possible. This allows a writer to navigate oceans of information by fashioning precise search terms, so he or she will emerge with a cogent body of notes that will save time when composition begins. Create a computer file into which you place all information relevant to the subject. Enter your sources (complete with the uniform resource locator (URL) if you are working on the internet) when you first encounter them. Working "backwards"—retrieving sources long after first consulting them—can be very difficult in a world that is drowning in information. As you compile source material, do not forget the scope and size of an assignment, as well as your deadline.

Once you have assembled an array of notes and sources, you begin to make this body of work your own by paraphrasing and, where appropriate, using direct quotation to tell the reader how a given source is thinking and feeling. In some contexts, direct quotation can be very useful and, with credit, it is not plagiarism. Be aware, however, that too much quotation from a single source may exceed "fair use" as defined by copyright law, and require written permission. Even short excerpts (usually more than two lines) of song lyrics and poetry may exceed fair use. Limits on prose are looser. The United States Copyright Law does not define "fair use" precisely. Direct quotation using internet sources is very easy (copy and paste), so do not be tempted to use it when your own words are more appropriate. Most faculty use a software program to discover plagiarism in a submitted paper. Students have received no grade for a plagiarized paper or even been dropped from a class or programs.

As you work your way through a body of notes, you will begin not only to paraphrase sources (or quote directly), but also to organize your work. Move each piece of information up if you have an idea of where it may fit, or down if you do not. Delete if information is not useful, if it repeats what you already have done, or if you do not have the word allowance to include so much detail. You do not need to be perfect at this stage, so don't agonize. You'll get another chance.

WRITERS' WORKING CONDITIONS

As a writer, you are what you read. Reading does more than supply information for writing projects. It teaches you subconsciously how to write. While reading, a writer is absorbing spelling, sentence structure, and other basics. Make time each day for pleasure reading.

Writing is work and, as such, requires time independent of other activities, including social media. In a world where everyone is expected to be "plugged in" all the time, carving out time for writing can be very difficult, but it is essential. Serious writers must spend a few hours each day alone with their keyboards. In our world of information overload, this can be a challenge.

A writer must learn to self-edit, and to act as a critic of his or her own work before submitting to editors or professors. With that in mind, many professional editors discourage "sloppy copies," the practice of handing rough work off so that someone else can correct errors. While such practice may fill a pedagogical purpose in elementary school, its use in a professional context is an indication that a writer may be ignorant of the basics of spelling and sentence composition. When submitting a paper in high school or college, the final copy is expected to be as close to perfectly crafted as possible.

Along the same line, be very wary of "auto-correct" in word-processing software. Machines cannot judge context, and results can be very humorous. In one instance, for example, a reference to Martin Luther's 95 theses (tacked to a church door in Wittenberg, Germany during 1517), came up "feces." Only a machine would make such an error. Only a human being could catch it. Proofread your own work carefully because your familiarity with the work may cause you to gloss over errors, reading what you meant to say not what you actually wrote. Never be afraid of asking someone to read your work. A fresh perspective may earn you a better response or grade.

YOUR SUBCONSCIOUS CAN WORK WITH YOU

Everyone who writes has been faced with a deadline, facing a blank screen, staring at a clock, worried that the creative "sap" no longer runs. The deadline, the blank screen, and the ticking clock (symbolic of the deadline, and impending failure) forms a negative feedback loop, otherwise known as "writer's block."

At this point, a writer can try to force the creative process, but this usually fails. The mind is an unruly partner, and trying to whip it into action does little but reinforce the block. It's time to work with the subconscious—take a walk, or a shower. Wash the dishes. Lay on the couch and close your eyes, and put yourself in a mode in which the subconscious will work on your problems. After that, go back to work.

Never be without a piece of scrap paper and a pen. Your subconscious may feed you an idea when you are required to be doing something else. Jot down a few key words that will stimulate memory when you can sit down at the keyboard. In this way, stray thoughts can be collected and elaborated later. These are the building blocks of effective composition.

—*Bruce E. Johansen*

Further Reading
LaRocque, P. *The Book on Writing: The Ultimate Guide to Writing Well*. Grey and Guvnor Press, 2013. LaRoque, a master writer, shares advice on the art and craft of composition.
Provost, G. *100 Ways to Improve Your Writing*. New American Library, 1985. Provost provides quick, breezy, instruction on writing; in a decades-old title that has not gone out of print, or out of style.
Strunk, W., Jr. and White, E. B., editors. *The Elements of Style*. 4th ed., Longman, 1999. A classic, erudite practical guide to style and the basics of English composition.
"Writing Skills: Skills You Need." www.skillsyouneed.com/writing-skills.html. Accessed 1 Sept. 2020.
Writing Skills: Success in 20 Minutes a Day. 5th ed., Learning Press, 2012. This workbook contains basic advice on how to develop writing skills in an academic context.
Zinsser, W. *On Writing Well: The Classic Guide to Writing Nonfiction*. 30th anniversary ed., 7th ed., revised and updated. HarperCollins, and Harper Perennial, 2006. This title (like Strunk and White) is a classic guide that focuses on writing quality.

PUBLIC SPEAKING

ABSTRACT

Public speaking permeates almost all aspects of our lives. Despite its significance, the fear it stirs in people leads many to try and avoid it; for some, at all costs! Through their avoidance people ultimately serve to only short change themselves. By choosing to confront the fear elicited from the thought of public speaking, over time it can be overcome. Exposure work is a strong ally in conquering the fear associated with public speaking.

INTRODUCTION

The thought of giving a speech or presentation in front of an audience makes most people want to run and hide. The comedian Jerry Seinfeld uses humor to emphasize how strongly people fear speaking in front of others, "According to most studies, people's number one fear is public speaking. Number two is death. Death is number two. Does that sound right? This means to the average person, if you go to a funeral, you're better off in the casket than doing the eulogy." While most people try to avoid public speaking at all costs, the reality is it is nearly impossible to completely avoid. The more that public speaking is avoided, the more anxious people feel when "forced" to make a presentation or speech. This chronic avoidance leads to missed opportunities and prevents personal growth.

In the profession of nursing, public speaking is expected. From interviews by a college admission panel to presenting your rationale for admission to a nursing program, you may be asked to go in front of groups of people and tell them why you want to be a

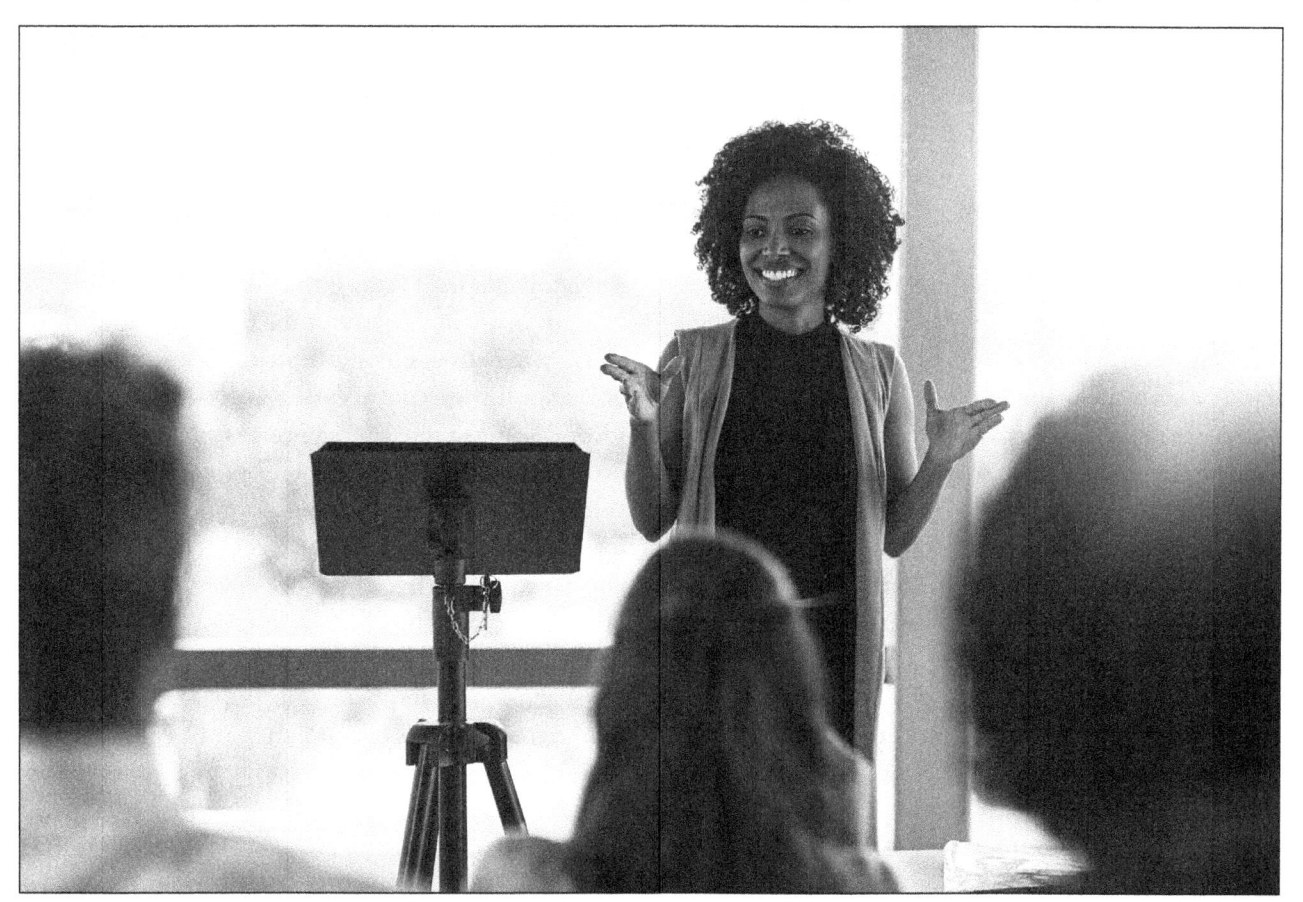

In nursing, public speaking is expected, from interviews by a college admission panel to presenting your rationale for admission to a nursing program. In nursing school, class projects presented to classmates, presentations of patient information to the faculty, and patient teaching sessions as part of a grade. Taking a job may require speaking with people in a group setting. For example, some hospitals ask job applicants to meet with potential colleagues, tell these colleagues why they might be a fit in their unit, and answer specific questions. Being comfortable in front of groups, whether small or large, is a necessary skill. (PeopleImages via iStock)

nurse. In nursing school, class projects presented to classmates, presentations of patient information to the faculty, and patient teaching sessions as part of a grade, are only a few examples of expected activities requiring public speaking. Taking a job may require speaking with people in a group setting. For example, some hospitals ask job applicants to meet with potential colleagues, tell these colleagues why they might be a fit in their unit, and answer specific questions. Being comfortable in front of groups, whether small or large, is a necessary skill.

The aim of this article is to highlight the prevalence and benefits of public speaking and to describe specific steps to transform public speaking from an anxiety provoking to enjoyable experience.

PUBLIC SPEAKING: MORE THAN GIVING SPEECHES

Public speaking includes but is broader than simply giving a speech to an audience; it refers to any time when a speaker orally communicates with an audience. The following are all examples of public speaking: speaking before a college admissions board, giving a class or work presentation, sharing a story to a group of people, reading aloud to others, speaking up during a team meeting to express your ideas, conducting a patient education program, giving a toast, and auditioning for a show. The range of activities that involve a public speaking component are numerous and span social, academic, and professional settings. Over the past few decades, the importance that employers place on applicants' public speaking abilities has increased substantially. Unfortunately, people's fear of public speaking has remained elevated.

OVERCOMING THE FEAR OF PUBLIC SPEAKING

There is an extensive body of literature that suggests the most effective way to overcome one's anxieties is to face the fear head on in a gradual and systematic fashion. This process is formally referred to as exposure work. For individuals who fear public speaking (which according to research is the majority of people) exposure work directly targets this fear. Since the main focus is to confront one's fear, at the beginning of the exposure people feel an increase in anxiety; this is an expected and necessary part of exposure work. However, the anxiety does decrease with repeated exposures, and the initial fear of public speaking lessens. As the anxiety lowers, one's self-confidence in their public speaking abilities typically increases.

While exposures are highly effective there are three key components that are important in order to truly benefit from them. The first two essential factors are the *frequency* and *consistency* of the exposure work, which determines both how quickly results are felt and how long the results last. Frequency refers to how often the exposures are conducted. Doing one presentation or answering a question in class once a month, or even once a week, will likely not lead to a significant reduction in one's anxiety of giving presentations or speaking up in class. When first starting out with exposure work, doing multiple exposures per day is important. The second aspect, consistency, refers to continuing to do the exposures on a regular basis. Doing five exposures on Monday but then waiting until the following Monday to do another five exposures has good frequency (five exposures per day vs. one exposure per day) but lacks the consistency (once a week vs. once a day). The reason that frequency and consistency are important is because the fear of public speaking has become so ingrained within the individual that in order to change one's perception of public speaking the person needs to create a new association of public speaking. This new perception is obtained through experience; the more often and more consistent the experiences occur the more quickly the new mindset becomes the natural way of thinking and believing.

DETERMINING WHERE TO START

The third key component for exposures relates to the systematic and gradual nature of the exposure work. For example, if an individual has a fear of public speaking then giving a presentation in front of an audience of 100 people would likely be far too overwhelming. Starting with this exposure would likely be too difficult to accomplish, and if attempted initially may lead to even more anxiety of public speaking. Depending on the individual's anxiety the presentation can start as basic as the following: presenting aloud to just oneself; looking at oneself in the mirror while presenting; presenting to one other person you feel comfortable with; presenting to a couple of people you feel comfortable with; presenting to someone you feel less comfortable with; presenting to a small group of people. If needed, the exposure presentations to others could start with having the audience member(s) initially not looking at the speaker during the presentation and then working up to having the audience face the presenter. Eventually the process could include having the audience member ask a question(s) after the presentation. For more difficult exposures, the questions can be more challenging or even express disagreement with an aspect of the presentation. The possible variations with creating the exposure hierarchy are countless and the key is for each person to develop their own hierarchy that has a range of exposures, including some that are anxiety provoking but manageable and others that initially would be extremely challenging or "impossible" for the person to complete. Starting with the more manageable items allows the person to gain a sense of mastery and accomplishment and eventually makes the initial "impossible" tasks seem less scary and more doable.

WHEN TO USE IMAGINAL EXPOSURES

Sometimes it may be impossible for the individual to make one or more presentations a day (or even a week) to audiences. In these situations, imaginal exposures can be used. For imaginal exposures the presenter should imagine they are standing in front of an audience. The key is for the person to truly immerse themselves in the situation by visually seeing and mentally and/or verbally describing all the details of the event. All five senses (sight, smell, hearing, taste, and touch) should be incorporated when visualizing and describing the situation; this is important as it helps increase how real the exposure feels.

Another time to use imaginal exposures is when the situation itself may be too overwhelming at first. For example, if the person has a fear of public speaking related to having conversations with a group of people, imaginal exposures would be a good place to start. The same rules apply here; the imaginal exposure should involve the person visualizing and describing the situation in as much detail as possible, which includes using the five senses. During the exposure the person should engage in an imaginal conversation in which the individual is an active contributor to the conversation.

REAL-LIFE IMPORTANCE

Public speaking is a skill. It is something that is learned and mastered. Ralph Waldo Emerson acknowledges how public speaking abilities are not inherent within an individual; he believed "All great speakers were bad speakers at first." Often times the biggest barrier to mastering the art of public speaking relates to individuals' fear of speaking in front of others and their resulting desire to minimize or avoid public speaking opportunities. It is very difficult to enjoy an activity whether it be socializing at a party, making a toast, or giving a speech or presentation when one is feeling high levels of anxiety. The good news is that by frequently confronting the fear in a systematic and consistent manner the anxiety related to public speaking scenarios decreases. By reducing the fear associated with these situations space opens up for the once present anxiety to be replaced with feelings of confidence, mastery, excitement, and happiness.

—*Kimberly Glazier and Stefan Leonte*

Further Reading

Adams, M. "Public Speaking 101–Become a Great Storyteller." *EDGE*, 2015, www.worldchampionsedgenet.com/resources/articles/becoming-a-great-storyteller/. This article emphasizes how learning to master the art of storytelling is integrally intertwined with becoming an exceptional public speaker. Specific strategies to increase one's storytelling abilities are outlined.

Branson, R. "Richard Branson on the Art of Public Speaking." *Entrepreneur*, 4 Feb. 2013, www.entrepreneur.com/article/225627. This article discusses the author's fear of public speaking. It also describes how he learned to overcome his fear, and how his ability to do so directly led to the elevated and international success of his company.

Quinn-Szcesuil, J. "How Can Public Speaking Help Your Career?" *Minority Nurse*, 2017, www.minoritynurse.com/how-can-public-speaking-help-your-career/. Accessed 30 Aug. 2020.

"Why Is Public Speaking Important?" *Writing Commons*, writingcommons.org/open-text/genres/public-speaking/844-why-is-public-speaking-important. Accessed 4 May 2015. This article describes the following three common types of public speaking: informative, persuasive, and entertaining. It also outlines the significant role that public speaking plays in all individuals' lives and highlights how building one's public speaking abilities simultaneously improves one's critical thinking abilities.

Zeoli, R. "Seven Principles of Effective Public Speaking." *American Management Association*, 16 Apr. 2014, www.amanet.org/training/articles/Seven-Principles-of-Effective-Public-Speaking.aspx. This article talks about how public speaking is a skill that is learned. It proceeds to outline seven key principles that help teach individuals how to improve their public speaking abilities.

NETWORKING

ABSTRACT

In today's competitive climate, networking is a valuable tool for young adults to develop. Networking opportunities can arise through social media, extracurricular activities, hobbies, and interests. The first step in networking is being aware of the opportunities that exist, so that they can help you with your future wants. Whether you are networking for a career goal, social interest, or college, this article will provide guidelines to help you navigate the process of using networking to attain your goals.

INTRODUCTION

Networking is a skill that many leaders learned early on. It can be practiced and learned in a variety of settings. The first thing to do to encourage networking is to pick a field, college, profession or interest that you would like to learn more about and find like-minded sites or individuals who can help you succeed in these fields. Networking is an important social skill, as it can help you meet individuals that can help you attain your professional and personal goals. Social connections can help you get access to resources or people that can help you get a job, get into the college of your dreams, or master a hobby. Seeking out networking opportunities can help you improve your resume or find a mentor in your field of interest. It can also help you develop social and communication skills.

There are many social media sites that contain blogs or chat rooms where you can communicate with people who share the same interests as you. If it is a specific college you want to go to, social networking can be a good way to start. A recent study has shown that 92 percent of teenagers go online daily, and in this decade, social media has become a requirement for succeeding at networking. Some online sites where young adults connect include Facebook, Tumblr, Instagram, Twitter, and others. It is very important to maintain a professional environment with everything you post regardless of site. Realize that your words, photos, and videos will be scrutinized carefully and that future job employers and college admission counselors will be viewing your postings. What you post and write can be used against you, so be very cautious with what you chose to put on social media. With that precaution in mind, online sites have proven to be a successful part of the networking process. In this day and age if you do not have access to social media, you are at a great disadvantage, and may be seen by some to be behind in technology.

Networking can help you create a career portfolio, and can give you access to leaders in your field of interest. One way to increase your chances of in-person networking is to attend career or college days. These usually occur at high schools, colleges, or at specific locations that are usually posted online. While you are at one of these events, ask about the possibility of shadowing a student, employee, or member of the faculty. This is a great way to further enhance your networking skills and gain valuable work experience.

In-person networking opportunities can teach you a lot about yourself and the way you handle the networking process. During the process you can evaluate yourself on how you associate with others. Body language is an important nonverbal communication skill that should be considered and developed. Remember to smile, focus, and maintain an open demeanor. Sit up straight, and try not to cross your hands in front of your chest or hunch. These nonverbal clues can all be learned or unlearned to help navigate the networking process. Wearing a name tag can also help at networking events, and can serve as a reminder to the person you are talking with. While you network in a social setting, remember to ask open-ended questions, as this allows the person you are talking with to share more about themselves. Listen carefully and with interest to what the person in front of you is saying. Jot down names, occupations, and the topics of conversation discretely during in-person networking or as soon as you leave the event. Keep a list of connections that may be helpful to you later in your college admissions process or employment.

Expressing yourself verbally, with clarity, is also a key part of the networking process. Many young adults have found something in common with the person they speak with, and this commonality can provide one with a serious connection that may be able to help in the future. At networking events, save business cards, attendee lists or pamphlets, and write follow up thank you notes if you spend a significant amount of time with a key individual. If it is a college event, try to schedule an interview with an alumni member before you leave. Remember that networking can provide you with an opportunity to meet a mentor who can help you with your goals. Networking opportunities can also arise through friends and family, so remember to let people know you are interested in a certain goal or college, and ask if they have any connections they might introduce to you.

Being a successful networker does mean you have to be present at events, and show up at meetings. These events provide you an excellent opportunity to meet people who have attained the goals you would like to. While at the events, walk around the room, and see if you know someone or see a familiar face. If not, go up to someone friendly, shake his or her hand, and introduce yourself and your grade level. If you recognize that this person is someone that is key in your field, be sure to express that you have read their article, social media post, or something that tells them you are aware of their importance and reputation. People love to talk about themselves and their accomplishments, and this will put you both at ease.

Realize that networking opportunities are available all over. At airports, cafes, or even your local coffee shop, you can run into a person who will help you advance your profession, or who knows something about the admission process of the college of your choice. For example, if you see someone with a college sweatshirt on, tell them you are applying to the school. Not all people attend the school on their sweatshirt, but many do, and it's a great way to meet a new contact. If you notice someone reading a nursing textbook, ask where they are going to school and let them know you are interested in the profession. Be sure to thank them if they take time to chat and if not, apologize for interrupting them. It is important to see networking as a valuable opportunity to help you attain your goals.

Always dress the part for a networking event. Wearing professional clothing is important. Depending on personal preferences and events, you can decide if you want to cover up identifying features such as tattoos or extra piercings. Some people are judgmental, and at an interview or networking event you are being judged and evaluated by the person in front of you. Remember to always act professionally at a networking event or interview. Show up on time and do not use questionable language, slang, or street terminology when communicating with the person you are interviewing or networking with, no matter how laid back you perceive them to be. When not attending a specific event, be sure when you are out in public and decide to interact with a potential contact, that you are neat and clean. First appearances are critical if you are going to ask their help later.

The hope is that after your networking opportunity or interview, you receive the job, volunteer opportunity, or college acceptance letter! Congratulations! At an appropriate time, you can then ask your network connection to write you a letter of recommendation for future employment or academic opportunities. This letter can prove your value and your connection with your networking contact. Ask for both a paper and electronic copy of the letter of recommendation, and be sure to save your electronic letters on your computer, and your print letters in a paper-based portfolio.

—*Bernadette Riley and Gina Riley*

Further Reading

"10 Tips for Effective Networking." *University of Maryland, Baltimore County*, careers.umbc.edu/students/network/networking101/tips/. Accessed 30 Aug. 2020.

Christian, C., and R. Bolles. *What Color Is Your Parachute for Teens: Discovering Yourself, Defining your Future*. 2nd ed., Ten Speed Press, 2010. A book about finding your strengths and interests at an early age, so that you can decide what type of schooling, job, or career is right for you. This book includes profiles of individuals who have leveraged their strengths to find their dream job.

Cohen, S., A. Dwane, P. deOliveira, and M. Muska. *Getting In! The Zinch Guide to College Admissions and Financial Aid in the Digital Age*. Cliff Notes, 2011. A short, well-researched, current guide for mastering the college admissions process. Includes information on college admissions offices, application guidelines, choosing the right college, athletic recruiting, and scholarship/financial aid opportunities. This book also contains helpful sections on college essay assistance and waiting for an answer after the application process.

Kouzes, J. M., and B. Z. Posner. *The Leadership Challenge: How to Make Extraordinary Things Happen in Organizations*. Jossey Bass, 2012. A book about how individuals can create positive change within their organization by engaging in practices of modeling, shared vision, challenge, action, and heart-based encouragement. Provides information on forward moving leadership, integrating tenets of intrinsic motivation and desires in planning and doing within corporations, companies, and nonprofit organizations.

Lenhart, A. "Teens, Social Media & Technology Overview–2015." *Pew Research Center*, www.pewinternet.org/2015/04/09/teens-social-media-technology-2015/. A review of social media and technology use in teenagers. Trends include increased use of smartphones and mobile devices, as well as continuing use of social media platforms like Facebook and Twitter. Use of Instagram, Snapchat, Tumblr, and Google+ is also discussed.

Rath, T. *Strengths Finder 2.0*. Gallup Publishing, 2007. This is a classic book about finding and leveraging your strengths in the classroom, at work, during interviews, and at home. Purchase of this book in electronic or print format comes with a code that allows you to take an online assessment that highlights your five signature strengths.

NURSING SPECIALTIES

One of the largest in this work, this section includes 23 specific types of nursing options available, from more general roles, like staff nurse, travel nurse, telehealth nurse, and nurse administrator to very specific ones, including neonatal, gerontological, wound care, clinical research, and palliative nurse. Settings vary as well, from large hospitals to small doctor's offices. In addition, this section includes important roles like transitional care from home into a nursing home for example, educator, continuing education coordinator and patient educator.

Staff Nurse and Primary Care Nurse	151
Nursing Administrator	152
Medical-Surgical Nurses and Perioperative Nurses	154
Obstetric and Neonatal Nurses	157
Perinatology	159
Pediatrics	162
Gerontological Nursing	170
Critical Care Nursing	173
Clinical Nurse Specialist (CNS)	176
Doctor's Office, Clinic Nurses, and Physician Assistants (PAs)	177
Nurse Practitioner (NP)	179
Nurse Anesthetist	181
Home Health Nurse and Public Health Nurse	184
Occupational Health	187
Transitional Care	189
Wound, Ostomy, and Continence (WOC) Nurse	191
Telehealth Nursing	192
Palliative Care and Hospice Nursing	194
Travel Nurse	198
Clinical Research Nurse	199
Case Management/Utilization Management and Care Navigation	201
Educators—Academic and Vocational Programs	203
Continuing Education Coordinator and Patient Educator	205

Staff Nurse and Primary Care Nurse

ABSTRACT

Staff nurses are registered nurses who work at a hospital, nursing home, or a similar institution. They provide general services to the patients that come in for treatment. Primary care nurses are nurse practitioners who work with specific patients over an extended period of time.

STAFF NURSE

The term staff nurse comprises a large range of healthcare workers, but it primarily refers to registered nurses (RNs) who are employed in a healthcare facility. This facility is usually a hospital but may also be a nursing home, outpatient clinic, or a similar setting. In general, staff nurses are responsible for working side-by-side with other healthcare professionals, including physicians, other nurses, and nurse assistants, in order to treat and manage the patients that are admitted to the institution. Staff nurses generally work in assigned shifts and are supervised by nurse managers or charge nurses.

Nurse managers are nursing professionals who are in charge of running individual units. They coordinate between all the different individuals working on their floor and upper management and are in charge of making sure the unit is performing up to standard. They generally do not see patients. Charge nurses are responsible for managing the nursing shifts in their unit. They perform administrative tasks such as creating schedules and help provide feedback on the performance of the nurses in their charge. They may also assist with direct patient care. One key difference between the two positions is that while charge nurses only manage the nurses in their unit, nurse managers supervise support staff and other non-nurses as well, in addition to performing more macro-level tasks, such as overseeing budgets.

The staff nurse, working under the supervision of these two professionals, is often the first person a patient encounters when admitted to the hospital. The staff nurse is charged with assessing the patient's condition and taking the patient's vital signs. The staff nurse may also administer medications and injections, help perform diagnostic testing, help draw up a care plan for the patients, and educate patients. They typically work in close cooperation with physicians and other healthcare professionals. Unlike nurses who work in a doctor's office setting and usually look after one patient at a time, staff nurses in hospitals generally care for multiple patients at a time. They also typically work much longer shifts, usually three twelve-hour shifts. As such, being a staff nurse can be a taxing and stressful job.

To secure a staff job at a hospital, the candidate will need to become an RN. This can be accomplished by completing a nursing program—earning an associate's degree, a bachelor's degree, or a diploma—and passing the certification exam, the NCLEX-RN (National Council Licensure Examination). Charge nurses typically have a bachelor's degree in nursing as well as at least three-to-five years experience working as an RN in a clinical setting. Nurse managers typically hold at least a bachelor's degree and frequently a master's degree, either an MSN (Master of Science in Nursing) or a degree in management.

PRIMARY CARE NURSE

Primary care nurses are advanced practice registered nurses (APRNs) who work with a specific patient or patients over an extended period of time. While physicians have traditionally served as a patient's primary care provider, with ongoing shortages of MDs, nurses and physician assistants have increasingly taken on this role. Primary care nurses may work in a number of settings including hospitals, private clinics or offices, nursing homes, or in private at-home care. The primary care nurse is charged with diagnosing patients, planning and implementing treatment strategies, educating the patient and their family about their condition and treatment, administering medication, and other related tasks.

Primary care is the first level of care that patients receive and primary care nurses are often the patient's first point of contact when they have medical concerns. Primary care nurses are typically licensed nurse practitioners. Not all nurse practitioners, though, are primary care nurses, as they can work in secondary and tertiary care as well, depending on their specialty.

To become a nurse practitioner, a candidate must first qualify as an RN, typically by earning a bachelor's of science in nursing (BSN) degree. They will then obtain either a master's degree or a doctorate. Increasingly, a doctorate is preferred. Most nurse practitioners who obtain a doctorate earn a Doctor of Nursing Practice (DNP). They may also earn a PhD in nursing, although this degree is primary for candidates who wish to pursue research or an academic career. The DNP program builds on the MSN degree and allows students to further specialize; students who are studying to be a nurse practitioner will focus largely on that practice. The program lasts from three to five years and is designed to prepare students in eight key competencies, including organizational and systems leadership, healthcare policy, and evidence-based practice. All DNP students are also required to fulfill 1,000 clinical practice hours.

After earning their degree, students must obtain certification as a nurse practitioner. This involves them passing an examination given by one of the two certification boards, the American Nurses Credentialing Center (ANCC) or the American Academy of Nurse Practitioners Certification Board (AAPCB). Candidates become certified in their specific area of professional interest. Those who wish to become primary care nurses may opt for the Adult-Gerontology Primary Care Nurse Practitioner Certification (ACPCNP-BC) or the Family Nurse Practitioner Certification (FNP-BC).

—*Andrew Schenker*

Further Reading

"Complete Job Description of a Staff Nurse." TopRNtoBSN.com. www.toprntobsn.com/job-description-staff-nurse/. Accessed 5 Oct. 2020.

Dunphy, Lynne M. *Primary Care: The Art and Science of Advanced Practice Nursing—An Interprofessional Approach.* 5th ed., F.A. Davis Company, 2019.

"Primary Care Nursing Careers & Salary Outlook." *NurseJournal.* 31 July 2020. nursejournal.org/primary-care-nursing/primary-care-nursing-careers-salary-outlook/.

"Registered Nurses." U.S. Bureau of Labor Statistics. *Occupational Outlook Handbook.* www.bls.gov/ooh/healthcare/registered-nurses.htm. Accessed 5 Oct. 2020.

"The Difference Between Nurse Manager vs. Charge Nurse: Leadership Roles in Healthcare." Maryville University. online.maryville.edu/vs/nurse-manager-vs-charge-nurse/. Accessed 5 Oct. 2020.

Nursing Administrator

ABSTRACT

Nurses who work in an administrative or supervisory role may assume a number of different jobs. Nurse mangers supervise nursing staff in a hospital setting and serve as a liaison between management and staff. Directors of nursing are nurses who organize and oversee nursing operations in a hospital or similar setting. Chief nursing officers are the top nursing administrators in their organization.

NURSE MANAGER

Nurse managers are nursing professionals who bridge the gap between beside nurses and nursing administration. According to the American Organization of Nurse Executives, "the nurse manager is responsible for creating safe, healthy environments that support the work of the healthcare team and contribute to patient engagement." Nurse managers are responsible for directing, supervising, and leading the staff of a hospital or medical facility, including nurses and support staff. They typically work in a hospital setting where they manage a specific unit or specialized floor.

Other settings in which a nurse manager might work include urgent care clinics, doctor's offices, nursing homes, or home healthcare.

Because of their managerial duties, nurse managers do not typically provide direct care to patients but may assist staff if needed. Instead, they are tasked with directing the nursing staff, overseeing patient care, and being involved in some budgetary and management decisions. Among the daily tasks that a nurse manager may perform are hiring, training, and evaluating staff members; serving as a liaison between nursing staff and administration; assisting with escalated situations; scheduling shifts; attending to paperwork; and reporting on finances. Nurse managers usually spend much of their time in an office setting rather than directly working in a clinical setting. They may also attend various administrative meetings and serve on committees.

Nurse managers may be advanced practice registered nurse (APRNs) in larger facilities, which means that they hold at least a master's degree. Some nurse managers may hold a bachelor's degree but this is becoming less common in urban settings. The first step towards becoming a nurse manager is to become an RN. This involves earning a bachelor's degree in nursing and then passing the licensing exam, the NCLEX-RN (National Council Licensure Examination). (Although some RNs may hold an associate's degree or a diploma, these are usually considered insufficient for becoming a nurse manager). After earning their bachelor's degree, candidates will typically gain several years of bedside experience before being appointed nurse manager or pursuing a master's degree. Many nurse managers hold an MSN (Master of Science in Nursing). Nurse managers may become licensed by taking a certification exam, either the Nurse Executive or Nurse Executive, Advanced certification, both offered through the American Nurses Credentialing Center (ANCC).

DIRECTOR OF NURSING

Directors of nursing, also known as nurse directors, are administrators who organize and oversee nursing operations in a hospital or similar setting. In some facilities, the top nursing executive may still be called the Director of Nursing. These nursing professionals advise administrators and other senior staff on questions of nursing service while serving as a liaison between nurses, management and administration. Directors of nursing typically work in an office and do not provide direct patient care. Although they frequently work in hospitals, they may also find employment in any number of other settings, including doctor's offices, long-term care facilities, insurance companies, healthcare companies, government agencies, and colleges and universities.

The specific tasks that a director of nursing performs may vary based on the size and type of the institution for which they work. Some common jobs they perform include supervising nursing staff, overseeing the department's budget, managing patient records, working on planning and development, overseeing inventory, resolving escalated situations, and reporting to high-level staff members. The director of nursing is a leadership role and those who take it on are expected to be adept at managing difficult situations and to be strong communicators.

Directors of nursing are RNs with a degree in nursing, usually at minimum a bachelor's degree with extensive experience or a postgraduate degree, and have passed the certification exam, the NCLEX-RN (National Council Licensure Examination). Many directors of nursing positions now require an advanced degree, typically an MSN (Master of Science in Nursing) or a master's degree in healthcare administration. Some directors of nursing go on to earn a Doctor of Nursing Practice (DNP) degree. Directors of nursing have several opportunities for certification, including the Nurse Executive Certification (NE-BC) through the American Nurses Credentialing Center (ANCC), the Director of Nursing Services (DNS-CT) credential though the American Association of Directors of Nursing Services (AADNS), and the Certified Director of Nursing (CDON) credential though the National Association of Directors of Nursing Administration in Long Term Care (NADONA LTC).

CHIEF NURSING OFFICER (CNO)
Chief nursing officers (CNOs), also known as chief nurse executives (CNEs) or vice presidents of nursing, are the top nursing managers in an organization. They are responsible for managing and coordinating the daily activities of the nursing department in the hospital or other organization in which they work. As in other nursing management positions, they serve as a liaison between nursing staff and administration. In addition to hospitals, CNOs may work in outpatient clinics, group physician practices, government agencies, and for healthcare companies.

CNOs perform a wide range of activities revolving around the management and administration of the nursing department and advising senior management as to how to best carry out the institution's nursing practices. Among the specific tasks a CNO might perform include managing nursing budgets, conducting performance assessments, planning new patient services, organizing and administering best practices in nursing care, representing nurses in board meetings and other settings, and educating staff. Although CNOs do not typically recruit and hire staff, they may manage the personnel that oversee hiring. In some settings, the CNO may be responsible for managing several nursing departments within the same healthcare system.

Before becoming a CNO, a candidate will typically have many years experience in the nursing field, including in management positions. Although a Bachelor of Science in Nursing (BSN) degree is the minimum requirement for the position, a master's degree is increasingly preferred. The accrediting body for hospitals and other health facilities, the Joint Commission, addresses these requirements in the Nursing Standards Chapter of their manual. A Master of Science in Nursing (MSN) is most often the standard degree for the job, though candidates may also be expected to have postgraduate schooling in management. To achieve this goal, a candidate may specialize in Nursing Administration or Leadership in Health Care Systems when earning their MSN or pursue a dual-degree program, either an MSN/MHA (Master of Health Administration) or an MSN/MBA (Master of Business Administration). Some larger organizations or more prestigious positions may require the candidate to hold a Doctor of Nursing Practice (DNP) degree.

—*Andrew Schenker*

Further Reading
"Chief Nursing Officer." Registered Nursing.org. www.registerednursing.org/specialty/chief-nursing-officer/. Accessed 6 Oct. 2020.
"Director of Nursing." Registered Nursing.org. www.registerednursing.org/specialty/director-of-nursing/. Accessed 6 Oct. 2020.
"Nurse Manager." Nurse.org. 9 July 9 2020. nurse.org/resources/nurse-manager/. Accessed 6 Oct. 2020.
"Nurse Manager: Leading the Nurse Profession into the Future." Duquesne University School of Nursing. onlinenursing.duq.edu/blog/roles-nurse-manager-leading-nursing-profession-future/. Accessed 6 Oct. 2020.
Roussel, Linda. *Management and Leadership for Nurse Administrators*. 8th ed., Jones & Bartlett Learning, 2020.
Ruesink, Megan. "What Does It Really Take to Be a Director of Nursing?" Rasmussen College. 21 June 2017. www.rasmussen.edu/degrees/nursing/blog/director-of-nursing/. Accessed 6 Oct. 2020.
"Standards." The Joint Commission. www.jointcommission.org/standards/. Accessed 10 Oct. 2020.

MEDICAL-SURGICAL NURSES AND PERIOPERATIVE NURSES

ABSTRACT
Medical-surgical nursing is the largest nursing specialty in the United States. Medical-surgical nurses provide a variety

of different nursing services for adult patients in a number of different settings. Perioperative nurses work specifically with patients who are having surgery or other invasive procedures.

MEDICAL-SURGICAL NURSING

Medical-surgical nurses, often referred to as med-surg nurses, are generalists. Working in a hospital, clinic, or other similar setting, these professionals are experts in a wide range of conditions. Med-Surg nurses are responsible for caring for the patients with both surgical and medical (nonsurgical) conditions. Typically, the patients treated by these professionals present a diverse array of conditions and ailments with which the med-surg nurse must be familiar. Their general duties include coordinating care plans for patients, educating patients about their conditions and care, working to implement care, and assessing the patient on a regular basis. They usually work under the supervision of a manager or charge nurse.

In the early history of the nursing profession, most nurses worked in hospital settings, performing bedside care. These nurses were considered medical-surgical nurses. As the profession grew, however, the role of the med-surg nurse expanded and became its own specialty. As a result, medical-surgical nurses today work in a large number of different settings, including clinics, emergency departments, nursing homes, health maintenance organizations (HMOs), home healthcare, telemedicine, and ambulatory nursing. Because of the variety of care provided by the med-surg nurse, it is often a position held by newly graduated nurses who have not yet specialized and who learn from the variety of conditions they encounter on the job. Nonetheless, many veteran nurses practice in a medical-surgical setting as well. According to the Academy of Medical-Surgical Nurses (AMSN), the professional association for the profession in the United States, medical-surgical nursing is the single largest nursing specialty in the country.

The educational requirements for becoming a medical-surgical nurse are the same as for other registered nurses (RNs). Candidates must first complete a nursing degree, either an associates' degree, a bachelor's degree, or a diploma. For many employers, the bachelor's degree program, BSN (bachelor of science in nursing), is increasingly preferred, and some medical-surgical nurses go on to complete a master's degree, too. After graduation, students must pass the certifying exam, the NCLEX-RN (National Council Licensure Exam-Registered Nurse), in order to practice. These new RNs then typically participate in a comprehensive orientation program or participate in an internship program for medical-surgical nursing before working on their own. All hospitals offer a comprehensive orientation program designed to certify skills and orient the new employee to policies and procedures. Some hospitals may offer an even more comprehensive internship designed to build on skills learned in nursing programs. After two years of employment, medical-surgical nurses are eligible to receive further certification in the form of the Certified Medical-Surgical Registered Nurse (CMSRN) credential, which is offered through the Medical-Surgical Nursing Certification Board (MSNCB) or the Medical-Surgical Nursing Certification (RN-BC), offered by the American Nurses Credentialing Center (ANCC).

PERIOPERATIVE NURSING

Perioperative nurses, also known as operating room (OR) nurses or surgical nurses, are RNs that assist during surgery or other invasive procedures. Perioperative nurses work in every type of surgical situation and they are charged with caring for patients before, during, and after the surgical procedure. They work in a variety of settings, including hospitals, clinics, and surgery centers—wherever surgeries or invasive procedures are performed. The exact nature of the tasks performed by perioperative nurses depends on the specific role and location of practice. Perioperative nurses are involved in the preoperative, intraoperative and postoperative process of patient care.

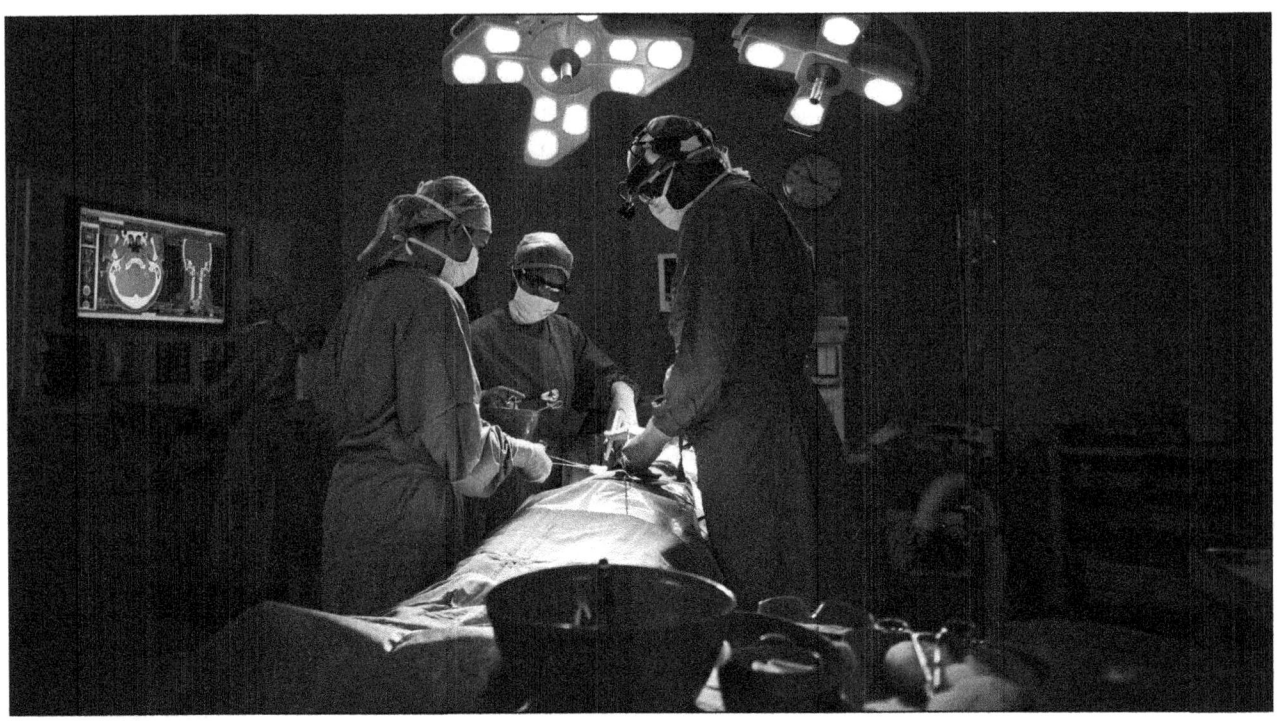

Perioperative nurses, also known as operating room nurses or surgical nurses, are registered nurses (RNs) that assist during surgery. Perioperative nurses work in every type of surgical situation. (shapecharge via iStock)

Generally speaking, there are four essential roles performed by perioperative nurses: scrub nurse, circulating nurse, RN first assistant (RNFA), and PACU (postanesthesia care unit) RN. The scrub nurse, responsible for selecting and passing instruments to the surgeon, works within the sterile field in the operating room. In conjunction with the circulating nurse, they set up the OR for the patient, choose instruments and supplies, and hand surgical instruments to the surgeon. The circulating nurse works outside the sterile field and is in charge of managing activities in the operating room. Among their tasks are inspecting surgical equipment, reviewing preoperative assessments with the patient and making sure consent forms are signed, and ensuring that surgical sterility is maintained. The RNFA works directly with the surgeon to assist in controlling bleeding, assists with suturing, observes for complications, and applies dressings and bandages. The RNFA also attends to the patient's care before, during, and after the surgery. Some surgeons provide their own RNFA who is credentialed by the hospital to assist the surgeon within the policies and procedures of the facility. The PACU nurse is responsible for the care of the patient immediately after surgery. They monitor the patient as they stabilize after the procedure and prepare them for transfer to another unit. The PACU in the past was also referred to as the recovery room. In addition to these four principal roles, a perioperative nurse may work as an operating room director, in which they manage the budget, staffing, and ordering of equipment for the OR; as a clinical educator; or as a researcher.

In order to become a perioperative nurse, a candidate must first fulfill the requirements for a RN, which include graduation from a nursing program (either with an associate's degree, a bachelor's degree, or a diploma) and passing the NCLEX-RN (National Council Licensure Examination) in order to become certified. After graduation and certification, nurses typically must complete an additional year of education or training in order to work as a perioperative nurse. This requirement can be carried out either by enrolling in a postbachelor's perioperative certificate program or by on-the-job training or internships offered by hospitals. The Association of periOperative Registered Nurses (AORN), the primary professional organization for perioperative nurses in the United States, also offers an online program, "Periop 101: A Core Curriculum." Many other programs, whether the on-the-job programs in hospitals or the certificate programs, are based on the standards set by AORN's course.

For perioperative nurses looking to advance their careers, there are several additional options. After they have completed at least two years and 2,400 hours of professional perioperative work, a nurse is qualified to pursue the Certified Perioperative Nurse (CNOR) credential. The CNOR is offered through the Competency and Credentialing Institute (CCI), requires passing a 185-question exam, and is valid for five years. In order to work as an RNFA, a nurse must complete a formal, accredited RNFA program. These programs typically last two to three semesters. After completion of the degree and 2,000 hours of documented practice as an RFNA, a nurse is eligible to pursue the Certified Registered Nurse Assistant (CRNFA) credential which is also offered through the CCI.

—*Andrew Schenker*

Further Reading

Academy of Medical-Surgical Nurses (AMSN), www.amsn.org. Accessed 29 Sept. 2020.

Association of periOperative Registered Nurses (AORN), www.aorn.org. Accessed 30 Sept. 2020.

"How to Become a Perioperative Nurse." *GraduateNursingEDU.org*, www.graduatenursingedu.org/perioperative/#:~:text=Perioperative%20nurses%20help%20plan%2C%20carry,%2C%20during%2C%20and%20after%20surgery. Accessed 29, 2020.

Ignatavicius, Donna D., et al. *Clinical Companion for Medical-Surgical Nursing: Concepts for Interprofessional Collaborative Care*. 9th ed., Elsevier, 2018.

"Medical-Surgical Nurse." *Registered Nursing.org*, www.registerednursing.org/specialty/medical-surgical-nurse/. Accessed 29 Sept. 2020.

"Periop 101: A Core Curriculum(tm) OR Course Outcomes." *Association of periOperative Registered Nurses (AORN)*, www.aorn.ort/education/facility-solutions/periop-101/course-outcomes.

"Registered Nurse First Assistant." *Nurse.org*, nurse.org/resources/rnfa-career-guide/. Accessed 29 Sept. 2020.

"Surgical Nurse." *Nurse.org*, nurse.org/resources/perioperative-surgical-nurse/. Accessed 29 Sept. 2020.

OBSTETRIC AND NEONATAL NURSES

ABSTRACT

Obstetric nurses are registered nurses (RNs) who care for mothers before, during, and after childbirth. Neonatal nurses work with newborn babies experiencing complications, helping new mothers to care for their infants. They may be RNs or, in the case of neonatal nurse practitioners, advanced practice nurses.

OBSTETRIC NURSING

Obstetric (OB) nurses, also known as perinatal nurses, provide care for patients during pregnancy, labor and childbirth. They typically work in the maternity unit of a hospital, an obstetric-gynecology (OB-GYN) office, a midwife practice, a private birthing center, or any other setting where women give birth or prepare to give birth. OB nurses are responsible for supporting and assisting expectant mothers during every stage of their pregnancy and into the early days of the postpartum period. During the period before the mother gives birth, the OB nurse will discuss the birthing process with the patient and provide education and support for the expectant mother. They will also either perform or assist a physician (obstetrician) in performing various prenatal exams and procedures. These may include pelvic exams, ultrasounds, mammograms, urine and blood samples, weight monitoring, and the administration of medicine. OB nurses may also meet with women who wish to become pregnant and offer advice and education to these patients as well.

During the birth, the OB nurse will typically be in the birthing suite where they perform two principal roles, as an assistant to the obstetrician and as a coach for the patient. Many hospitals utilize private birthing suites for low-risk deliveries meant to feel like home where women stay during labor, deliver in the room and then stay for a while after birth before moving to a nursing unit. High risk births, such as those requiring cesarean sections (C-sections) will be done in a surgical suite or special delivery room. Among the specific tasks an OB nurse performs during delivery are preparing the mother for delivery, starting an intravenous (IV) drip, labor coaching, noting complications and reporting them to the doctor, and administrating ordered medication. Following the delivery, the OB nurse will closely monitor the mother and baby for a few hours before they are sent to postpartum care. They will monitor the vital signs of both baby and mother and manage any complications that may have occurred. They may also assist the mother with breastfeeding or bottle feeding with formula.

In postpartum care, the OB nurse will help the mother recover from the labor, while educating her about newborn care. The nurse will also administer medication and any necessary shots, monitor any swelling or bleeding, and draw blood for tests for the mother. They will also clean, weigh, and administer medication as ordered to the newborn child. The obstetric nurse may continue to care for the mother after she is discharged from the hospital, conducting follow-up visits and seeing after the continued health of both mother and child. Some OB nurses continue to provide routine care for mothers through menopause.

OB nurses are RNs, which means they have completed a nursing program—earning either an associate's degree, a bachelor's degree, or a diploma—and passed a certifying exam, the NCLEX-RN (National Council Licensure Examination-Registered Nurse).

Before practicing as an OB nurse, the candidate will typically gain clinical experience working in women's health. After working in the field for two years, nurses are eligible for official certification. The credential offered to OB nurses is the Inpatient Obstetric Nursing certification which is granted by the National Certification Corporation (NCC).

Nurse midwives are nursing professionals who provide a wide range of health services for women, especially during and after pregnancy. Among the services performed by a nurse midwife are delivering babies, providing surgical assistance to physicians during C-section births, performing gynecological exams, and offering family planning services and prenatal care. In some cases, nurse midwives may serve as a woman's primary maternity care provider. Certified nurse midwives are advanced practice registered nurses (APRNs) and have completed graduate coursework, either at the master's or doctorate level, and have passed the Certified Nurse Midwife (CNM) examination.

NEONATAL NURSING
Neonatal nurses work with newborn infants experiencing one or more birth issues that require critical care. The infants may be premature, have birth defects, have infections, may be born addicted, or suffer other acute conditions. Neonatal nurses typically work in a hospital or clinic, but may also work in a community center or other related setting. Some neonatal nurses work in a hospital's neonatal intensive care unit (NICU) and are known as NICU nurses.

The neonatal period refers to the first month of a child's life, but neonatal nurses may care for their patients for longer than that period. Some neonatal nurses continue to care for patients who experience long-term illness for a number of years after birth. Neonatal nurses observe newborns closely to determine if their behavior is normal or if it requires intervention. Neonatal nurses perform a variety of duties, which may include administrating medication, resuscitating infants, or helping the mother breastfeed her child. They may also perform administrative work such as dividing patient loads and reviewing notes.

Neonatal nurses are RNs. The RN may be a graduate of an associate's degree program or a diploma nursing program, but a bachelor's degree is becoming increasingly preferred. After completing their education, candidates must then pass the NCLEX-RN licensing exam. To become a neonatal certified nurse, nurses must also earn a neonatal care certificate, either the RNC Certification for Neonatal Intensive Care (RNC-NIC) or the Critical Care RN (Neonatal) certification, as well as certification in neonatal resuscitation. To become a neonatal nurse practitioner, candidates must complete either a master's or doctorate program in nursing and earn state certification in the state in which they wish to practice.

—*Andrew Schenker*

Further Reading
"A Day in the Life of an Obstetric Nurse." *City College*, www.citycollege.edu/ob-nurse/. Accessed 1 Oct. 2020.
Flavin, Brianna. "The Info You Need to Know About Being a Neonatal Nurse." *Rasmussen College*, 20 Jan. 2020, www.rasmussen.edu/degrees/nursing/blog/being-a-neonatal-nurse/.
"How to Become a Neonatal Nurse Specialist or Practitioner." *All Nursing Schools*, www.allnursingschools.com/specialties/neonatal-nursing/. Accessed 1 Oct. 2020.
Murray, Sharon, et al. *Foundations of Maternal-Newborn and Women's Health Nursing*. 7th ed., Elsevier, 2019.
"Obstetrics (OB) Nurse." *RegisteredNursing.org*, www.registerednursing.org/specialty/obstetrics-ob-nurse. Accessed 1 Oct. 2020.

PERINATOLOGY

ABSTRACT
Perinatology is the branch of medicine dealing with the fetus and infant during the perinatal period (from the twenty-eighth week of gestation to the twenty-eighth day after birth).

A perinatal nurse provides care from preconception to pregnancy and the weeks following birth, often teaching what to expect during pregnancy, types of childbirth available, postpartum issues, and care of the baby.

SCIENCE AND PROFESSION
Practitioners of perinatal medicine include physicians and advanced practice nurses with a specialty in perinatology (neonatal and pediatric nurse practitioners). They then complete additional training specifically related to the perinatal period (defined variously as beginning from twenty to twenty-eight weeks of gestation and ending one to four weeks after birth). The emphasis of perinatology is on a time period rather than on a specific organ system. The principal event of the perinatal period is birth. Prior to delivery, the perinatologist is concerned with the physiological status and well-being of both mother and fetus. Immediately after delivery, the perinatologist strives to maximize the newborn's chances for survival.

The perinatal nurse may work in a variety of diverse settings, including clinics, medical offices, and hospitals. Working in labor and delivery nursing units, antepartum and postpartum units, teaching labor and delivery classes are just a few opportunities for careers in perinatal nursing. The perinatal nurse works in collaboration with advanced practice nurses and physicians to support the care continuum around pregnancy and childbirth.

DIAGNOSTIC AND TREATMENT TECHNIQUES
Prior to the birth, several diagnostic procedures are commonly employed by the perinatologist: ultrasonography, the measurement of fetal activity, and the evaluation of fetal lung maturity. Ultrasonography uses sound waves to create images. Sound waves are transmitted from a transducer that has been placed on the skin. Waves that are sent into the body reflect off internal tissues and structures, and the reflections are received by a microphone. Sound travels through

tissues with different densities at different rates, which are characteristic for each tissue.

Computers interpret the reflected sounds and convert them into an image that can be viewed. The images must be interpreted or read by someone with specialized training, usually a radiologist. Ultrasound does not involve radiation so it is not harmful to the fetus. Because sound waves are longer than radiation, the image generated is not as clear as that obtained with electromagnetic waves such as those from a computed tomography (CT) scan or a conventional X-ray.

The measurement of fetal activity is important in evaluating fetal health. Fetal movement is normal; the earliest movement felt by the mother is called quickening. The diminution or cessation of fetal movement is indicative of fetal distress. Accordingly, movement is monitored by reports from the mother, palpation by the clinician, and ultrasound: Mothers report movements, individuals examining pregnant women can apply their hands to the abdomen and feel fetal movements, and ultrasonography can show breathing and other movements in real time using continuous video records of fetal movements.

Fetal lung maturity is assessed by measuring the relative amounts of lecithin and sphingomyelin in amniotic fluid. The concentration of lecithin increases late in fetal development, while sphingomyelin decreases. A lecithin-sphingomyelin ratio that is greater than two indicates sufficient fetal lung maturity to ensure survival after birth.

Labor and delivery are the primary events of the perinatal period. The perinatal nurse is actively in-

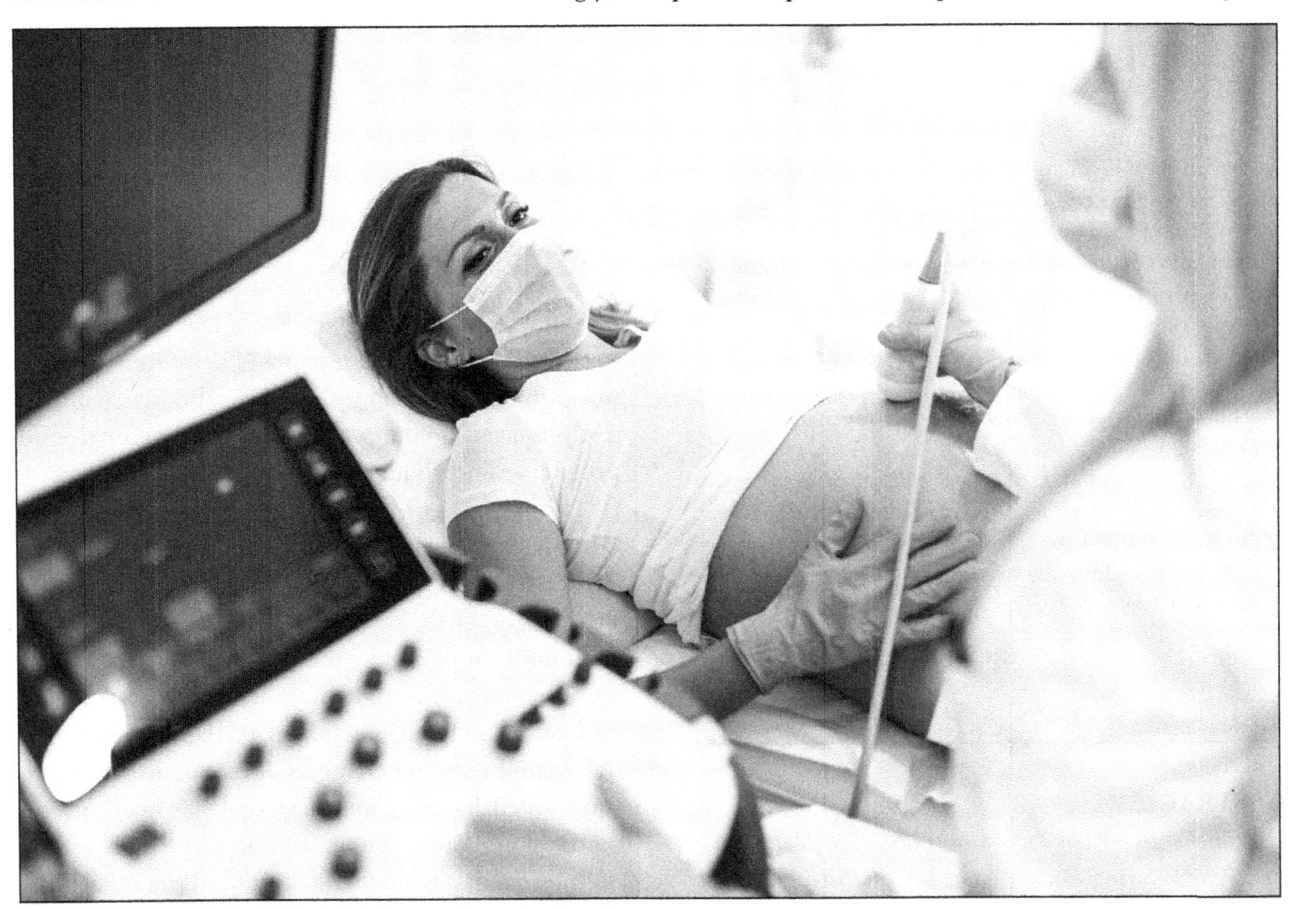

A pregnant woman gets an ultrasound (nito100 via iStock)

volved in assessing and monitoring status of the woman in labor. Factors that can lead to difficulties include abnormalities of the placenta and prematurity. The placenta can be abnormally located (placenta previa) or can separate prematurely (placenta abruptio). Normally, the placenta is located on the lateral wall of the uterus. Placenta previa is defined as a placenta located in the lower portion of the uterus. The placenta is compressed by the fetus during passage through the birth canal. This compression compromises the blood supply to the fetus, which causes ischemia and can lead to brain or other tissue damage or to death. This condition is usually managed by a cesarean section. Placenta abruptio refers to a normal placenta that separates prior to fetal delivery. This condition is potentially life-threatening to both mother and fetus; immediate hospitalization is indicated.

Prematurity is defined as delivery before the fetus is able to survive without unusual support. Premature infants are placed in incubators. A lack of body fat in the infant leads to difficulty in maintaining a normal body temperature; special heating is provided to offset the problem. Lung immaturity may require mechanical assistance from a respirator. An immature immune system makes premature infants especially susceptible to infections; strict isolation precautions and prophylactic antibiotic therapy address this problem.

Many factors contribute to increasing the risks normally associated with pregnancy and delivery: maternal size and age; drug, tobacco, or alcohol use; infection; medical conditions such as diabetes mellitus and hypertension; and multiple gestations. A woman with a small pelvic opening may be unable to deliver her child normally; the solution in this case is a cesarean section. The risk of genetic abnormalities increases with advancing maternal (and, to a lesser degree, paternal) age. Counseling prior to conception is indicated. Once an older woman becomes pregnant, amniotic fluid should be obtained to test for genetic abnormalities. The degree of surveillance is dependent on maternal age: The recommended frequency of medical checks increases for older women.

Alcohol intake during pregnancy can result in an infant who is developmentally disabled; smoking during pregnancy frequently leads to an infant with a low birth weight. Drug usage during pregnancy can lead to anatomic or mental impairment. Avoiding the use of all substances is the easiest way to eliminate problems completely; any drug should be used only under the guidance of a physician. Some viral infections such as German measles (rubella) early in pregnancy can cause birth defects. Immunization prior to conception will avoid these problems.

Diabetes mellitus can cause abnormally large intrauterine growth and babies (frequently more than 10 pounds and referred to as macrosomic) who are too large for normal delivery. Diabetes that commonly develops during pregnancy is called gestational diabetes. Medical monitoring to detect diabetes early is prudent. Appropriate medical management of preexisting diabetes minimizes problems associated with pregnancy. A macrosomic infant must be delivered with a cesarean section. Hypertension can also develop during pregnancy. Like diabetes, it can compromise both mother and fetus. Appropriate and aggressive medical management, sometimes including complete bed rest, is needed to control high blood pressure during pregnancy. Multiple gestations (such as twins or triplets) strain the supply of maternal nutrients to the developing fetuses. Because space is limited, multiple fetuses are usually smaller than normal at birth.

Rhesus disease, also known as Rh incompatibility, can complicate pregnancy. It can occur only in the child of a father whose blood type is Rh-positive and a mother whose blood type is Rh-negative, and it affects the blood supply of a fetus. The treatment includes the identification of both maternal and paternal blood types and the administration of Rho(D) immune globulin to the mother at twenty-six weeks of gestation and again immediately after birth. An affected infant may require blood transfusions; in a severe case, transfusions may be needed during pregnancy.

PERSPECTIVE AND PROSPECTS

Management of a pregnancy requires specialized skills. As the number of risk factors related to either mother or fetus increases, the problems associated with pregnancy also increase. The care of a pregnant woman and her fetus requires input from many individuals with specialized training. Consequently, perinatology is very much a team effort. Together, the team members can ensure a safe journey through the perinatal period for a pregnant woman and a healthy transition to life outside the womb for a newborn infant.

—*L. Fleming Fallon, Jr.*

Further Reading

Bradford, Nikki. *Your Premature Baby: The First Five Years.* Firefly Books, 2003.

Creasy, Robert K., and Robert Resnik, editors. *Maternal-Fetal Medicine: Principles and Practice.* 5th ed., W. B. Saunders, 2004.

Cunningham, F. Gary, et al., editors. *Williams Obstetrics.* 23rd ed., McGraw-Hill, 2010.

Martin, Richard J., Avroy A. Fanaroff, and Michele C. Walsh, editors. *Fanaroff and Martin's Neonatal-Perinatal Medicine: Diseases of the Fetus and Infant.* 2 vols. 9th ed., Mosby/Elsevier, 2010.

Moore, Keith L., and T. V. N. Persaud. *The Developing Human.* 9th ed., Saunders/Elsevier, 2013.

"Perinatal Nurse." *Johnson & Johnson Nursing*, nursing.jnj.com/specialty/perinatal-nurse. Accessed 3 Sept. 2020.

"Perinatal Nurse." *Nursing Explorer*, www.nursingexplorer.com/careers/perinatal-nurse. Accessed 3 Sept. 2020.

"Pregnancy and Perinatology Branch (PPB)." *National Institute of Child Health and Human Development*, 30 Nov., 2012.

Ruhlman, Michael. *Walk on Water: Inside an Elite Pediatric Surgery Unit.* Viking-Penguin, 2003.

Sadler, T. W. *Langman's Medical Embryology.* Lippincott Williams & Wilkins, 2014.

"Women's Health Perinatal Nursing Care Quality Measures." *The Association of Women's Health, Obstetric and Neonatal Nurses (AWHONN)*, awhonn.org/womens-health-perinatal-nursing-care-quality-measures/. Accessed 3 Sept. 2020.

PEDIATRICS

ABSTRACT

Pediatrics is the field of medicine devoted to the care of children from birth through childhood, puberty, and adolescence. The specialty focuses on the physical, psychosocial, developmental, and mental health of children usually under the age of eighteen. In some cases, individuals over the age of eighteen, such as children with developmental delays or mental retardation may be better served by a pediatrician or in a pediatric unit.

SCIENCE AND PROFESSION

Pediatrics is one of the widest-ranging medical specialties, embracing virtually all major medical disciplines. Some pediatricians, physicians with additional training, are generalists, and others specialize in pediatric cardiology, pediatric endocrinology, pediatric gastroenterology, pediatric oncology and hematology, pediatric dermatology, pediatric emergency medicine, or pediatric surgery.

A pediatric nurse is a registered nurse (RN) or an advanced practice nurse (APRN) with special training in pediatrics. There are also pediatric nurse practitioners (PNP) who are RN's with advanced degrees that allow them to prescribe medicines, perform developmental screenings, and administer immunizations.

Pediatric nurses work in a variety of settings. Hospitals and health systems, physician offices, clinics, surgical centers and any health facility that provides care for children. Neonatal intensive care units (ICUs), pediatric critical care units and pediatric on-

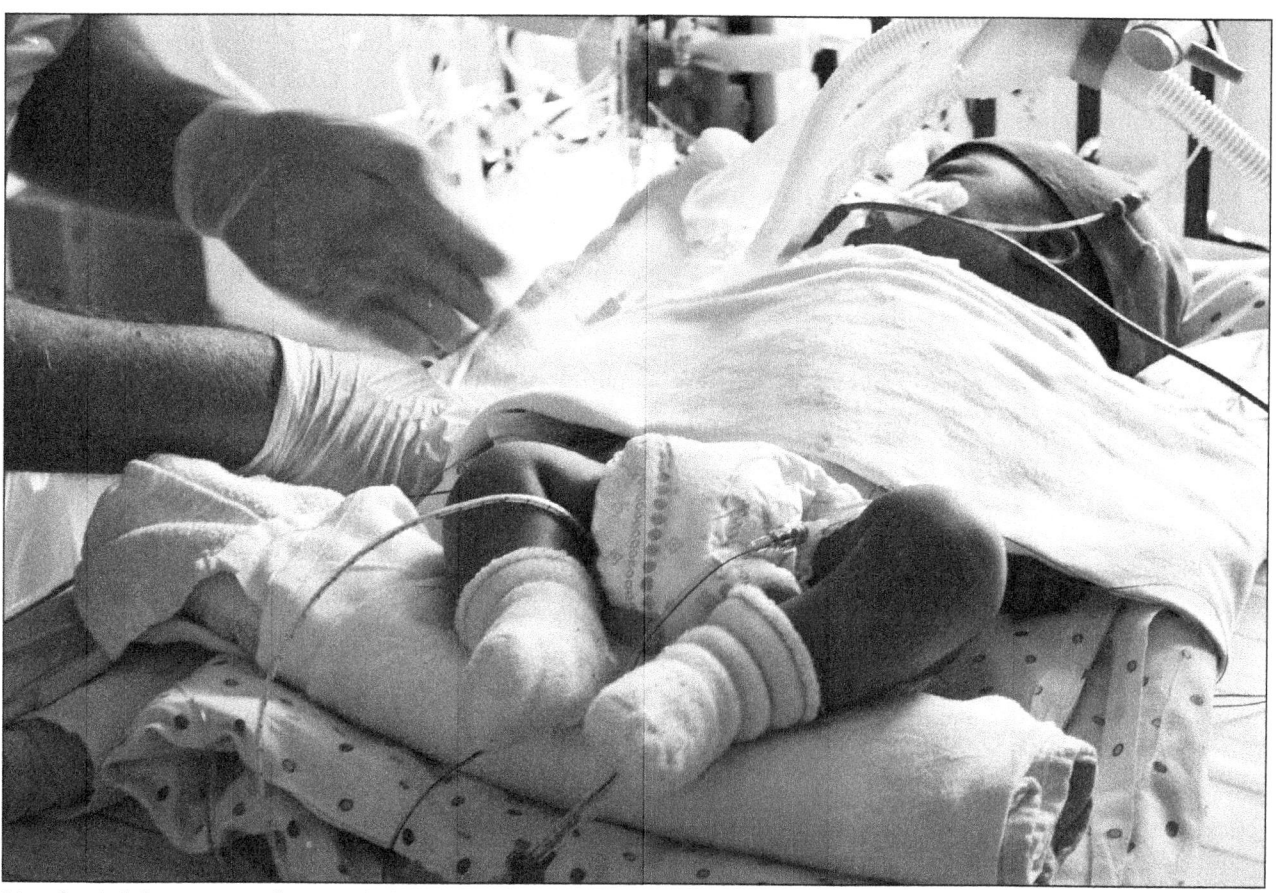

Many hospitals have a neonatology unit for babies who are born prematurely, who have disease conditions or birth defects, or who have low birth weight. All these infants may require short-term or prolonged care. (FroggyFrog via iStock)

cology units all require nurses committed to caring for children. Almost every specialty in adults can be found in children and the complexity of their care is often more difficult. Some physicians state that eight hours of care in a child is equivalent to twenty-four hours of care in an adult. Children respond more quickly to treatment and also crash more quickly, meaning they will get sicker faster.

The practice of pediatrics begins with birth. Most babies are born healthy and require only routine medical attention. Many hospitals, however, have a neonatology unit for babies who are born prematurely, who have disease conditions or birth defects, or who have low birth weight, weighing less than 5.5 pounds (2,495 grams) (even though they may be full-term babies). All these infants may require short-term or prolonged care by pediatricians in the neonatology unit.

Doctors and nurses specializing in neonatology, including advanced practice nurse practitioners with specialty certification in pediatrics or neonatology, have radically improved the survival rates of premature and low-weight babies. In neonatal care of the premature newborn, the infant may have to be helped to breathe, fed through tubes, and otherwise maintained to allow it to develop.

The problems of premature babies usually center on the fact that they have not fully developed physically, although other factors may also be involved, such as the health and age of the mother, undernourishment during pregnancy, lack of prenatal care, anemia, high blood pressure, abnormalities in the mother's reproductive organs, infectious disease, or physical trauma or injury to the mother. A past record of infertility, stillbirths, abortions, and other premature births may indicate that a pregnancy will not go to full term.

Low birth weight in both premature and full-term babies is directly related to the incidence of disease and congenital defects. Low-birth-weight infants have a 50 percent higher chance of experiencing developmental problems, including hearing and vision problems and chronic conditions such as heart disease later in life. Recent studies also indicate an increase in neurological problems such as attention-deficit hyperactivity disorder and autism spectrum disorder in these children.

Because the lungs are among the organs that develop late in pregnancy, many premature infants are unable to breathe on their own. Some premature babies are born before they have developed the sucking reflex, so they cannot feed on their own.

Hundreds of congenital diseases can be present in the neonate. Some are apparent at birth; some become evident in later years. Some may be life-threatening to the infant or become life-threatening in later years. Others may be harmless.

The child may be born with an infection passed on from the mother, such as rubella (German measles) or human immunodeficiency virus (HIV). Rubella may also infect the child in the womb, causing severe physical deformities, heart defects, cognitive delays, deafness, and other conditions.

Genital herpes affects about 2,000 newborns in the United States each year and may cause serious complications. A herpes infection during the second or third trimester of a woman's pregnancy may increase the chance of preterm delivery or cesarean section.

Group beta strep (GBS) infections are another serious problem for one of every 2,000 newborns in the United States. GBS infection may cause sepsis (blood infection), meningitis, and pneumonia. Pregnant women are tested for GBS infection during pregnancy, typically at thirty-five to thirty-seven weeks. With a course of antibiotics, a woman who tested positive for GBS infection has only a one in 4,000 chance of delivering a baby with GBS infection, compared to a one in 200 chance without antibiotics.

Among the most prevalent congenital birth defects is cleft lip and palate. Cleft lip occurs when the upper lip does not fuse together, leaving a visible gap that can extend from the lip to the nose. Cleft palate occurs when the gap reaches into the roof of the mouth.

Various abnormalities may be present in the hands and feet of neonates. These can be caused by congenital defects or by medications given to the pregnant mother. Arms, legs, fingers, and toes may fail to develop fully or may be missing entirely. Some children are born with extra fingers or toes. In some children, fingers or toes may be webbed or fused together. Clubfoot is relatively common. In this condition, the foot is twisted, usually downward and inward.

Many congenital heart defects can afflict the child, including septal defects (openings in the septum, the wall that separates the right and left sides of the heart), the transposition of blood vessels, the constriction of blood vessels, and valve disorders. Newborns are screened for congenital heart defects before leaving the hospital after birth. Congenital disorders of the central nervous system include spina bifida, hydrocephalus, cerebral palsy, and Down syndrome.

Spina bifida is a condition in which part of a vertebra (a bone in the spinal column) fails to fuse. As a result, nerves of the spinal cord may protrude through the spinal column. This condition varies considerably in severity; mild forms can cause no significant problems, while severe forms can be crippling or life-threatening. In hydrocephalus, sometimes called "water on the brain," fluid accumulates in the infant's cranium, causing the head to enlarge and putting great pressure on the brain. This disorder, too, can be life-threatening.

Cerebral palsy is caused by damage to brain cells that control motor function in the body. This damage can occur before, during, or after birth. It may or may not be accompanied by mental disability. Many children with cerebral palsy appear to have below-average intelligence because they have difficulty speaking, but, in fact, their intelligence may be normal or above normal.

Down syndrome (trisomy 21) is one of the most common chromosomal anomalies detected at birth, affecting one in 691 infants born to mothers. It is caused by an extra chromosome passed on to the child. The distinct physical characteristics of Down syndrome include a small body, a small and rounded head, oval ears, and an enlarged tongue. Mortality is high in the first year of life because of infection or other disease.

Cystic fibrosis is one of the most serious genetic disorders of white children. Because the lungs of children with this disease cannot expel mucus efficiently, it thickens and collects, clogging air passages. The mucus also becomes a breeding ground for bacteria and infection. Other parts of the body, such as the pancreas, the digestive system, and sweat glands, can also be impaired. A common congenital disorder among African American children is sickle cell disease. It causes deformities in red blood cells that clog blood vessels, impair circulation, and increase susceptibility to infection.

One of the major problems of infancy is sudden infant death syndrome (SIDS), in which a baby that is perfectly healthy, or only slightly ill, is discovered dead in its crib. In 2011 in the United States, over 2,200 infant deaths were reported as SIDS, according to the US Centers for Disease Control and Prevention. The cause is not known. The child usually shows no symptoms of disease, and autopsies reveal no evidence of smothering, choking, or strangulation. Research indicates that rebreathing of carbon dioxide as well as exposure to secondhand cigarette smoke and other forms of indoor air pollution may greatly increase the risk of SIDS.

Infectious diseases are more prevalent in childhood than in later years. Among the major diseases of children (and often adults) throughout the centuries have been smallpox, malaria, diphtheria, typhus, typhoid fever, tuberculosis, measles, mumps, rubella, varicella (chickenpox), scarlet fever, pneumonia, meningitis, and pertussis (whooping cough). In more recent years, HIV and hepatitis infection have also become significant threats to the young.

Certain skin diseases are common in infants and young children, such as diaper rash, impetigo, neonatal acne, and seborrheic dermatitis, among a wide variety of disorders. Fungal diseases of the skin occur often in the young, usually because of close contact with other youngsters. For example, tinea pedis (athlete's foot), tinea cruris (jock itch), and tinea corporis (a fungal infection that occurs on nonhairy areas of the body) are spread by contact with an infected playmate or by the touching of surfaces that harbor the organism. Similarly, parasitic diseases such as head lice, body lice, crab lice, or scabies are easily spread among playmates. Some skin conditions are congenital. Between 20 and 40 percent of infants are born with, or soon develop, skin lesions called hemangiomas. They may be barely perceptible or quite unsightly; they generally resolve by the age of seven.

One form of diabetes mellitus arises in childhood, insulin-dependent diabetes mellitus (IDDM) or type 1. In the healthy individual, the pancreas produces insulin, a hormone that is responsible for the metabolism of blood sugar, or glucose. In some children, the pancreas loses the ability to produce insulin, causing blood sugar to rise. When this happens, a cascade of events causes harmful effects throughout the body. In the short term, these symptoms include rapid breathing, rapid heartbeat, extreme thirst, vomiting, fever, chemical imbalances in the blood, and coma. In the long term, diabetes mellitus contributes to heart disease, atherosclerosis, kidney damage, blindness, gangrene, and a host of other conditions.

Cancer can afflict children. One of the most serious forms is acute lymphocytic leukemia. Its peak incidence is between three and five years of age, although it can also occur later in life. Leukemia is characterized by the overproduction of white blood cells (leukocytes). In acute lymphocytic leukemia, the production of lymphoblasts, immature cells that ordinarily would develop into infection-fighting lymphocytes, is greatly increased. This abnormal proliferation of immature cells interferes with the normal production of blood cells, increasing the child's susceptibility to infection.

In addition to the wide range of diseases that can beset the infant and growing child, there are many other problems of childhood that the parent and the pediatrician must face. These problems may involve physical and behavioral development, nutrition, and relationships with parents and other children.

Both parents and pediatricians must be alert to a child's rate of growth and mental development. Failure to thrive in infancy may indicate a range of physical problems, such as gastrointestinal, endocrine, and other internal disorders. In three-quarters of these cases, however, the cause is not a physical disorder. The child may simply be underfed because of neglect. Failure to thrive is seen often in babies who are reared in institutions where the nursing staff does not have time to caress and comfort infants individually.

Similarly, later in childhood, failure to grow at a normal rate can be caused by malnutrition or psycho-

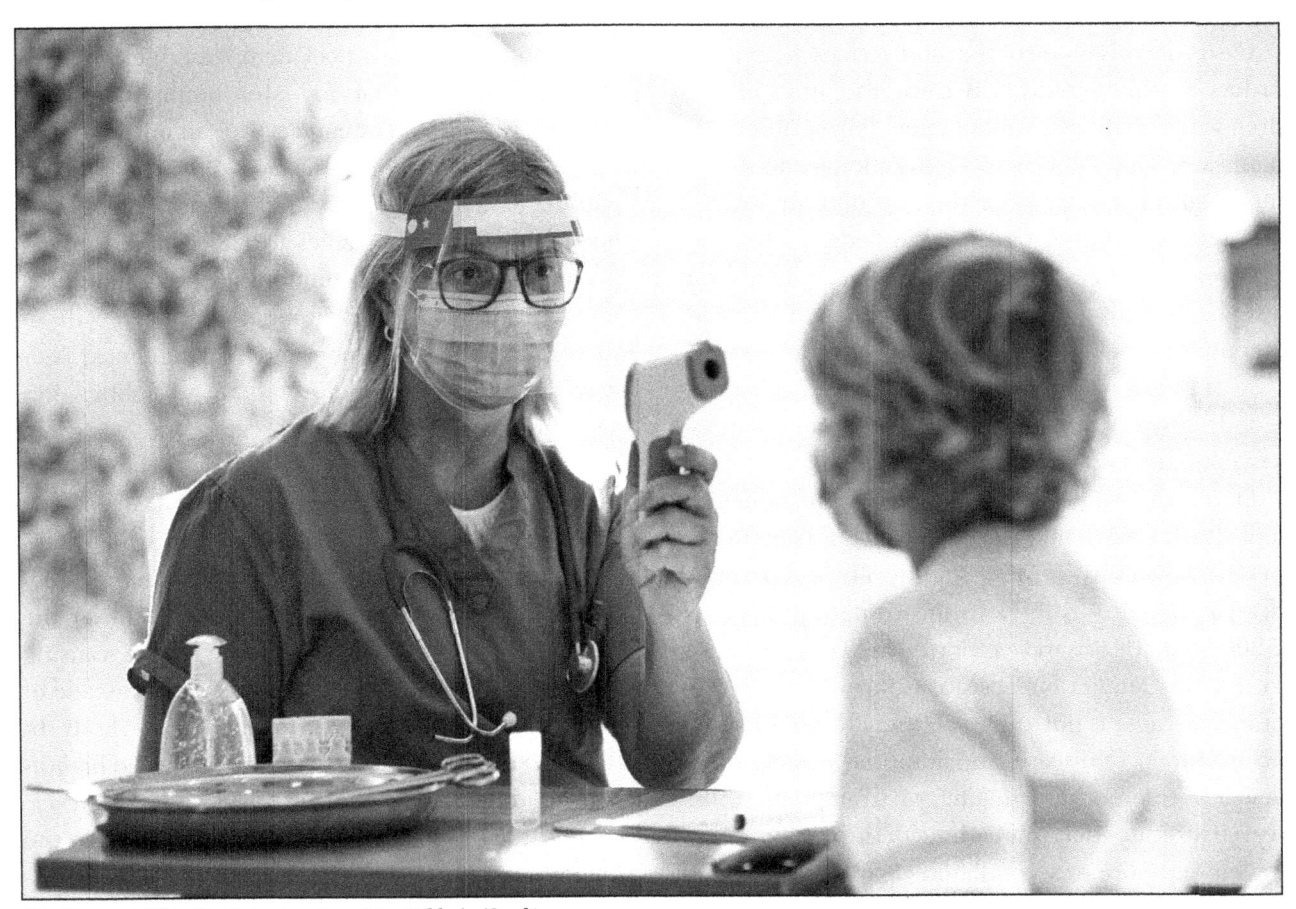

Checking a child patient's temperature (FamVeld via iStock)

logical factors. It could also be attributable to a deficiency in a hormone that is the body's natural regulator of growth. If this hormone is not released in adequate supply, the child's growth is stunted. An excess of this hormone may cause the child to grow too rapidly. Failure to grow normally may also indicate an underlying disease condition, such as heart dysfunction and malabsorption problems, in which the child does not get the necessary nutrition from food.

The parent and pediatrician must also ensure that the child is developing acceptably in other areas. Speech and language skills, teething, bone development, walking and other motor skills, toilet habits, sleep patterns, eye development, vision, and hearing have to be evaluated regularly.

Profound intellectual disability is usually evident early in life, but mild to moderate disability may not be apparent until the child starts school. Slowness in learning may be indicative of intellectual disability, but this judgment should be carefully weighed, because the real reason may be impaired hearing or vision, neglect, or an underlying disease condition. The diagnosis of developmental disabilities and neurological disorders, such as autism spectrum disorder and attention-deficit hyperactivity disorder (ADHD), has greatly increased in recent years and poses a special challenge to both parents and pediatricians.

The battery of diseases and other disorders that may beset a child remains more or less constant throughout childhood. Puberty, however, begins hormonal changes that trigger new disease threats and vast psychological upheaval. As early as eight years of age in girls and after ten or eleven years of age in boys, the body begins a prolonged series of changes that changes the child into an adult.

Hormones that were previously released in minimal amounts course throughout the body in great quantities. In boys, the sex hormones are called androgens. Chief among them is testosterone, which is secreted primarily by the testicles. It causes the sexual organs to mature and promotes the growth of hair in the genital area and armpits and on the chest. Testosterone also enlarges the larynx (voicebox), causing the voice to deepen.

Girls also produce some testosterone, but estrogens and other female sex hormones are the major hormones involved in puberty. They cause the sexual organs to mature, the hips to enlarge and become rounded, hair to grow in the genital area and armpits, the breasts to enlarge, and menstruation to begin.

Many disease conditions can arise in association with the hormonal changes that occur during puberty, such as breast abnormalities and genital infections. Far and away the most common medical disorder at this time, however, is acne. Acne is a direct result of the rise in testosterone that occurs during puberty. About 85 percent of teenagers experience some degree of acne, and about 12 percent of these will develop severe, deep acne, a serious condition that can leave lifelong scars.

Important psychological changes also occur during puberty. The personality can be altered as the developing child begins to crave independence. Ties to the family weaken, and the teenager becomes closer to his or her peer group. Sexual feelings can be strong and difficult to repress. In modern society, this can be the time when the teenager begins to experiment with tobacco, alcohol, drugs, or other means of achieving a "high," although in some groups the use of these substances begins much earlier.

Substance abuse is a major problem throughout society, but it is particularly devastating among young people. Sexual activity among teenagers is widespread and, combined with inadequate education about health issues and limited access to care, has led to significant medical problems. The incidence of sexually transmitted infections (STIs) is higher among teenagers than any other group. Teenage pregnancy is also a challenging issue in modern society. If the pregnant teenager who continues her pregnancy is from a disadvantaged family background, she is even more likely than other teen mothers to receive little or

167

no prenatal care. Risks of delayed or absent prenatal care can include a fetus that is not properly nourished. Additional risks can arise from a mother who smokes, drinks alcohol, or takes drugs throughout the pregnancy. In these cases, the child often may be born prematurely, with all the physical problems that premature birth involves. Hospital care of these infants is extremely costly.

DIAGNOSTIC AND TREATMENT TECHNIQUES
Infectious diseases passed from the mother to the newborn child are a particular challenge. In some cases, such as with GBS and herpes infections, appropriate antibiotics and antiviral agents can be given. In others, such as with babies born with HIV, support measures and medications that help prevent the progress of the disease are the only procedures available.

Many birth defects and deformities can be repaired or ameliorated. Disorders such as cleft lip or palate, deformities of the skeletal system, heart defects, and other physical abnormalities often can be remedied by surgery. Certain structural malformations may require prosthetic devices and/or physical therapy. Poor or disadvantaged children may struggle if birth defects are not treated.

The treatment of spina bifida depends on the seriousness of the condition; surgery may be required. With hydrocephalus, medication may be helpful, but most often a permanent shunt is implanted to drain fluids from the cranium. Before this technique was developed, the prognosis for babies with hydrocephalus was poor: More than half died, and a great many suffered from mental disability and physical impairment. Today, 70 percent or more live through infancy. Of these, about 40 percent have normal intelligence.

There are no cures for cerebral palsy, but various procedures can improve the child's quality of life, exercise and counseling among them. Neither is there a cure for Down syndrome. If intellectual disability is profound, the child may require institutionalized care. When a child with Down syndrome can be cared for at home in a loving family, his or her life can be improved.

SIDS continues to be a problem both in hospitals and in the home. The American Academy of Pediatrics' Back to Sleep campaign, in which parents are encouraged to place babies on their backs for sleeping, has been extremely successful, however, and has resulted in a decrease in the incidence of SIDS by 70 to 80 percent.

Managing the infectious diseases of childhood is one of the major concerns of pediatric providers, who are often called on to treat infections, for which they have a wide variety of antibiotics and other agents. Pediatric providers also seek to prevent infectious diseases through immunization and vaccination. Medical authorities now recommend routine vaccination of all children in the United States against diphtheria, tetanus, pertussis, measles, mumps, rubella, poliomyelitis, pneumococcal pneumonia, *Hemophilus influenzae*, varicella, hepatitis A and B, and human papillomavirus. Vaccines are also available against rabies, influenza, cholera, typhoid fever, plague, and yellow fever; these vaccines can be given to the child if there is a danger of infection. Vaccines for diphtheria, tetanus, and pertussis are generally given together in a combination called the DTaP vaccine. Measles, mumps, and rubella vaccines are also given together as the MMR vaccine. Repeated doses of some vaccines are necessary to ensure and maintain immunity.

Skin disorders of childhood, including teenage acne, are usually treated successfully at home with over-the-counter remedies. As with any disease, however, a severe skin disorder requires the attention of a trained provider.

Patients with diabetes mellitus type 1 are dependent on insulin throughout life. It is necessary for the pediatrician or attending nurse to teach both the parent and the patient how to inject insulin regularly, often several times a day. Furthermore, patients must monitor their blood and urine constantly to deter-

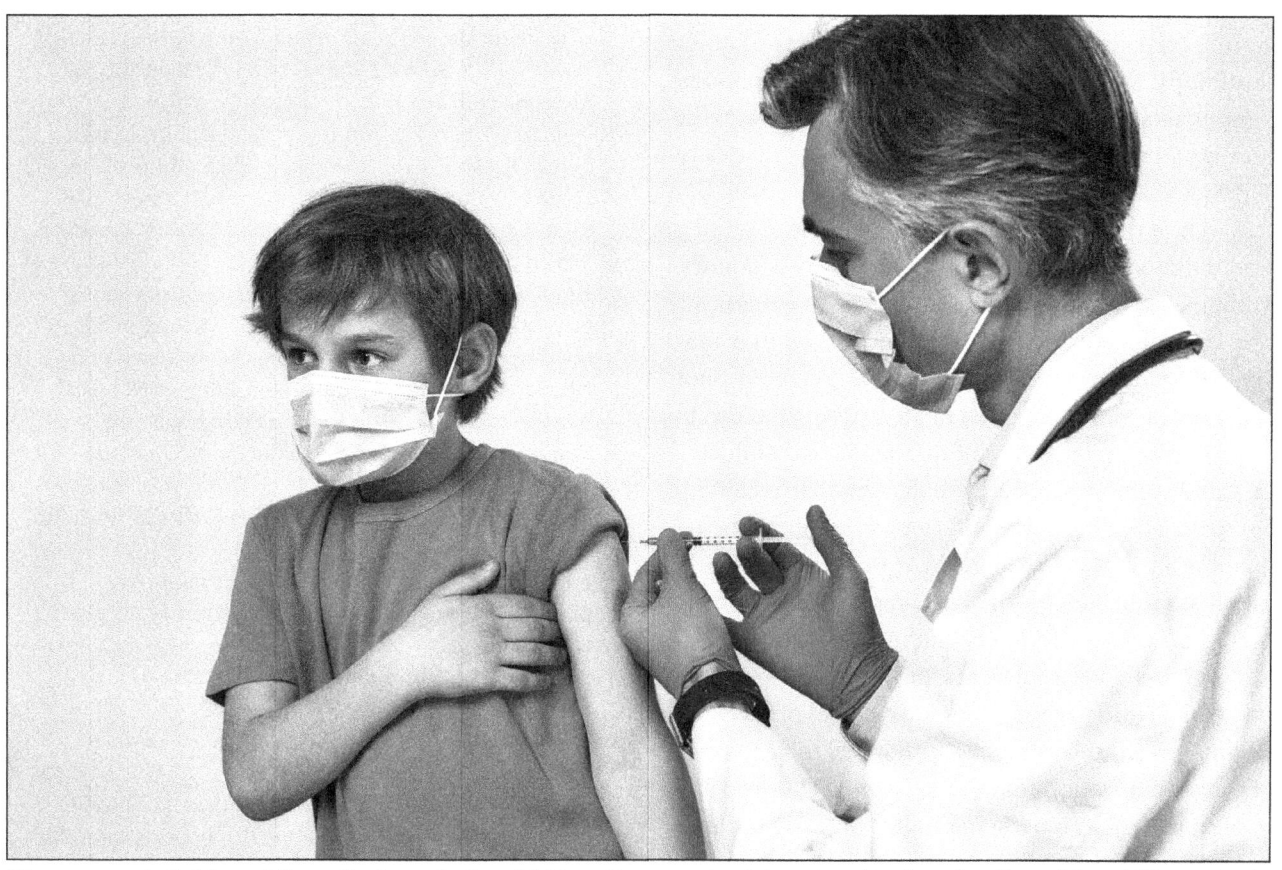

Diseases are controlled through the routine immunization of children. Programs educate parents and teachers about the need for a child to receive the full dosage of vaccine. (LanaStock via iStock)

mine blood sugar levels. They must also adhere to stringent dietary regulations. This regimen of diet, insulin, and constant monitoring is often difficult for the child to learn and accept, but strict adherence is vital if the patient is to fare well and avoid the wide range of complications associated with diabetes.

Other serious conditions are now considered to be treatable. Modern pharmacology has greatly improved the prognosis of children with leukemia. Similarly, many children with growth disorders can be helped by treatments of growth hormone. Medications and other treatment modalities for the mental disorders of childhood have improved in recent years. Children with intellectual disabilities can often be taught to care for themselves, and some even grow up to live independently.

Children with behavioral problems may be helped by clinicians specializing in child psychology or psychiatry. The problems of sexuality, sexually transmitted infections, and pregnancy among teenagers have provoked a nationwide response in the United States among medical and sociological professionals. Safe-sex programs have been launched, and clinics specializing in counseling for teenage girls are in operation to stem the rise in teenage pregnancies.

PERSPECTIVE AND PROSPECTS

Pediatrics affects virtually every member of society. Because pediatric nursing is diverse, the role of the nurse varies with site of employment. New treatments and techniques are growing daily. Surgical advances are addressing congenital defects, complexities of operating on babies and children, and a variety of other conditions. Diseases that once raged through populations of all ages are now being controlled through the routine immunization of children. Some diseases of childhood are not yet controllable by vaccines, but research in this area is ongoing.

Childhood health is directly related to economics. Middle-class and upper-class children have ready access to professional care for any problems that may arise. The medical and psychological needs of poor children, however, are often neglected. In an effort to improve the medical care of disadvantaged children, organizations may repair birth defects such as cleft lip and palate free of charge and some vaccines are being made available at low or no cost to poor and working-class families. There is still a gap in healthcare between socioeconomic levels that must be addressed.

Programs educate parents and teachers about the need for a child to receive the full dosages of vaccines. Computerized records allow authorities to keep track of the immunization status of individual children and to alert their parents when a follow-up inoculation is due. Most school districts require a certain panel of shots before a child can enter school. Many public health departments, in addition to private practice physician offices, provide these injections.

The psychological problems of impoverished children are at least as serious as the bodily diseases that threaten them. They may live in a universe of violence, deprivation, child neglect and abuse, and drug addiction, and they might lack a stable family environment and opportunities for advancement. Pediatric providers at all levels can advocate for these youth by becoming involved in medical, psychological, and sociological outreach programs to help disadvantaged children.

—*C. Richard Falcon and Lenela Glass-Godwin*

Further Reading

Hall, Laura J. *Autism Spectrum Disorders: From Theory to Practice*. 2nd ed., Pearson, 2012.

Hay, William W., Jr., et al., editors. *Current Diagnosis and Treatment: Pediatrics*. 22nd ed., Lange Medical Books/McGraw-Hill, 2014.

Kliegman, Robert M., and Joseph St. Geme, editors. *Nelson Textbook of Pediatrics*. 21st ed., Saunders/Elsevier, 2020.

Larsen, Laura. *Childhood Diseases and Disorders Sourcebook*. 3rd ed., Omnigraphics, 2012.

"List of Nursing Organizations." *Nurse.org*, nurse.org/orgs_shtml. Accessed 2 Sept. 2020. A listing of all nursing organizations, including the Academy of Neonatal Nursing, National Association of Neonatal Nurses, National Association of Pediatric Nurse Practitioners, National Association of School Nurses, and others.

Litin, Scott C., editor. *Mayo Clinic Family Health Book*. 4th ed., HarperResource, 2009.

"Pediatric Nurse." *Nurse.org*, nurse.org/resources/pediatric-nurse/#what-is-a-pediatric-nurse. Accessed 2 Sept. 2020.

Price, Debra, and Julie Gwin. *Pediatric Nursing*. 11th ed., Saunders, 2011.

Sanghavi, Darshak. *A Map of the Child: A Pediatrician's Tour of the Body*. Henry Holt, 2003.

Zitelli, Basil J., Sara McIntire, and Andrew J. Nowalk. *Zitelli and Davis' Atlas of Pediatric Physical Diagnosis*. 6th ed., Saunders, 2012.

GERONTOLOGICAL NURSING

ABSTRACT

As individuals age, their bodies undergo many changes and may require medical care to treat various conditions associated with the aging process such as vision loss, heart problems, cancer, Alzheimer's disease, and dementia. Gerontological nursing, formerly known as geriatric nursing, is a field of healthcare in which nurses specialize in the care of elderly individuals (people over the age of sixty-five) and recognize their unique needs. These nurses also work with the families of aging individuals to ensure that patients receive adequate care. Gerontological nursing continues to expand in the United States because of the growing population of aged individuals. Gerontological nurses work in a variety of settings including hospitals and medical centers, assisted living facilities such as nursing homes, and private homes.

OVERVIEW

Gerontological nurses are trained in general nursing duties, but they also have specialized training in caring for older patients who are more likely to suffer from multiple ailments. These nurses spend time with both aging individuals and their families or care workers. They interact with patients, families, staff at hospitals and care facilities, therapists, social workers, pharmacists, and others. They can advise families on long-term care options and connect them with the services they may need. Because the elderly population typically takes multiple medications, gerontological nurses need to be aware of possible drug interactions, be able to monitor patients for any issues, and work with physicians to adjust medications as needed.

All nurses must be able to handle the busy and demanding industry of caring for people. Elderly individuals require more care than younger patients do and may need assistance with simple self-care tasks. This requires physical strength to help a person stand up, walk, dress, bathe, and perform other activities. Many gerontological nurses are versed in insurance plans and premiums to help patients understand their coverage and work with their insurance companies.

Gerontological nurses must prepare themselves for the emotional toll that caring for aging individuals takes not only on them but also on families and other caretakers. Many elderly patients are near the end of

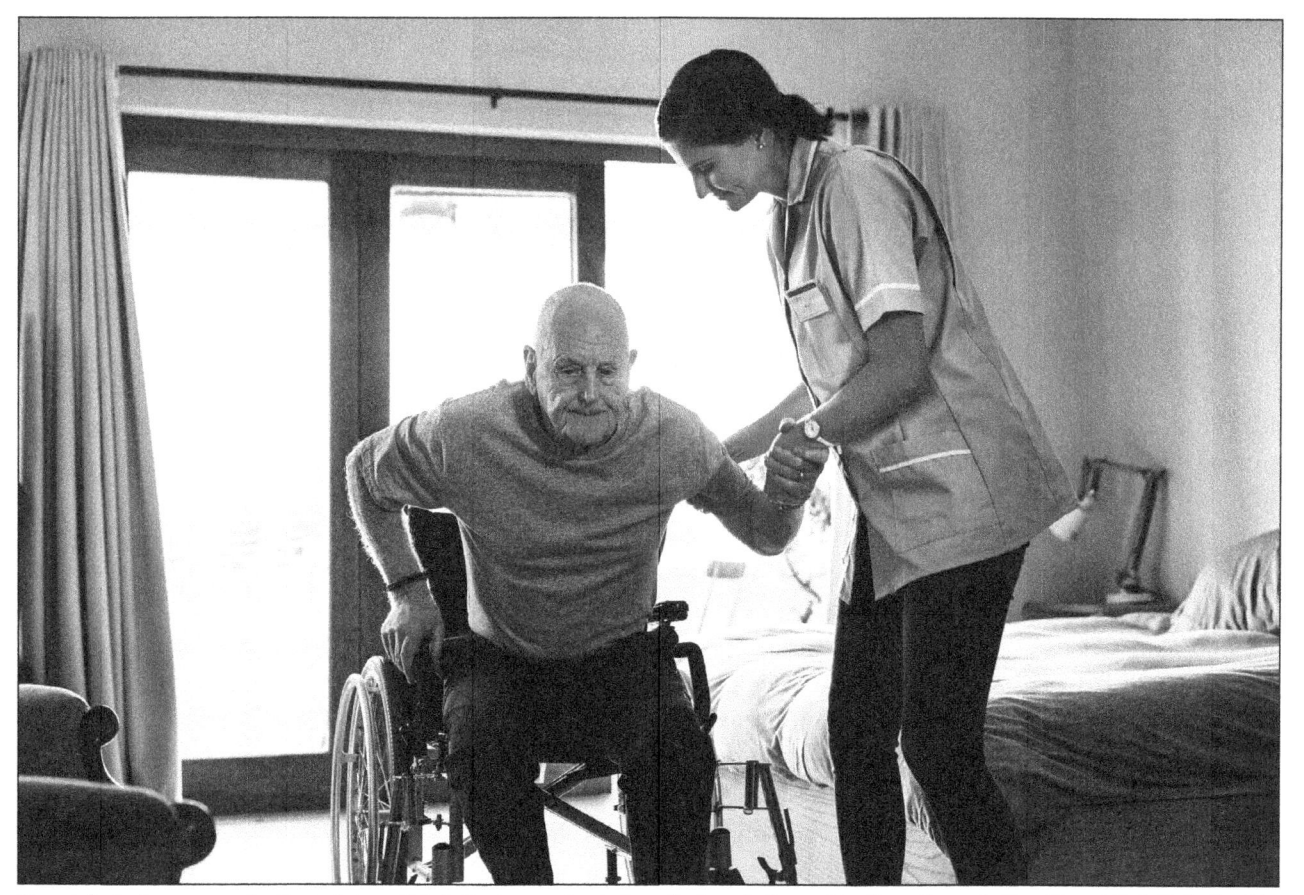

Gerontological nurses require physical strength to help a person stand up, walk, dress, bathe, and perform other activities. (Dean Mitchell via iStock)

their lives; some are in pain or feel frustrated, sad, or angry, while others are content or happy. Therefore, gerontological nurses should be caring, patient, empathetic, sensitive, compassionate, and understanding. These personality traits are necessary to help them deal with patients' varying moods. Gerontological nurses also must be prepared to discuss sensitive issues, such as end-of-life options and rights, with both patients and their families. They should be aware that sometimes people are not prepared to discuss these issues or may not agree with what a nurse has to say. In addition, gerontological nurses have to be able to deal with patients' deaths.

Gerontological nurses can work in numerous settings, such as doctors' offices, medical centers and hospitals, and nursing homes. They may serve as aids in private homes to care directly for elderly individuals or to teach families how to care for their elderly relatives. Some may work as liaisons or advocates for patients or their families, especially those who need help understanding medical jargon and treatment plans. These nurses may help patients and families make health decisions and can calm fears regarding certain procedures and treatments.

Various degrees and certifications are required for a career in gerontological nursing. Degrees include an associate of science in nursing (ASN) or associate degree in nursing (ADN), a bachelor of science in nursing (BSN), and a master of science in nursing (MSN). Other educational paths include licensed practical nurse (LPN) or licensed vocational nurse (LVN), and registered nurse (RN) programs. Individuals may pursue clinical nurse specialist (CNS) or nurse practitioner (NP) programs at the master's degree level, which may provide advanced knowledge of gerontological nursing. Several certifications exist, but they require the attainment of certain degrees, such as a BSN; completion of programs, such as an RN program; specific hours of practice and continuing education; and years of experience in the general nursing/gerontological nursing fields.

THE TOPIC TODAY
As of the twenty-first century, the baby boomer generation makes up a substantial part of the US population. Members of this generation, born between 1946 and 1964, were the result of a surge in births following World War II (1939–1945). This generation greatly influenced the country's economy; however, as its members have begun to age and require more care, they have put a strain on the healthcare industry. In addition, medical advances and technology have helped people to live longer, but not necessarily healthier, lives which is also straining healthcare.

The longer individuals live, the greater the chances are that they will need assistance with day-to-day living activities, such as bathing, toileting, eating, getting out of bed, dressing, managing medications, handling finances, driving, and shopping. Elderly people are more likely to acquire certain chronic physical and mental illnesses or other cognitive conditions associated with old age. Some of these medical conditions include vision or hearing loss/changes, arthritis, sleep changes/disorders, cancer, diabetes, osteoporosis, cardiovascular disease, stroke, Alzheimer's disease, and dementia. While some of these conditions may be managed by the patient and require only minimal care, others require around-the-clock care. Older people also tend to take multiple medications to treat their ailments and depend on medical services more than younger patients do.

TRENDS AND ISSUES
According to the 2010 US Census, the number of people over the age of one hundred increased by 68.5 percent since 1980, while the general population increased by only 36.3 percent. In addition, the World Health Organization (WHO) has estimated that the world's population over the age of sixty will increase from 11 percent to 22 percent by 2050. The growing elderly population has increased the demand for healthcare professionals trained in gerontology. This job field will continue to rise in the future because ag-

ing individuals will continue to require special care to treat their unique needs. However, although the need for gerontology nurses is growing, there continues to be a nursing shortage in the United States, with only 1 percent of registered nurses and 3 percent of advanced practice registered nurses certified in gerontology in 2016. This shortage is exacerbated by a high turnover rate for gerontology nurses.

The growing aging population also will have an impact on families, whose members may be forced to take on caretaker roles. In the 2010s, a growing number of elderly patients were choosing to age in their homes instead of moving to retirement or assisted living facilities. In these cases, gerontological nurses are trained to work with family members on how to best care for elderly loved ones. This also creates the need for gerontology nurses to be able to adapt to different settings. Trends in gerontology nursing have also been changing toward positive aging and chronic disease management, which includes helping patients be active in their own care and creating personalized proactive care plans.

—*Angela Harmon*

Further Reading

"Baby Boomer." *Investopedia*, www.investopedia.com/terms/b/baby_boomer.asp. Accessed 4 Jan. 2017.

"Becoming a Geriatric Nurse." *EveryNurse.org*, everynurse.org/becoming-a-geriatric-nurse. Accessed 4 Jan. 2017.

Bragg, Elizabeth J., and Jennie Chin Hansen. "Ensuring Care for Aging Baby Boomers: Solutions at Hand." *Generations*, 8 June 2015, www.asaging.org/blog/ensuring-care-aging-baby-boomers-solutions-hand.

"Day in the Life of a Geriatric Nurse Practitioner". *Nurse Practitioner Schools*, www.nursepractitionerschools.com/blog/day-in-life-geriatric-np. Accessed 4 Jan. 2017.

Donaldson, Rebecca. "Challenges of Geriatric Care Nursing." *Relias Academy*, 4 Oct. 2016, blog.reliasacademy.com/challenges-of-geriatric-care-nursing/.

Fagin, Claire, and Patricia Franklin. "Why Choose Geriatric Nursing?" *Geriatric Nursing*, Sept./Oct. 2005, www.nsna.org/Portals/0/Skins/NSNA/pdf/Imprint_SeptOct05_geriatric_fagin.pdf.

"How to Become a Geriatric Nurse." *All Nursing Schools*, www.allnursingschools.com/articles/geriatric-nurse. Accessed 4 Jan. 2017.

Katz, Katy. "Everything You Need to Know about Becoming a Geriatric Nurse." *Rasmussen College*, 5 Sept. 2013, www.rasmussen.edu/degrees/nursing/blog/everything-you-need-know-about-becoming-geriatric-nurse.

"Overview of Aging." *Geriatric Nursing*, 2018, geriatricnursing.org/overview-of-aging/. Accessed 12 Oct. 2018.

Stone, Robyn I., and Linda Barbarotta. "Caring for an Aging America in the Twenty-First Century." *Generations*, 9 June 2011, www.asaging.org/blog/caring-aging-america-twenty-first-century.

"Three Influential Trends in Gerontology." *Stenberg College*, 29 July 2015, www.stenbergcollege.com/blog/therapeutic-recreation/3-influential-trends-in-gerontology/.

CRITICAL CARE NURSING

ABSTRACT

Critical care nursing involves providing medical care for patients with life-threatening health problems, such as severe trauma, heart attack, or stroke. Critical care registered nurses (RNs) may also be known as intensive care unit (ICU) nurses, and are dedicated to the care of patients and families in the acute care phase of illness. Critical care nursing is among the oldest of nursing specialties, having begun to develop during the 1950s. Critical care nurses may work in emergency rooms, pediatric intensive care units (ICUs), burn units, cardiovascular and cardiac critical care units and other sites of acute care, as well as in many types of facilities.

BACKGROUND

The nursing profession and the care of critically ill patients have existed since ancient times. For centuries, many nurses in Europe were Roman Catholic nuns.

This began to change when a number of military hospitals opened in England during the nineteenth century to treat soldiers. As a result, increased attention was focused on treating severe wounds of war.

A number of prominent individuals, including nurses Florence Nightingale and Clarissa "Clara" Harlowe Barton, advanced the profession in the United States during the nineteenth century. Nightingale famously developed better patient care during the American Civil War, while Barton founded the American Red Cross after the war. They and others drew attention to the need to train nurses in patient care, and some schools operated by and for nurses opened in the late nineteenth century. Modernization in the nursing profession began early in the twentieth century as nursing schools came under the control of hospitals, allowing trainees to gain hands-on experience. Nursing became even more important in many countries during the First and Second World Wars. British nurses served on the battlefields with British troops, and many American women who volunteered to travel overseas as nurses gained critical care experience during the war.

Critical care nursing developed quickly in the latter half of the twentieth century. Prior to 1953, hospitals did not operate units dedicated to critically ill patients. Dr. William McClenahan recognized the importance of such units, and he persuaded hospital administrators in Chestnut Hill, Pennsylvania, to create units to meet the needs of these patients. McClenahan faced a number of obstacles in his efforts. Administrators were concerned about the expense of such units. They also were unwilling to treat men and women together in the same room, because until that time, women and men were housed in different wards. He overcame these arguments and the unit, once established, performed well beyond his expectations. The success of this first ICU prompted other hospitals to open their own.

By the late 1960s, 90 percent of American hospitals with at least five hundred beds had ICUs. Advances in

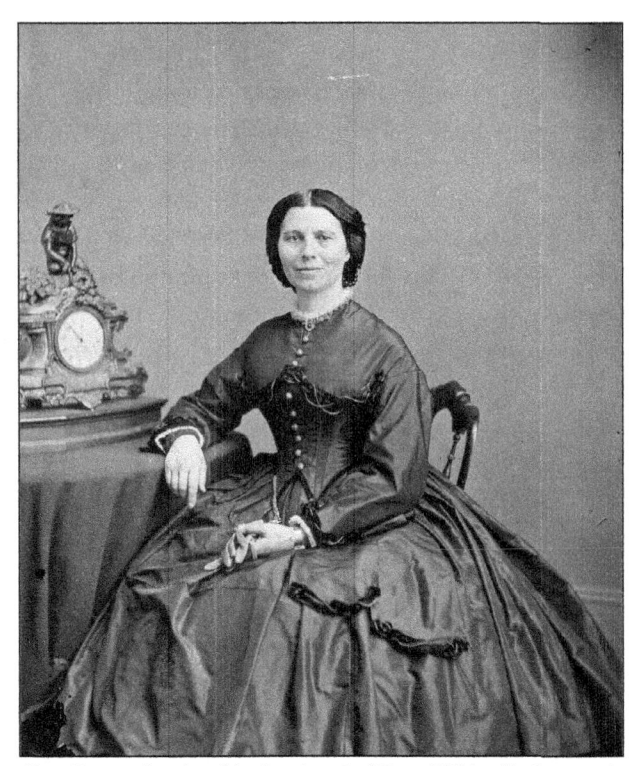

Clara Barton, founder of the American Red Cross (Wikimedia Commons)

medical care meant that the staffs of these units had to be trained properly to work with equipment such as cardiac monitors and provide cardiopulmonary resuscitation (CPR) and other care. The high concentration of critically ill patients required medical personnel who could make quick decisions about care under pressure.

Nurses in these ICUs organized into a group, the American Association of Critical-Care Nurses (AACN), which was founded as the American Association of Cardiovascular Nurses in 1969 before changing its name two years later. This organization established standards of care, education standards, and a certification exam. The AACN Certification Corporation was established in 1975 to provide and renew certification. The first journals, including *Critical Care Nurse* and *Advanced Critical Care*, were launched during the 1980s. As of 2014, the AACN reported membership of more than one hundred thousand nurses.

Medical advances and the creation of critical care units contributed to changes in the role of nurses. A variety of specialty nurse training programs and certifications developed. Nurses took on greater roles in patient care as the late twentieth century progressed. They moved from assisting doctors to shouldering responsibility for duties previously in the control of physicians, such as performing some procedures.

OVERVIEW

Critical care nurses must be experienced registered nurses (RNs). Some facilities may have degree requirements, or seek those attaining Certified Critical Care Nurse designation, available through the AACN. All critical care nurses must work within their scope of practice based on education and the nurse practice acts of the locale.

Critical care nurses may be employed in emergency rooms and critical care wards, as well as in doctor offices, walk-in clinics, and other facilities. They may have a variety of duties, depending on the situation and institution where they work. Critical care nurses may assess patient conditions, treat injuries, provide life support, assist physicians, record vital signs, ensure medical equipment is functioning, administer medications, order tests, and offer education and support to families. They work closely with other members of critical care teams.

Nurses trained in critical care may specialize. For example, modern technology has provided the means to care for premature and critically ill newborns.

Neonatal intensive care nurses specialize in monitoring and caring for these tiny patients, and are trained to help educate parents on assuming care as infants' conditions improve. The care nurses provide includes medical care as well as infant care, such as comforting babies and recording their progress. Other critical care nurses may work in pediatric intensive care, general intensive care, or cardiac care units, for example.

The demand for critical care nurses is generally high, although need from region to region varies considerably. An aging population in the United States as the baby boomers retire has led to greater need for medical care of all types. According to the *Atlantic*, the number of senior citizens in the United States is predicted to increase by 75 percent between 2010 and 2030, resulting in sixty-nine million seniors. About eighty-eight million Americans are expected to be age sixty-five or older in 2050. Older adults frequently have at least one chronic condition. A twenty-first-century shift toward providing home care to greater numbers of patients has led many in the healthcare industry to predict that patients treated in hospitals would be the sickest of the sick. Such a shift is expected to increase demand for critical care nurses.

—*Josephine Campbell*

Further Reading

"Acute, Critical Care Nursing: The Frontlines of Patient Care." *Minority Nurse*, 30 Mar. 2013, minoritynurse.com/?s=critical+care+nursing. Accessed 4 Jan. 2017.

Aitken, Leanne, et al. *ACCCN's Critical Care Nursing*. 3rd ed., Elsevier Australia, 2015.

Bisk Education. "Nursing Careers: Critical Care Nurse." *Villanova University*, www.villanovau.com/resources/nursing/icu-critical-care-nursing-job-description/#.WGwLalMrKpo. Accessed 4 Jan. 2017.

"Complete History of AACN." *American Association of Critical-Care Nurses*, www.aacn.org. Accessed 3 Sept. 2020.

Fairman, Julie, and Joan E. Lynaugh. *Critical Care Nursing: A History*. U of Pennsylvania P, 2000.

Grant, Rebecca. "The U.S. Is Running Out of Nurses." *Atlantic*, 3 Feb. 2016, www.theatlantic.com/health/archive/2016/02/nursing-shortage/459741/.

"The History of Nursing." *Nursing School Hub*, www.nursingschoolhub.com/history-nursing/. Accessed 4 Jan. 2017.

Sederstrom, Jill. "7 Specialties Lead Demand for Nurses." *Healthcare Traveler*, 22 Apr. 2013, healthcaretraveler.modernmedicine.com/healthcare-trav eler/content/tags/american-association-critical-care-nurses/7-specialties-lead-demand?page=full.

Urden, Linda D., et al. *Priorities in Critical Care Nursing.* 7th ed., Elsevier Health Sciences, 2015.

CLINICAL NURSE SPECIALIST (CNS)

ABSTRACT

A clinical nurse specialist (CNS) is an advanced practice registered nurse (APRN) who serves as an expert in a specific area of nursing. While a CNS may serve as a direct care provider, they are primarily concerned with designing and implementing programs of patient care and coming up with solutions to problems in the healthcare field.

WHAT IS A CLINICAL NURSE SPECIALIST (CNS)?

A clinical nurse specialist is a nursing professional who is an expert in a specific area of clinical expertise. There are five criteria of specialization for a CNS. They may work with a specific population, they may specialize in a specific type of care, they may specialize in a specific type of medical problem, they may have a specific medical subspecialty, or they may work in a specific setting. Within their specialty, CNSs perform a wide variety of services. According to the American Association of Critical-Care Nurses (AACN), CNSs are "responsible for diagnosis and treatment of health/illness states, disease management, health assessment, screening and promotion, and prevention of illness and risk behaviors among patients, families, groups, and communities."

In their role as a direct care provider, the CNS is similar to a nurse practitioner. CNS's meet with patients and perform health assessments, may order diagnostic and lab tests, but do not generally prescribe medications. While nurse practitioners operate more or less autonomously (depending on the state they practice in), CNSs often work with other providers and have less autonomy in their treatment of patients. They are more likely to serve as a consultant or supervisor than as a patient's principal care provider. CNSs also serve as an important liaison between the healthcare team and the patient and their family and they frequently advise other nurses and use their expertise to influence patients' care.

The clinical nurse specialist is not focused primarily on the specifics of patient care, but on the larger macrolevel picture of a group of patients, the healthcare system and administration. Within an individual hospital or other healthcare organization, a CNS will often be responsible for researching, developing and maintaining specific policies, procedures, and standards to improve the level of care offered in the institution. Often, the CNS serves in a consultation role, either for a specific hospital or for other healthcare companies or institutions, using their expertise to improve healthcare delivery. They are also often heavily involved in research, carrying out studies to bring new areas of knowledge into clinical practice.

Clinical nurse specialists, in short, are charged with using their expertise to design and implement methods for improving the healthcare services offered by a specific institution or to a specific population. According to research carried out by the AACN, the practice of clinical nurse specialists has had numerous positive outcomes in the healthcare field. These include reduced hospital costs and length of stay for patients, reduced frequency of emergency room visits, improved pain management practices, increased patient satisfaction with nursing care, and reduced medical complications in hospitalized patients.

A related profession to the clinical nurse specialist is the clinical nurse leader (CNL), which is a relatively new nursing position, having been initiated in 2003. The CNL is a master's-prepared nurse who is responsible for planning and implementing a patient's care within a clinical environment. They are also responsible for more managerial-oriented tasks such as developing improvement strategies, facilitating team communication, and implementing specific solutions in their medical environment. Unlike the CNS, who is concerned with macrolevel nursing, the CNL is focused on the specifics of a much smaller environment, for example, a single hospital unit. Compared to the specialized CNS, the CNL is far more of a generalist.

HOW TO BECOME A CLINICAL NURSE SPECIALIST

Clinical nurse specialists are advanced practice registered nurses (APRNs) which means they hold either a master's degree or a doctorate. Usually this means a master of science in nursing (MSN) degree or a doctor of nursing practice (DNP), with the latter increasingly preferred. Before earning these degrees, a candidate will usually qualify as a registered nurse by obtaining a nursing degree (whether an associate's degree, a bachelor's degree, or a diploma), and pass a certification exam, the National Council Licensure Exam-Registered Nurse (NCLEX-RN). After completing their graduate coursework, CNSs then obtain certification in their area of specialization through certifying boards such as the American Nurses Credentialing Center (ANCC), the American Association of Critical-Care Nurses (AACN) and other professional organizations. The ANCC only offers one certification for CNSs, in adult gerontology, so CNSs who wish to be certified in pediatric or neonatal care will have to do so through the AACN. CNSs in oncology, for example, apply for Advanced Oncology Certified Clinical Nurse Specialist (AOCNS) designation through the Oncology Nursing Certification Corporation.

Clinical nurse leaders (CNL) typically hold an MSN (master of science in nursing) degree. They must earn this degree from a master's program that meets specific curricular guidelines for becoming a CNL as established by the AACN. CNLs then earn their certification through the Clinical Nurse Leader Certification Program. This program, which involves completing a three-hour computer-based exam, is administered by the Commission on Nurse Certification (CNC), an autonomous arm of the AACN. There are currently no provisions for state licensure of CNLs.

—*Andrew Schenker*

Further Reading
Bell, Linda, editor. *AACN Scope and Standards for Acute Care Clinical Nurse Specialist Practice*. American Association of Critical-Care Nurses, 2014.
"Clinical Nurse Leader (CNL) Job Description." *GraduateNursingEDU.org*, www.graduatenursingedu.org/clinical-nurse-leader/. Accessed 1 Oct. 2020.
"Clinical Nurse Specialist: Education Requirements, Career Paths, & Job Outlook." 1 Oct. 2020, www.allnursingschools.com/clinical-nurse-specialist/.
Duffy, Melanie, et al. *Clinical Nurse Specialist Toolkit: A Guide for the New Clinical Nurse Specialist*. 2nd ed., Springer Publishing Company, 2016.
Fulton, Janet S., et al. *Foundations of Clinical Nurse Specialist Practice*. 3rd ed., Springer Publishing Company, 2020.
"What Is a Clinical Nurse Specialist (CNS)?" *MSNEDU.org*, 1 Oct. 2020, www.msnedu.org/clinical-nurse-specialist/.

DOCTOR'S OFFICE, CLINIC NURSES, AND PHYSICIAN ASSISTANTS (PAs)

ABSTRACT
Nurses that work in doctor's offices and clinics can be either licensed practical or vocational nurses (LPN/LVNs) or registered nurses (RNs). They perform a variety of tasks, helping the physician deliver routine healthcare to their patients. A physician assistant (PA) also works under the supervision of a physician, but is given more autonomy to examine, diagnose, and treat patients.

DOCTOR'S OFFICE AND CLINIC NURSES
Although a high percentage of nurses tend to work in hospitals, the nursing profession is one that allows practitioners to seek employment in any number of settings. Among the more common are doctor's offices and clinics. Nurses who work in these settings carry out their practice under the supervision of phy-

sicians and sometimes supervising nurses. While nurses who work in hospital settings often deal with more significant illnesses and injuries, those who work in doctor's offices and clinics deal more with routine checkups and preventative care. They often build long-term relationships with patients in a way that is not possible in a hospital setting.

Like hospital nurses, doctor's office and clinic nurses perform a wide range of duties. They are often the first point of contact with a patient, as they take them to the exam room, take their vitals and history, and prepare them for the physician's visit. Among their other tasks are administering vaccinations and other shots, performing blood work, carrying out diagnostic tests such as electrocardiograms (ECGs) and peak flows, and assisting physicians in the performance of their duties. They may also assist in any surgeries performed in the office and the clinic, including setting up sterile fields and working directly with the physician performing the surgery.

In addition to working directly with patients, nurses in doctor's offices and clinics perform a number of other tasks. These may include medical coding, calling patients to notify them of test results, answering patient calls, calling insurance companies for authorization, calling in prescription orders to pharmacies, and managing charts. In a clinic setting, the nurse may also focus more on an educational role, speaking directly with patients to inform them about topics such as nutrition, blood pressure management, and the specifics of their condition. Nurses in clinic settings also tend to be more autonomous than those in either doctor's offices or hospitals, particularly since many clinics tend to be understaffed.

Nurses that work in doctor's offices and clinics may be either LPNs, LVNs, or RNs. The nurse in a physician office works under the licensure of the physician. RNs may take on more of a supervisory role and may oversee LPNs depending on the staff makeup of the individual office or clinic. To become an LPN or LVN, an individual must complete an LPN or LVN program. Programs are typically offered through community colleges or vocational schools and last about twelve to eighteen months. RNs must complete a more intensive program, either an associate's degree, a bachelor's degree, or a diploma program, although a bachelor's is increasingly preferred. After completing their coursework, LPNs and LVNs and RNs must pass the licensure exam, the NCLEX (National Council Licensure Exam (NCLEX) before they are allowed to practice. The exam differs depending on whether the candidate is seeking to become an LPN (NCLEX-PN) or an RN (NCLEX-RN).

PHYSICIAN ASSISTANTS

Physician assistants are professionals who practice medicine under the direction and supervision of physicians, surgeons, and other healthcare workers. The degree of this supervision varies according to the laws of each individual state, but physician assistants are generally tasked with examining, diagnosing, and treating patients. The position dates back to the 1965 when the Duke Medical Center started a program to assist Vietnam veterans who had served as medics during the war in their transition to civilian life. Other programs launched shortly afterward and the field has continued to grow since then. With an increasing need for healthcare providers in the United States, the field is more in demand than ever.

Physician assistants work in all areas of medicine and the specific nature of their work depends on their specialty. However, among the most common tasks they perform include taking patient histories, performing physical exams, ordering laboratory and diagnostic tests, prescribing medications, and developing and overseeing patient treatment plans. From here, the tasks differ widely. A physician assistant who works in surgery, for example may close incisions and provide direct patient care before, during, and after the procedure. In some areas, particularly in underserved communities, physician assistants may serve as a patient's primary care provider, although, depending on the specific laws of the state in which they practice, they may still work under a supervising physician. More than half of physician assistants work in doctor's offices, about a quarter work in hospitals, and about eight percent are employed by outpatient care centers.

To become a physician assistant, a candidate must attend an accredited master's degree program specifically tailored to the profession. Before applying, candidates will have typically earned a bachelor's degree and will have completed two years of college coursework in basic and behavioral sciences. Many programs also require prior healthcare experience, including hands-on patient care. Master's programs typically last twenty-six months (three academic years) and include both classroom instruction and clinical rotations. Coursework typically includes classes in anatomy, biochemistry, pharmacology, clinical laboratory science, and medical ethics among other areas of study. Students typically complete 2,000 hours of clinical work. After graduating, students are eligible to take the Physician Assistant National Certifying Exam (PANCE). Students who pass this exam are eligible to use the title Physician Assistant-Certified or PA-C. To maintain certification, PAs are required to complete 100 hours of continuing medical education every two years and take a recertification exam, the Physician Assistant National Recertifying Exam (PANRE) every ten years. Before they can practice, PAs must also obtain a license in the individual state in which they plan to practice.

—*Andrew Schenker*

Further Reading

Ballweg, Ruth, et al. *Physician Assistant: A Guide to Clinical Practice*. 6th ed., Elsevier, 2017.

"Hospital Nursing vs. Clinical Nursing." *RegisteredNursing.org*, www.registerednursing.org/hospital-vs-clinic/. Accessed 2 Oct. 2020.

"How to Become a Clinic Nurse." *Study.com*, study.com/articles/How_to_Become_a_Clinic_Nurse.html#:~:text=Clinic%20nurses%20are%20usually%20licensed,and%20help%20with%20patient%20education. Accessed 2 Oct. 2020.

Kokemuller, Neil. "The Pros of Being a Nurse in a Doctor's Office." *Chron*, work.chron.com/pros-being-nurse-doctors-office-1988.html. Accessed 2 Oct. 2020.

"Physician Assistants." US Bureau of Labor Statistics. *Occupational Outlook Handbook*, www.bls.gov/ooh/healthcare/physician-assistants.htm#tab-1. Accessed 2 Oct. 2020

Nurse Practitioner (NP)

ABSTRACT

A nurse practitioner (NP) is an advanced practice registered nurse that performs a variety of tasks including assessing patient needs, performing and interpreting diagnostic and laboratory tests, diagnosing disease, and devising and carrying out treatment plans. Many NPs serve as their patient's primary care providers.

THE JOB OF A NURSE PRACTITIONER

The role of NP was first defined in 1965 and has evolved steadily since. The doctor and nurse team of Henry Silver and Loretta Ford created the first formal graduate certificate program for NPs, but graduates were limited in the level of care they could provide to patients. Beginning in 1971 as a response to a national shortage of doctors, US Secretary of Health, Education, and Welfare Elliot Richardson formally recommended expanding the role of NPs to allow them to serve as primary care providers. This recommendation was implemented and today an increasing number of patients look to NPs as their general practitioners.

The specific function of a nurse practitioner differs by specialization and by the laws of the state in which he or she practices. The majority of NPs (about 55 percent) work as family nurse practitioners (FNPs). These professionals focus on health promotion and disease prevention and often serve as the primary care provider for a wide range of the population.

Among the duties carried out by FNPs are diagnosing illnesses, including conducting lab and diagnostic tests as well as physical examinations; designing and supervising both pharmacological and nonpharmacological treatment plans; and counseling patients and their families.

The nurse practitioner's scope of practice is dictated by the specific laws of the state in which they work. Although they hold prescriptive privileges throughout the country, they are only granted full practice rights in twenty-two states (plus Washington, DC, Guam, and the Northern Mariana Islands). In these states, these nurses are granted autonomy under their regional state boards of nursing to assess patients, diagnose conditions, order diagnostic exams, and provide treatment without the supervision of a physician. In sixteen states (plus Puerto Rico, American Samoa, and the US Virgin Islands), NPs are subject to reduced practice, which means that the nurse must be supervised by another healthcare provider in at least one element of their practice. In the remaining twelve states, NPs are guided by restricted practice guidelines. This means that they must be supervised or delegated by a physician.

If the majority of NPs take on a broad range of patients by serving as family nurse practitioners, then the rest of the professionals who work in the field specialize in a specific population or area of practice. Apart from FNPs, the most common specialty for NPs is adult gerontology, where they work with elderly and aging populations. Other common specialties in the field include acute care NPs who handle emergency and sudden-onset conditions, pediatric NPs, women's health NPs, psychiatric and mental health NPs, and neonatal NPs. In addition, many NPs subspecialize in a specific condition, environment, population, or clinical focus. Examples of subspecialties include allergies and immunology, emergency room, hospice, pediatric oncology, orthopedics, sports medicine, travel, and urology.

BECOMING A NURSE PRACTITIONER

Working as a nurse practitioner requires a minimum of a master's degree. Many nurse practitioners hold doctorates and nursing organizations have increasingly expressed a preference for the industry standard for all advanced practice registered nurses (APRN), including nurse practitioners, to shift towards the doctorate degree. For example, in 2004, the member schools of the American Association of Colleges of Nursing (AACN) voted to endorse the *Position Statement on the Practice Doctorate of Nursing* which called for the minimum educational requirement for advanced nursing to be moved from master's to doctorate-level by 2015. Although this has not yet happened, it may in the future as professional organizations such as the American Association of Nurse Anesthetists and the National Association of Clinical

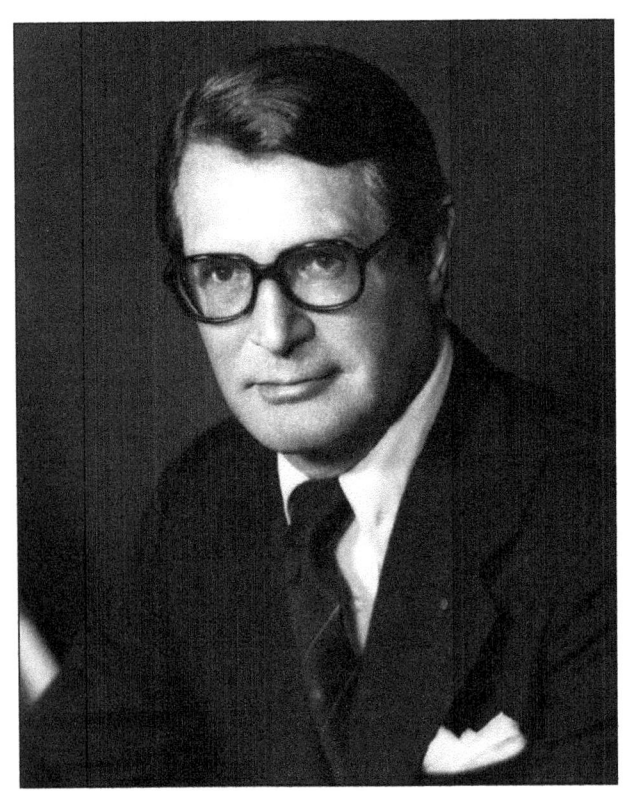

In 1971, U.S. Secretary of Health, Education, and Welfare Elliot Richardson formally recommended expanding the role of NPs to allow them to serve as primary care physicians. (Wikimedia Commons)

Nurse Specialists have echoed the AACN's call in recent years.

Nurse practitioners typically become a licensed registered nurse (RN) first. Becoming an RN requires the candidate to earn an associate's or bachelor's degree in nursing or an equivalent diploma. Master's and doctoral programs, though, typically prefer a bachelor's degree so those nursing students who want to go on to become an advanced practice nurse will usually earn a BSN (Bachelor of Science in Nursing) degree. After completion of their degree program, registered nurses must pass the National Council Licensure Examination (NCLEX-RN).

Once a potential nurse practitioner has qualified to practice as a registered nurse, he or she will then go on to earn an advanced degree, either a master's degree or a doctorate. Nursing candidates who pursue the former path earn a master of science in nursing (MSN) degree. The MSN program can vary in length from one year to several years. MSN students take both generalized coursework in areas such as advanced health assessment, advanced pharmacology, and nursing research, as well as in the specific area in which they want to specialize.

Most nurse practitioners who obtain a doctorate earn a doctor of nursing practice (DNP). They may also earn a PhD in nursing, although this degree is primary for candidates who wish to pursue research or an academic career. The DNP program builds on the MSN degree and allows students to further specialize; students who are studying to be a nurse practitioner will focus largely on that practice. The program lasts from three to five years and is designed to prepare students in eight key competencies, including organizational and systems leadership, healthcare policy, and evidence-based practice. All DNP students are also required to fulfill 1,000 clinical practice hours.

After earning their degree, students must obtain certification before they can practice as nurse practitioners. They can earn this certification through one of two organizations, the American Nurses Credentialing Center (ANCC) or the American Academy of Nurse Practitioners Certification Board (AAPCB). The ANCC offers four different certifications for nurse practitioners—granting licensure for family practice, adult gerontology (both general and acute practice), and psychiatric-mental health practice—while the AAPCB offers three.

The primary professional organization for nurse practitioners in the United States is the American Association of Nurse Practitioners (AANP). The AANP was founded in 2013 when two older organizations, the American Academy of Nurse Practitioners and the American College of Nurse Practitioners, merged. The organization's mission is to "empower all NPs to advance quality healthcare through practice, education, advocacy, research, and leadership." It has over 113,000 members.

—*Andrew Schenker*

Further Reading

American Association of Nurse Practitioners (AANP), www.aanp.org/. Accessed 25 Sept. 2020.

"Nurse Anesthetists, Nurse Midwives, and Nurse Practitioners." US Bureau of Labor Statistics, *Occupational Outlook Handbook*, www.bls.gov/ooh/healthcare/nurse-anesthetists-nurse-midwives-and-nurse-practitioners.htm. Accessed 25 Sept. 2020.

Santana, Nadia. *The Ultimate Nurse Practitioner Guidebook: A Comprehensive Guide to Getting Into and Surviving Nurse Practitioner School, Finding a Job, and Understanding the Policy that Drives the Profession*. Peter Lang Publishing, 2018.

"What Is a Nurse Practitioner?" *Nurse Practitioner Schools*, www.nursepractitionerschools.com/faq/what-is-np/. Accessed 25 Sept. 2020.

Nurse Anesthetist

ABSTRACT

Nurse anesthetists are advanced practice registered nurses (APRNs) who administer anesthesia and other medications and monitor patients who receive anesthesia. Certified regis-

tered nurse anesthetists (CRNAs) in the United States have a minimum of a master's degree and often a doctorate and have additional passed a certification exam.

WHAT IS A NURSE ANESTHETIST?

Nurse anesthetists, known in the United States as CRNAs, are nursing professionals who administer anesthetics and other medicine to patients in a variety of settings. Although doctors (anesthesiologists) are often in charge of providing and monitoring anesthetics in urban settings, in rural hospitals and the US Armed Forces, it is almost always a CRNA who performs this task. But CRNAs are not limited to these settings and work in medical and surgical hospitals, critical access hospitals, mobile surgery centers, outpatient care centers, nursing research facilities, and private medical offices of all types. In addition to clinical practice, CRNAs can also work in a managerial role in any of these settings, for numerous governmental agencies, or for professional testing organizations, among other employers.

For CRNAs who do work in clinical practice, their primary task to provide care before, during, and after surgical and other medical procedures, as well as helping with pain management. They work as part of a surgical team that may include surgeons, anesthesiologists, dentists, and other medical professionals. Their first task is to talk with the patient, discussing any medications they may be taking or any allergies or illnesses they have that may interfere with the administration of anesthesia. During this conversation, the CRNA also educates the patient about the process so

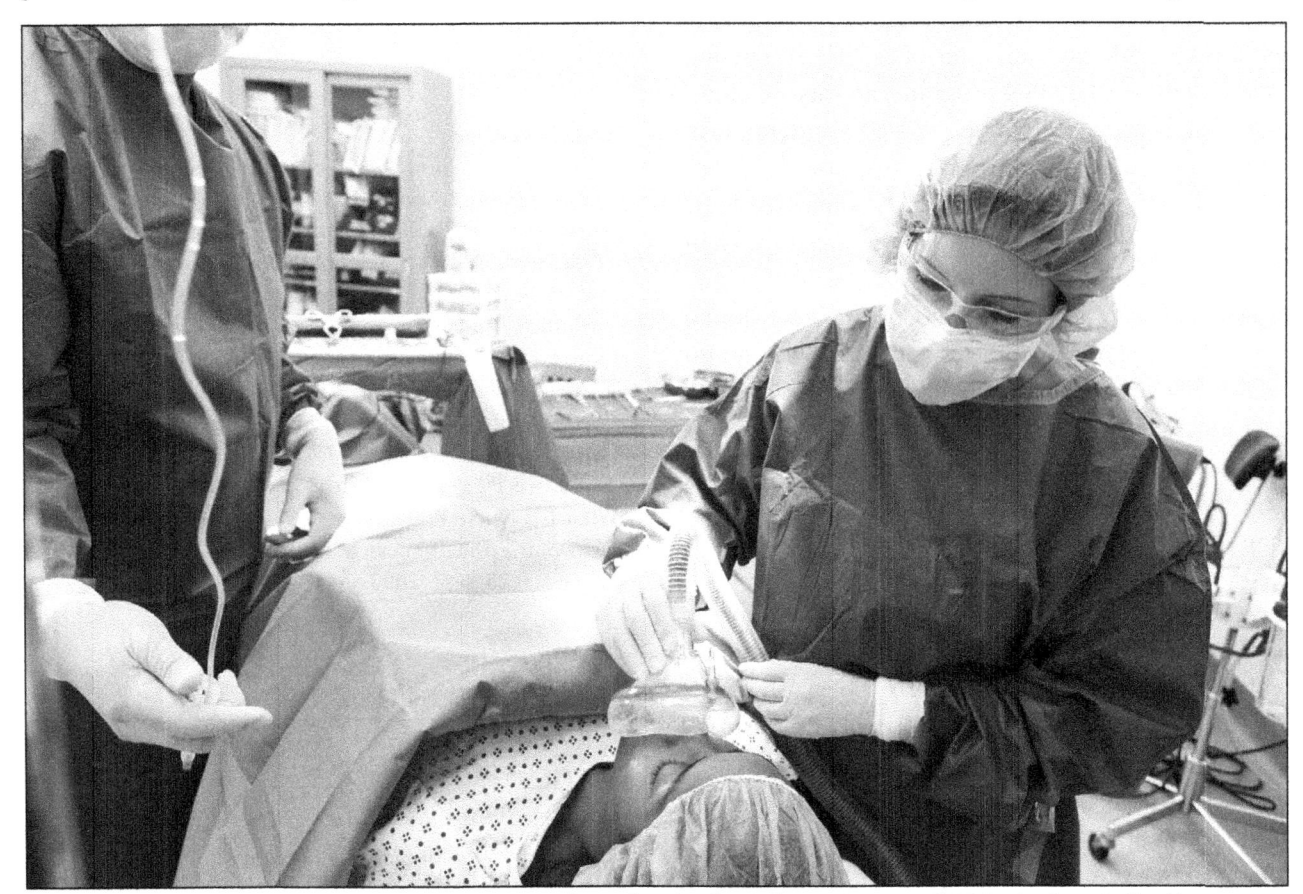

An anesthesiologist is seen sedating her patient before a surgical procedure in a hospital operating room. (SDI Productions via iStock)

that they can be an informed patient. The nurse anesthetist than administers the precise dosage of anesthesia needed, either general or local, monitoring the patient throughout the surgical procedure to make sure they are reacting properly to the dosage. They may make adjustments to the anesthesia during the procedure.

After the procedure, the CRNA facilitates the patient's reemergence from the anesthesia, conducts a postanesthesia evaluation, educates the patient about recovery and pain management, and discharges the patient from postanesthesia care. Other tasks that a CRNA may perform include prescribing medication, providing critical care or emergency services, and ordering and interpreting diagnostic and laboratory tests. Many states allow CRNAs to work independently, although others require a doctor's supervision or a collaborative agreement with a doctor.

HISTORY OF THE PROFESSION

The first nurses to administer anesthesia practiced during the US Civil War, when extreme numbers of casualties led to a greater need for anesthesia administrators. After the war, many Catholic nuns established of hospitals across the country and the Sisters themselves were often trained in providing anesthesia. The first notable nurse anesthetist in the postwar period was Sister Mary Bernard who began practicing at St. Vincent's Hospital in Erie, Pennsylvania in 1887. Soon after, Agnes Magaw began working as a nurse anesthetist for Dr. Charles Mayo at St. Mary's Hospital in Rochester, Minnesota. The Mayo family then founded the Mayo Clinic and Magaw continued to work for Charles Mayo where she became a pioneer in anesthesiology, developing the drip mask method, and documenting the administration of 14,000 administrations of anesthesia without incident.

As nurse anesthesia developed as a profession, the medical establishment began to fight back, claiming that doctors had a sole right to administer anesthesia. In 1934, a group of prominent Los Angeles physicians filed suit against a nurse anesthetist, claiming she had violated the California Medical Practice Act. The case made it to the California Supreme Court who ruled against the doctors, granting a legal precedent for nurses to administer anesthesia. Numerous legal challenges have continued into the twenty-first century, including as recently as 2012 in *California Society of Anesthesiologists v. Brown*, but CRNAs have continued to legally uphold their right to practice. Today, there are about 45,000 CRNAs employed in the United States who administer 49 million anesthetics to patients each year.

BECOMING A NURSE ANESTHETIST

To become a certified registered nurse anesthetist, a candidate must first become licensed as a registered nurse. Registered nurses (RN) in the United States hold an associate's degree, a bachelor's degree, or a diploma. Most graduate programs in nursing prefer that admitted applicants hold a bachelor's degree, so students wishing to become an advanced practice registered nurse (APRN) such as a nurse anesthetist will typically earn a bachelor of science in nursing (BSN) degree. After completing their degree, registered nurses are required to complete the NCLEX-RN (National Council Licensure Examination-Registered Nurse) before they are licensed to practice.

After becoming licensed, CRNA candidates must work as a registered nurse, usually in a critical care setting, for a minimum of a year, but often up to three. After that, they can apply to an accredited nurse anesthesia program. Currently, the minimum educational requirement for a nurse anesthetist is an MSN (master of science in nursing) degree, although many nurse anesthetists choose to earn a doctorate degree, usually a DNP (doctor of nursing practice). Many observers in the field believe that the minimum requirement for practice will switch to a doctorate degree in the future. Master's programs usually take two years to complete and doctorate programs three years. All programs offer clinical experience and have a regulated curriculum that requires studies in seven specific areas including anesthesia pharmacology, pain management, and statistics and research.

After graduation, the candidate must complete a certifying exam in order to practice. The exam, known as the National Certification Examination (NCE), is offered by the National Board of Certification and Recertification for Nurse Anesthetists (NBCRNA). In order to remain certified, nurse anesthetists are required to earn continuing education credits through the NBCRNA's Continued Professional Certification (CPC) Program. Nurse anesthetists are evaluated for continued certification on an eight-year cycle.

The primary professional organization for CRNAs in the United States is the American Association of Nurse Anesthetists (AANA). The AANA was founded in 1931 and today counts over 53,000 members, including student members. The AANA is responsible for certifying nurse anesthesia programs and, according to its mission statement, is "dedicated to advancing its members' profession and patient safety through advocacy, evidence-based practice standards, professional development, and commitment to innovation, collaboration and diverse ideas, experiences, and beliefs."

—*Andrew Schenker*

Further Reading
American Association of Nurse Anesthetists (AANA), www.aana.com. Accessed 28 Sept. 2020.
Bankert, Marianne. *Watchful Care: A History of America's Nurse Anesthetists*. Continuum International Publishing Group, 1989.
Nagelhout, John C., and Sass Elisha. *Nurse Anesthesia*. 6th ed., Elsevier, 2018.
"Nurse Anesthetist." *Nurse.org*, nurse.org/resources/nurse-anesthetist/. Accessed 28 Sept. 2020.
"Nurse Anesthetists, Nurse Midwives, and Nurse Practitioners." US Bureau of Labor Statistics, *Occupational Outlook Handbook*, www.bls.gov/ooh/healthcare/nurse-anesthetists-nurse-midwives-and-nurse-practitioners.htm. Accessed 28 Sept. 2020.

Home Health Nurse and Public Health Nurse

ABSTRACT
Home health nurses are nurses who specialize in caring for patients in their homes when patients and their families are unable to provide the necessary level of care themselves. They may be registered nurses (RNs), licensed practical nurses (LPNs), or certified nurse assistants (CNAs). Public health nurses, also known as community nurses, work with whole communities, providing health education, increased access to care, and direct healthcare services.

HOME HEALTH NURSING
Home health nursing is a rapidly growing field that is only expected to become more in-demand as the US population continues to age. Home health nurses provide one-on-one care to patients in their homes. Typically, these patients require more care than they or their families are capable of providing. Many patients that use home health nursing are elderly, disabled, or terminally ill, but some may require home nursing on a more temporary basis, for example, someone who is recovering from an injury. Although home health nurses work in the patient's home, they are often based at a facility where they report before going to the assigned home. This facility may be a home health agency, a hospice organization, a retirement community, or an insurance company.

Professionals who work as home healthcare nurses have different levels of education which determine the level of care they can provide. (RNs who work as home healthcare nurses can provide the widest range of services. They administer medication, take vital signs, perform physical assessments, perform lab tests, assist with daily activities and mobility, and develop care plans in concert with a physician. LPNs may also work in home healthcare and perform many of the same duties as RNs but typically do not perform physical assessments, perform lab tests, or develop care plans. Certified nursing assistants (CNAs) work-

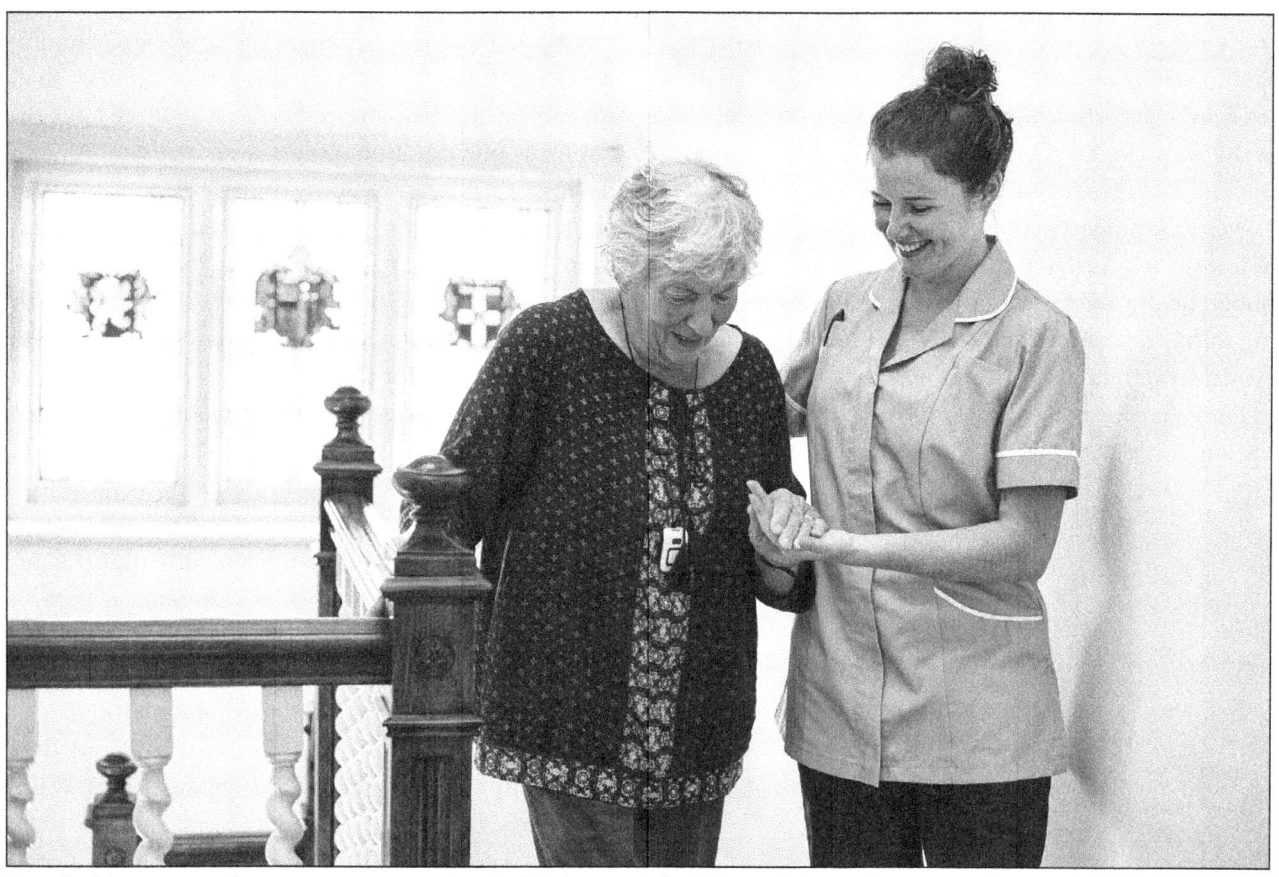

Home health nurses provide one-on-one care to patients in their homes. As the U.S. population continues to age, this is an increasingly in-demand field of nursing. (sturti via iStock)

ing in home healthcare are limited to taking vital signs and assisting with daily activities and mobility. They are typically supervised by an RN to whom they report any concerns. Home healthcare nurses may work with a single patient on a long-term basis or see multiple patients at once. They may also specialize in a specific area of home healthcare, such as gerontology, pediatrics, wound care, community health, and psychiatric or mental health.

Educational requirements for home health nurses vary by position. RNs must complete an associate's degree, a bachelor's degree, or a diploma program and then pass a certifying exam, the National Council Licensure Exam-Registered Nurse (NCLEX-RN). LPNs complete a training program, which is usually offered through a vocational/technical school or community college and then pass a certifying exam, the NCLEX-PN. CNAs complete a briefer and less intensive training program of their own. Home health nurses looking to advance in their field can obtain a master of science in nursing (MSN) degree and become certified as a clinical nurse specialist (CNS). The American Nursing Credentialing Center (ANCC) formerly offered a specific Home Health Clinical Nurse Specialist Certification (HHCNS-BC), but this is now only available for renewal for those who have already earned it.

PUBLIC HEALTH NURSING

Public health nursing, also known as community health nursing, is defined by the American Public Health Association as the "practice of promoting and protecting the health of populations using knowledge from nursing, social, and public health sciences." Public health nursing as a community practice dates back to 1893 when the nurse and reformer Lillian Wald, who coined the term "public health nursing," opened the Henry Street Settlement on New York's Lower East Side to provide healthcare and education to low-income residents of the neighborhood. Today, public health nurses continue the tradition by working with communities to improve the health resources available to them.

Public health nurses are RNs who typically work in settings such as public or government health departments, occupational health facilities, schools, community clinics, and voluntary organizations. Rather than treat individual patients, public health nurses more often focus on education, policy, and advocacy. Among the tasks that they may perform are to design and carry out health education campaigns, arrange for immunizations and screenings, monitor health trends in specific communities, develop policy, and work with governmental authorities at all levels to improve access to health services for their communities. Public health nurses working in government organizations usually take on more of an administrative role than those in other settings. Nurses who are employed in underserved communities, for example, often work directly with members of that community. Although this involvement is commonly in an educational capacity, in some low-income and rural communities, public health nurses may also provide direct healthcare services, such as preventive care and immunizations.

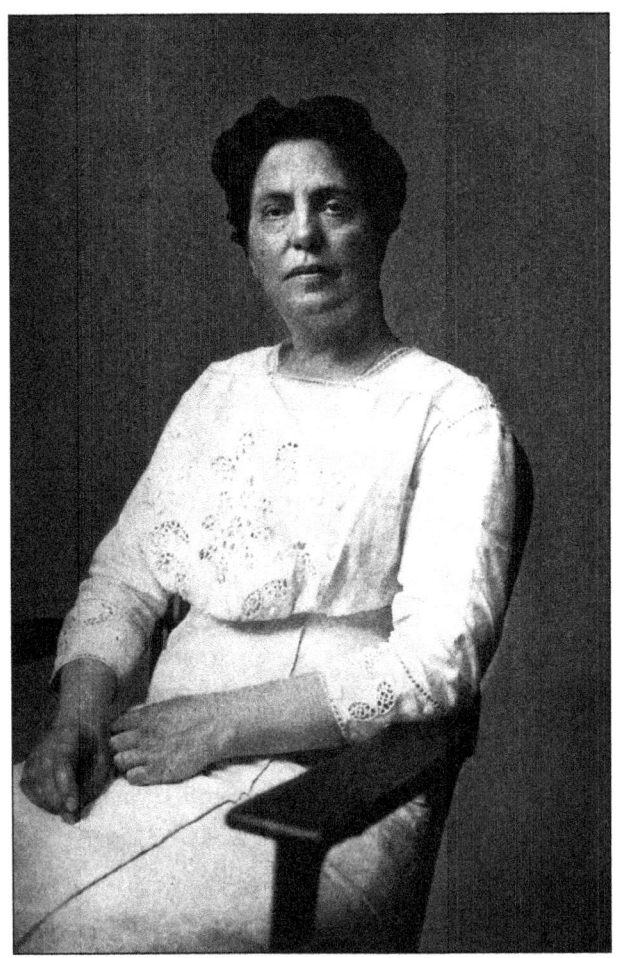

Public health nurses are RNs, which means they have completed a program in nursing (either at the associate's, bachelor's, or diploma level) and passed a certification exam (NCLEX-RN). Depending on the specific nature of the public nurse's job, a postgraduate degree may also be required, particularly if the nurse works in a supervisory role. Many colleges offer a degree in public health at the Master's level. Public health nurses might also seek out a certification in public health. The American Nursing Credentialing Center (ANCC) used to offer a specific Advanced Public Health Certification (PHNA-BC), but this is now only available for renewal for those who have already earned it. More general public health certifications are available through the National Board of Public Health Examiners (NBPHE) for those enrolled in or completing graduate level classes that reflect a core of public health courses or have a master's or PhD degree or a bachelor's degree with five years' experience in the public field.

—*Andrew Schenker*

Lillian Wald, who coined the term "public health nursing," opened the Henry Street Settlement on New York's Lower East Side to provide health care and education to low-income residents of the neighborhood. (Wikimedia Commons)

Further Reading

"5 Places Where Public Health Nurses Work." *Nurse Journal*, 3 June 2020, nursejournal.org/public-health-nursing/5-places-where-public-health-nurses-work/.

"Home Health Nurse." *Registered Nursing.org*, www.registerednursing.org/specialty/home-health-nurse/#:~:text=Home%20health%20nursing%20is%20a,unable%20to%20care%20for%20themselves. Accessed 30 Sept. 2020.

"How to Become a Home Health Nurse." *All Nursing Schools*, www.allnursingschools.com/specialties/home-health-nurse/. Accessed 30 Sept. 2020.

Marrelli, Tina M. *Home Care Nursing: Surviving in an Ever-Changing Care Environment.* Sigma Theta Tau International, 2017.

Macarthur, Sam. "What Is a Certification in Public Health?" *MPH online*, www.mphonline.org/cph-mph-credential-explained/. Accessed 30 Sept. 2020.

"Public Health Nurse." *ExploreHealthCareers.org*, explorehealthcareers.org/career/nursing/public-health-nurse/#:~:text=While%20most%20nurses%20care%20for,and%20increase%20access%20to%20care. Accessed 30 Sept. 2020.

Stanhope, Marcia, and Jeanette Lancaster. *Public Health Nursing: Population-Centered Health Care in the Community*. 10th ed., Elsevier, 2020.

Occupational Health

ABSTRACT

Occupational health is the application of healthcare that focuses on injury and illness prevention and the treatment of injuries that can occur in the workplace or that result from a person's employment. An occupational health nurse provides services for workers and community groups, often in a business or factory setting and is concerned with a safe working environment, employees' overall health and fitness for work, and helping the employer decrease health-related costs in the business. Emergent care is also part of the role if an employee is injured on the job.

SCIENCE AND PROFESSION

The discovery that eighteenth-century chimney sweeps were prone to developing testicular cancer is often cited as the first example of an acknowledged occupational illness. In fact, physicians and other healthcare professionals had been aware for many centuries that certain jobs were linked to particular medical disorders: millers developed coughs, and hat makers became mentally unbalanced. Textbooks urged physicians to consider a patient's occupation both in diagnosing and in treating illness. The emergence of occupational health as a distinct specialty within the medical professions is, however, a relatively recent phenomenon.

The Industrial Revolution brought with it not only the separation of one's home life from one's work life but also an increased risk of injury from factory machinery. Spinning jennies, power looms, mill wheels and belts, and early assembly line processes all carried the risk of accidental amputations, mangled limbs, and other permanently crippling injuries. Not surprisingly, much of the early emphasis of occupational health focused on safety. While company doctors treated the injured workers, engineers sought ways to reduce the job hazards.

By the twentieth century, several different but related specialties had evolved that focused on different aspects of occupational health. Industrial hygienists combine training in engineering and public health and attempt to improve safety in the workplace by providing education and training for workers and by redesigning the work area to eliminate hazards. Doctors of occupational medicine are employed by both government and industry to diagnose and to treat occupational illnesses and work-related disabilities. In addition to diagnosing and treating work-related injuries and illnesses, occupational healthcare providers may provide preemployment physical examinations, health screenings, and health promotion education and risk management programs based on occupational hazards and outcomes of trends of injuries or risks identified in the workplace. Public awareness of occupational health issues has led to the passage of legislation creating such agencies as the United States

Occupational Safety and Health Administration (OSHA). All occupational health specialists in the United States must work within guidelines established by OSHA. There is a high cost to society from such disabilities as the black lung disease suffered by coal miners and the toxic or radioactive exposure experienced by workers ranging from hospital laboratory technicians to pipefitters and welders. As a result, occupational health has become an ever-expanding, complex, and important medical specialty.

DIAGNOSTIC AND TREATMENT TECHNIQUES
Because occupational health problems can affect any part of the human anatomy, their diagnostic and treatment techniques are drawn from all areas of medical science. If a worker is injured on the job or suffers from an easily recognizable problem, such as a repetitive motion disorder, diagnosis and treatment can be quite straightforward. In the case of repetitive motion, problems such as carpal tunnel syndrome, which is sometimes experienced by word processing operators, might be treated by advising patients to change their work posture, providing them with splints to align the wrists and hands properly, employing corrective surgery to alleviate pain, and redesigning the work site to prevent future problems. The treatment for many on-the-job injuries will also include an extensive course of physical and rehabilitative therapy to allow the worker to return to work eventually, either at the old job or at a new one.

Many occupational health problems, however, are not as readily diagnosed as carpal tunnel syndrome. The industrial hygienist and the doctor of occupational medicine often must rely on the expertise of epidemiologists and toxicologists to determine the substances to which occupational exposure may be responsible for a worker's ill health. In cases in which workers complain of vague symptoms such as chronic fatigue, nausea, or neuropathy (loss of nerve function), an accurate diagnosis can prove elusive. The medical literature contains numerous examples of occupational illnesses that mimicked other common disorders. For example, doctors misdiagnosed a cosmetologist as suffering from multiple sclerosis (a degenerative disease of the central nervous system) when she was actually experiencing nerve damage caused by many years of exposure to the chemical solvents used to apply and remove artificial fingernails. Because many occupational illnesses can take years or even decades to appear, in some cases an accurate diagnosis may never be achieved. Once a diagnosis is made, treatment for an occupational illness caused by exposure to chemicals, for example, can be as simple as assigning the worker to tasks that eliminate exposure or as technologically sophisticated as using dialysis or chemical chelation to remove toxins from a patient's blood.

PERSPECTIVE AND PROSPECTS
Occupational health is one of the most challenging specialties in modern medicine. Practitioners must combine skills and knowledge gleaned from a wide spectrum of related skills. The proliferation of technologically complex methods and materials in the workplace has resulted in occupational exposures and illnesses that were unknown until the twentieth century. At the time that occupational health first emerged as a distinct concern in the medical community, industrial hygiene focused almost exclusively on safety in the workplace. If the factory could be designed so that workers did not risk losing a limb whenever they operated machinery, the hygienist could feel a sense of accomplishment.

Workplace safety remains a concern in occupational health, but obvious hazards such as poorly lit work areas or exposed moving parts on machines have been joined by a host of subtler threats to workers' well-being. Epidemiologists and toxicologists have linked on-the-job exposure to dust, heavy metals, radiation, solvents and other chemicals, and even blood-borne pathogens to a host of cancers, disabling diseases, reproductive problems, and other concerns.

Yet, not only must the industrial hygienist and doctor of occupational medicine worry about protecting workers from these physical hazards, but the modern occupational health specialist must also be concerned with the long-term effects of repetitive motions, noise exposures, and even emotional stress. As the influence of workers' jobs on those workers' health and on the health of their families is recognized as a major factor in a family's overall well-being, the importance of the occupational health specialist becomes increasingly obvious within modern society. Occupational health specialists employed in government, industry, and private practice, each approaching the question of worker wellness from a slightly different perspective, all fill a vital and expanding niche in modern medical practice.

The regulatory agency OSHA was created by Congress with the Occupational Safety and Health Act of 1970 to ensure safe work environments free of hazards that could cause death or serious physical harm to employees. It has the authority to fine or charge employers who do not follow safety regulations. The National Institute of Occupational Safety and Health (NIOSH), also created in 1970, conducts research and advises OSHA on issues related to hazards in the workplace.

—Sharon W. Stark and Nancy Farm Mannikko

Further Reading

American Association of Occupational Health Nurses. Resources, aaohn.org. Accessed 3 Sept. 2020.

Caplan, Robert D., et al. *Job Demands and Worker Health: Main Effects and Occupational Differences*. U of Michigan P, 1980.

Cralley, Lester V., and Patrick R. Atkins, editors. *Industrial Environmental Health: The Worker and the Community*. 2nd ed., Academic, 1975.

Gatchel, Robert J., and Izabela Z. Schultz. *Handbook of Occupational Health and Wellness*. Springer, 2012.

Guzik, Arlene. *Essentials for Occupational Health Nursing*. Wiley-Blackwell, 2013.

Koren, Herman. *Illustrated Dictionary and Resource Directory of Environmental and Occupational Health*. 2nd ed., CRC, 2005.

Levy, Barry S., et al., editors. *Occupational Health: Recognizing and Preventing Disease and Injury*. 5th ed., Lippincott, 2006.

Morgan, Monroe T. *Environmental Health*. 3rd ed., Thomson, 2003.

Occupational Health. *World Health Organization*, 2015.

"Occupational Health Nurse." Explore Health Careers, explorehealthcareers.org/career/nursing/occupational-health-nurse/. Accessed 3 Sept. 2020.

Sadhra, Steven S., and Krishna G. Rampal, editors. *Occupational Health: Risk Assessment and Management*. Blackwell Scientific, 1999.

Sellers, Christopher C. *Hazards of the Job: From Industrial Disease to Environmental Health Science*. U of North Carolina P, 1999.

Smedley, Julia, et al., editors. *Oxford Handbook of Occupational Health*. 2nd ed., Oxford UP, 2012.

TRANSITIONAL CARE

ABSTRACT

Transitional care is a generally compact period of healthcare, approximately 30 days, in which its principal focus is a smooth transition among various healthcare settings or from one level of care to another. Examples of this transition of care can be seen when a patient transfers from different floors within a hospital or a patient is discharged from an inpatient hospital setting to a rehabilitation center, skilled nursing facility (SNF) or nursing home. Some hospitals have a Transitional Care Unit where patients reside until appropriate skills are mastered or a transfer to another site can take place. Nurses are assigned to Transitional Care to facilitate the flow of patients between sites or to a Transitional Care Unit to care for the patient awaiting transfer.

KEY COMPONENTS

During a transition of care, there are several key components of patient information that must be communicated. The nurse is responsible for a significant portion of this communication. This data is crucial to ensure a smooth transition for both patient and providers. The communication of this vital information can be transmitted through face-to-face communication, a telephone conversation, a secured electronic medical record, or by the patient's paper medical record. The following is essential information needed in a transition of care:

- Current diagnoses
- Past medical history
- Past surgical history
- Medications
- Allergies
- Advanced directives
- Baseline physical and cognitive assessments
- Lab and imaging results
- Rationale and goals of care for the transfer

It is also important to note that contact information for both caregivers and providers should be included whenever possible to ensure that any gaps in information can be filled. There may be situations where other pertinent patient information may need to be included to ensure a transition of care is not fragmented and missing significant components.

CHALLENGES

Patient care has changed immensely over the past decade. It is rare that one practitioner cares for a patient across the continuum of medical settings. It is now more common for a practitioner to care for their patients in a single, specific setting. For example, a primary care provider may only see their patients in a clinical outpatient setting. If their patient is admitted to the hospital, a provider within the hospital will then most likely take over the patient's care. Furthermore, this patient may then be transferred to an outpatient setting such as a SNF, where another provider then takes over the patient's care. A transfer to a nursing home also involves a new set of providers. This is a common example of transitional care across healthcare settings. Each of these transfers has the potential to leave out crucial patient information. This can lead to medical oversights and mistakes including repeat lab tests, unnecessary diagnostic imaging, and medication errors.

The nurse plays an integral role in communication during the transitional care process. The ability to organize data into understandable components, provide both an oral and written report, gather necessary written materials to transition with the patient, schedule the transfer, and notify all involved parties of the place, date and time of transfer, including the family and significant others.

Transitional care that is well executed can reduce unnecessary healthcare costs and mistakes. This transition of care must include several key components of the patient's current medical state and past medical history. Cooperation among providers and clear communication between all of those involved in the patient's care can create a more optimal transition of care for patients, caregivers, and providers. The nurse must take an active role in the transitional care of the patient.

—*Carly A. Gray and Geraldine Marrocco*

Further Reading

Coleman, E. A. "Falling Through the Cracks: Challenges and Opportunities for Improving Transitional Care for Persons with Continuous Complex Care Needs." *Journal of the American Geriatrics Society*, vol. 51, 2003, pp. 549–55.

Coleman, E. A., and R. Berenson. "Lost in Transition: Challenges and Opportunities for Improving the Quality of Transitional Care." *Annals of Internal Medicine*, vol. 140, 2004, pp. 533–36.

Naylor, Mary. "A Decade of Transitional Care Research with Vulnerable Elders." *Journal of Cardiovascular Nursing*, vol. 3, 2000, pp. 88–89.

"What Is Transitional Care Management?" *Keystone Health*, keystone.health/what-is-transitional-care-management. Accessed 2 Sept. 2010.

Wound, Ostomy, and Continence (WOC) Nurse

ABSTRACT
A wound, ostomy, and continence (WOC) nurse is a nursing professional who specializes in the treatment of patients with acute and chronic wounds, bladder or bowel diversions, and urinary or bowel incontinence conditions.

WOUND, OSTOMY, AND CONTINENCE NURSING

WOC nursing is the branch of nursing that deals with both the acute and rehabilitative needs of patients with select disorders of the gastrointestinal, genitourinary, and skin systems. Among the numerous conditions WOC nurses treat are fistulas, ostomies, drains, pressure injuries, abdominal stomas, and wounds of all kinds. Fistulas are abnormal connections between two body parts—for example an artery and a vein or a blood vessel and an organ—which are usually caused by an injury or as a complication from surgery. Ostomies are surgical procedures in which bodily waste is redirected through a surgically created opening into either an outside prosthetic (an "ostomy bag") or an internally created pouch. When the bodily waste is directed outward, it is usually through an opening known as an abdominal stoma. Ostomies are performed as a result of any number of conditions that require waste diversion, including cancer, inflammatory bowel disease, incontinence, birth defects, and severe abdominal or pelvic trauma. The most common types of ostomies are the colostomy, in which a portion of the rectum or colon is removed and the remaining colon is brought to the abdominal wall to create a stoma; a urostomy, in which urine is diverted away from a diseased or defective bladder; and an ileostomy, in which an opening is created from the ileum, the lowest part of the small intestine. WOC nurses must be well-trained to care for patients having any of these procedures.

WOC nurses practice in a variety of settings, including hospitals, long-term care facilities, outpatient clinics, acute care facilities, or as home healthcare workers. They may be employed full-time by one of these facilities, may be self-employed, or may work on contract for services. Among the other tasks that WOC nurses may perform include supporting primary care providers in both inpatient and outpatient settings; educating patients and families on how to manage their wounds, ostomies, and continence problems; working as case managers; and acting as a liaisons between manufacturers, primary care providers, and patients. Among the specialized knowledge that WOC nurses possess are an in-depth understanding of dressings, skin care products, specialized beds and mattresses, incontinence supplies, and pouching systems.

BECOMING A WOUND, OSTOMY, AND CONTINENCE NURSE

In order to become a WOC nurse, a candidate must first be licensed as a registered nurse, meaning that they have completed a degree program in nursing and have passed the NCLEX-RN (National Council Licensure Examination for Registered Nurses). From there, candidates must complete additional education focused on wounds, ostomies, and/or continence care. This education may take several forms and a few universities offer specific instruction in all three clinical areas of WOC nursing. These institutions are accredited by the WOCN (Wound, Ostomy, and Continence Nurses) Society, which is the largest and most recognized organization for WOC nurses with over 5,000 members. Most WOC nurses will go on to complete a written WOC certification examination. These examinations are offered through the Wound, Ostomy and Continence Nursing Certification Board (WOCNCB). Nurses who wish to focus more on wound treatment may opt for the Certified Wound Specialist (CWS) certification which is offered through the American Academy of Wound Management (AAWM).

Opportunities for further professional growth are offered through the WOCN.

—*Andrew Schenker*

Further Reading

"Become a WOC Nurse." *WOCN: Wound, Ostomy, and Continence Nurses Society*, www.wocn.org/become-a-woc-nurse/. Accessed 24 Sept. 2020.

Quinn-Szcesuil, Julia. "What Does a WOC Nurse Do?" *Minority Nurse*, Apr. 2019, minoritynurse.com/what-does-a-woc-nurse-do/.

"What Is an Ostomy?" *United Ostomy Associations of American, Inc.*, www.ostomy.org/what-is-an-ostomy/. Accessed 25 Sept. 2020.

"WOC Nurses." *Nursing2020*, journals.lww.com/nursing/fulltext/2003/01001/woc_nurses.18.aspx. Accessed 24 Sept. 2020.

TELEHEALTH NURSING

ABSTRACT

Telehealth nursing, or telenursing, is the practice of specially trained nurses using audio and video technology and advanced digital and optical communications to deliver healthcare. This type of healthcare is usually in the form of care management for emergent or chronic conditions, coordination of care, and health maintenance services. It is beneficial to both the patient and the nurse; the patient benefits from increased access to healthcare services, while the nurse benefits from a more flexible and less physically stressful work environment. It is predicted that telehealth nursing will become more widespread in the future.

BACKGROUND

Telehealth nursing is a subfield of a medical practice area known as telehealth or telemedicine. This refers to any healthcare delivered through some form of communication other than personal contact. The field is as old as the telephone. Within a few years of the first telephone patent being issued in 1876, at least one medical journal, *The Lancet*, was advocating the use of the telephone for physician-patient consultations to eliminate the need for some in-person appointments. Since that time, physicians and their nurses have frequently used the telephone to assess basic health issues, answer questions about medications and side effects, and reassure anxious patients. Twenty-four-hour access to nurse-staffed helplines has been a staple of health insurance benefits for many years.

What has brought the concept to the forefront is the increased availability and capability of new technology that can be used in the twenty-first century. Instead of merely listening to a parent describe his or her child's rash, for instance, a telehealth nurse, or telenurse, can use a video link to see it. This allows the nurse to use a wider range of training and experience to determine whether a situation is serious enough to require the in-person attention of a medical practitioner or whether another remedy can be recommended.

Telenurses can use technology to have virtual consultations with patients who need assistance with health improvement programs such as smoking cessation or weight loss. The connection can help patients stay on track with their efforts, provide encouragement and support, and help the nurse identify any potential issues that are arising. Prenatal patients and new mothers also benefit from these consultations.

Technology exists that allows a patient to connect in-home monitoring equipment, such as blood pressure devices and blood glucose monitors, to a computer that can communicate with the nurse's computer. The nurse has direct access to the readings and can determine whether a patient's condition is under control or is in need of some adjustment or care. Telenurses can provide guidance and assurance to patients managing complex and chronic conditions, helping to improve their health outcomes while also reducing the number of in-person visits these patients need. Telenurses can be valuable in helping senior patients with multiple health issues and patients

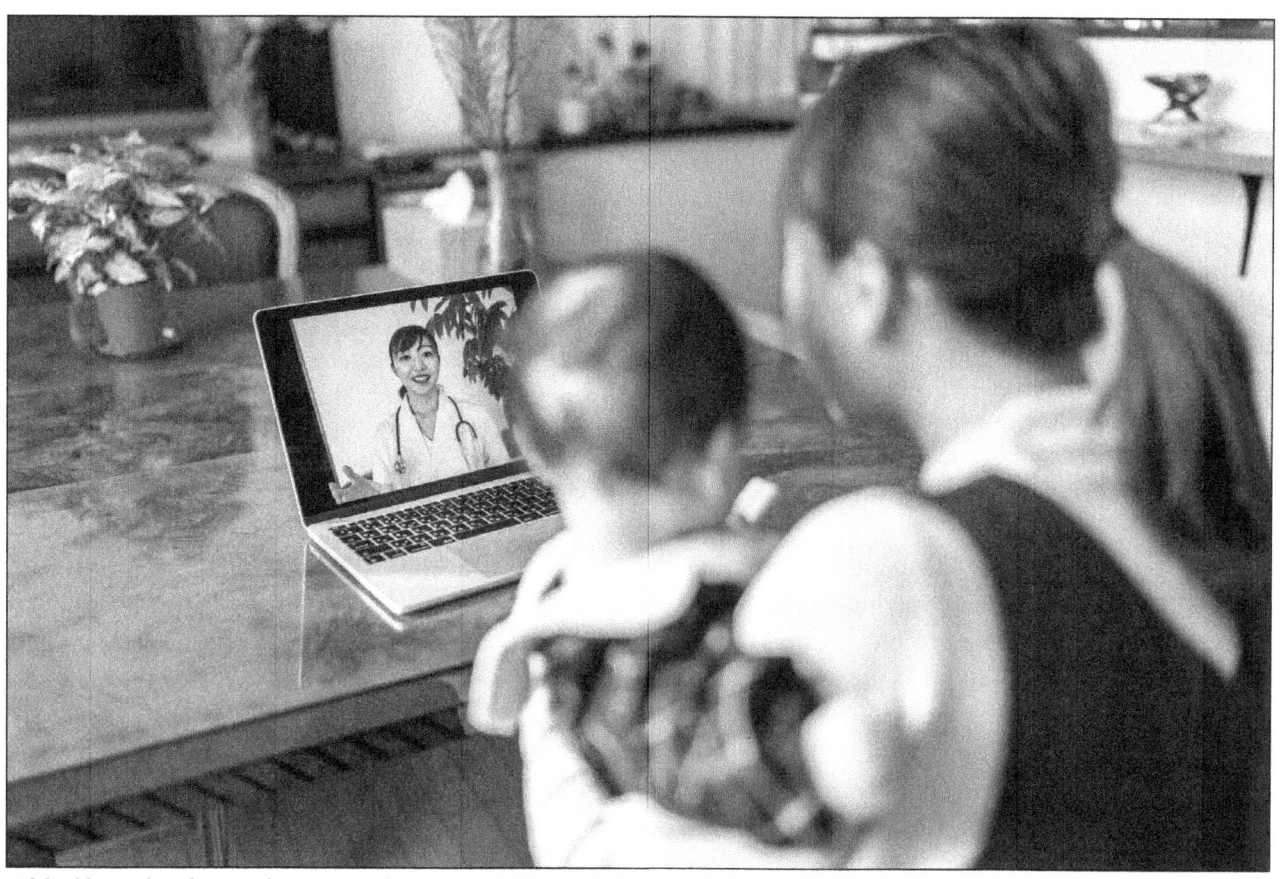

Telehealth, or telemedicine, refers to any health care delivered through some form of communication other than personal contact. Here, a patient confers with their medical professional over video chat. (recep-bg via iStock)

with illnesses such as multiple sclerosis, hepatitis, acquired immunodeficiency syndrome (AIDS), and other serious conditions to manage their conditions.

Improved technology allows telehealth nurses to access far more patient records than any single nurse in a physician's office could. Records from several associated offices or from many offices within an insurance network can be accessed from a single call center. This allows the nurse to provide more personalized care and to keep better records of the care administered via telenursing. The result is an improved patient experience that can often yield better outcomes. Fewer nurses are able to provide better care to more patients than would be possible if each office had to staff its own call center or if patients had to come in for in-person visits.

OVERVIEW

Telehealth nursing is evolving from simply answering questions about medications or the possible causes of symptoms to being an integrated part of healthcare management for many patients. Nurses working in this capacity can develop ongoing connections with patients that allow them to develop a better perspective on how a patient's treatment is progressing, what problems the patient is experiencing with his or her treatment, and other information that can help the physician and the patient's entire healthcare team provide better care. The technology-based consultations can provide more frequent interactions with patients who live in remote areas or who have barriers to coming to the physician's office, such as mobility or transportation issues.

Telenurses can serve as health coaches for people endeavoring to improve their health or for people recovering from life-altering medical situations, such as heart attacks or strokes. They often help to coordinate care for patients who see several physicians for multiple conditions, such as a patient with diabetes who needs to see a cardiologist for heart concerns, an ophthalmologist to monitor potential vision problems, and a podiatrist for proper foot care. Telenurses can serve as educators for people learning to cope with new illnesses or recovering from surgical procedures. In most cases, all of these efforts can be done with fewer staff and at a lower cost than in-person care would require.

The practice of telehealth nursing provides some benefits for nurses, too. For many telehealth nurses, the job provides shorter, more regular work hours. Telenursing can allow for more focused specialization if the nurse so desires. It can allow the nurse to develop better relationships with patients in his or her caseload. Telenursing can also provide a way for nurses who have problems with the physical aspects of nursing—long hours of standing, lifting patients, and so on—to continue practicing their skills.

While telenursing has many advantages, it also raises some concerns. Nurses sometimes worry that telenursing will eliminate jobs in the future. Others fear that the trend will lead to less personal healthcare, where in-person visits with nurses or physicians are the exception instead of the norm. Other concerns include the possibility of increased medical errors, the potential for medical problems to be missed by the lack of personal contact, and the greater possibility of electronic records theft and resulting medical fraud.

Reimbursement for telehealth services vary greatly by payer, state, practice and services and are constantly changing. For example, Medicare reimburses for telehealth services offered by a healthcare provider at a distant site to a patient in a health professional shortage area and receiving virtual care at a recognized site. Working with a reputable provider will encourage appropriate reimbursement for telehealth.

—*Janine Ungvarsky*

Further Reading

Barrett, David. "Should Nurses Be at the Forefront of Telehealth?" *The Guardian,* 20 Jan. 2014, www.theguardian.com/healthcare-network/2012/jan/20/nurses-needed-at-telehealth-forefront.

Bunn, Jennifer. "Telehealth—the Future of Healthcare?" *Ausmed,* 26 Oct. 2016, www.ausmed.com/cpd/articles/telehealth.

Edmunds, Marilyn W., et al. "Telehealth, Telenursing, and Advanced Practice Nurses." *Journal of Nursing Practices,* Apr. 2010, www.medscape.com/viewarticle/719335.

Llewellyn, Anne. "Beyond the Bedside: The Role of Telehealth Nursing." *Nursetogether.com,* 23 June 2014, www.nursetogether.com/beyond-bedside-role-telehealth-nursing/.

Taylor, Goldie. "The Evolution of Telehealth Nursing." *Minority Nurse,* 8 Apr. 2016, minoritynurse.com/the-evolution-of-telehealth-nursing/.

"Telehealth Nursing Practice." *American Academy of Ambulatory Care Nursing,* www.aaacn.org/telehealth.

"Telemedicine Reimbursement Guide." *eVisit,* evisit.com/resources/telemedicine-reimbursement-guide/.

PALLIATIVE CARE AND HOSPICE NURSING

ABSTRACT

End-of-life care is an important part of the nursing care continuum. The goal of palliative care is to relieve suffering and improve quality of life for patients with an advanced or chronic illness that may eventually lead to death and provide support to their families during the journey. Disease treatment continues during palliative care. Hospice differs in that it focuses on pain and symptom management in the terminal phase of illness without active treatment of the underlying disease. The nursing roles require similar skills.

PALLIATIVE CARE

Patients with active, progressive or advanced diseases who need assistance with the relief and prevention of suffering and help to enhance their quality of life are candidates for palliative care. It is a holistic, interdisciplinary specialty that utilizes multiple healthcare providers to deliver needed care. The World Health Organization (WHO) defines palliative care as an approach to assist patients and families by early identification and assessment leading to treatment of pain, and physical, spiritual, and psychosocial problems when faced with a life-threatening illness. It is an ongoing process with no time limit. Examples of diseases in adults and children that may benefit from palliative care are congestive heart failure (CHF), chronic obstructive pulmonary disease (COPD), cancer, congenital defects, and neurological deficits. Palliative care does not in any way hasten or postpone death, it merely manages the journey to provide the best quality of life until a terminal diagnosis occurs. Palliative care programs may be available through the local hospital, a home care facility, or a hospice.

HOSPICE CARE

Hospice care focuses on the patient with an advanced, life-limiting illness and their caregivers. It provides compassionate care in the last stages of incurable disease when treatment options fail. The goal is to provide the patient with a good death, meaning comfort, quality of life, and dignity in their last days. Referral

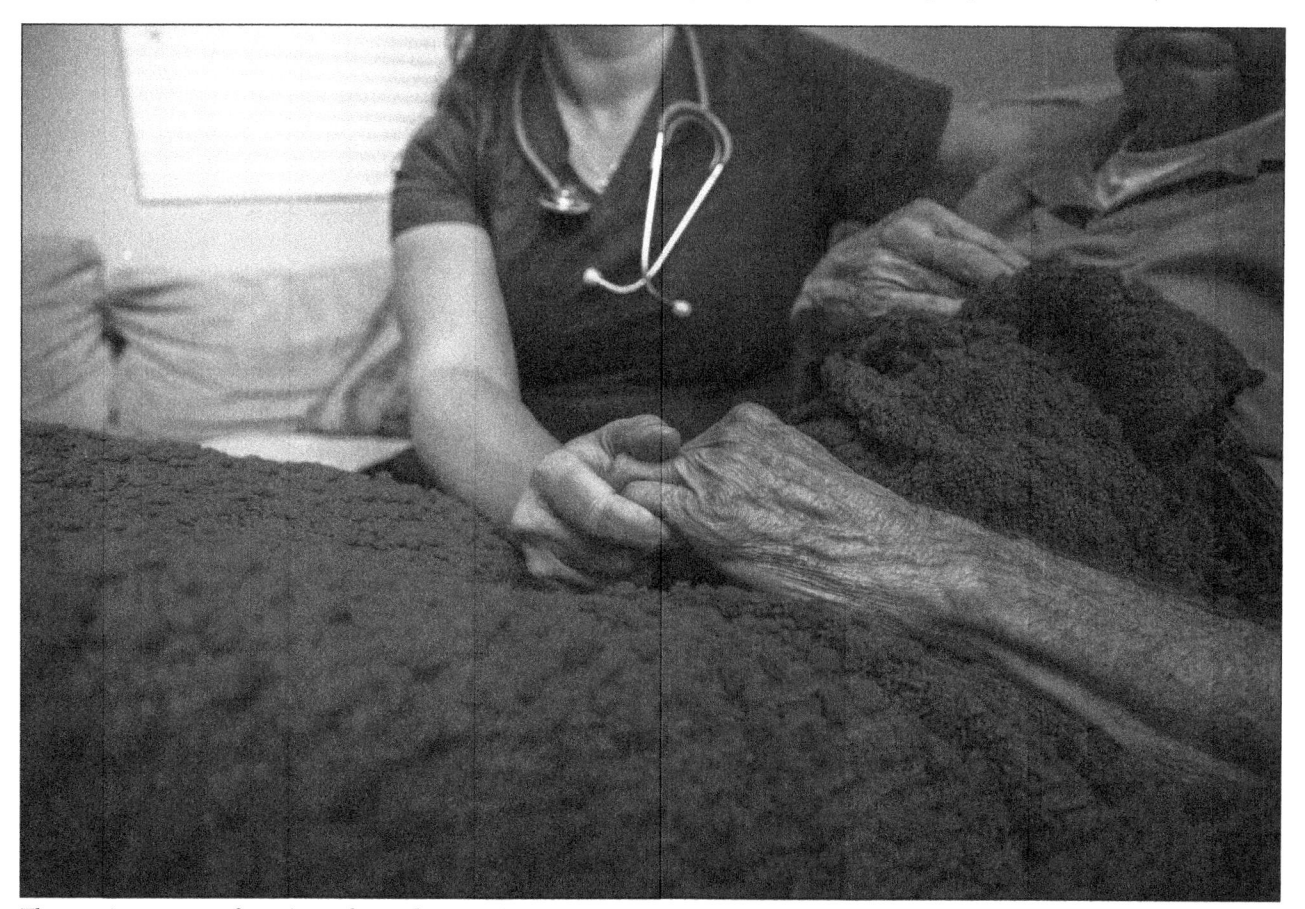

The commitment to care for patients who are dying requires compassion, communication skills, strength, and willingness to engage with the patient over a long period of time. (Lpettet via iStock)

to hospice, often after a period of palliative care, occurs when treatment can no longer control or cure disease. The life expectancy of a person referred to hospice care is usually six months or less. Choosing hospice care is a family decision made in consultation with the patient's doctor. Unfortunately, referrals to hospice care often come too late. Patients and families may not want to give up on treatment and doctors may not be willing to admit there is nothing more to do for the patient. Patients admitted to hospice care can always leave and return to active treatment if a new treatment becomes available. With the advent of palliative care, referrals to hospice may be managed more appropriately as more healthcare providers are involved with the patient. Hospice care may be provided in the home or an inpatient hospice facility that is free-standing or part of a hospital.

PROGRAM COMPONENTS

Both palliative care and hospice care focus on the patient and family or caregivers. The programs offer support systems during what can be a difficult time for all involved. This support encourages the patient to live as actively as possible with the best quality of life both during the chronic disease state and ultimately, the terminal disease state. Family and caregiver support are available in conjunction with the patient and in groups that focus on their particular issues and concerns. Special groups for children of parents experiencing palliative or hospice care is often available. Bereavement support, the period of time after the patient has died, is often provided.

A team approach is used in palliative and hospice care programs. Care may include physical care such as that provided by home healthcare nurses, hospice nurses or nurses assigned to a palliative or hospice care unit. Emotional and spiritual care is provided by trained staff or counselors and chaplains or other spiritual leaders. The patient's doctor is active with the patient in palliative care as treatment for the disease is continuing, but often a specially trained hospice physician takes over the care of the patient when a referral to hospice is made as active treatment ceases and the focus is on comfort measures and pain management.

THE PALLIATIVE CARE NURSING ROLE

Palliative care (PC) nurses have the primary contact with the patient and family as they navigate through their disease. When a referral to palliative care is made, the PC nurse must be able to educate the patient and family to the definition of palliative care, clearly explain that treatment will continue, and that the role of palliative care is to assist the patient, family, and caregivers through what can be a trying time. PC nurses are instrumental as they offer advice, provide emotional support, arrange or provide physical comfort measures and support the staff that are providing ongoing disease treatment for the patient. PC nurses must be knowledgeable in pain and symptom management, psychosocial and spiritual care, grief and loss issues, end-stage disease process, and strong communication skills to deliver a sometimes difficult message. Working in this specialty may be stressful. PC nurses work in many settings, including hospitals, nursing homes, physician offices and home healthcare or hospice. While there may be a palliative care unit, most PC nurses work as part of a team that sees patients wherever they are admitted. Hospital PC nurses generally do not see the patient in the home setting unless the hospital also provides home health. Transitioning the patient between care settings is often needed and the PC nurse will have an active role in insuring care continuity.

The demand for PC nurses is expected to increase as patients age, chronic illness can be managed for longer periods of time and the healthcare community recognizes the need for care management through the disease. The process of dying will always occur, creating an ongoing demand for palliative care services. Most PC nurses are registered nurses with a bachelor of science in nursing (BSN) or a master of science in nursing (MSN). The Hospice and Palliative Credentialing Center provides five certification examinations for registered nurses, advanced practice nurses, pediatric palliative nurses, nursing assistants, and those dealing with perinatal loss. Requirements vary by state and employer. The average salary for a palliative care nurse is similar to that of a staff nurse, varies by location, and may range from $45,000 to $70,000.

THE HOSPICE NURSING ROLE

The hospice nurse provides care for the patient, family and caregiver at the end of the patient's life. The hospice nurse (HN) may be employed in a variety of settings including hospitals, inpatient and outpatient hospice settings or home healthcare. As with palliative care nurses, many are credentialed registered nurses but may also be Certified Hospice and Palliative Nursing Assistants (CHPNA). Hospice nurses generally work with terminally ill patients to ensure an optimal quality of life with the least amount of pain for as long as possible.

While some hospitals have an inpatient hospice service, many hospices are freestanding entities or not for profit foundations. The hospice nurse is hired to provide direct, hands-on care to terminally ill patients. The HN may also provide a respite, or rest period, for family and caregivers when the patient is receiving hospice care in the home. When the hospice is a nonhospital-based organization, the roles of the HN are varied. Some of the roles include patient intake or admission, case management, home visits, triage, hospital liaison, and management of the hospice. When considering employment in a hospice setting, the same skill set as a palliative care nurse is necessary with the addition of dealing with the patient, family and caregiver at the moment of death. The salary range varies with geographic location and hospice setting. Generally, hospital-based hospice programs will pay better than smaller, free-standing hospice programs. Salaries are dependent on role, education, certification, and other factors.

SUMMARY

Palliative care and hospice are an increasing part of end of life care as patients are living longer with both chronic and terminal diseases. When a nurse chooses the specialties of palliative care and hospice care, the demands are significant but the rewards are worth it if you talk to nurses in this field. The commitment to care for patients who are in the dying process and up to death requires compassion, communication skills, strength, and willingness to engage with the patient over a longer period of time than what a staff nurse in the hospital is able to provide.

—*Patricia Stanfill Edens*

Further Reading

Center to Advance Palliative Care, www.capc.org. Accessed 11 Sept. 2020.

Edens, Pat Stanfill, and Catherine D. Harvey. "Developing and Financing a Palliative Care Program." *American Journal of Hospice and Palliative Medicine*, vol. 25, no. 5, Oct./Nov. 2008.

"Palliative Care Nurse Job Description and Salary Information." *Jacksonville University*, www.jacksonvilleu.com/blog/nursing/palliative-care-nurse-job-description-salary-information/. Accessed 11 Sept. 2020.

"Understanding the Role of a Hospice Nurse." *Crossroads Hospice*, www.registerednursing.org/specialty/hospice-nurse/ on Accessed 11 Sept. 2020.

"What Is Hospice Care?" *American Cancer Society*, www.cancer.org/treatment/end-of-life-care/hospice-care/what-is-hospice-care.html. Accessed 11 Sept. 2020.

"What Is Hospice Nursing?" *RegisteredNursing.org*, www.registerednursing.org/specialty/hospice-nurse/. Accessed 11 Sept. 2020.

"What Is Palliative Care?" *International Association for Hospice and Palliative Care*, hospicecare.com/what-we-do/publications/getting-started/5-what-is-palliative-care. Accessed 11 Sept. 2020.

"WHO Definition of Palliative Care." *World Health Organization*, www.who.int/cancer/palliative/definition/en/. Accessed 11 Sept. 2020.

Travel Nurse

ABSTRACT

A travel nurse is a registered nurse (RN) who works short-term stints at hospitals, clinics, and other healthcare facilities. Rather than hire on for a full-time, permanent position, these nursing professionals often move from location to location on short contracts, filling in where they are needed.

WHAT IS A TRAVEL NURSE?

The implementation of nurse-patient (N-P) ratios, a standard that defines how many patients each nurse cares for, is an idea that has gained prominence in recent years. N-P ratios ensure that nurses are able to provide an adequate level of care to every patient assigned to their care. As of 2020, California is the only state that has enacted nurse-patient ratio legislation for all hospital care units, although several other states have enacted lesser measures and many individual hospitals have their own criteria regarding nurse-patient ratios. Because of the implementation of these policies, as well as a general shortage of nurses, many facilities do not have the nursing staff to properly provide appropriate levels of care. For hospitals and other healthcare facilities looking for a safe way to overcome this shortage, turning to the services of a travel nurse is an increasingly common solution.

A travel nurse is an RN who works for an independent staffing agency that has contracted with a facility to provide nurses to make up for shortages in the facility's staffing plan. The agency assigns the travel nurse to a specific hospital or clinic where he or she will fill in, often on a thirteen-week contract. Not all contracts are this length and contracts can often be extended, but the thirteen-week period has become the industry standard. The travel nurse has a good deal of flexibility in determining which assignments he or she accepts and many people in the profession enjoy the sense of self-determination that the arrangement provides.

Once the nurse accepts an assignment, he or she travels to the location where the job is to be performed. Travel expenses are usually reimbursed and housing is generally provided. Travel nurses perform the same tasks as RNs who work for a single institution which include assessing a patient's healthcare needs, planning and carrying out treatment plans, collaborating with physicians and other nurses, and educating patients and families about the patients' conditions and treatments. Travel nurses may also work in any number of specialty areas such as intensive care units, emergency rooms and cardiac units, and their specific tasks may be tailored to these specialties.

In addition to normal, domestic situations, travel nurses may opt to work less typical assignments. Among these jobs are rapid response or crisis assignments. These jobs may involve responding to a natural or man-made disaster such as a hurricane or tornado. More often, they involve working at a hospital that has seen a sudden spike in intake or has opened a new unit and finds itself rapidly understaffed. Nurses who take on these kinds of assignments typically work for a shorter period of time than thirteen weeks and are often paid more than the typical travel nurse. They are required to arrive quickly at the job site, usually within two weeks. In addition, some travel nurses accept assignments abroad and these usually last from one to two years. They may serve impoverished and underserved populations or respond to disasters or outbreaks of disease.

BECOMING A TRAVEL NURSE

Travel nurses must be certified RNs. This means that they must first earn a degree in nursing, either a bachelor's degree, an associate's degree, or a diploma. Many healthcare facilities to which a travel nurse might be assigned may prefer the nurse to have a bachelor's degree, and so students who wish to become a travel nurse often opt for a BSN (bachelor of science in nursing) degree. After earning their degree, the RN must then pass the NCLEX-RN (National Council Licensure Exam-Registered Nurse) exam in order to obtain certification and legally practice.

Before signing up with a travel nurse agency, candidates are typically expected to work for at least one year (and sometimes two) as a RN, either in their specific area of specialty or in acute care. Additional certification may be recommended in line with the nurse's specific specialty. All RNs must be licensed in their state of practice. The Enhanced Nursing Licensure Compact (eNLC), with thirty-three states currently participating, allows nurses to hold a license in a participating state without having to obtain a separate license to practice when moving state to state. A travel nurse with a compact nursing license must still obtain a new state license for states not participating in the eNLC through a process known as reciprocity, or licensing though endorsement. The RN is responsible for researching licensing requirements prior to accepting a travel nurse position. The agency cannot apply for the license for a nurse, but can assist with the process.

—*Andrew Schenker*

Further Reading
"A Primer for Getting Your Nursing License in Another State." *Travel Nursing*, www.travelnursing.com/news/career-development/a-primer-for-getting-your-nursing-license-in-another-state/. Accessed 30 Sept. 2020.
Kleinfield, Sonny. *Becoming a Nurse*. Simon & Schuster, 2020.
"Travel Nurse." *Registered Nursing*, www.registerednursing.org/specialty/travel-nurse/. Accessed 29 Sept. 2020.
"What Is Travel Nursing?" *Nurse.org*, nurse.org/articles/how-to-make-the-most-money-as-a-travel-nurse/. Accessed 29 Sept. 2020.

CLINICAL RESEARCH NURSE

ABSTRACT
A clinical research nurse is responsible for the care of patients participating in a research trial. Clinical research nurses are generally registered nurses with additional training and certifications related to the research process.

INTRODUCTION
When a patient enters a clinical research trial, a clinical research nurse focuses on the patient's care. A clinical research trial or protocol looks at new ways to prevent, detect, or treat disease. When a patient voluntarily enters a clinical trial, it helps physicians and researchers learn more about the disease and improve care for future patients. Types of clinical trials may include the understanding of a disease by studying patterns and cause and effects (epidemiology), the understanding of human behavior (behavioral), they may look at how people access healthcare and services (health services) and participate in protocols that evaluate an intervention on outcomes (clinical trial).

The clinical research nurse is a registered nurse with additional training, education and often certifications. In 2016, the American Nurses Association (ANA) formally recognized clinical research nursing as a specialty. Clinical research nurses are specially trained to protect research subjects while maintaining the integrity of the research protocol. A research protocol is basically a road map of the research that will take place to validate an assumption that a treatment is effective. The International Association of Clinical Research Nurses (IACRN) focuses on defining, validating and advancing the specialty. Certification such as that provided by the Association of Clinical Research Professionals (ACRP) results in increased job responsibility, greater career advancement, more employment opportunities, and recognition of excellence in the field.

DUTIES OF CLINICAL RESEARCH NURSES
Duties of clinical research nurses (CRN) varies from center to center and hospital to hospital based on the types of research being conducted, the complexity of clinical trials, and the numbers of patients accrued annually. For example, a hospital conducting nursing

research will not have the complexity of a cancer center focusing on extensive pharmaceutical interventions and pharmacokinetics. Research nurses will encounter differing levels of complexity in the research arena but all require a strict attention to detail and a commitment to patient safety.

Clinical research nurses see patients, help define criteria in the trial, write standard operating procedures to ensure consistency between staff, evaluate research methods, and assist physicians and advanced practice nurses with procedures. The CRN may draw lab work, administer investigational drugs, and interview patients about symptoms and side effects. Accurate data collection is the foundation for a strong clinical trial outcome. Research nurses may also be involved in identifying and recruiting patients to studies, obtaining informed consent, providing education, and communicating with the principal investigator and physicians involved in the research.

Clinical research nurses are responsible in conjunction with the principal investigator for the quality, honesty and integrity of clinical trials. They ensure that trials are conducted in compliance with local, state, federal, and international regulations. In particular, attention to detail is critical related to clinical trials that will be submitted to the Food and Drug Administration (FDA).

JOB DESCRIPTION AND SALARY

Job descriptions for clinical research nurses are fairly similar across settings of practice. Providing clinical and administrative nursing support for research trials, studies, and projects; recruiting and screening potential study participants; performing assessments, evaluations, and administering medications and research instruments; and collecting data are primary functions. Other functions vary by setting and may include assisting with surgical procedures and other invasive procedures; providing patient and family education; coordinating with other healthcare professionals; and taking direction from the clinical investigators responsible for the study.

Salaries vary by location and type of organization. Ranges from $48,000 to $80,000 and higher may be seen across the United States. Most often clinical research nurses are considered exempt employees, meaning they are paid a salary and are not eligible for overtime pay. The hours are often daytime, Monday through Friday with occasional weekend work depending on patient needs and protocol design.

A clinical research nurse is responsible for supporting primary or clinical investigators. There are also nursing researchers that conduct their own clinical trials or studies. These nurses generally have a masters in nursing degree or PhD, with training in developing and writing research studies.

SUMMARY

Achieving registered nurse status opens doors to additional areas of practice, including clinical research. The clinical research nurse is instrumental to the future of advances in medicine as new drugs, agents and equipment rapidly increase and must be tested on human subjects. Protecting patients by ensuring research quality and safety will directly impact their care. All patients should be offered the opportunity to participate in research studies.

—*Patricia Stanfill Edens*

Further Reading

"Certifications." *The Association of Clinical Research Professionals*, acrpnet.org/certifications/. Accessed 11 Sept. 2020.

International Association of Clinical Research Nurses, iacrn.org. Accessed 11 Sept. 2020.

"Job Description: Clinical Research Nurse I." Human Resources. *Emory University*, apps.hr.emory.edu/JobDescriptions/class.jsp?code=PF02. Accessed 11 Sept. 2020.

"NIH Clinical Research Trials and You." *National Institutes of Health*, www.nih.gov/health-information/nih-clinical-research-trials-you. Accessed 11 Sept. 2020.

Roberts, K., S. Gelder, and H. Wild. "Clinical Research Nurse Interns: The Future Research Workforce." *Nursing Research*, vol. 24, no. 2, 18 Nov. 2016, pp. 6–7.

"Steps to Becoming a Clinical Trials Research Nurse—Education and Experience." *MHAOnline*, www.mhaonline.com/faq/how-do-I-become-a-clinical-trials-research-nurse. Accessed 11 Sept. 2020.

CASE MANAGEMENT/UTILIZATION MANAGEMENT AND CARE NAVIGATION

ABSTRACT

Case management and care navigation are two types of nursing roles that practice across the continuum of care. The goal of case management is to provide the correct level of care for the correct amount of time for the patient. Determining the correct reimbursement and resource utilization for the hospital is utilization management. The goal of care navigation is to provide direction for patients in managing their decisions about the multiple points of care needed in order to receive knowledgeable, timely, and seamless treatment. The nursing roles in case management and care navigation achieve similar outcomes for the patient with the nurse serving as an advocate for patient treatment and outcomes of care. Both of these roles work closely with many different types of healthcare professionals to provide a seamless healthcare experience for the patient.

CASE MANAGEMENT/UTILIZATION MANAGEMENT

Case management as defined by the American Nurse Credentialing Center, part of the American Nurses Association, is "a dynamic and systematic collaborative approach to provide and coordinate health services to a defined population. Nurse case managers actively participate with their clients to identify and facilitate options and services for meeting individuals' health needs with the goal of decreasing fragmentation and duplication of care and enhancing quality, cost-effective clinical outcomes." Utilization management achieves both quality outcomes and cost containment in a complex health system that has ongoing cost inflation. Utilization management functions are conversations and documentation between the hospital nurse case manager providing services and the insurance company paying for the services. The case manager is the contact point during the hospital stay to provide the insurance company with the level and progress of care along with the patient's discharge plan during the patient's hospital admission. The nurse case manager is the central point of contact with the hospital team, balancing resources and costs for patients and advocating a seamless and timely experience without delay among physicians, multiple healthcare workers, and insurance companies.

CARE NAVIGATION

Care Navigators may also be called patient navigators who are registered nurses in the hospital setting that provide assistance to the individual who is facing significant health problems that require complex management and coordination. In some instances outside of the hospital, patient navigators may be used to assist an individual to get medical appointments made, arrange transportation and may even accompany them as a patient advocate. Hospital care navigators are skilled in being a liaison between the patient and their caregivers, physicians and family members to effectively communicate, facilitate, explain, and support the patient's needs to achieve outcomes of recommended treatment.

Early identification of a potentially terminal diagnosis is a situation that requires understanding of what order and choices of treatments occur. Cancer is one example of a disease process that requires complex treatments. The experienced cancer care navigator can provide information to the patient and family that will reassure, support and assist them to "navigate" the many different treatments and side effects that may result. Patients undergoing treatments need to know the resulting impact on their appearance. Care navigators work with patients to provide the emotional support during treatment and prepare them for ongoing management of the disease process. The nurse navigator makes the cancer journey more understandable while providing emotional support to the patient and family.

PROGRAM COMPONENTS

Both case management and care navigation have a focus on the patient, family, and caregivers. The programs offer the patient a seamless and coordinated experience in a complex and increasingly fragmented healthcare system. While the hospital setting is the most common location for these programs, both case management and care navigation can also be individually offered as a health insurance benefit. Recent healthcare legislation such as the Affordable Care Act (ACA) has opened the door for formally recognizing and reimbursing these services. Facilitating the most efficient pathway to achieving health and autonomy for the individual is the goal of both programs through advocacy, assessment, planning, communication, education, managing resources, and facilitating services.

Case management has some differences from care navigation. Case management is a care delivery model and serves the hospitalized individual by managing activities between multiple disciplines. Case management functions include direct communication across the payer, primary care physician, and other health service professionals, especially nursing, to identify an appropriate discharge plan, length of stay, and posthospital services. From admission through postdischarge, case managers must follow legal and regulatory guidelines established by the government and payers.

Care navigators do have overlapping components with the bedside nurse but also cross departments as the patient moves through the disease process. They complement care delivery and work closely with the physician to provide an ongoing understanding by individuals about their treatments and conditions. Simply put, care navigators explain treatment options, provide advice and support to the patient during their experience. Acting as a guide to the patient and their family decreases the confusion and creates an environment for making decisions needed for care and treatment.

THE NURSING ROLE IN CASE MANAGEMENT/UTILIZATION MANAGEMENT

Preparing for a nurse case manager role has increasingly required a bachelor's degree and in some instances, postgraduate education or certification in case management. Regardless of academic credentials, nurse case managers need clinical expertise, effective communication, and problem-solving skills as well as a broad understanding of today's healthcare system. Nurse case managers see the bigger picture of health across multiple groups of people or population health. Critical-thinking skills and knowledge of medical necessity for different levels of care are two very important roles for the nurse case manager and utilization management case manager. Utilization management (UM) case managers need skills to communicate with payers, manage resource use, and act as a liaison between physicians, their orders and the payer. Case managers are also employed by insurance companies and partner with the hospital UM case manager to manage resources needed for payment of care.

As healthcare costs continue to rise and life expectancy increases, the case manager role will continue to be needed in the healthcare industry. Currently, the demand is greater than the supply. Preparation to become a case manager is provided in baccalaureate nursing programs. Case management certification is offered by both the American Nurses Credentialing Center through the Case Management Society of America and the American Case Management Society. The salary range will vary but pays more than a bedside nurse dependent on the role, education, certification, and other factors.

THE NURSING ROLE IN CARE NAVIGATION

When a new and complex diagnosis is made for a patient, a care navigator is assigned to support and guide the patient throughout their treatment. Nurse care navigators are trained in psychosocial skills in addition to their basic nursing education, which are used in interactions with patients. Experienced nurse navigators and professional nurse consultants are responsible in their facilities for designing protocols and guidelines. Active discussions during ongoing professional conference call meetings facilitate teamwork, efficiency, and improve patient outcomes for this role. Nurse navigators actively reach out on behalf of their patients to facilitate communication between providers; prevent delays in treatment; manage and monitor patient symptoms; offer psychological support; and recommend resources to use. As their role of one point of contact for the patient who has multiple clinicians and settings to deal with, care navigators can manage information and, with active listening and patience, reassure patients. The role of a care navigator enables the nurse to practice at his or her highest level of expertise. Nursing care navigators pursue additional education and experience in their chosen field which can result in salary increases based on geographic location and type of hospital setting.

SUMMARY

Nursing case management and care navigation both provide support to patients in the delivery of care. With today's healthcare continually changing and increasing in complexity, both of these roles allow patients the choice, autonomy, and support to pursue their health. The rewards of serving in one of these roles is seen with the rise of patient-centered and value-based care, which continues to allow nurses to be at the forefront of influencing the delivery of healthcare in the United States.

—Carol A. Beehler

Further Reading

"Care Management: Implications for Medical Practice, Health Policy and Health Services Research." *Agency for Healthcare Research and Quality*, www.ahrq.gov/ncepcr/care/coordination/management.html. Accessed 20 Oct. 2020.

"Definition and Philosophy of Case Management." *Commission for Case Manager Certification*, ccmcertification.org/about-ccmc/about-case-management/definition-and-philosophy-case-management.

Kelly, K.J., S. Doucet, and A. Luke. "Exploring the Roles, Functions, and Background of Patient Navigators and Case Managers: A Scoping Review." *International Journal of Nursing Studies*, vol. 98, Oct. 2019, pp. 27–47.

Leonard, Margaret, and Elaine Miller. *Nursing Case Management*. ANCC, Credentialing Knowledge Center, 2009.

White, P., and M.E. Hall. "Mapping the Literature of Case Management Nursing." *Journal of Medical Library Associations*, vol. 94, Suppl. 2, Apr. 2006, pp. E99–E106.

Zander, Karen. *Case Management Models, Best Practices for Health Systems and ACO's*. 2nd ed., HCPro, 2017,

Zangerle, Claire, M. "What Are the Roles and Responsibilities of a Case Manager in a Hospital Setting?" *Nursing Management*, vol. 46, no. 10, Oct. 2015, pp. 27–28.

EDUCATORS—ACADEMIC AND VOCATIONAL PROGRAMS

ABSTRACT

Nurse educators are registered nurses (RNs), often with advanced education, who teach students in a nursing program or academic setting. In addition to advanced education, clinical experience is a necessary part of teaching.

EDUCATORS IN THE ACADEMIC SETTING

Nurse educators are vital to training and educating the next generation of nurses. The job outlook is excellent, as nursing care is a growing need as the population ages and new treatments and diseases emerge. The average salary in an academic setting such as a community college or college offering bachelors' degrees is $50,000 to $80,000 and varies with locale, education, experience and courses taught. Higher salaries are paid to nurses with a doctoral degree or who take on additional administrative duties. Faculty may work a full-time academic position with a nine-month academic year appointment and have both teaching and clinical responsibilities or they may serve as adjunct, or part-time faculty, and teach one or two courses or supervise students only in the clinical setting. Faculty are often paid less than nurses caring for patients. Daytime hours during the week often compensates for the lower salary. Faculty do not generally work twelve-hour shifts or on weekends.

Educators are asked to develop lesson plans, also known as curriculum guides, teach both classroom courses and their clinical applications, oversee students in the clinical setting while students are providing patient care, and model nursing behaviors including ethics, confidentiality and patient safety. Faculty members may teach entry level courses such as fundamentals of nursing or focus on specialization in areas such as pediatric nursing, cardiac nursing or critical care nursing. Nurse educators must stay current in their knowledge of nursing and be prepared to take continuing education courses, read and research advances in nursing and often are required to publish articles and conduct nursing research as a part of their academic appointment. Nursing faculty actively involved in nursing research are providing the foundation for the profession going forward.

Teaching aspiring students in an entry level nursing program is the most often role for academic nurse faculty, but faculty are also needed in advanced degree programs such as master's in nursing, doctorate in nursing practice and specialty areas such as anesthesia and midwifery. The more advanced the level of education, the more education the faculty member is expected to have in order to teach at this level. For example, teaching in a nurse practitioner (NP) program would most likely require both an advanced degree and certification as an NP.

There is a high demand for nursing faculty in the academic setting. The US Department of Labor reports that in 2020, a million new and replacement nurses are needed. The American Association of Colleges of Nursing reported that 65,000 qualified applicants were denied admission to a nursing program due to a shortage of faculty. Educators must have knowledge and clinical expertise, strong communication and public speaking skills, an ability to communicate complex concepts clearly, and a desire to help others gain skills to provide care to a vulnerable patient population.

EDUCATORS IN THE VOCATIONAL SETTING

Nurse educators with a focus on licensed practical nurse (LPN) or licensed vocational nurse (LVN) education may work in a variety of settings including vocational centers and private educational facilities. Licensed practical nursing programs may also be located in some community colleges. The program generally lasts one year. Nurse educators with a role in LPN education require, at minimum, a bachelor's in nursing degree from an accredited college of nursing. RNs without a bachelor's degree are prohibited from becoming LPN instructors, but may be able to be a certified nursing assistant (CNA) instructor. Instructors must have appropriate clinical experience in addition to education and experience on a medical-surgical or general nursing care floor is always desirable.

The role of an LPN/LVN instructor requires classroom instruction but has a significant amount of clinical work usually in the hospital or nursing home setting. Classes taught may include anatomy and physiology, nutrition, health assessment, microbiology and hands-on skills such as vital signs and assisting the patient with activities of daily living. Salary is dependent on locale, education, experience, and employer.

—Patricia Stanfill Edens

Further Reading

"About the Nursing Shortage." *American Association of Colleges of Nursing*, www.aacnnursing.org/News-Information/Nursing-Shortage-Resources/About. Accessed 22 Sept. 2020.

"Education Resources." *American Association of Colleges of Nursing*, www.aacnnursing.org/Teaching-Resources. Accessed 22 Sept. 2020.

"Licensed Practical/Vocational Nurses: A Place on the Team." *American Association of Occupational Health Nurses*, vol. 65, no. 4, 2017, pp. 154–57.

"LPN Instructor Careers with BSN." *Practical Nursing.org*, www.practicalnursing.org/lpn-instructor-careers-bsn. Accessed 22 Sept. 2020.

"Nurse Educator." *ExploreHealthCareers.org*, explorehealthcareers.org/career/nursing/nurse-educator/. Accessed 22 Sept. 2020.

"Nurse Educators." *National League for Nursing (NLN)*, www.nln.org. Accessed 22 Sept. 2020.

"Nursing Vocational School Program Information." *Study.com*, 23 Apr. 2020, study.com/nursing_vocational_school.html.

CONTINUING EDUCATION COORDINATOR AND PATIENT EDUCATOR

ABSTRACT

The field of nursing is an evolving profession as new technology becomes available, and new studies are published. Not only is it important to continue your education after you graduate, in most facilities, it is required so that nurses can provide the most up-to-date, high-quality patient care. Some states require formal continuing education for renewal of the nursing license. Education is not only important for the nurse, but also the patient. Nurses educate patients on a regular basis in order for the patient to continue to better their health.

STAFF EDUCATION: ORIENTATION

When a nurse is first hired, whether experienced or as a new graduate, the nurse must attend an orientation. Orientation is hospital specific with the goal of providing a basic overview of hospital policies. This orientation is usually a one to two-week period with different interactive classes. Speakers from multiple departments in the hospital may provide information about their location and function. For example, pharmacy, laboratory and blood bank, radiology, and other departments may come and present a brief overview of their services.

After the classroom orientation, the nurse will then go through orientation with a preceptor (an experienced nurse who usually has at least one year of experience) on the unit assigned to the new employee. This time is used to acquaint the nurse with the hospital, the different policies and procedures and ensure the nurse can provide safe, appropriate care to the patient. The length of this type of orientation varies based on the nurse's experience and the type of nursing care needed to be provided. A specialty floor like an intensive care unit (ICU) or bone marrow transplant unit will have unit specific competencies the nurse must complete before the nurse is allowed to exit the orientation phase. For example, a Bone Marrow Transplant Nurse would need to learn how to properly infuse the cellular infusion. An intensive care nurse would need to learn how to titrate medications, and how to monitor certain machines like ventilators. Most newly hired nurses have a checklist of certain skills and experiences tailored to the unit they have been hired for hat they must obtain before they can exit orientation.

The length of time a nurse is in orientation varies by hospital, unit assignment, and patient acuity. Nurses new to the profession will generally receive a longer clinical orientation after the classroom orientation as hands on patient care requires skills that may not have been learned during the nursing program.

CONTINUED AND CONTINUING EDUCATION

The medical field is a continuously evolving profession. Nursing is no different. Per regulatory guidelines, nurses must be competent in certain skills.

Hospital facilities must be able to provide documentation of nurses' skills, often as a part of the hospital accreditation process by outside agencies such as The Joint Commission, the accrediting agency for healthcare providers. Most hospital facilities have designated departments to ensure education requirements are met in a timely manner. For example, most nursing education departments have cardiopulmonary resuscitation (CPR) instructors for required re-certifications. This department is also responsible for educating nurses on new techniques, new equipment, and new policies. Classes are offered at times convenient to all shifts and schedules and are often required as a condition of employment.

The field of nursing operates on evidenced based practice. Practices change over time and in order for all nurses to be knowledgeable of this information, the education department creates certain educational tools to disperse to nurses. For example, it was once taught that when a nasogastric tube (NGT) was placed in a patient, an accurate way to confirm placement in the stomach was simply to place a stethoscope onto the patient's stomach while simultaneously injecting air into the NGT to listen for correct placement. It has now been proven, that although you may still hear the air passing through, the NGT could still be located in the patient's lungs. It is now best practice to obtain an X-ray in order to confirm that the NGT is in the stomach before using. Education departments would have been responsible for relaying this information so that this practice was changed within the facility, and were responsible for maintaining documentation that all nurses had been educated on this change.

In addition to the continued education of employed nurses, a more formal continuing education outside the hospital may be required in certain states for re-licensure as a registered nurse. For example, some states require continuing education related to domestic violence and human immunodeficiency virus (HIV)/Acquired immunodeficiency syndrome (AIDS) or may state an hourly requirement of continuing education united (CEUs) allowing the nurse to select the topics most needed based on employment such as recognizing child abuse. These courses provide CEUs that are recognized by both the employer and the state as meeting rigorous education standards that may also include testing. The CEU was created in 1970 after a US Department of Education Task force in conjunction with the International Association for Continuing Education and Training (IACET) studied noncredit continuing education activities. The CEU provides a standard unit of measure; 10 hours of contact learning equals one CEU. Only organizations who meet strict criteria may grant CEUs. For example, major medical centers and teaching hospitals may offer CEU courses while other hospitals may need their employees to receive CEUs at off-site facilities. The CEU is a standard manner to quantify education and training activities. CEU programs also consider diversity or providers and take into consideration the adult learner. In addition to state licensing requirements, CEUs may also be required for professional memberships and certification.

PATIENT EDUCATION

Educating patients and families plays an important role in the field of nursing. Whether in a hospital setting or outpatient clinic setting, it is vital to educate patients or families in order to have success at preventing further complications and so the patient and family can continue the plan of care after leaving the hospital. Patient education may help patients and families deal with the crises of acute and chronic diseases, help them learn self-care and how to gather information and how to develop strategies to promote optimal health.

For example, patients who have been diagnosed with diabetes will need to be educated on the disease itself, the proper technique to check their glucose, the proper way of self-administering insulin if needed and signs and symptoms to watch for if glucose levels get too high or low. Some facilities may have specific patient educators hired to teach this information, but nurses must be prepared to fulfil this role when needed. All staff nurses will be involved in educating patients and families in hospital and other healthcare provider settings. This education may involve teaching about what drugs the patient is receiving in the hospital, why coughing and deep breaths are important after surgery, and why keeping the bedrails up is important to prevent falls. For more formal patient education, a registered nurse with a bachelor of science in nursing is often required and a master of science in nursing is often preferred. Patient Educators may focus on one specific area or several closely related areas. For example, Diabetes Educators help the newly diagnosed patient deal with a complex disease management process.

SUMMARY

Many professions require ongoing education after the basic education process, but no where is this more important than with nursing. Because of the rapid advances in healthcare and medicine, continual learning is critical to optimal outcomes for the patient. Educating patients and families is an integral part of the nursing process whether at the bedside or in more formal classes.

—*Olivia Poteete Kerstens*

Further Reading

"About the CEU." *International Association for Continuing Education and Training*, www.iacet.org/standards/ansi-iacet-2018-1-standard-for-continuing-education-and-training/continuing-education-unit-ceu/about-the-ceu/. Accessed 18 Sept. 2020.

"Orientation Process." Nurse Educator Resource Center. *Vanderbilt University Medical Center*, www.vumc.org/nerc/35825. Accessed 18 Sept. 2020.

"Nursing Continuing Education Requirements by State." *AACEUS: Online Continuing Education for Healthcare Professionals*, www.aaaceus.com/state_nursing_requirements.asp. Accessed 18 Sept. 2020.

"Patient Education Coordinator." *Daily Nurse*, dailynurse.com/patient-education-coordinator/. Accessed 18 Sept. 2020.

Qulehsari, M. Q., et al. "Lifelong Learning Strategies in Nursing: A Systemic Review." *Electron Physician*, vol. 9, no. 10, 2017, pp. 5541–50, www.ncbi.nlm.nih.gov/pmc/articles/PMC5718860/.

Specific Nursing Care

With over 30 essays, this section includes a great variety of ways that nurses can use their skills and talents. From pain management, meditation, biofeedback, and guided imagery to diet-based therapies, exercise-based therapies, art therapy, and robotics, this section explores dozens of specific ways nurses can care for their patients. Also included in this section are essays on health organizations such as the NIH and the Office of Cancer Complementary & Alternative Medicine, and genetic counseling.

Dying, Death, and Grief	211
Pain Management	217
National Institutes of Health (NIH)	221
Health Promotion	226
Diet-Based Therapies	230
Exercise-Based Therapies	232
Education and Training of CAM Practitioners	237
Integrative Medicine	242
Internet Medicine	246
Internet and Health Information	*250*
Office of Cancer Complementary and Alternative Medicine (OCCAM)	252
Office of Dietary Supplements (ODS)	253
Self-Care	255
Spirituality and CAM	257
Relaxation Response	260
Relaxation Therapies	262
Meditation	267
Transcendental Meditation (TM)	270
Mind-Body Medicine	273
Guided Imagery	275
Natural Treatments for Stress	276
Natural Treatments for Well-Being	280
Therapeutic Touch (TT)	282

Reiki	285
Rolfing	289
Art Therapy	290
Music Therapy	293
Biofeedback	297
Nursing Care Plan	301
Genetic Counseling	303
Robotics in Healthcare	307
Bioinformatics	312
Popular Health Movement	314

Dying, Death, and Grief

ABSTRACT
Understanding the stages of grief allows the healthcare practitioner to better provide care for patients. End-of-life care, palliative care, and hospice care are all components of providing the continuum of care from diagnosis to death.

INTRODUCTION
Medicine determines that death has occurred by assessing bodily functions in either of two areas. Persons with irreversible cessation of respiration and circulation are dead; persons with irreversible cessation of ascertainable brain functions are also dead. There are standard procedures used to diagnose death, including simple observation, brain-stem reflex studies, and the use of confirmatory testing such as electrocardiography (ECG or EKG), electroencephalography (EEG), and arterial blood gas analysis (ABG).

Between 60 and 75 percent of all people die from chronic terminal conditions. Therefore, except in sudden death (as in a fatal accident) or when there is no evidence of consciousness (as in a head injury which destroys cerebral functions while leaving brain-stem reflexive functions intact), dying is both a physical and a psychological process. In most cases, dying takes time, and the time allows patients to react to the reality of their own passing and the family to begin the grieving process. Often, patients react by becoming vigilant about bodily symptoms and any changes

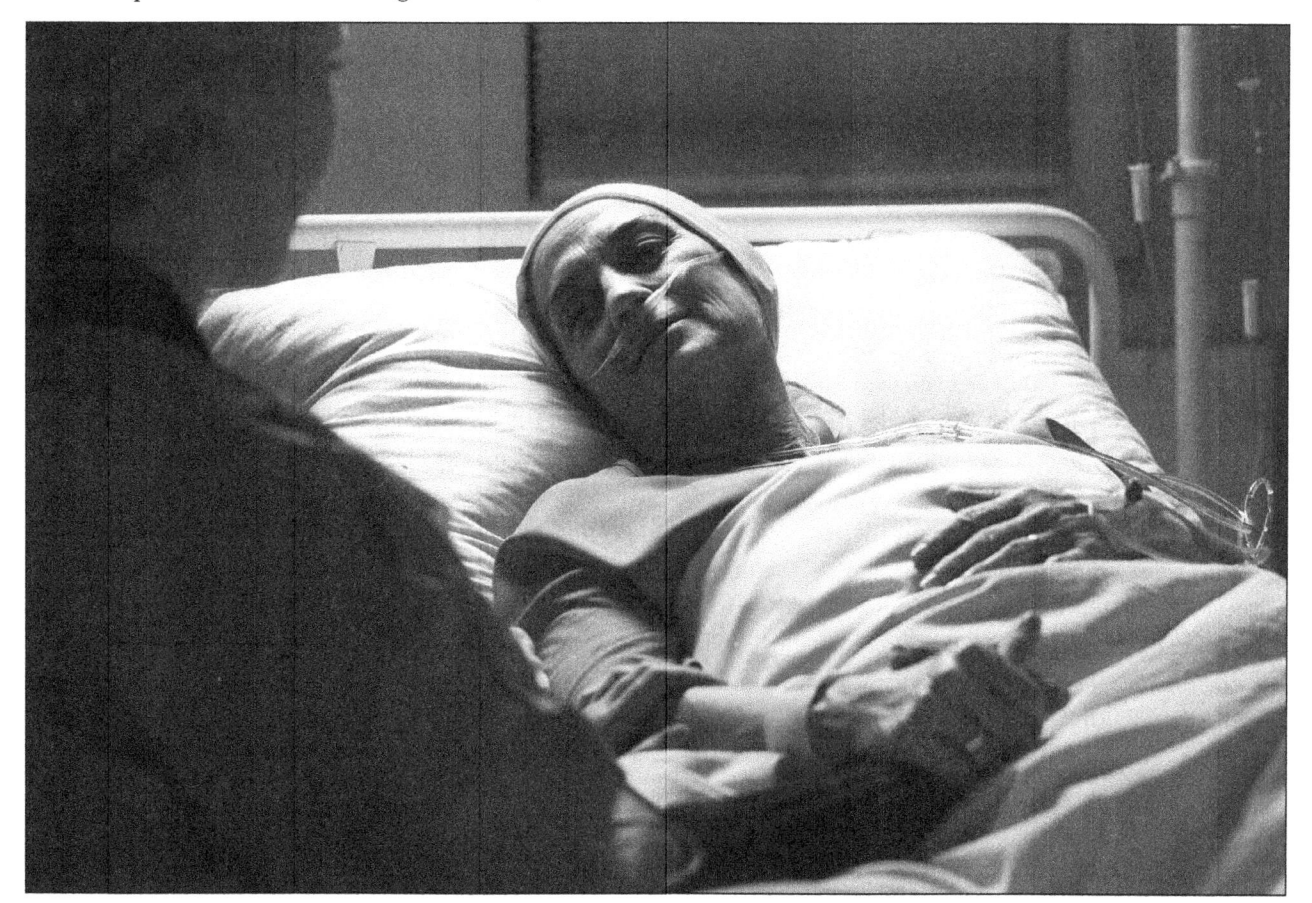

Medicine has come to acknowledge that physicians should understand what it means to die. Indeed, while all persons should understand what their own deaths will mean, physicians must additionally understand how their dying patients find this meaning. (Katarzyna Bialasiewicz via iStock)

in them. They also anticipate changes that have yet to occur. For example, long before the terminal stages of illness become manifest, dying patients commonly fear physical pain, shortness of breath, invasive procedures, loneliness, becoming a burden to loved ones, losing decision-making authority, and facing the unknown of death itself. Families and friends may begin to separate from the patient prematurely as they process the dying of their loved one.

As physical deterioration proceeds, all people cope by resorting to what has worked for them before: the unique means and mechanisms which have helped maintain a sense of self and personal stability. People seem to go through the process of dying much as they have gone through the process of living—with the more salient features of their personalities, whether good or bad, becoming sharper and more prominent. People seem to face death much as they have faced life.

ELISABETH KÜBLER-ROSS: ON DEATH AND DYING

In 1969, psychiatrist Elisabeth Kübler-Ross published the landmark *On Death and Dying*, based on her work with two hundred terminally ill patients. Though the work of Kübler-Ross has been criticized for the nature of the stages described and whether or not every person experiences every stage, her model has retained enormous utility to those who work in the area of death and dying. Technologically driven, Western medicine had come to define its role as primarily dealing with extending life and thwarting death by defeating specific diseases. Too few physicians saw a role for themselves once the prognosis turned grave. In the decades that followed the publication of *On Death and Dying*, the profession has reaccepted that death and dying are part of life and that, while treating the dying may not mean extending the length of life, it can and should mean improving its quality.

Kübler-Ross provided a framework to explain how people cope with and adapt to the profound and terrible news that their illness is terminal. Although other physicians, psychologists, and thanatologists have shortened, expanded, and adapted her five stages of the dying process, neither the actual number of stages nor what they are specifically called is as important as the information and insight that any stage theory of dying yields. As with any human process, dying is complex, multifaceted, multidimensional, and polymorphic.

The nurse may be exposed to a variety of patients in varying stages of dying. From the terminal cancer patient to the patient with a chronic disease such as liver failure or congestive heart failure, understanding how to support and care for dying patients is a critical nursing skill. In addition to direct patient care, understanding how to support the family and friends of the patient is also essential. Family and friends will need support after the patient's death and many hospitals and organizations provide bereavement groups to assist in their adaptation to the loss of their loved one.

COMPLICATIONS AND DISORDERS

Kübler-Ross defined five stages of grief. Denial is the first stage defined by Kübler-Ross, but it is also linked to shock and isolation. Whether the news is told outright or gradual self-realization occurs, most people react to the knowledge of their impending death with existential shock: Their whole selves recoil at the idea, and they say, in some fashion, "This cannot be happening to me." Broadly considered, denial is a complex cognitive-emotional capacity that enables temporary postponement of active, acute, but in some way detrimental, recognition of reality. In the dying process, this putting off of the truth prevents a person from being overwhelmed while promoting psychological survival. Denial is truly a mechanism of defense.

Many other researchers, along with Kübler-Ross, report anger as the second stage of dying. The stage is also linked to rage, fury, envy, resentment, and loathing. When "This cannot be happening to me" becomes, "This is happening to me. There was no

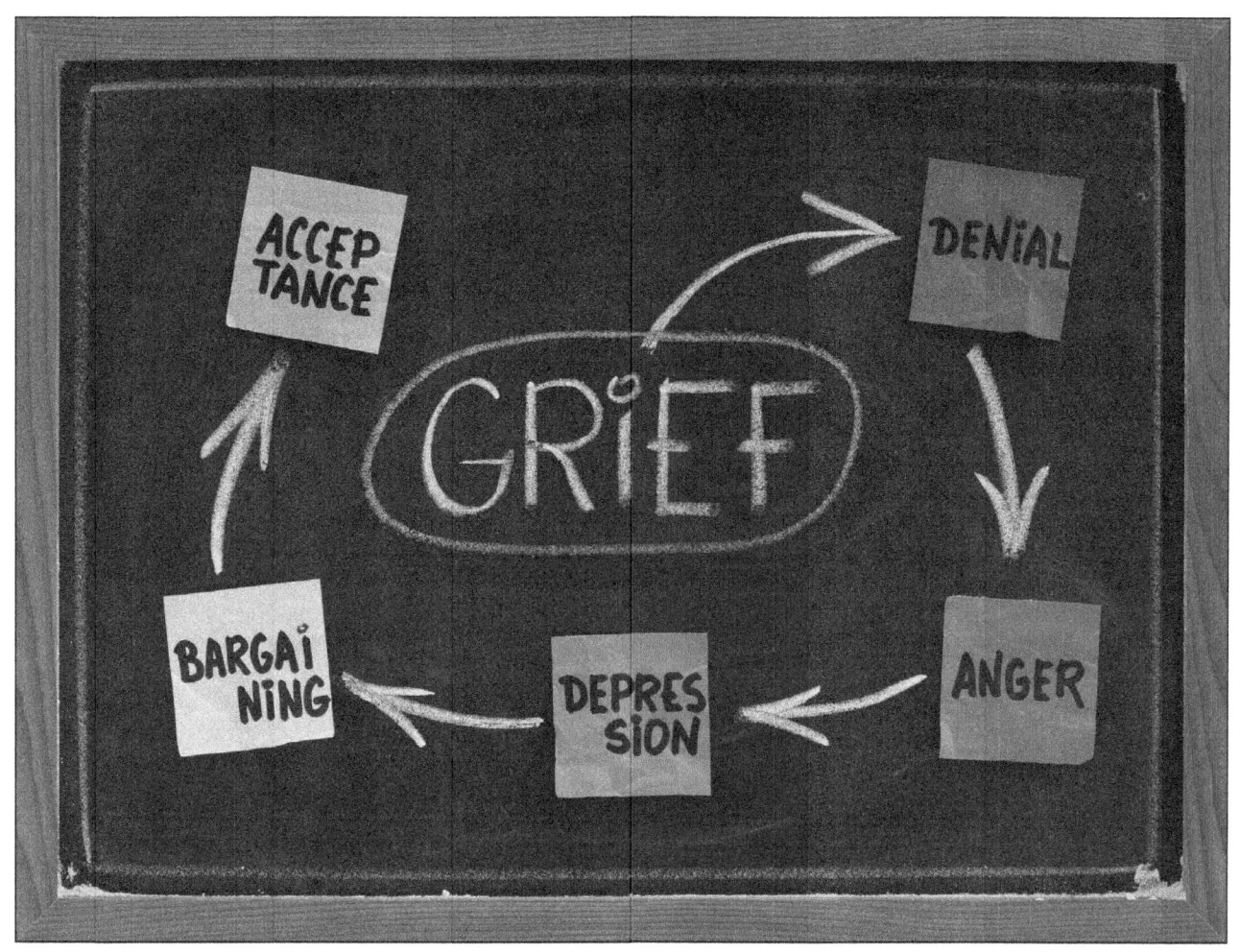

Kübler-Ross's Five Stages of Grief (Marek Kuliasz via iStock)

mistake," patients are beginning to replace denial with attempts to understand what is happening to and inside them. When they do, they often ask, "Why me?" Though it is an unanswerable question, the logic of the question is clear. People, to remain human, must try to make intelligible their experiences and reality. The asking of this question is an important feature of the way in which all dying persons adapt to and cope with the reality of death.

People react with anger when they lose something of value; they react with greater anger when something of value is taken away from them by someone or something. Rage and fury, in fact, are often more accurate descriptions of people's reactions to the loss of their own life than is anger. Anger is a difficult stage for professionals and loved ones, more so when the anger and rage are displaced and projected randomly into any corner of the patient's world. An unfortunate result is that caregivers often experience the anger as personal, and the caregivers' own feelings of guilt, shame, grief, and rejection can contribute to lessening contact with the dying person, which increases his or her sense of isolation.

Bargaining is Kübler-Ross's third stage, but it is also the one about which she wrote the least and the one that other thanatologists are most likely to leave unrepresented in their own models and stages of how people cope with dying. Nevertheless, it is a common phenomenon wherein dying people fall back on their faith, belief systems, or sense of the transcendent and the spiritual and try to make a deal—with god, life, fate, a higher power, or the universe. They ask for more time to help family members reconcile or to achieve something of importance. They may ask if they can simply attend their child's wedding or graduation or if they can see their first grandchild born.

At some point, when terminally ill individuals are faced with decisions about more procedures, tests, surgeries, or medications or when their thinness, weakness, or deterioration becomes impossible to ignore, the anger, rage, numbness, stoicism, and even humor will likely give way to depression, Kübler-Ross's fourth stage and the one reaction that all thanatologists include in their models of how people cope with dying.

The depression can take many forms, for indeed there are always many losses, and each loss individually or several losses collectively might need to be experienced and worked through. For example, dying parents might ask themselves who will take care of the children, get them through school, walk them down the aisle, or guide them through life. Children, even adult children who are parents themselves, may ask whether they can cope without their own parents. They wonder who will support and anchor them in times of distress, who will (or could) love, nurture, and nourish them the way that their parents did. Depression accompanies the realization that each role, each function, will never be performed again. Both the dying and those who love them mourn.

Much of the depression takes the form of anticipatory grieving, which often occurs both in the dying and in those who will be affected by their death. It is a part of the dying process experienced by the living, both terminal and nonterminal. Patients, family, and friends can psychologically anticipate what it will be like when the death does occur and what life will, and will not, be like afterward. The grieving begins while there is still life left to live.

Bereavement specialists generally agree that anticipatory grieving, when it occurs, seems to help people cope with what is a terrible and frightening loss. It is an adaptive psychological mechanism wherein emotional, mental, and existential stability are painfully maintained. When depression develops, not only in reaction to death but also in preparation for it, it seems to be a necessary part of how those who are left behind cope to survive the loss themselves. Those who advocate or advise cheering up or looking on the bright side are either unrealistic or unable to tolerate the sadness in themselves or others. The dying are in the process of losing everything and everyone they love. Cheering up does not help them; the advice to "be strong" only helps the "helpers" deny the truth of the dying experience.

Kübler-Ross's fifth stage, acceptance, is an intellectual and emotional coming to terms with death's reality, permanence, and inevitability. Ironically, it is manifested by diminished emotionality and interests and increased fatigue and inner (many would say spiritual) self-focus. It is a time without depression or anger. Envy of the healthy, the fear of losing all, and bargaining for another day or week are also absent. This final stage is often misunderstood. Some see it either as resignation and giving up or as achieving a happy serenity. Some think that acceptance is the goal of dying well and that all people are supposed to go through this stage. None of these viewpoints is accurate. Acceptance, when it does occur, comes from within the dying person. It is marked more by an emotional void and psychological detachment from people and things once held important and necessary and by an interest in some transcendental value (for the atheist) or god (for the theist). It has little to do with what others believe is important or "should" be done. It is when dying people become more intimate with themselves and appreciate their separateness from others more than at any other time.

END-OF-LIFE CARE

End-of-life care, including palliative care and hospice care, achieved greater prominence as the needs of terminally ill patients, family members and friends were recognized. Hospice care is medical care to manage the person with terminal illness to live a comfortable life as long as possible. Referral of a patient to hospice care usually occurs with six months or less to live according to the physician, the patient is rapidly declining despite medical treatment, or the patient chooses to end treatments in favor of a more comfortable life. The limitations to referral to hospice is that the physician and family must estimate how long the patient has to live. Some patients are referred to hospice and live only a week or two and some patients may live beyond the six months of expected life. Predicting death is an inexact science. In part because referral to hospice is inexact, palliative care emerged as a precursor to hospice care in 1999 with the creation of the Center to Advance Palliative Care (CAC).

The Center to Advance Palliative Care (CAPC), established in 1999, is a national organization that began as a part of the Icahn School of Medicine at Mount Sinai in New York City. CAPC emerged to improve the care of people living with serious illness and their families. More recently the Joint Commission, an organization responsible for accrediting hospitals and healthcare providers, mandated palliative care service availability as a necessary intervention. Intervention with the patient and family often occurs well prior to the end of life with the purpose of assisting the patient and family to transition through a serious or life-threatening disease. A patient with chronic obstructive lung disease (COPD) or congestive heart failure (CHF) may live for a significant length of time with proper medical management. Helping the patient deal with limitations of their disease while maintaining quality of life is often a goal of palliative care. Working with the family and friends of the patient living with a chronic, life-threatening disease allows them to begin to accept and make plans for the future as the patient progresses in the illness long before a referral to hospice is appropriate.

GRIEVING

While patients grieve their impending loss of life as they progress through the stages of grief, family and friends will experience grief after the loss of a loved one. Grieving is the usual, expected reaction to loss. After a loss, a normal process occurs in grieving, involving feelings such as anger and sadness, followed by reassessment and reorganization of oneself and one's perspective. Some bereaved individuals experience prolonged or extreme grief reactions, commonly referred to as "complicated grief." In these cases, grief may be associated with depression, physical illness, and heightened risk of mortality. Some losses, such as miscarriage or loss of a lover, are not widely recognized, leading to an experience known as "disenfranchised grief."

Much of life depends on successful adaptation to change. When that change is experienced as a loss, the emotional and cognitive reactions are properly referred to as "grief." When the specific loss is acknowledged by a person's culture, the loss is often met with rituals, behaviors that follow a certain pattern, sanctioned and choreographed within the culture. The term "bereavement" is applied to the loss of a significant person (such as a spouse, parent, child, or close relative or friend). In this case the grief and the sanctioned rituals are referred to as "mourning," although some writers use the terms "mourning" and "grieving" as synonyms.

THE GRIEF PROCESS

The grief process is complex and highly individualized. It is seldom as predictable and orderly as the stages presented by Bowlby and Kübler-Ross might imply. Studies conducted by psychologist Janice Genevro in 2003 and Yale University researchers in 2007, as well as a survey of Canadian hospices in 2008, contradict the stage theory of grief altogether and suggest that grief is actually a complex mix of recurring emotions and symptoms that eventually alleviate. The duration of intense grief is quite variable, which can be a source of frustration to bereaved individuals who just want to know when their intense grief will end. Some people take a while to fully realize their loss. In a process known as "denial" or "disbelief," the grieving itself may be delayed. In a normal grief process, bereaved people eventually reach acceptance and accomplish reassessment and reorganization of their lives.

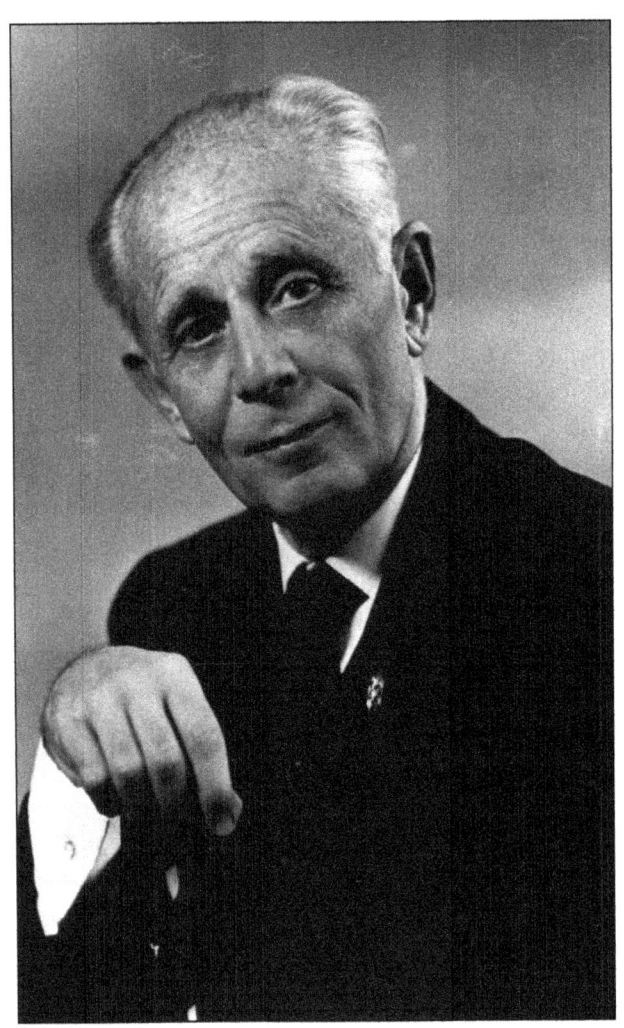

Hans Selye (Wikimedia Commons)

Grieving is the psychological, biological, and behavioral way of dealing with the stress created when a significant part of the self or prop for the self is taken away. Austrian endocrinologist Hans Selye made a vigorous career defining stress and considering the positive and negative effects that it may have on a person. He defined stress as "the nonspecific response of the body to any demand made upon it." Clearly any significant change calls for adjustment and thus involves stress. Selye indicated that what counts is the severity of the demand, and this depends on the perception of the person involved.

CONCLUSION
Dying, death, and grief are highly individualized. While defined guidelines such as Kübler-Ross and others assist in understanding the processes, assessing and getting to know the individual patients and families is necessary to provide them the best possible support. Prompt recognition of needs for support and care is critical. Palliative care emerged, in part, to help patients and their families earlier in the chronic or terminal illness process as hospice referrals often came too late to provide needed support. Helping patients and families move through the illness continuum is an important part of healthcare and especially nursing care.

—*Paul Moglia, Everett J. Delahanty Jr.,
Allyson Washburn, and Patricia Stanfill Edens*

Further Reading
"Coping with the Loss of a Loved One." *American Cancer Society*, www.cancer.org/treatment/end-of-life-care/grief-and-loss.html. Accessed 1 Sept. 2020.
Becker, Ernest. *The Denial of Death*. Free Press, 1997. Written by an anthropologist and philosopher, this is an erudite and insightful analysis and synthesis of the role that the fear of death plays in motivating human activity, society, and individual actions. A profound work.
Center to Advance Palliative Care, www.capc.org. Accessed 1 Sept. 2020. Content and tools designed to enable

healthcare practitioners to provide support to patients and families living with serious or terminal illnesses.

Cook, Alicia Skinner, and Daniel S. Dworkin. *Helping the Bereaved: Therapeutic Interventions for Children, Adolescents, and Adults*. Basic Books, 1992. Although not a self-help book, this work is useful to professionals and nonprofessionals alike as a review of the state of the art in grief therapy. Practical and readable. Of special interest for those becoming involved in grief counseling.

Corr, Charles A., Clyde M. Nabe, and Donna M. Corr. *Death and Dying, Life and Living*. 6th ed., Wadsworth/Cengage Learning, 2009. This book provides perspective on common issues associated with death and dying for family members and others affected by life-threatening circumstances.

Edens, Pat Stanfill, and Catherine D. Harvey. "Developing and Financing a Palliative Care Program." *American Journal of Hospice and Palliative Medicine*, vol. 25, no. 5, Oct./Nov. 2008.

Forman, Walter B., et al., editors. *Hospice and Palliative Care: Concepts and Practice*. 2nd ed., Jones and Bartlett, 2003. A classical text that examines the theoretical perspectives and practical information about hospice care. Other topics include community medical care, geriatric care, nursing care, pain management, research, counseling, and hospice management.

Kübler-Ross, Elisabeth, editor. *Death: The Final Stage of Growth*. Reprint. Simon & Schuster, 1997. A psychiatrist by training, Kübler-Ross brings together other researchers' views of how death provides the key to how human beings make meaning in their own personal worlds. Addresses practical concerns over how people express grief and accept the death of those close to them, and how they might prepare for their own inevitable ends.

Kushner, Harold. *When Bad Things Happen to Good People*. 20th anniv. ed., Schocken Books, 2001. The first of Rabbi Kushner's works on finding meaning in one's life, it was originally his personal response to make intelligible the death of his own child. It has become a highly regarded reference for those who struggle with the meaning of pain, suffering, and death in their lives.

"What Are Palliative Care and Hospice Care?" National Institute on Aging. *National Institutes of Health*, www.nia.nih.gov/health/what-are-palliative-care-and-hospice-care. Accessed 1 Sept. 2020.

"What Is Hospice?" *Hospice Foundation of America*, hospicefoundation.org/Hospice-Care/Hospice-Services. Accessed 1 Sept. 2020.

Pain Management

ABSTRACT

Managing patient pain is an important part of nursing care. Poor management of pain may result in less than optimal outcomes, especially after surgery or in acute illnesses such as cancer. Poor pain management is due to failure to assess initial pain, failure to have a pain management component in the medical and nursing plan of care, lack of documentation, fear of patient addiction, and lack of knowledge about the role pain plays in recovery. Pain is the most common reason people seek medical care. Nurses must assess and document pain in their patients.

PAIN MEDICATION

Pain relievers are divided into categories. Over-the-counter (OTC) medicines such as acetaminophen (Tylenol) and nonsteroidal anti-inflammatory drugs (NSAIDs) such as aspirin, naproxen (Aleve) and ibuprofen (Advil, Motrin) are available without a prescription although a physician may recommend an OTC medicine to the patient. Prescription pain relievers include corticosteroids, antidepressants, anticonvulsants (antiseizure), prescription dose ranges (higher than OTC doses) for NSAIDs, lidocaine patches and opioids. Recently, opioids have received attention for abuse, but they are instrumental in managing acute pain such as immediately after surgery or in cancer patients. Opioids may include codeine, fentanyl, hydrocodone-acetaminophen combinations, morphine, oxycodone and oxycodone-acetaminophen combinations. Opioids are extremely addictive and doctors try to use the least dose necessary to control pain and also seek alternatives to prescribing this class of drugs.

All drugs should be used for the shortest amount of time to minimize side effects and, in the case of addictive drugs like opioids, minimize the chance of dependency. Sides effects for each drug are available in the information packets supplied with the product or from the pharmacy. Drowsiness, dizziness, nausea, constipation and difficulty urinating, itching, stomach distress up to and including bleeding, fatigue, addiction and other side effects may occur with both OTC and opioid use. There are alternatives to drug therapy for pain management in select cases.

PAIN MANAGEMENT INDUSTRY

An entire industry has developed around the management of, particularly, chronic pain. Patients with acute inflammatory pain or painful neuropathies do not necessarily warrant opioids. A variety of approaches are being tried to minimize the risk of addiction and abuse while still achieving pain control. Anesthesia based pain management managed by physicians uses a combination of approaches including drugs, nerve blocks and injections. Chiropractors may employ therapeutic ultrasound, transcutaneous electrical nerve stimulation and manual adjustment for neck and back pain. Radiologists may be involved in direct injection of agents such as corticosteroids into joints for pain relief from arthritis or tendonitis. Depending on the cause and site of the pain, a variety of other medical specialties and health professionals may be consulted to better manage pain.

NONMEDICATION INTERVENTIONS

For people with mild to moderate chronic pain, medication may offer relief. However, many people find they can gain long-term control over their pain through complementary methods, such as heat or cold application, music, relaxation, exercise, meditation, acupuncture, and a positive attitude.

"For the vast majority of people who have chronic pain, there just are not any pharmacologic or physical interventions that can totally eliminate the pain," says University of Washington (Seattle) pain management expert Dennis C. Turk.

"Pain is a chronic condition, just like hypertension or diabetes," Turk explains. "When you have a chronic condition, you need to do more things for yourself. It is going to last a long time. It is best to help yourself and learn to self-manage and control your pain."

OPTIONS

In addition to traditional pain relievers, nondrug methods of pain relief may help a person gain that control. Some techniques—such as imagery and the use of hot and cold—relax the muscles, help one sleep, and distract one from symptoms. Other techniques, such as music, films, and recorded comedy routines, can take one's mind off physical complaints, as does losing oneself in a good book.

While some remedies require little expertise or help from others, some may require instruction from a professional. Ronald Glick, the director of the University of Pittsburgh Pain Evaluation and Treatment Center, recommends that patients seek advice from a chronic pain specialist who can coordinate all aspects of management, including physical therapies and psychological techniques. While these pain relief techniques help many people with chronic pain, they are not cures for pain.

Heat and cold. "The most important thing about heat and cold is that it gives a sense of control," Turk says. "They are things you can do yourself to help relieve the pain, which can immediately reduce the emotional stress."

Direct application. "Heat and cold can be quite helpful for people with musculoskeletal conditions," says Turk. "Something as simple as a bag of frozen peas wrapped in a towel can be a useful self-management technique that relieves muscle tension in the back, neck, and shoulders." Most people are familiar with holding an ice pack on a twisted ankle or lying on a heating pad for a sore back. However, hot and cold treatments can be used in other ways. Moist heat can be applied with a warm towel or through a soak in a bath tub. An elastic bandage can hold an ice pack in place. A paper cup filled with water and kept in the freezer becomes a tool for localized cold massage, while iced wash cloths can cover a larger area.

Relaxation. "Relaxation response" is a term coined by Herbert Benson of the Mind-Body Medical Institute in Boston. It is an array of beneficial physiologic effects associated with focused relaxation, some of which may mitigate the perception of pain. For best results, one should make relaxation a part of one's daily routine.

There are a number of ways to invoke the relaxation response, and many audiotapes are available to help. One popular approach is to assume a comfortable position, take several deep breaths, and then focus on breathing, or on a word or a sound, while passively avoiding intruding thoughts.

Muscle relaxation exercises. Progressive muscle relaxation is a technique that may be effective for both muscle spasm pain and stress reduction. "Relaxation skills are useful in reducing muscle tension and can help reduce frustration and some of the stress," says Jennifer Markham of the University of Pittsburgh Pain Clinic. Progressive muscle relaxation involves focusing attention on each muscle group until it feels heavy and relaxed. One usually begins in the feet and gradually progresses upward.

Imagery exercises. Imagery, which often accompanies the management of pain through relaxation, allows one to visualize what it would be like to "let the pain go." If one knows what is causing the pain—for instance, a pinched nerve in the spine—the idea is to picture the encroaching vertebral space opening and freeing the trapped nerve. By calling on a variety of senses, one can go to a favorite place, such as the beach or the mountains. Music, nature sounds, and instructional tapes make it easier for beginners to escape to a mental paradise.

"Relaxation techniques redirect your thinking from physical pain and onto something else," says Penney Cowan, founder and executive director of the American Chronic Pain Association. "Imagining the beach, the sun on your face, and the warmth of the sand helps divert your mind from how much your head is hurting."

Biofeedback. Biofeedback offers a measurable response to relaxation and imagery techniques. Through the use of sensors connected to a computer, one receives visual or auditory cues that indicate an increase or decrease in muscle tension, heart rate, and skin temperature. Using this feedback, one trains oneself to control body functions not normally thought about. Biofeedback may be useful in chronic pain or other conditions associated with muscle spasm or tension, such as some headaches.

Exercise. Although one may not feel like getting off the couch because of the pain, exercising within the confines of one's physical limitations can decrease pain. The reasons for this are complex, but one prominent theory is that exercise releases endorphins, which are natural pain-relieving chemicals in the brain. "Exercise is absolutely critical," says Turk. "The type of exercise will depend on the condition, but as a general rule of thumb, the more active you remain and the more you use your muscles, the better off you're going to be."

A physical therapist can tailor an initial exercise plan based on a person's capacity to exercise and then gradually make recommendations for increasing how much to do and for how long. Pain experts recommend pacing activities. Overdoing it on good days can cause more pain later. Experts recommend reducing exercise during a flare-up of pain, but it is important to resume an exercise routine as soon as possible.

Acupuncture. Acupuncture is a form of Chinese medicine. It involves insertion of very thin needles into the skin at different and specific points on the body. It has been shown to be effective for the treatment of chronic back pain. It requires several treatments, usually between two and five, before a response can be seen. Results of acupuncture also largely depend on the skills of the acupuncturist.

Cognitive Behavioral Therapy for Pain

Pain is a normal, protective reaction to an injury or illness. It is the body's signal that it is time to take care of a problem. Chronic pain is pain that continues for weeks, months, or years. It may be related to such chronic illnesses as arthritis, disorders of the nerves, or cancer pain. It may begin with an injury or short illness but continue even when the physical damage is no longer evident.

For many persons, chronic pain management includes tackling only the physical symptoms of pain, but many cognitive, behavioral, and emotional aspects can hamper or help healing. How you think and feel about your health or illness will impact your recovery and how much the pain will interfere with your everyday life.

Negative thought patterns like "I'll never get better" or "This pain stops me from doing everything" may influence the decisions you make about your healthcare. If you feel there is little to no chance of successful treatment, you may be less likely to seek beneficial treatment or may continue with unsuccessful treatments. However, if you believe success is possible, you are more likely to participate in seeking and completing recovery treatments.

Stress also can be a major part of a pain cycle. Managing any chronic condition is stressful enough on its own. Aside from the stress of the illness itself, financial concerns and strained relationships secondary to the illness can add to stress. This regular stress stimulates physical responses in the body, which can increase pain and delay healing.

Identifying these factors, learning more positive thought patterns, and developing better communication techniques can be important in managing chronic pain. Cognitive behavioral therapy (CBT) is a specialized form of therapy designed to help one take these steps.

A common assumption is that people with chronic pain are only imagining their pain. However, part of CBT is to help acknowledge that the pain is real and to develop healthy thought patterns to manage it. The therapy will be based on your specific need, but it often involves creating realistic beliefs about pain, treatment options, and outcomes. Your therapist will help you to develop positive thinking and self-talk, reduce behaviors that continue an illness-way-of-life, increase positive behaviors that get you toward your goal, improve communication skills with family and medical team, and develop pain-management skills.

The overall goal is to replace ways of living that do not work with methods that do. The changes will help you gain more control over your life, instead of living solely through what pain you have.

CBT may be done in a one-on-one or group setting, depending on your needs. Your therapy may also include other persons, such as a spouse or other family members. Most often, the treatment is short-term, lasts between six to twenty sessions, and requires practice and homework to be most effective.

Chronic pain is often caused or exacerbated by a combination of issues, some of which can be immediately addressed, while others may take longer to resolve. CBT, in the meantime, can play a role in helping you manage pain and improve your quality of life. It will help you develop the skills to reshape your thinking, so that you can improve your treatment effects and decrease new cycles of pain.

—Pamela Jones and Rosalyn Carson-DeWitt

Meditation. The benefits of meditation go beyond relaxation response. Daily meditation may be an excellent tool in fighting chronic pain. There are a variety of different meditation techniques, and one should choose a mediation style that is comfortable. Meditation is not a religious practice and can be done easily in the privacy of one's home.

Hypnotherapy. Hypnosis has nothing to do with popular images of stage performance. It was first utilized as a therapeutic modality more than one hundred years ago, and it is a technique that can be useful in chronic pain management. Hypnotherapy is performed by a trained and licensed therapist. The exact way that hypnosis works is not fully understood. It is known, however, to induce a state of focused awareness, which can alleviate many forms of pain.

Attitude and communication. How one thinks about one's aches and discomforts, one's level of anxiety and depression, one's expectations, and one's ability to cope determines how much pain one feels. Cognitive-behavior modification techniques help change unhealthy attitudes and habits that can develop when pain is chronic.

A person should concentrate on his or her abilities and find pleasure in the things he or she can do rather than dwelling on activities that have become difficult because of pain. One should communicate with family members. "Psychology helps people begin to understand they do have some control, even if they don't have a magic wand to make the pain go away," says Markham. "When they realize they have some control [over their pain], it gives them hope."

SUMMARY

Pain can be a debilitating part of injury and illness. Managing pain requires a careful assessment of causes and a detailed plan for pain management. Pain management may be drug therapies or interventions, including those considered complementary and alternative in nature. Regardless of the pain management strategy, the least invasive approach is indicated that still allows patients to tolerate their pain and continue with activities of daily living.

—*Debra Wood, Steven Bratman, Brian Randall, and Patricia Stanfill Edens*

Further Reading

Gatlin, C. G., and L. Schulmeister. "When Medication Is Not Enough: Nonpharmacologic Management of Pain." *Clinical Journal of Oncology Nursing*, vol. 11, 2007, pp. 699–704.

King, N. B., and V. Fraser. "Untreated Pain, Narcotics Regulation, and Global Health Ideologies." *PLoS Medicine*, vol. 10, no. 4, 2013www.ncbi.nlm.nih.gov/pmc/articles/PMC3614505.

Lee, H., K. Schmidt, and E. Ernst. "Acupuncture for the Relief of Cancer-Related Pain." *European Journal of Pain*, vol. 9, 2005, p. 437.

"Opioid Misuse and Addiction." National Institutes of Health. US National Library of Medicine. *Medline Plus*, medlineplus.gov/opiodmisuseandaddiction.html. Accessed 16 Sept. 2020.

"Pain Relievers." National Institutes of Health. US National Library of Medicine. *Medline Plus*, medlineplus.gov/painrelievers.html. Accessed 16 Sept. 2020.

Rydholm, M., and P. Strang. "Acupuncture for Patients in Hospital-Based Home Care Suffering from Xerostomia." *Journal of Palliative Care*, vol. 15, 1999, p. 20.

"Treatment Options for Chronic Pain." *American Society of Regional Anesthesia and Pain Medicine*, www.asra.com/page/46/treatment-options-for-chronic-pain. Accessed 16 Sept. 2020.

Wright, L. D. "Meditation: A New Role for an Old Friend." *American Journal of Hospice and Palliative Care*, vol. 23, 2006, pp. 323–27.

NATIONAL INSTITUTES OF HEALTH (NIH)

ABSTRACT

The National Institutes of Health (NIH) is one of the eleven agencies constituting the US Department of Health and Human Services.

HISTORY AND MISSION

The NIH is a US federal agency that occupies a multi-building campus in Bethesda, Maryland. It consists of a variety of offices, institutes focused on specific medical problems, research laboratories and centers, a center for scientific review, and a national medical library. Its main goal is to discover knowledge that will improve the state of public health for all persons, especially those in the United States. This goal extends to all medical conditions afflicting men, women, and children of all ethnic backgrounds. It also extends to seeking knowledge in areas of basic biological research, clinical research, and research on policy and practice in healthcare.

The National Institute of Health (precursor to the NIH) was formally established by the Ransdell Act of 1930, which bestowed the name on what was formerly called the Hygienic Laboratory (HL) of the Marine Hospital Service (MHS) in New York. The Ransdell Act also allowed for the establishment of fellowships for basic medical and biological research. The very beginnings of the NIH extend back to 1887, however, when basic laboratory work into medical problems was pursued by the MHS, the founding body of the United States Public Health Service (PHS). The MHS was formed in 1798 to provide hospital care for seamen, but by the 1880s it had shifted its focus to screening ship passengers for infectious diseases capable of starting epidemics.

New European research in the 1880s suggesting that microorganisms caused such diseases spurred American interest in medical research and helped form the original HL. Work by the HL continued, with the laboratory eventually moving from the MHS to its own Washington, DC, campus. The study of microorganisms continued, extending from study of individual persons to studying the effects of bacteria on water and air pollution. Progress for such work was rewarded in 1901 with governmental money for the construction of a building (completed in 1904) to house the HL and further foster work focused on advancing the public health. Because the value of such work was not well established, however, no permanent funding was provided, leaving the organization subject to ongoing evaluation and supplemental funding.

In 1902 the MHS was reorganized and renamed the Public Health and Marine Hospital Service (PH-MHS); in 1912 it adopted the shortened name of the Public Health Service (PHS). During the intervening time, the HL continued its work and expanded to work in chemistry, pharmacology, zoology, immunology, and the regulation and production of vaccines and antitoxins. Additionally, new scientific staff were added to the staff of medical doctors already on board. Changes in the mission of the organization in 1912 also opened the door for the pursuit of research on noncontagious diseases and water pollution. This work continued during World War I in the form of examining sanitation, anthrax outbreaks, smallpox, tetanus, influenza, and other combat-related conditions. The success of the PHS's work in these areas caught the attention of legislators and resulted in the Ransdell Act of 1930, which established both the National Institute of Health and the practice of setting aside public monies for funding medical research. In 1937, the National Cancer Institute (NCI) was created. In 1944, the PHS formally designated the NCI as a component of the NIH, setting the pattern of a problem-focused structure within the NIH that continues to the present.

World War II led the NIH to focus almost exclusively on war-related problems. This involved examinations of fitness for military service and issues such as dental problems and syphilis. The effects of hazardous substances and conditions on workers in war industries; risks armed service professionals faced from lack of oxygen, cold temperatures, and blood clots while flying; burns, shock, bacterial infections, and fever; and the development of vaccines and therapies for tropical diseases such as malaria also composed much of its work during this time.

Successes established during the wars by such medical research led the PHS to take the 1944 Public Health Service Act to Congress. This act led to grant-funding mechanisms being extended from the NCI alone to the entire National Institute of Health. Additionally, an increasing public interest in health organizations caused Congress to create additional institutes for research on mental health, dental diseases, and heart disease between 1946 and 1949. In 1948, the National Heart Act allowed for the formal pluralization of the National Institutes of Health, rather than a singular institute with the NCI as a sub-institute. The Public Health Service Act of 1944 also provided funding for the Warren Grant Magnuson Clinical Center, which opened in 1953 to focus exclusively on clinical research on health.

From this point forward, each of the individual institutes now composing the NIH came into being. By 1960 there were ten institutes, and by 2017 there were twenty-seven institutes and centers. As different health interests develop and advances in medical knowledge are needed, the NIH has responded by allocating its resources to pursue goals in those areas. This has been done both by developing institutes and also by creating specialized offices to pursue contemporary medical problems.

Illness and medicine know no boundaries, however, so the NIH has also maintained an interest in global public health issues. Such interest was formally shown in 1947, when grants were first awarded to investigators abroad. Similarly, in 1968, the John E. Fogarty International Center (FIC) was created to coordinate international research efforts, involving liaisons with the World Health Organization and a variety of international research organizations. The FIC also supports language translation, documentation, and reviews of new health findings. It facilitates biomedical communications through its maintenance of the National Library of Medicine (NLM), MEDLINE, CATLINE, AIDSLINE, and numerous other databases for researchers, physicians, and the public at large. Similarly, focused consensus development conferences, where investigators and clinicians from around the world can meet to evaluate new and existing therapies, are another way in which international interests are pursued.

In keeping with its practical focus, the NIH has strived to seek out knowledge that yields new drugs, devices, and procedures that are useful not just for the government but for the public at large as well. In 1986, the Technology Transfer Act allowed for a partnership between NIH-funded research and the private sector. Encouraging researchers to examine possible commercial and practical applications of basic medical research to wide-reaching clinical or research use benefits overall scientific and health progress. Partnering with business allows private industries to take over the process of marketing and developing products in a manner more affordable to them than to the government, allowing the government to focus on development while benefiting through the use of the eventual marketed products.

ORGANIZATIONAL STRUCTURE AND METHOD

The NIH is organized to accomplish its goals by using its offices, institutes, and research centers. Research is conducted on the NIH campus in its own funded laboratories as well as in the labs of scientists supported by NIH funding, who are stationed in institutes of higher education, teaching hospitals, and research institutions in the United States and other countries. In addition to supporting ongoing research, the NIH also supports research infrastructure by maintaining a library and a variety of printed and electronic resources to facilitate communication among its researchers, the larger scientific community, policymakers, and the public. Scientific research also is supported through development of one of the most valuable resources known to medicine: new researchers. The NIH sponsors a variety of training programs focusing on medical training and research in order to keep a large body of high-quality scholars and investigators in development. Such programs extend from career development for postdoctoral researchers and predoctoral training, to high school-level learning in the sponsoring of internships and other learning experiences for teenagers interested in medical science careers.

Funding for research and training programs outside the NIH campus and research centers is facilitated through grant proposal programs that distribute federal tax monies devoted to such endeavors. Applicants to such programs are able to submit independent proposals for work related to the goals of the NIH that they believe is demanded by the state of science and knowledge. They are also able to submit proposals in response to program announcements and calls for proposals on specific topics as outlined by the institutes and offices of the NIH. Many different grant mechanisms exist for such proposals, including grants supporting the work of individual trainees, training programs for cohorts of researchers at different stages of career development, the ongoing work of career scientists, small grants for new or experimental work, focused projects, and even centers of research excellence where many researchers focus on the same topic of study. In addition, grant support is offered to sponsor conferences and academic meetings on special topics in health research and training.

To receive this funding, those wishing to be considered must submit proposals for confidential peer review through the Center for Scientific Review (CSR), which is part of the NIH structure. Proposals are reviewed by panels of experts who evaluate the research plans, goals, staff, environment, and overall innovation and merit of the work proposed. In addition, ethical considerations about the proposed research are reviewed and considered for both animal welfare and the welfare of human research participants. Emphasis on issues of medical ethics had been a long-standing issue for research. It was, however, highlighted in the 1960s, when grantees receiving NIH grant monies were required to state the ethical principles guiding their research on humans, and in 1979, when written guidelines for research on human subjects were established. Once through peer review, proposals are reviewed again by a national advisory council to determine the priority of the work in addressing the goals of the NIH and its institutes and offices. After the proposals are approved by this council for advancement, the individual institutes (sometimes cooperating with specific NIH offices) work to fund them with the monies allotted. Unfortunately, not all proposals can be funded. It should be noted that even after funding, the work of the NIH continues so as to ensure that proper research ethics are followed through the life of the research.

Research funded by the NIH is facilitated by the various institutions and research offices that fall under its organizational umbrella, each focusing on a discrete area of health interest. Some of the institutions involved include the National Cancer Institute (NCI); the National Eye Institute; the National Heart, Lung, and Blood Institute; and the National Human Genome Research Institute. Also included are the National Institutes on Aging, Alcohol Abuse and Alcoholism, Allergy and Infectious Diseases, Arthritis and Musculoskeletal and Skin Diseases, Child Health and Human Development, Deafness and Other Communication Disorders, Dental and Craniofacial Research, Diabetes and Digestive and Kidney Diseases, Drug Abuse, Environmental Health Sciences, Mental Health, Minority Health and Health Disparities, and Neurological Disorders and Stroke.

In addition to these institutes, the NIH has numerous offices focusing on specific issues or populations that need to be addressed in health research. These offices focus on contemporary issues of importance for research and include the Offices of Technology Transfer, AIDS Research, Research on Women's Health, Behavioral and Social Sciences Research, Dietary Supplements, Rare Diseases, Science Policy,

Biotechnology Activities, Science Education, and Information Technology. There are also offices that focus on the management of research, specific organizational issues at the NIH, or the communication of information from the NIH to members of the public. These include the Offices of Intramural Research, Extramural Research, Program Evaluation and Performance, Human Resources, Financial Management, Acquisition and Logistics Management, Management Assessment, and Communications and Public Liaison as well as the NIH Legal Advisor and the Freedom of Information Act Office.

For a full listing of components of the NIH, go to www.nih.gov.

PERSPECTIVE AND PROSPECTS

The NIH has been responsible for supporting some very influential research for more than one hundred years, garnering more than eighty Nobel Prizes for NIH-supported work. More vaccines against infectious diseases are available than ever before. The successful mapping of the human genome has set the stage for enhanced genetic testing and the development of gene therapies. Substantial decreases in mortality rates have been achieved for heart disease and strokes. Survival rates for individuals afflicted by cancer have increased, as have survival rates for infants with respiratory distress syndrome. Recovery from spinal cord injuries has been enhanced so as to lessen the probability of long-term disability. Advances in the pharmacological and behavioral treatment of mental health problems such as depression, anxiety, bipolar disorders, and schizophrenia have been achieved. Preventive approaches in dentistry have been highly successful in stopping and slowing dental problems.

Given such successes, billions of dollars of federal tax monies continue to be devoted to the NIH budget to foster continued scientific advances. New work focused on improving prevention, screening, assessment, diagnosis, and treatment for conditions such as AIDS, alcoholism and drug dependence, Alzheimer's disease, arthritis, blindness, communication disorders, diabetes, heart disease, kidney disease, lung cancer, lupus, mental illnesses, Parkinson's disease, stroke, and other persisting conditions continues on a daily basis. While great successes have been achieved to date, new research is needed that will focus on specialized approaches that may enhance health for women, minorities, youth, and the elderly. The combination of these needs, past successes, and governmental commitment to improving the state of the public health ensures that the NIH will continue onward with its mission for the foreseeable future.

In December 2015, after more than ten years of little to no change in the NIH's budget, President Barack Obama signed a bill into law that provided an extra $2 billion in the organization's budget for 2016. This move proved that the importance of the work done by NIH is recognized by both major political parties. In FY 2020, the approved budget amount was $41.68 billion.

—*Nancy A. Piotrowski*

Further Reading

"About NIH." US Department of Health and Human Services. *National Institutes of Health*, www.nih.gov/about-nih. Accessed 2 Sept. 2020.

Garrett, Laurie. *Betrayal of Trust: The Collapse of Global Public Health*. Hyperion, 2001.

Guest, Charles, et al. *Oxford Handbook of Public Health Practice*. 3rd ed., Oxford UP, 2013.

Kelly, Nora. "What's Next for the National Institutes of Health?" *The Atlantic*, 13 Jan. 2016, www.theatlantic.com/politics/archive/2016/01/national-institutes-of-health-congress-budget/423837/.

Lee, Philip R., and Carroll L. Estes, editors. *The Nation's Health*. 7th ed., Jones and Bartlett, 2003.

"List of NIH Institutes, Centers, and Offices." US Department of Health and Human Services. *National Institutes of Health*, 8 Feb. 2017, www.nih.gov/institutes-nih/list-nih-institutes-centers-offices. Accessed 2 Sept. 2020.

Shnayerson, Michael, and Mark J. Plotkin. *The Killers Within: The Deadly Rise of Drug Resistant Bacteria*. Little, 2003.

Tikkanen, Roosa and Melinda K. Abrams. "U.S. Health Care from a Global Perspective, 2019: Higher Spending, Worse Outcomes?" *The Commonwealth Fund*, www.commonwealthfund.org/publications/issue-briefs/2020/jan/us-health-care-global-perspective-2019. Accessed 2 Sept. 2020.

HEALTH PROMOTION

ABSTRACT

Health promotion programs focus on keeping people healthy. Choosing healthy behaviors and making changes to develop or maintain health enhances quality of life. Disease prevention as a part of healthy behaviors may reduce the risk of developing some preventable diseases or better managing chronic diseases. Screening for disease is an active measure in health promotion. Stress reduction refers to a set of procedures with the goal of decreasing bodily and mental tension by increasing rest and coping skills.

SOCIAL DETERMINANTS OF HEALTH

Health promotion focuses on modifiable risk factors and behaviors. Depending on where individuals live, risk behaviors may include smoking, high stress levels, lack of exercise, and eating a poor diet. Economic, social, cultural, and political conditions also are determinants of health. Economics plays a significant role when, for example, there is insufficient money to purchase healthy food or individuals are living in a setting without access to fresh foods. Adequate screening for disease including tests such as blood work, mammography, and blood pressure monitoring are important.

Nurses are just some of the health professionals actively involved in screening programs, smoking cessation programs and stress reduction programs. Typically, a call to your physician or local hospital can help identify resources for health promotion activities. Watch for public service announcements, health fairs and media campaigns designed to raise awareness of healthy behavior. Education for healthy eating, exercise, and smoking cessation are often available free or at reduced rates in hospitals and organizations in the local area. Public health departments and even local churches may routinely hold health promotion activities, including for example, free dental clinics, free monitoring for diabetes and other activities.

SCREENINGS

Health must be monitored to identify diseases and health conditions before there are signs and symptoms. A variety of screening tests may be used to find certain types of cancer, high blood pressure, high cholesterol, diabetes, weak bones or osteoporosis, depression, and other mental health conditions and sexually transmitted diseases. The need for screenings generally increases with age, but individuals and their doctors need to discuss needed tests. Talking with family members is also recommended to determine if there are diseases that run in the family such as diabetes or colon cancer. There are a variety of screenings that you should discuss with your physician such as the need for mammography (breast cancer), colonoscopy (colon and rectal cancer, polyps), blood work to look for human immunodeficiency virus (HIV) or acquired immunodeficiency syndrome (AIDS), Hepatitis C, prostate cancer (prostate specific antigen [PSA] blood test and digital rectal examination), blood sugar, and A1C to look for evidence of diabetes and others.

Most screenings are minimally invasive, meaning there are relatively minor risks. You and your doctor should discuss risks and potential benefits of screening. The Affordable Care Act requires most insurance plans to cover screening tests. Some hospitals and health systems may also offer free or reduced rate screenings at various times during the year.

SMOKING

Smoking is the strongest risk factor for chronic diseases including heart disease and cancer. Cigarette smoking has long been known to have adverse effects. Smokers get more wrinkles than nonsmokers and brown/black discoloration of teeth so they tend to look older than their chronological age. They also are more likely to develop worsening of age-related problems such as gum disease, loss of teeth, and alteration in sense of smell and taste. Loss of teeth leads to difficulty chewing, which in turn leads to difficulties with digestion. Most people who lose teeth eventually develop loss of the bone that should support their teeth, making it increasingly difficult to fit dentures.

Smokers are ten times more likely to get lung cancer than nonsmokers. Lung cancer is now the number one cause of cancer death in women, as well as in men. In addition to lung cancer, smokers have a higher incidence of cancers of the head and neck, esophagus, colon, rectum, kidney, bladder, and cervix. Smokers are three to six times more likely to have a heart attack than are nonsmokers. In older people, the major risk factor for disease of the coronary arteries is hypertension, but smoking is still significant, especially when combined with other risk factors for heart disease, such as diabetes or high cholesterol. Smoking and diabetes are also the two most important risk factors for diseases of the veins and arteries of the lower leg. Those who continue to smoke once these diseases develop are much more likely to require limb amputation than those who quit. Smokers may develop chronic obstructive pulmonary disease (COPD), which includes emphysema and chronic bronchitis, and are eighteen times more likely than nonsmokers to die of diseases of the lungs other than cancer. Older smokers also show a decrease in muscle strength, agility, coordination, gait, and balance. The changes in these areas make them seem older than their actual age.

Smoking has long been thought to be associated with peptic ulcer disease. In addition, smoking makes the symptoms of many diseases worsen or increases the risk of complications in patients with allergies, diabetes, hypertension, and vascular disease. Male smokers are at greater risk of experiencing sexual impotence. Female smokers tend to experience an earlier menopause, bone loss called osteoporosis and are therefore at increased risk for hip fracture than nonsmokers. Smokers are more likely to develop glaucoma than nonsmokers. (Studies completed in 1996 indicated an increased risk with smoking for macular degeneration, the leading cause of blindness in older adults. The evidence is mixed on smoking and Alzheimer's disease, but a 1998 study contradicted earlier work and found that the risk is greater in smokers than in nonsmokers.) Finally, smokers are at greater risk of death or injury caused by cigarette-related fires.

Cigarette smoking tends to speed up the processes in the liver for breaking down, using, and eliminating medications, both nonprescription and prescription. This means that medications may not perform as expected in the body. Smokers may need to take medications more frequently or in greater doses than nonsmokers, so it is important for healthcare providers to know that a person smokes. The drugs known to be affected by smoking include sedatives, narcotic and synthetic narcotic painkillers, certain antidepressants, anticoagulant medications, asthma medications, and certain blood pressure medications. These changes are of particular concern in the older population for a number of reasons. First, older people (whether smokers or nonsmokers) tend to need more medications than younger people. With each additional drug, the risk of serious drug interaction and other adverse effects increases. Second, changes in body composition and function that alter the metabolism of drugs come with age, making medication use somewhat riskier in older persons, in terms of adverse effects and complications. The additional changes associated with smoking increase these risks significantly.

The dangers of passive smoking are well documented. More than fifty compounds in secondhand smoke are identified as carcinogens in humans. The effects seem to be more harmful in children than in adults, but adults who are affected are at increased risk for cancer, heart disease, noncancerous lung diseases, and allergies.

SMOKING CESSATION
Numerous studies have shown that smoking cessation has health benefits in as little as one year, such as reducing the risk of heart attack and coronary artery disease. Within two years of smoking cessation, the risks of stroke and diseases of the blood vessels in the lower leg are reduced as well. Even though chronic lung disease is not reversible, those who quit smoking slow the decline in lung function considerably. Risks for cancers also decrease significantly with smoking cessation and are similar to the cancer risk for nonsmokers in ten to thirteen years. These findings indicate that it is worthwhile even for older people to give up smoking. An average forty-year-old gains approximately nine additional years of life by quitting smoking, and a sixty-year-old gains approximately three additional years.

Because smoking is an addiction, it may be difficult to quit, particularly after years of cigarette use. Most smokers have to stop several times before quitting permanently. Setting a quit date, attending support group meetings, taking it one day at a time, undergoing hypnosis, making a contract with a friend or a healthcare provider, substituting carrot sticks for cigarettes, increasing exercise (particularly swimming), and breathing deeply all seem to be helpful techniques. Nicotine replacement systems are available in the United States on a nonprescription basis, but it is important for older people, particularly those with health problems or who are taking multiple medications, to consult a healthcare professional prior to using them. It is also important that anyone using these aids stop smoking completely. Continuing to smoke while using nicotine replacement could potentially cause toxicity, and it decreases the success of cessation attempts, since the behavior of smoking is still present. Two nonnicotine-containing medications are available by prescription for smoking cessation: bupropion SR (Wellbutrin, Zyban) and varenicline (Chantix). Both medications significantly increase the success rates at the end of treatment and one year later. The mechanism of action is by stimulating chemical messengers in the brain that are affected by nicotine.

Electronic cigarettes are used as a tool for smoking cessation. It is a battery-powered device that can deliver nicotine without the combustion or smoke. Use and awareness of e-cigarettes has dramatically increased over the past few years. Studies have suggested that physical and behavioral stimuli, such as holding a cigarette, can reduce the craving to smoke. Recent findings suggest that individuals who used e-cigarettes reduced the number of tobacco cigarettes they smoked. These findings suggest that the e-cigarettes may be an important tool for reducing the harm that tobacco cigarettes can cause. Unfortunately, the benefits and risks of electronic cigarette as of 2013 are still uncertain. More studies are needed for further investigation of their safety and efficacy.

STRESS
Stress can exacerbate difficulties in daily functioning, slow recovery from mental or physical problems, and impede immunological functioning. Stress reduction techniques represent a cluster of procedures that share the goal of reducing bodily and emotional tension: physical therapies, exercise, biofeedback training, meditation, hypnosis, psychotherapy, relaxation training, stress inoculation therapy, and medications. Stress reduction can be implemented by individuals using exercise, meditation, and other noninvasive interventions, or under the guidance and supervision of licensed doctors and health professionals.

Biofeedback training, meditation, hypnosis, and relaxation training all focus on inducing relaxation or altered consciousness by shifting a person's attention. Meditation is a focused thinking exercise involving a quiet setting and nonjudgmental mindfulness of the thoughts that arise. Meditation may also involve the repetition of a word or phrase called a mantra. By blocking distracting thoughts and refocusing one's attention, meditation reduces anxious thinking and promotes clarity. It is useful for anxiety, minor concentration difficulties, and daily relaxation.

Hypnosis involves the use of suggestion or concentrated attention to induce a sleeplike state, or trance. Hypnosis can be induced by a hypnotist or via self-hypnosis. Hypnotic states are characterized by increased suggestibility, ability to recall forgotten events, decreased pain sensitivity, and increased vasomotor control. The ability to be hypnotized varies from person to person based on susceptibility to suggestion and psychological needs. Hypnosis is used as a brief therapy targeting such problems as insomnia, pain, panic, addiction, and sexual dysfunction.

Relaxation training involves three primary methods: autogenic training, which involves such techniques as head, heart, and abdominal exercises; progressive relaxation, which involves becoming aware of tension in the various muscle groups by relaxing one group at a time in a specific order; and breathing exercises. Relaxation training is best learned when a therapist trains an individual in person and then the exercises are practiced independently. Relaxation can be practiced several times daily, as well as in response to stressful events. High blood pressure, ulcers, insomnia, asthma, drug and alcohol problems, spastic colitis, tachycardia (rapid heartbeat), pain management, and anxiety disorders are treated with relaxation training.

Psychotherapy is a common treatment for stress implemented by psychiatrists, psychologists, social workers, psychiatric nurses, and counselors. Not only does it help individuals to sort out their problems mentally but it is also an effective stress management strategy. Psychotherapy helps individuals learn new coping skills and identify unhealthy and unhelpful thought patterns that are contributing to or exacerbating one's stress levels. When individuals analyze their lifestyles and life events, stress-inducing behaviors and life patterns can be explored and targeted for modification. Stress inoculation therapy is a specific type of psychotherapy involving techniques that alter patterns of thinking and acting. It comprises three steps: education about stress and fear reactions, rehearsal of coping behaviors, and application of coping behaviors in stress-provoking situations. It is useful for treating anxiety disorders related to stress.

For individuals with posttraumatic stress disorder, an anxiety disorder, or acute stress disorder, drugs may be used to promote stress reduction alongside other relaxation techniques. Medications should not be used unless the severity of one's distress cannot be managed by psychological therapy. These drugs can provide overall bodily relaxation, induce rest, or decrease the anxious thinking that exacerbates stressful experiences. Sedatives, tranquilizers, benzodiazepines, beta-blockers, and barbiturates are examples of such drugs, although most should only be used in the short term and under the monitoring of a medical professional. Additionally, physical therapies and exercise are recommended for stress reduction. Baths (hydrotherapy), massages, yoga, and aerobic exercise are effective elements of a stress reduction program.

PERSPECTIVE AND PROSPECTS

Being healthy at any age is vitally important. Appropriate screening programs, decided upon in conjunction with the physician and nationally recognized schedules, can identify diseases prior to the development of signs and symptoms of disease which enhances health and response to treatment. Stopping smoking is the single best activity to improve health. Stress reduction techniques evolved from ancient meditation practices and simpler methods of pain management can contribute to overall well-being. For a more in-depth health promotion plan, the individual and the physician should consider family history, current physical condition, factors such as weight, age, sex, and activity levels and overall health behaviors and screening results in determining the best plan for a healthy life.

—*Nancy A. Piotrowski, Rebecca Lovell Scott, and Patricia Stanfill Edens*

Further Reading

"Coping with Stress." US Department of Health and Human Services. *Centers for Disease Control and Prevention*, 2 Oct. 2015.

Davis, Martha, Elizabeth Robbins Eshelman, and Matthew McKay. *The Relaxation and Stress Reduction Workbook*. 6th ed., New Harbinger, 2008.

"Defining Health Promotion and Disease Prevention." *Rural Health Information Hub*, www.ruralhealthinfo.org/toolkits/health-promotion/1/definition. Accessed 2 Sept. 2020.

"Get Screened." US Department of Health and Human Services. *Office of Disease Prevention and Health Promotion*, health.gov/myhealthfinder/topics/doctor-visits/screening-tests/get-screened. Accessed 2 Sept. 2020.

"Manage Stress." US Department of Health and Human Services. *HealthFinder.gov*, 30 July 2015.

Manning, George, Kent Curtis, Steve McMillen, and Bill Attenweiler. *Stress: Living and Working in a Changing World*. 3rd ed., Savant Learning Systems, 2016.

"Mindfulness-Based Stress Reduction (MBSR) Information." *National Center for Complementary and Integrative Health*, n.d. Accessed 17 May 2016.

Parles, Karen, and J. H. Schiller. *One Hundred Questions and Answers about Lung Cancer*. 2nd ed., Jones and Bartlett, 2010. A patient-oriented guide that covers a range of topics related to lung cancer.

Seaward, Brian Luke. *Managing Stress: Principles and Strategies for Health and Well-Being*. 8th ed., Jones and Bartlett Learning, 2013.

"Stress: How to Cope Better with Life's Challenges." American Academy of Family Physicians. *FamilyDoctor.org*, Nov. 2010.

"Stress Management." *American Heart Association*, n.d. Accessed 17 May 2016.

Tummers, Nanette E. *Stress Management: A Wellness Approach*. Human Kinetics, 2013.

DIET-BASED THERAPIES

ABSTRACT

Diet-based therapies involve using special dietary interventions to improve health, increase longevity, and prevent and treat specific health conditions and diseases.

OVERVIEW

Diet-based therapy uses specialized dietary regimens to promote wellness and to prevent and treat specific diseases. A healthy eating plan includes vegetables, fruits, whole grains, fat-free or reduced fat dairy, lean meats, poultry, fish and limits saturated and trans fats, sodium, and added sugars. No single food can prevent cancer; however, a diverse and healthy diet may reduce cancer risk. Reducing obesity may prevent heart and other diseases. A healthy diet provides energy to stay active and nutrients for growth and repair of cells. Diet therapies are more likely to be effective if practiced as a preventive measure against disease or if started early after the onset of disease. A poor diet may raise the risk of dying from heart disease, stroke, and type 2 diabetes.

Humans need a balanced diet to be healthy. As a component of disease treatment, physicians may prescribe a special diet that must be carefully followed. While nurses often answer diet-related questions, an important part of the healthcare team is the Registered Clinical Dietitian who assesses the patient's therapeutic nutritional needs, develops and implements nutrition programs, and may even teach healthy cooking classes. Working closely with the doctor, staff and the patient, they provide an individualized diet plan, counseling, and education to meet patient's dietary needs.

MECHANISM OF ACTION

Individuals may react differently to dietary interventions based on a variety of factors. Genetic factors, other health behaviors such as smoking and levels of physical activity must all be factored in to determine results of dietary therapies. Before undertaking any diet therapy, the patient should discuss the plan with the physician. Physicians may recommend specific diets or may recommend that the person see a registered clinical dietitian. Extreme diets that omit complete classes of food are not always safe and should be undertaken only in consultation with the physician. Diet information must be critically evaluated before undertaking any specific diet. A healthy diet, appropriate exercise and maintaining an appropriate body weight are always a good idea.

USES AND APPLICATIONS

Diets have been an important part of healthcare management over the years. Diets have been used to treat a variety of diseases, for example, hypertension. One of the most important science based-diets designed to control blood pressure is the Dietary Approaches to Stop Hypertension (DASH) diet, which is promoted by the National Heart, Lung, and Blood Institute, part of the National Institutes of Health (NIH).

The DASH diet is a plan that is low in saturated fats, cholesterol, and total fat. It emphasizes the intake of fruits, vegetables, fat-free or low-fat milk and milk products, whole grain products, fish, poultry, and nuts. The diet is low in lean red meat, sweets, added sugars, and sugar-containing beverages. It is rich in potassium, magnesium, calcium, protein, and fiber.

Type 2 diabetes is another chronic disease that can be partially controlled by diet. The ideal diabetic meal consists of a combination of foods, such as bread, products that are high in fat, dairy items that provide protein, and starchy vegetables. Most of the protein in a diabetic diet comes from chicken, fish, lean beef, or dairy. Servings and portions in diabetic diets depend on a person's level of physical activity.

Cardiovascular diseases can also be prevented and controlled by diet. Histological studies show that vascular injury accumulates from adolescence, making it extremely important to monitor one's lifestyle and diet from childhood to prevent a heart condition in the future. Any diet designed to control or prevent cardiovascular disease most be low in saturated fats (less than 7 percent of the daily diet) and low in cholesterol (less than 300 milligrams [0.06 tsp] per day for healthy adults and less than 200 milligrams [0.04 tsp] per day for adults with high levels of low-density lipoprotein (LDL), or bad, cholesterol).

The American Cancer Society recommends that people with cancer not undertake a dietary program as an exclusive or primary means of treatment. The cancer patient should discuss any dietary changes with the physician or medical oncologist before beginning any changes.

SCIENTIFIC EVIDENCE

There are multiple studies that support the use of diet therapies in disease management. NIH studies have demonstrated that a low level of salt combined with the DASH diet is effective at lowering blood pressure. The effect of this combination (at a sodium level of 1,500 milligrams per day [.3 tsp]) was an average blood pressure reduction of 8.9/4.5 millimeters of mercury (systolic/diastolic) in normal subjects. Persons in the studies who were hypertensive experienced an average reduction of 11.5/5.7 millimeters of mercury.

Studies have shown higher rates of heart disease in people who eat more saturated fats. A low intake of saturated fats will reduce LDL (bad) cholesterol and triglycerides in the blood. The Diabetes Prevention Program demonstrated that losing weight and increasing exercise decreased the risk of diabetes by 58 percent, even more than a prescription drug. The American Cancer Society states staying at a healthy weight, staying active throughout life, following a healthy eating plan and minimizing alcohol intake may greatly reduce a person's risk of developing or dying from cancer.

CHOOSING A PRACTITIONER
Registered clinical dietitians are educated and qualified to diagnose eating disorders and design diets to treat specific medical conditions and diseases in conjunction with physicians and nurses. For example, diet restrictions related to diabetes as prescribed by the physician and poor eating habits or loss of appetite from cancer noted by the nurse. Dietitians most often practice in hospitals and formal health settings. Most states require licensure to practice as a registered clinical dietitian. Nutritionists are most likely found in schools, hospitals, cafeterias, long-term care facilities, and athletic organizations to deal with general nutritional aims and behaviors. The educational program is more rigorous for Registered Clinical Dietitians often requiring a grade point average (GPA) of 3.0 to enter the program. A nutritionist takes courses at the college level related to science and nutrition but often anyone giving nutrition device may choose to call themselves a nutritionist because they are giving dietary advice. A registered dietitian nutritionist must have a master's degree and 1,200 hours of supervised practice.

SAFETY ISSUES
When beginning a therapeutic diet that involves a dramatically different way of eating, people should receive expert supervision so that they can avoid nutritional deficiencies. Discussing diet changes with the physician is very important. The physician may recommend a consultation with a registered clinical dietitian or nutritionist before undertaking any diet modifications.

The human body, which needs carbohydrates, fats, and proteins for healthy function, burns its own reserves of energy in the absence of calorie intake. Fasting for extended periods leads to starvation, dehydration, and eventual death. Diets based on one type of food, such as those based solely on fruits, can cause protein deficiencies, which inhibit growth and development in children. Fruit-based diets can also cause deficiencies in vitamin D, vitamin B_{12}, calcium, iron, zinc, and essential fatty acids.

—*Fernando J. Ferrer and Patricia Stanfill Edens*

Further Reading
"American Cancer Society Updates Guideline for Diet and Physical Activity." *American Cancer Society*, 9 June 2020, www.cancer.org/latest-news/american-cancer-society-updates-guideline-for-diet-and-physical-activity.html.
"DASH Diet: Healthy Eating to Lower Your Blood Pressure." *Mayo Clinic*, www.mayoclinic.org/healthy-lifestyle/nutrition-and-healthy-eating/in-depth/dash-diet/art-20048456. Accessed 24 Aug. 2020.
"DASH Ranked Best Diet Overall for Eighth Year in a Row by *U.S. News and World Report*." *National Institutes of Health*, www.nih.gov/news-events/news-releases/dash-ranked-best-diet-overall-eighth-year-row-us-news-world-report. Accessed 24 Aug. 2020.
"Food and Nutrition Information Center." US Department of Agriculture. *National Agricultural Library*, www.nal.usda.gov/fnic. Accessed 24 Aug. 2020.
"How Dietary Factors Influence Disease Risk." *National Institutes of Health*, www.nih.gov/news-events/nih-research-matters/how-dietary-factors-influence-disease-risk. Accessed 24 Aug. 2020.
Rock, C. L., and C. Thomson, et al. "American Cancer Society Guideline for Diet and Physical Activity for Cancer Prevention." *CA: A Cancer Journal for Clinicians*, 9 June 2020, acsjournals.onlinelibrary.wiley.com/doi/full/103322/caac.21591. Accessed 24 Aug. 2020.

EXERCISE-BASED THERAPIES

ABSTRACT
Exercise-based therapies are physical activities performed to enhance overall health and wellness and to treat specific medical disorders.

OVERVIEW
According to a 2008 Centers for Disease Control and Prevention (CDC) health study, 7 percent of those sur-

veyed engaged in what is considered exercise-based complementary and alternative medicine (CAM) activities. While these activities may be considered outside the scope of conventional exercise practices in some instances, exercise is an integral part of disease management. For example, cardiac rehabilitation utilizes a modified therapeutic exercise plan to enhance recovery. Cancer patients are encouraged to exercise within their limits to relieve symptoms and create a general feeling of well-being. Rehabilitation services are often provided after injury to restore function and improve abilities related to activities of daily living. The physician and rehabilitation professionals decide a plan of care based on individual patient's need. Yoga is often recommended to reduce joint pain and increase joint flexibility and function. There are also psychological benefits to exercise, including stress relief and reduced tension. Therapeutic exercise and targeted activities are an important component of healthcare.

Although pain relief was the most common reason for its use, exercise-based CAM is used throughout the spectrum of medical conditions. A survey of the medical literature revealed seven exercise-based CAM activities, namely yoga, Tai Chi, qigong, Pilates, the Alexander technique, the Feldenkrais method, and the Trager approach. With an estimated twenty-one million adult participants in the United States in 2012, according to the survey conducted by the National Center for Complementary and Integrative Health and the CDC's National Center for Health Statistics, yoga is the most popular exercise-based CAM activity. A five-thousand-year-old practice that

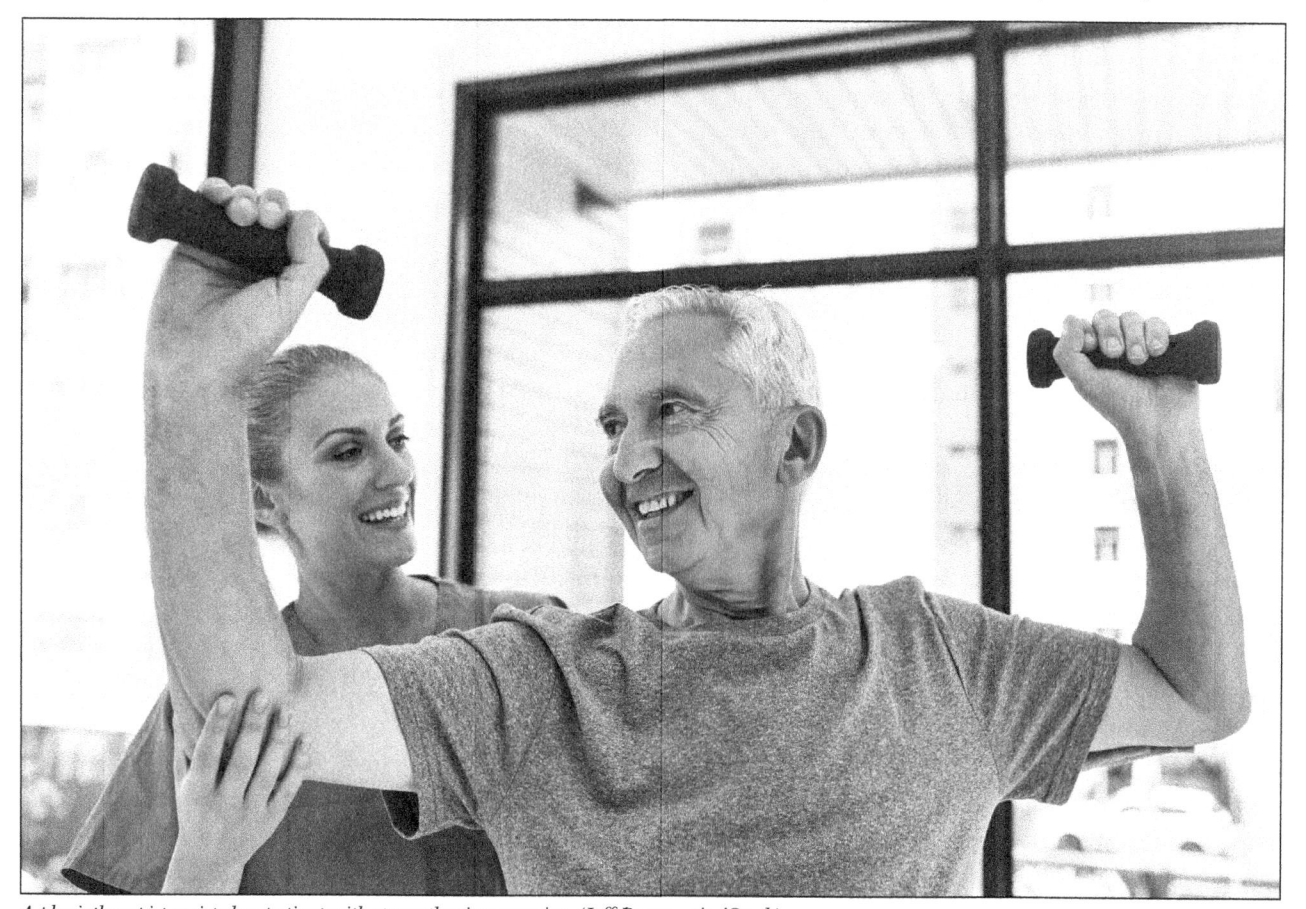

A physiotherapist assists her patient with strengthening exercises (Jeff Bergen via iStock)

originated in India, yoga seeks to integrate the mind, body, and spirit through physical poses, breathing exercises, meditation, and spiritual philosophy.

Pilates is another popular exercise system in the West. This one-hundred-year-old form of exercise is designed to strengthen core muscles while focusing on posture and proper breathing. Often, props and apparatus are used.

Tai Chi, originally conceived as a martial art in China five hundred years ago, is now practiced primarily for general physical fitness. Although many forms exist, in the West, Tai Chi uses a series of slow, graceful movements to enhance strength, stamina, and balance. Tai Chi is part of a larger, five-thousand-year-old system of traditional Chinese mental, spiritual, and physical training called qigong. Other components of qigong include physical poses, meditation, and breathing exercises.

The Feldenkrais method, the Alexander technique, and the Trager approach are lesser known exercise-based CAM activities. These are movement therapies in which practitioners are guided in their posture and physical actions to improve balance, reduce pain, and increase emotional well-being.

MECHANISMS OF ACTION
Prescribed rehabilitative plans focus on a specific patient need such as enhanced physical fitness, heart strength and recovery, and work in varying ways. Four of the seven forms of exercise-based CAM can be considered forms of general physical exercise. Yoga, Pilates, Tai Chi, and qigong involve various degrees of cardiovascular, strength, and flexibility training. They promote stamina, bone health, healthy weight, muscle tone, balance, and strength. Yoga, Tai Chi, and qigong also involve meditation. Although scientific research is ongoing, it appears that meditation decreases heart rate, increases blood flow to the organs, and improves mood regulation because of changes in the nervous system. No clinical data are available to determine the exact mechanism of action of the Alexander technique, the Feldenkrais method, or the Trager approach.

USES AND APPLICATIONS
Prescribed exercise is designed to restore function to a specific body part, increase stamina and enhance recovery and return to normal life. Exercise-based CAM is most commonly used to improve and maintain overall fitness. Other common therapeutic uses are to reduce stress, relieve pain, and improve flexibility. Exercise-based CAM experts claim, however, that these exercise systems are helpful in treating a variety of conditions, such as asthma, osteoporosis, menstrual pain, depression, cancer, high blood pressure, diabetes, arthritis, insomnia, neuromuscular disorders, fatigue, attention deficit disorder, gastrointestinal disorders, infertility, sinusitis, and heart disease.

SCIENTIFIC EVIDENCE
Multiple studies have demonstrated that exercise as part of lifestyle modification or as a prescribed rehabilitation plan is important to restoring optimal function and quality of life. Diabetic patients are encouraged to participate in moderate exercise, for example. Rehabilitation after a knee replacement is necessary to achieve optimal function. Determining whether exercise-based CAM is effective in the management and prevention of illness is challenging. A limited number of well-designed clinical trials are available. The wide variety of practices within these different styles makes obtaining a consensus difficult.

In 2010, several large, well-designed studies showed that Tai Chi and qigong were beneficial in preventing osteoporosis in postmenopausal women and in treating hypertension and heart disease. Additionally, these studies suggest that Tai Chi may be effective in enhancing the immune system of the elderly.

A review of the medical literature reveals promising evidence that yoga may help treat a variety of medical conditions, including mood disorders, hypertension, insomnia, back pain, and osteoporosis, and may im-

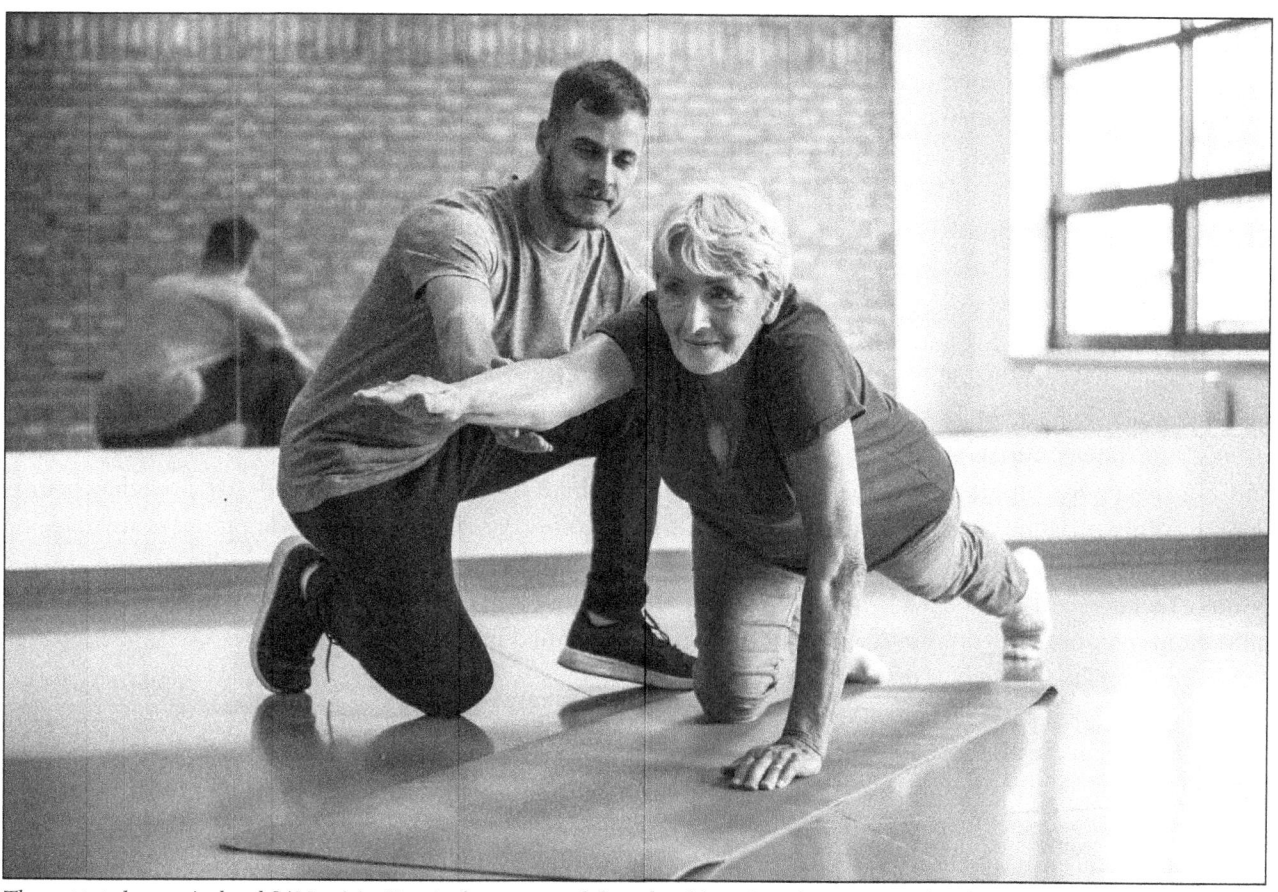

The most popular exercise-based CAM activity, Yoga is often recommended to reduce joint pain and increase joint flexibility and function. (izusek via iStock)

prove overall physical conditioning. In a 2008 randomized clinical trial in the journal *Menopause*, yoga reduced hot flashes in women by 30 percent. Furthermore, numerous studies have demonstrated that yoga diminishes sex performance anxiety and enhances female sexual desire. Many health practitioners use yoga in conjunction with conventional medicine in the treatment of cancer to reduce anxiety, pain, and insomnia, although scientists continue to debate the exact mechanisms of action involved.

A gap in the literature exists regarding the use of Pilates in treating medical conditions. Experts do agree that Pilates is effective in improving strength, flexibility, and balance. Although experts in the Feldenkrais method, the Alexander technique, and the Trager approach claim that their movement exercises reduce pain, prevent injury, and improve balance, no well-designed clinical trials have been conducted to determine their efficacy.

With regard to other medical claims about exercise-based CAM, no well-designed randomized controlled trials are available; a review of the medical literature did not support the claims.

CHOOSING A PRACTITIONER

Most hospitals and physician practices either provide or have access to robust rehabilitation programs, including physical therapists, exercise physiologists, occupational therapists and others. When undertaking a therapeutic exercise program, the physician will write a referral or prescription for licensed practitioners to provide care. When undertaking an exercise program on your own begin by talking with the physician about any potential issues or limitations that might influence response or be detrimental to your physical condition. Exercise programs outside the healthcare setting may not be as aware of physical limitations related to disease and may push people beyond their capabilities.

Hundreds of exercise-based CAM instructor-training programs have been established in the United States. None, however, include provider licensing requirements. Standards of certification for yoga instruction are largely based on the style of yoga studied and practiced. One program, the Yoga Alliance, is a nonprofit organization in the United States that maintains standards for yoga teacher-training programs. Teacher certification with this program requires a minimum of two hundred hours of training.

Several Tai Chi and qigong organizations provide teacher certification in the United States. Various levels of certification are offered based on hours of training and desired goals. Hundreds of Pilates training programs have been established in the United States too. Although licensing is not required, the Pilates Method Alliance offers a national teacher's certification program through written examination. Instructors of the Feldenkrais method, the Alexander technique, and the Trager approach are required to complete two- to-four-year training programs that encompass four hundred to sixteen hundred hours of class and fieldwork for certification.

SAFETY ISSUES

A therapeutic exercise program, one that is prescribed by a physician and conducted by a licensed rehabilitation professional, takes into consideration the patient's medical condition, existing health status, and other factors designed to enhance a safe and quality outcome. No exercise program should be undertaken without first discussing it with a healthcare provider if there are any health issues that might cause safety issues. Exercise-based CAM is generally considered safe for those without serious health conditions or injuries. Persons with spine or joint disease, uncontrolled blood pressure, or severe balance abnormalities should avoid some exercise-based CAM activities. Although uncommon, spine and joint injuries have occurred during CAM exercise activities. To avoid such injuries, participants should adhere to the directions of a certified instructor. Pregnant women, who should exercise caution when considering CAM, typically require modification of certain practices. All potential participants, especially if pregnant, looking into exercised-based CAM as a form of therapy should consult with their healthcare providers before joining any exercise-based program. It is advisable to choose a certified provider. Typically, a national association that confers the certification will have a list of qualified providers.

—*Marie President*

Further Reading

Barnes, P. M., B. Bloom, and R. L. Nahin. "Complementary and Alternative Medicine Use Among Adults and Children: 2007 United States." *National Health Statistics Reports*, vol. 12, pp. 1–23.

Carson, C., S. Lasker-Hertz, and P. Stanfill-Edens. "Exercise for Cancer Patients." www.oumedicine.com/docs/ou-medicine/exercisecancerpatients.pdf?sfvrsn=2. Accessed 25 Aug. 2020.

Jahnke, R., et al. "A Comprehensive Review of Health Benefits of Qigong and Tai Chi." *American Journal of Health Promotion*, vol. 24, no. 6, 2010, pp. 1–25.

Nagel, Denise. "Health Benefits of Tai Chi and Qiqong." *TheHuffingtonPost.com*, 23 June 2015.

"Nationwide Survey Reveals Widespread Use of Mind and Body Practices." National Center for Complementary and Integrative Health. *National Institutes of Health*, 10 Feb. 2015.

"Rehabilitation." *World Health Organization*, www.who.int/health-topics/rehabilitation#tab=tab_1. Accessed 25 Aug. 2020.

"What Is Cardiac Rehabilitation?" *American Heart Association*, www.heart.org/en/health-topics/cardiac-rehab/what-is-cardiac-rehabilitation. Accessed 25 Aug. 2020.

Yang, K. "A Review of Yoga Programs for Four Leading Risk Factors of Chronic Diseases." *Evidence-Based Complementary and Alternative Medicine*, vol. 4, no. 4, 2007, pp. 487–91.

EDUCATION AND TRAINING OF CAM PRACTITIONERS

ABSTRACT

If complementary and alternative forms of therapy or CAM is used in conjunction with conventional medicine, it is considered complementary. For example, using acupuncture to help with cancer treatment side effects is considered complementary medicine. When providers offer both traditional medicine and complementary medicine, it is called integrative medicine. If nonmainstream practice is used in place of conventional medicine, it is considered alternative and may involve nontested therapies. The shortage of clinical research studies related to complementary and alternative therapies make it difficult to quantify their advantages in use.

OVERVIEW

The education and training of practitioners of CAM are widely varied, as these practices encompass any type of therapy that is not considered conventional or scientifically proven. Many of these therapies, however, have a long history in other cultures. CAM education and training may involve rigorous courses of study similar to those for a medical degree or for postdoctoral training. However, some CAM education consists of only minimal training, such as a six-week course that leads to a certificate. Even within the same discipline, training and certification requirements may vary widely from state to state, because there is no national regulatory body to oversee the process.

The education and training of CAM practitioners are the focus here, so the discussion will cover only those areas of unconventional therapy with standard educational or training programs. Covered here are acupuncturists, chiropractors, homeopaths, massage therapists, naturopaths, and integrated medicine programs that combine conventional medicine with CAM practice.

Many other types of CAM practitioners, such as aromatherapists, crystal therapists, reflexologists, reiki practitioners, and native or indigenous healers, study for long periods with experienced experts in their field. However, no particular training programs, educational courses, recognized requirements, or state or national certifications are available in the United States for these practitioners.

PRACTITIONERS

Acupuncturist. Acupuncture is a standard accepted practice in the Chinese medicine tradition; however, it is relatively new in the United States and, as such, varies from state to state in education and certification requirements and venues. About forty states have established criteria for persons seeking to practice acupuncture. Nonmedical professionals, to become licensed as an acupuncturist, must take a four-year course of study and a board examination. Persons with a medical background, such as medical doctors, dentists, nurses, and chiropractors, must often complete a rigorous course of study too, including classroom study (a minimum of three hundred hours) and clinical acupuncture practice, before becoming licensed.

Courses in acupuncture focus on anatomy, physiology, and other areas that are typical for any type of medical practice. Courses also include detailed study of the nervous and vascular systems so that a practitioner has a thorough understanding of needle insertion and the body's reaction to it. A practitioner of acupuncture may also be trained in other aspects of Chinese traditional medicine.

Two bodies certify and accredit acupuncture colleges and practitioners in the United States: The Accreditation Commission for Acupuncture and Oriental Medicine and the American Board of Medical Acupuncture. These organizations provide continuing education and examinations for practitioners

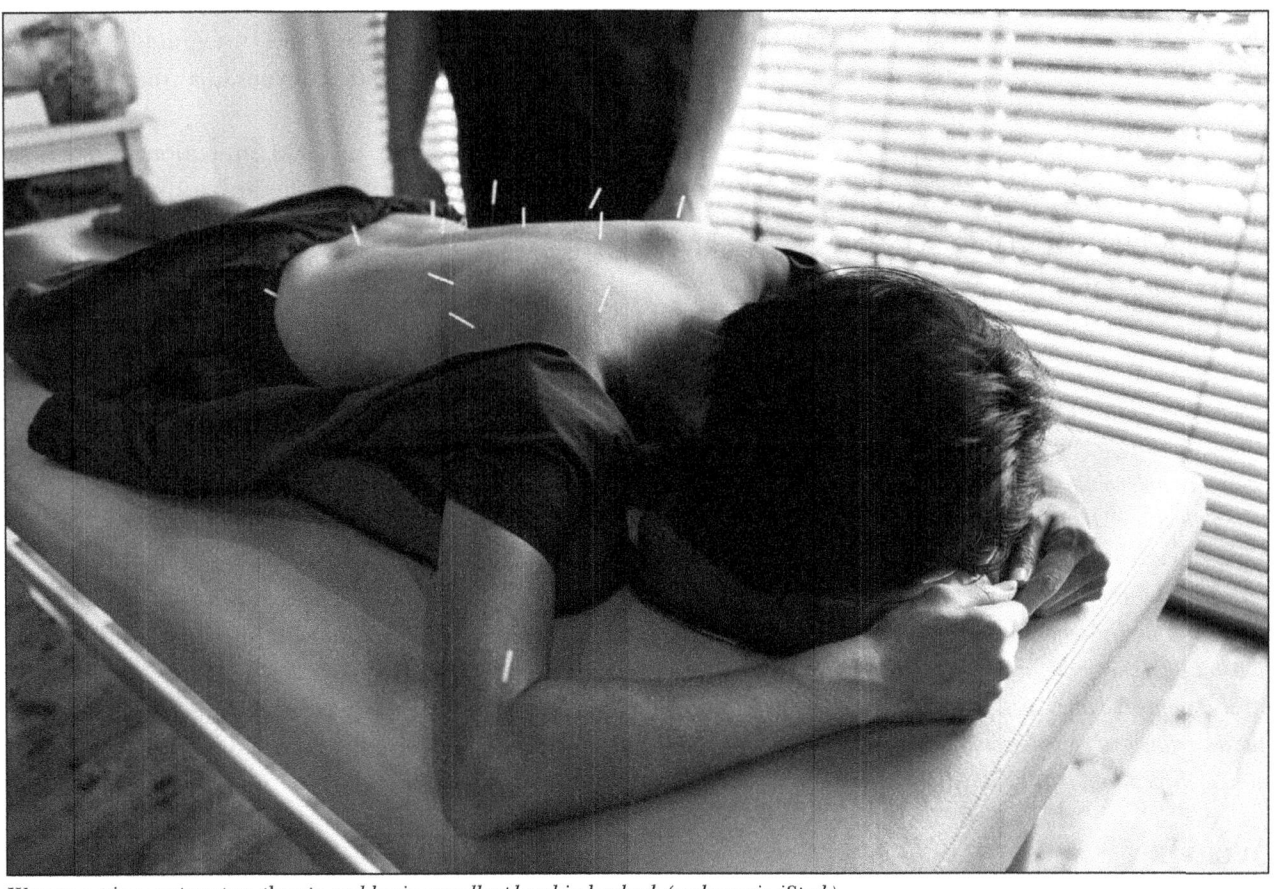

Woman getting acupuncture therapy and having needles placed in her back (andresr via iStock)

and oversight for educational programs in the United States. They also provide standards for acupuncturists trained in other countries who wish to practice in the United States.

Chiropractor. This branch of CAM may be one of the most highly regulated in the United States. The Council on Chiropractic Education (CCE) is an accreditation body for chiropractic schools, and its accreditation criteria are recognized by the US Department of Education. CCE regulates all training programs for chiropractors. The American Chiropractic Association, a leading professional organization for chiropractors, provides continuing medical education and other resources to practitioners.

A chiropractic training program must include a minimum of 4,200 hours of class time, laboratory work, and clinical experience and must include courses in orthopedics, neurology, and physiotherapy (all with a focus on clinical practice of manipulation and spinal alignment). Chiropractors may also pursue studies in a specialty, such as orthopedics, sports medicine, or rehabilitation.

After completion of a doctor of chiropractic (DC) program, student practitioners must pass a four-part examination from the National Board of Chiropractic Examiners and must pass a state examination to be licensed. In some areas, the state examination takes the place of the national examination.

Homeopath. The education and training of a homeopath can take varied courses. Programs designed for medical doctors or others with medical training tend to focus on homeopathy and its application, assuming that those with a medical degree would already have a basic background in medicine and medical practice. Other courses, geared to those who do not have a medical background, focus more on medical education, such as anatomy and physiology, but also train students in homeopathy practices and principles.

A few states in the United States offer training in homeopathy (Arizona, California, Colorado, Florida, Massachusetts, and Utah, and the District of Columbia). Admission requirements for courses of study vary widely; some require a medical doctor (MD) or similar degree, and others enroll students with little or no medical background. Because homeopathy itself is not regulated in the United States, anyone can use the word "homeopath" to describe themselves or their type of work. However, a person cannot identify himself or herself as a homeopathic doctor or imply to the public that he or she is practicing medicine if he or she does not hold a medical license.

Several programs offer homeopathic education, but no single certification is recognized throughout the United States. Each state has its own standards for licensing this type of care. Some homeopaths are licensed in a conventional type of medicine and may hold a degree as an M.D. or as a nurse practitioner. In Arizona, Connecticut, and Nevada, MDs and DOs (doctors of osteopathy) can be licensed as homeopathic physicians. Homeopathic assistants, who practice under the supervision of a homeopath, are licensed in Arizona and Nevada.

Organizations such as the Council for Homeopathic Certification and the American Board of

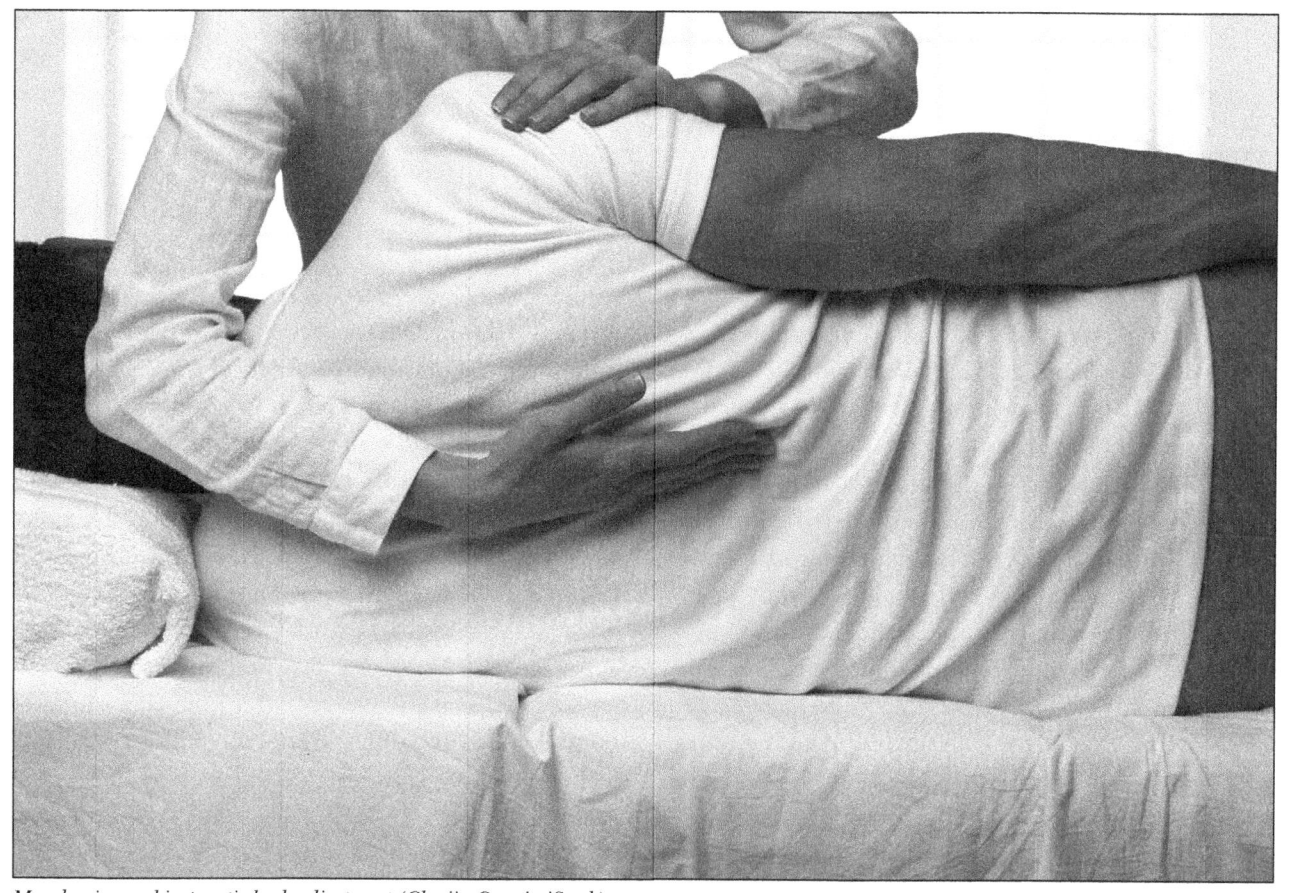

Man having a chiropractic back adjustment (ChesiireCat via iStock)

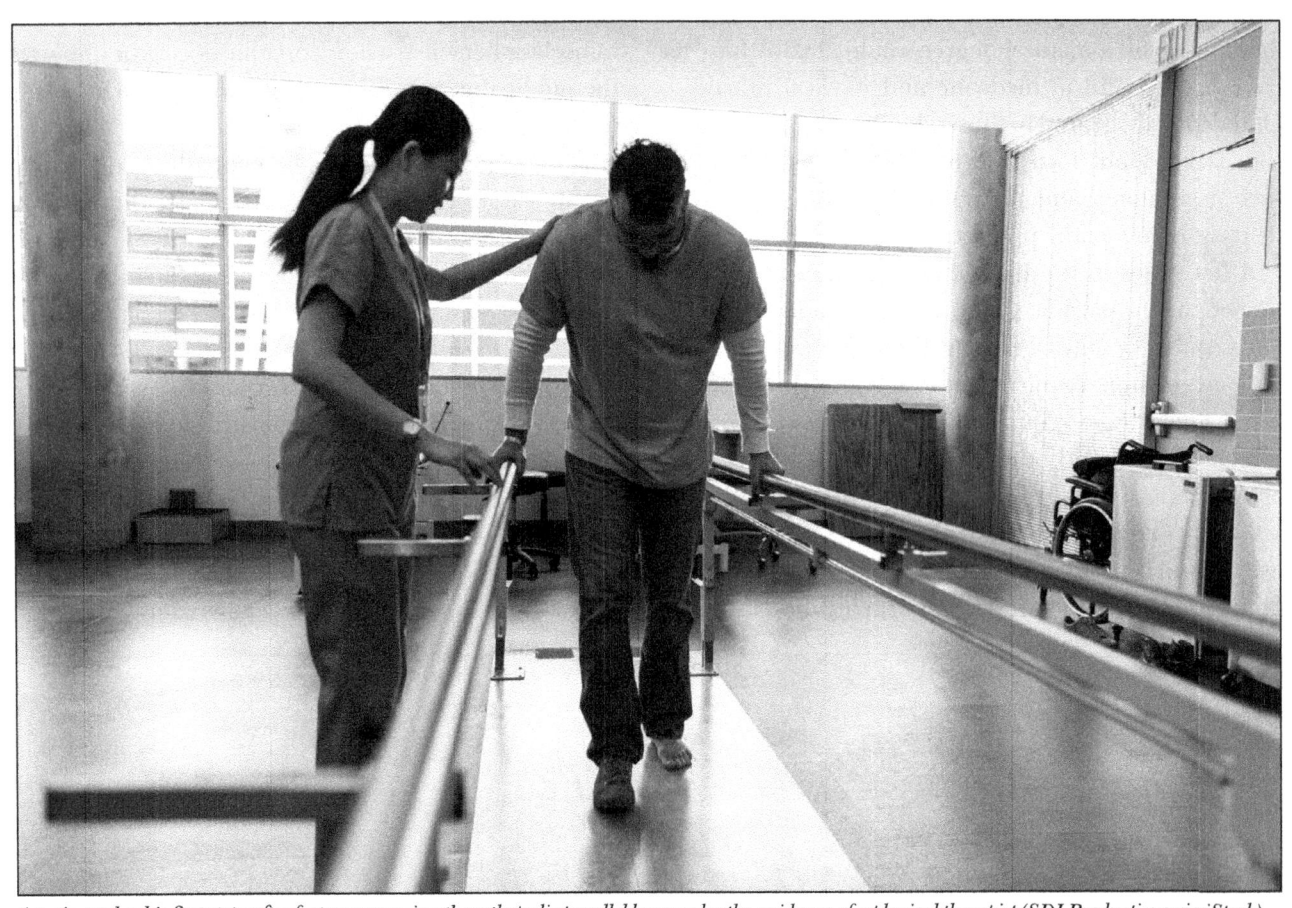

A patient takes his first steps after foot surgery using the orthopedic parallel bars under the guidance of a physical therapist (SDI Productions via iStock)

Homeotherapeutics offer certifications to homeopaths who have completed certain requirements: for example, MDs or DOs who pass oral and written exams in homeopathy. Upon completing these exams, the successful candidate is awarded a diplomate of homeotherapeutics (D.Ht.). Even though the Department of Education does not recognize any one organization as a certifying body, homeopathic practitioners use the standards upheld by these organizations to maintain competency and to encourage self-regulation.

Massage therapist. Most US states regulate the practice of massage therapy in some way with a type of governing board providing certification or licensure. Usually, a massage therapist must complete some course of training and pass a board examination to be licensed. However, the requirements vary widely from state to state. Education provided in massage therapy schools typically requires about five hundred hours of study and involves courses in anatomy, physiology, motion and body mechanics, and clinical massage practice. Licensure also may involve passing a nationally recognized test, such as the National Certification Examination for Therapeutic Massage and Bodywork or the Massage and Bodywork Licensing Examination.

Naturopath. There are two basic types of naturopath: traditional and naturopathic physicians. Education and training for traditional naturopaths vary from nondegree certificate programs to undergraduate degree programs. After completion of a degree program, a traditional naturopath can certify with the American Naturopathic Medical Certificate Board and become a naturopathic consultant. Traditionally, these types of naturopaths do not practice medicine and thus do not require a license.

A naturopathic physician must have a doctor of naturopathic medicine (ND, or NMD in Arizona) degree from an accredited school of naturopathic medicine. Only four schools in the United States (in Washington, Oregon, Arizona, and Connecticut) are accredited for this type of education. The ND involves four years of graduate-level study in a standard medical curriculum, with added courses in natural therapeutics. Practitioners must then pass a state board licensing examination. (In the state of Utah, naturopathic doctors must complete a residency before starting a practice.)

Practitioners often work as primary care clinicians, but some states do not recognize the DM degree, so practitioners in these areas cannot legally practice medicine. Generally, they may still practice traditional naturopathic medicine. Two states, South Carolina and Tennessee, specifically prohibit the practice of naturopathy in any form.

The Council of Naturopathic Medical Education is a governing body that provides accreditation for education in naturopathy. The American Naturopathic Certification Board provides testing and continuing education for this profession.

CAM EDUCATION AND TRAINING IN MAINSTREAM INSTITUTIONS

As the practice of CAM becomes more widespread and integrated into society, many medical colleges in the United States have begun to offer courses in CAM. One area of complementary medicine that is often taught in integrative medicine courses is pain management. CAM courses often teach conventional physicians how CAM methods can be incorporated into, and can truly complement, conventional medicine.

The University of Arizona College of Medicine teaches a program of integrative medicine that critically examines branches of alternative medicine and trains clinicians in practices that it finds helpful and that cause no harm. Other such programs include Mayo Clinic Complementary and Integrative Medicine, the Integrative Medicine Program at MD Anderson Cancer Center, and University of Michigan Integrative Medicine.

—*Marianne M. Madsen*

Further Reading

American Academy of Acupuncture, medicalacupuncture.org. The American Academy of Medical Acupuncture (AAMA) is the professional society of physicians (MDs and DOs) in North America who have incorporated acupuncture into their traditional medical practice.

American Association of Naturopathic Physicians, naturopathic.org.

American Chiropractic Association, www.acatoday.org. Chiropractic is a healthcare profession that focuses on disorders of the musculoskeletal system and the nervous system, and the effects of these disorders on general health in a holistic manner.

American Institute for Homeopathy, homeopathyusa.org/homeopathic-medicine.html.

American Massage Therapy Association, www.amtamassage.org.

"Complementary, Alternative or Integrative Health: What's in a Name?" National Center for Complementary and Integrative Health. *National Institutes of Health*, www.nccih.nih.gov/health/complementary-alternative-or-integrative-health-whats-in-a-name.

"Integrative Medicine." *Psychology Today*, www.psychologytoday.com/us/basics/integrative-medicine. Accessed 24 Aug. 2020.

National Center for Complementary and Integrative Health. *National Institutes of Health*, nccih.nih.gov. Conducts and supports research and provides information about complementary health products and practices. Accessed 24 Aug. 2020.

Tierney, Gillian. *Opportunities in Holistic Health Care Careers*. Rev. ed. McGraw-Hill, 2007. This book addresses the job outlook, educational requirements, regulation, and salaries for many CAM practitioners.

INTEGRATIVE MEDICINE

ABSTRACT
Integrative medicine is a relationship-centered care system that combines mainstream medical and alternative therapeutic methods to potentiate the body's innate capacity to heal.

OVERVIEW
According to Andrew Weil, a prominent physician and a proponent of this system, integrative medicine (IM) works with the body's natural potential for healing. In the human body, many pathways and mechanisms serve to maintain health and promote healing. The IM perspective recognizes that treatment, often a combination of allopathic and alternative medicine, should unblock and enhance these mechanisms.

In practice, the therapeutic process addresses the whole person and relies on the main pillars of a person's well-being: mind, body, spirit, and community. This paradigm emphasizes the importance of a sound physician-patient relationship for a successful healing process. Developing rapport and empathy greatly facilitates the efficacy of lifestyle changes and the use of therapies such as pharmaceuticals, homeopathy, dietary supplements, traditional Chinese medicine, Ayurveda, manual methods, mind/body techniques, and movement therapy.

Until the 1970s, little was done to connect traditional, ancient healing modalities to biomedicine. At that time, the holistic health movement in the United States and in Western Europe started a "dynamic alliance" of therapists, including American Indian healers, yoga teachers, and homeopaths. Modern medicine began taking steps to reduce the use of technology and the disconnect from the patient, while rediscovering more natural, less invasive avenues of healing.

The Consortium of Academic Health Centers for Integrative Medicine (later renamed the Academic Consortium for Integrative Medicine and Health), founded in 2000, brings together many highly esteemed academic medical centers dedicated to promoting IM through educational opportunities, health policies, research, and collaborative initiatives.

MECHANISM OF ACTION
Integrative medicine combines conventional medical treatments with carefully selected alternative therapies that are proven to be safe and effective. The goal of the integrative movement is to bring back the art of healing and to address the root of the pathological process, not just the symptoms. In addition to acquiring the foundations of medical knowledge, physicians should be able to release, explore, and exploit the intrinsic healing responses of the body. Practitioners are therefore encouraged to become familiar with, and critically assess, the modalities of complementary and alternative medicine (CAM).

Core areas of education include the philosophy of science, cross-cultural medicine, principles of mind/body medicine, self-healing, and spirituality. The practitioner's ability to self-explore and maintain his or her own health balance are considered essential for the therapeutic act. The physician strives to become a partner and a mentor, who understands the important coordinates of his or her patient's life events, culture, beliefs, and relationships. By acknowledging a person's uniqueness, the processes of health maintenance and healing are tailored to best address a person's background and conditions. Matching the patient's belief system can, especially in chronic illness, lead to the activation of an internal healing response, often known as the placebo effect. This response can ultimately result in enhanced health.

USES AND APPLICATIONS
Overall, IM is a combination of art and science that seeks health maintenance and disease prevention and treatment using the most natural, least invasive interventions available. Virtually all categories of disorders, and especially chronic diseases, can benefit from an integrated approach.

Cardiovascular disorders. Cardiovascular disorders such as congestive heart failure, coronary artery disease, hypertension, and peripheral vascular disease can be treated with conventional methods and with lifestyle modifications, nutrition, dietary supplements (omega-3 fatty acids, coenzyme Q_{10}, carnitine, arginine, hawthorn, and garlic), relaxation, meditation, and hydrotherapy. Primary prevention is critical in coronary artery disease and hypertension.

Cancer. Cancer can be treated with the synergistic reduction of the sequellae and by limiting the toxicity or trauma of conventional therapies and by alleviating psychological distress. Nutritional changes, dietary supplements (vitamins, immunomodulators, ginger, marijuana, and St. John's wort), acupuncture, mind/body techniques, and group support are often recommended. Preventive approaches (for breast cancer, for example) involve lifestyle changes (exercise, nutrition, limiting toxins, and breast-feeding), botanicals (seaweed, rosemary, and green tea), and mind/body methods.

Endocrine and metabolic disorders. Endocrine and metabolic disorders are also amenable to integrated therapies. Insulin resistance is often treated with metformin hydrochloride, lifestyle changes, and a low-carbohydrate diet. Supplements such as chromium, vanadium, alpha-lipoic acid, American ginseng, and fenugreek can provide benefits too. In persons with diabetes mellitus, essential care includes diet, exercise, and pharmaceuticals. Dietary supplements, such as vitamins, bilberry, and *Ginkgo biloba*, and mind/body techniques (e.g., relaxation and yoga) may mitigate vascular disease and even lower glucose levels. Alternative therapies to consider in persons with hypothyroidism include dietary supplements such as vitamins, zinc, selenium, and traditional Chinese botanicals, and practices such as yoga. Pharmaceuticals are available for the treatment of osteoporosis, and vitamin D, ipriflavone, and exercise constitute useful adjuvants.

Gastrointestinal disorders. Gastroesophageal reflux, peptic ulcer disease, and irritable bowel syndrome can be treated with lifestyle changes and with botanicals (licorice, chamomile, and marshmallow root), homeopathics, and mind/body therapies (including stress management and guided imagery).

Neurological disorders. Stroke, multiple sclerosis, Alzheimer's disease, Parkinson's disease, seizures, and migraine have been linked to oxidative stress, neurotoxic factors, and inflammatory processes. Thus, they can greatly benefit from integrative methods. The complementary therapies include, but are not limited to, dietary and nutritional supplementation (omega-3 fatty acids, glutathione, coenzyme Q_{10}, alpha-lipoic acid, N-acetylcysteine, niacin, vitamins, melatonin, and magnesium), herbal supplementation (*Ginkgo biloba*, milk thistle, turmeric, vinpocetine, and skullcap), meditation, yoga, and exercise.

Asthma and allergies. Asthma and allergies respond well to alternative methods that include nutritional and environmental changes, exercise, botanicals (ginkgo, coleus, licorice, kanpo, bioflavonoids, and stinging nettle), vitamins and minerals, homeopathics, massage, inhalation, breathing techniques, and mind/body therapy.

Upper respiratory infections and sinusitis. Upper respiratory infections and sinusitis can be treated with pharmaceuticals, dietary changes, hydration, steam inhalation, supplements (vitamins, antioxidants, zinc, magnesium, garlic, and echinacea), and homeopathic remedies.

Depression and anxiety. Depression and anxiety represent a spectrum of disorders ideally suited for IM. In addition to pharmaceuticals, persons can benefit from lifestyle changes, physical activity, nutritional remedies (omega-3 fatty acids, B vitamins, folic acid, and hydroxytryptophan), botanical remedies (St. John's wort, kava kava, and ginkgo), psychotherapy, relaxation training, yoga, acupuncture, and transcranial stimulation.

Pain. Pain management represents a challenge for both the physician and the person in pain. Truly integrating allopathic and alternative medicines can offer relief and reduce frustration. Reassurance and lifestyle changes are often the first step of the therapeutic plan. A vast array of useful approaches includes pharmacotherapy, exercise, supplements (arnica and omega-3 fatty acids), homeopathy, manual methods, acupuncture, transcutaneous nerve stimulation, and mind/body therapy. Surgery is considered after conservative therapies have failed. The issue of chronic pain and opioid addiction had grown especially concerning by the end of the second decade of the twenty-first century, and health experts were consistently seeking complementary and integrative methods for treating this pain to minimize reliance upon such drugs, particularly for military veterans. In 2017, the US Department of Veterans Affairs, the US Department of Health and Human Services, and the US Department of Defense announced that they had formed a partnership to fund at least twelve research projects valued at millions of dollars dedicated to researching the efficacy of nondrug pain management treatments such as mindfulness and massage.

Pregnancy and menopause. The integrative approach to pregnancy and menopause reaches beyond the use of combined mainstream and alternative therapies. These conditions require a careful initial encounter and subsequent consideration of the mind, body, spirit, and community context. The patient-practitioner interaction is oriented toward health rather than disease, and listening to the person seeking care is essential. In pregnancy especially, the need for noninvasive, natural approaches becomes crucial. Nausea and vomiting, for example, are treated with supplements (vitamin B_6, red raspberry leaf, ginger root, and chamomile), homeopathics, acupuncture, and mind/body therapies.

Alcoholism and substance abuse. Therapeutic options for alcoholism and substance abuse include botanicals (valerian, kudzu, kava kava), acupuncture, mind/body therapies, and spirituality. The options also include twelve-step programs.

SCIENTIFIC EVIDENCE

Integrative practice is committed to the scientific method and is rooted in evidence. At the same time, the integrative practitioner aims to transcend the confines of "scientific truth" and connect with the people he or she serves on multiple levels.

A number of CAM therapies have proved effective as complements to conventional medical treatments. These CAM therapies include dietary and herbal supplements, acupuncture, manual therapy, biofeedback, relaxation training, and movement therapy. When a strong evidence base is developed for a particular complementary method, it can become part of the integrative armamentarium. After it reviewed the evidence base, for example, the Society for Integrative Oncology supported the use of acupuncture in cases in which cancer-related pain is poorly controlled.

According to the American Academy of Pediatrics, a review conducted in 2002 found more than fourteen hundred randomized-control trials of pediatric CAM; the quality of these trials was determined to be as good as those focusing on conventional therapies. It is important to note that different levels of evidence are required to prove the safety and efficacy of complementary therapies, depending on the goals of the treatment. Lower levels of evidence (that is, nonrandomized and observational studies) are acceptable for preventive or supportive goals and for noninvasive approaches. Furthermore, integrating represents more than combining; it involves holistic treatment and the synergistic application of an array of treatments. Thus, the extent of the combination or integration varies. This leads to unique challenges for the scientific validation of integrative methods. Traditional research models often appear inadequate. More studies are needed that examine the appropriateness and manner of integration for specific diseases and conditions. In acknowledgment of the increased recognition and implementation of the interdisciplinary approach of integrative medicine, the National Institutes of Health's National Center for Complementary and Alternative Medicine, long responsible for spearheading and funding major research projects on the subject, was renamed as the National Center for Complementary and Integrative Health in 2014.

CHOOSING A PRACTITIONER

A large number of medical schools in the United States have courses in CAM. Integrative medicine centers and fellowship programs exist at many prominent universities and hospitals in the United States, including the University of Arizona, Duke University, Harvard University, the University of Michigan, and the Mayo Clinic. These centers tend to be directed by conventional physicians (doctors of medicine and doctors of osteopathy) and staffed by various practitioners.

The American Board of Integrative Medicine, a member board of the American Board of Physician Specialties, establishes standards for the application of IM principles and offers certification. Even so, qualified IM practitioners are still difficult to find, and the demand greatly exceeds the supply. Oftentimes, the collaboration between conventional physicians of various specialties and certified CAM practitioners provides the foundation and benefits of integrative care. The American Holistic Medical Association maintains a directory of integrative and holistic practitioners holding relevant degrees.

SAFETY ISSUES

When implemented by physicians and CAM practitioners who are well versed in the integrative method, IM is safe and beneficial.

—*Mihaela Avramut*

Further Reading

American Association of Integrative Medicine, www.aaimedicine.com. Promotes the development of IM.

American Board of Integrative Holistic Medicine, integrativeholisticdoctors.org. Establishes and maintains standards of care.

American Holistic Medical Association, www.holisticmedicine.org. Promotes holistic and integrative principles.

Baer, Hans. *Toward an Integrative Medicine: Merging Alternative Therapies with Biomedicine*. Altamira Press, 2004. A comprehensive overview of the holistic movement and its journey into mainstream medicine.

Consortium of Academic Health Centers for Integrative Medicine, www.imconsortium.org. Advances the principles and practice of integrative healthcare within academic institutions.

"Federal Agencies Partner for Military and Veteran Pain Management Research." US Department of Health and Human Services. *National Center for Complementary and Integrative Health*, 20 Sept. 2017, www.nccih.nih.gov/news/press-releases/federal-agencies-partner-for-military-and-veteran-pain-management-research.

Kurn, Sidney, and Sheryl Shook. *Integrated Medicine for Neurologic Disorders*. Health Press, 2008. Review of nutritional and herbal therapies for practitioners who treat persons with neurological disorders.

Leis, A. M., L. C. Weeks, and M. J. Verhoef. "Principles to Guide Integrative Oncology and the Development of an Evidence Base." *Current Oncology*, vol. 15, suppl. 2, 2008, pp. S83–S87. Discusses the need for evidence to support the overall practice of integration and the challenges posed by the validation process.

Rakel, David, editor. *Integrative Medicine*. 2nd ed., Saunders/Elsevier, 2007. An authoritative textbook that discusses the philosophy and method of integrative medicine and details therapeutic modalities for numerous diseases and conditions.

Rees, L., and A. Weil. "Integrated Medicine [Editorial]." *British Medical Journal*, vol. 322, 2001, pp. 119–20. Defines the basic tenets of IM.

Internet Medicine

ABSTRACT
The use of web-based and other electronic long-distance communication technologies for health information, assessment, service delivery, training, and public health administration is becoming more widespread.

SCIENCE AND PROFESSION
The internet is a computer-based tool that is facilitating communication among vast numbers of individuals, groups, businesses, and governments. In addition to facilitating purely social and business-related ventures, the internet is proving to be a valuable tool for improving the state of public health. This is because a new type of medical care and medical services has developed. These services, typically called telehealth, telemedicine, and e-medicine, use the internet as a key tool in their dispensation, organization, and evaluation of healthcare services. Telehealth is defined as the use of electronic information and telecommunications technology to support long-distance clinical healthcare and other activities. Education, public health and public administration may also utilize a telehealth strategy. Telehealth is different than telemedicine because its application is far broader than just the remote clinical medical service provided within telemedicine.

Such services have taken the form of a variety of healthcare-related websites that provide services once available only through a face-to-face visit with a doctor or other health or social services professional. The websites are valuable in that they provide almost instantaneous information and other communications assistance to patients, their families, treatment professionals, trainers, trainees in the healthcare and social service professions, and medical researchers.

In terms of assisting patients, internet-based medical approaches provide a variety of services to individual internet users. First, they provide a wealth of information on different symptoms and medical conditions. They also allow for screening of such conditions to see if they warrant further attention from medical professionals and advice on how to handle minor health ailments and medical emergencies. They also help consumers to find medical advice, healthcare providers, self-help or support groups, and therapy over the internet, all of which may or may not be supervised by medical professionals. Finally, they can give patients and their families information on different treatment options, including common procedures, the latest in alternative medicine, and even current clinical trials information.

Internet medicine can also be very helpful for family members of individuals having medical problems. Often, family members do not know how best to help their significant others in times of medical need. To meet this need, websites may post a wide variety of information that can help people understand the conditions, the requirements of treatment, the limits of treatment, and things they can do to be helpful to the ill family member. Additionally, websites sometimes offer lists of resources for family members.

Healthcare and social service providers also find the internet beneficial for their work. For some, it might be as simple as using the internet to schedule appointments, or to communicate test results, reminder information about treatment procedures, or appointment reminders via email with clients. For others, it might involve using special websites to conduct assessments of clients for the purpose of tracking their treatment success or progress. Professionals may also use telemedicine in order to learn about new treatments and procedures, or to learn about new drugs and other pharmaceutical products. In addition, healthcare and social service providers may benefit their general practice by using the internet to keep abreast of new clinical trials to test state-of-the-art treatments, changes in licensing laws affecting their practice, and the development of new healthcare databases for tracking, triage, and communication with insurance companies. Specialist referrals via telemedicine are also possible so that primary care doctors and the patient may visit with a specialist not available in their community. Nurse practitioners and patients in outlying clinics may also communicate with the physicians in medical centers using telemedicine. Providers are using the internet more and more for health services delivery.

Healthcare providers in training and their trainers also benefit greatly from telemedicine. To trainees living in remote areas or those who might be highly mobile, such as those in the armed forces, the internet provides immediate access to large online libraries, knowledgeable online teachers, and databases full of important medical information. Both long-established and new institutions interested in telemedicine increasingly are translating typical face-to-face training approaches into distance-based training programs utilizing the internet. Encyclopedias, descriptions of techniques, pictures of what different conditions might look like both inside and outside the body, and even video of actual procedures are available online. Similarly, instruction in the use of such material is available online through training programs that lead to certificates of training and actual accredited degrees, ranging from bachelor's to doctoral degrees and postdoctoral training. In addition to helping individuals who are at remote locations, such material also can be used to reach a larger number of trainees than might typically be able to observe or attend such training. The increased ability to teach, show procedures, or give supervision at a distance us-

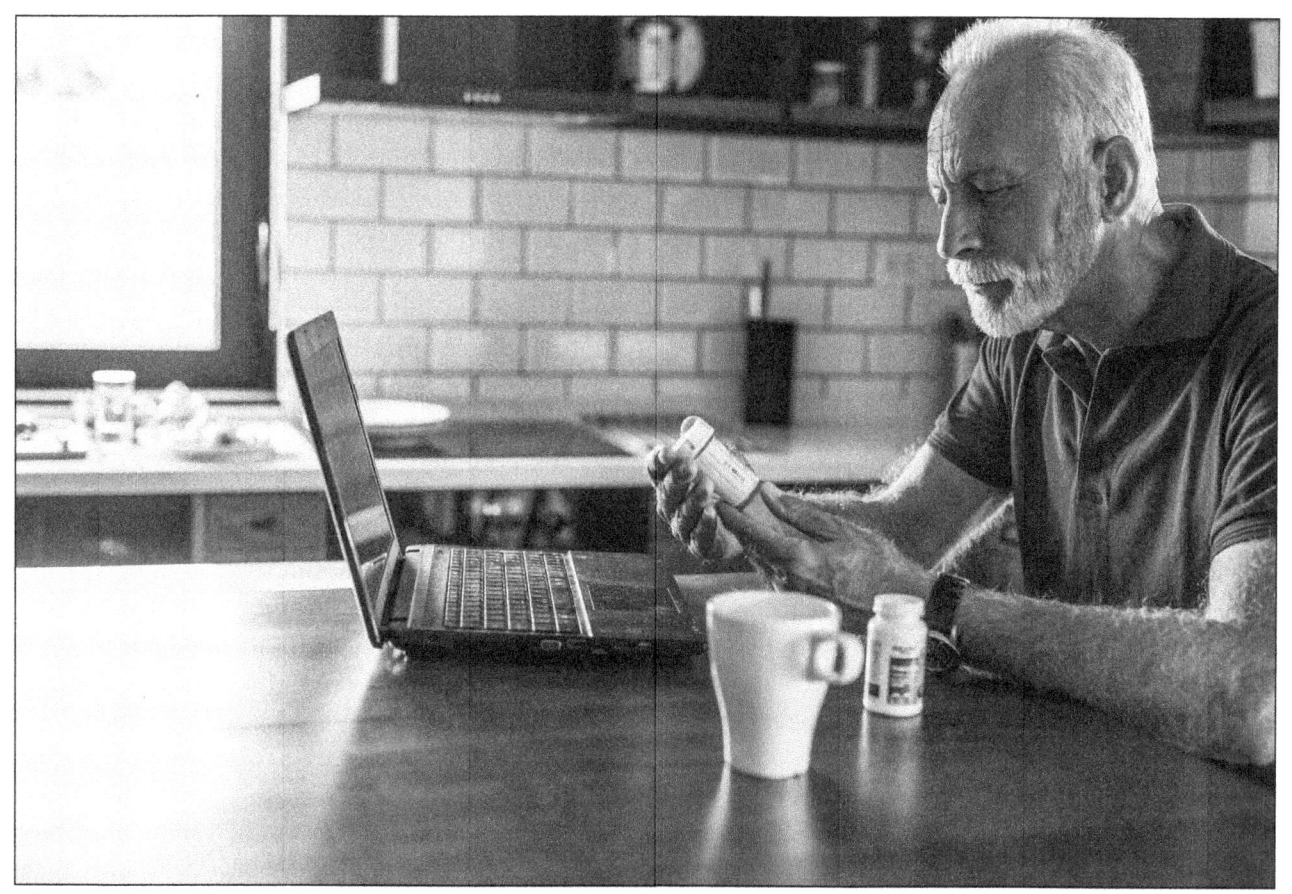

The internet has made it easier for the average person to seek medical information (blackCAT via iStock)

ing pictorial, written, oral, and video information greatly facilitates continuing education and improvement of general healthcare practice. It also helps to facilitate the evaluation of those practices and training sessions. Since all of the work takes place over the internet, different aspects of the work can be monitored and evaluated electronically.

Much of the evaluation of this kind of information is done by researchers who are studying client, trainer, provider, or even healthcare system behavior and organization. This is done by evaluating information, also known as data, in individual sessions or visits to websites, as well as by examining data that are collected over time, across multiple visits. For instance, a person might first go to a website for information on a specific medical condition and then, at a later time or times, come back and look up different treatment approaches, or visit online discussion groups. What they do from time to time would be evaluated by researchers to see how individuals use the site, how long they stay on it, or what things they try searching for that may not yet be on the site. The process of watching behavior over time is called tracking. Tracking allows researchers to profile the users of websites to learn more about their behavior, usually for the purpose of predicting their behavior and response to treatment. The information gathered by creating tracking databases of what happens with website users can be used to improve services and to decrease long-term healthcare service, training, and administration costs on a continuing basis.

Because of all the data being collected on how individuals are using different websites or other internet-based services, there has been some concern over the individual's right to privacy and the protection of the information collected. For instance, some people have been concerned that if they are searching for information related to the human immunodeficiency virus (HIV) or substance use, they might be identified as being at risk for having that condition whether they do or not. Furthermore, many individuals do not want that information linked to their identities or medical records. They may be wishing to avoid solicitation of business from sellers of medical services or products because of their association with the condition; they do not want their personal information sold for that purpose to the providers of such products or services. On the other hand, they may also wish to maintain privacy and keep their information confidential so as to avoid having any threat to their future insurability or their ability to get healthcare coverage. As an example, if a healthcare provider such as a health maintenance organization (HMO) tracked users' informa- tion on a website and discovered, through the database, that someone who was now applying for coverage had certain medical conditions, that person might have a greater risk of being refused coverage if his or her time on the website was not completely anonymous. Given these concerns, users of internet medicine need to understand that there are differences between the terms privacy, confidentiality, and anonymity, as well as in the legal issues and protections one can exercise when using this type of medicine. Each website may be operating under different constraints, and so it is always important for users of these services to be sure they understand how the websites handle privacy. Finding out how a website protects or does not protect the privacy of its users is the only way users can determine how safe it is to reveal confidential information when they use a specific website.

DIAGNOSTIC AND TREATMENT TECHNIQUES
One of the biggest opportunities offered by internet medicine is that of increasing the ability of individuals to do self-screening for medical conditions to see if they need medical assistance. Likewise, the ability of service providers to do screening and assessment for a larger number of people is increased relative to what can be done in person. This is because the assessments can be administered via the computer, saving valuable provider time. Additionally, assessments can be completed online and sent to providers in advance

for immediate evaluation. While it may be some time before conclusive diagnoses can be offered via online technology, such advances are not far off; the differences between online and in-person assessments are being studied.

Intervention via the internet is also much improved because large quantities of information can be dispensed electronically, printed out by clients or their families, or distributed to large numbers of individuals. Such informational interventions can be important for facilitating proper compliance with medical prescription regimens, helping clients to avoid bad drug interactions, or providing reminders about other things needed to facilitate wellness. Informational interventions can also be used for primary prevention, or preventing problems from happening in the first place. By providing suggestions for problem prevention, much suffering could be spared and many healthcare dollars can be saved. This is especially true for teenagers and college-age populations, who are often savvy web users.

Treatment also takes place on the internet via simultaneous online interactions such as in chat rooms, communicating via videoconferencing as in a normal conversation but using video cameras, and simple asynchronous email between the client and the provider. Generally this type of treatment is a complement to face-to-face treatment. For instance, some HMOs use online support groups as additional treatment for persons already receiving therapy. Others are using programs such as self-guided online courses that clients can work through to benefit their health. In general, practitioners are permitted to do this so long as they are properly licensed. This usually requires being licensed by the state in which they are practicing and/or where the client is receiving the services.

PERSPECTIVE AND PROSPECTS

The internet continues to grow on a daily basis, with an increasing number of computer owners and websites taking advantage of its capabilities. Communications technologies are also improving constantly, allowing for almost instant individual communication of written, oral, and visual information at distances and speeds that were inconceivable in the past. As a result of these developments, as well as increases in healthcare costs and the potential economic and health benefits provided by internet medicine, this specialty area is here to stay. Commitments by governments to examine such developments in health-care underscore this likelihood. In 1998, for example, the Health Resources and Service Administration of the United States Department of Health and Human Services established the Office for the Advancement of Telehealth. This office is devoted to advancing the use of telehealth and internet-based medicine to facilitate improvement in the state of public health and research on public health. The ability of such approaches to provide more services with streamlined administrative procedures and decreased costs holds much promise for improving the state of public health.

—*Nancy A. Piotrowski*

Further Reading

American Telemedicine Association. *American Telemedicine Association*, 2012.

Cullen, Rowena. *Health Information on the Internet: A Study of Providers, Quality, and Users*. Praeger, 2006.

Davis, James B., editor. *Health and Medicine on the Internet: A Comprehensive Guide to Medical Information on the World Wide Web*. 4th ed., Practice Management Information, 2003.

Hadeed, George, et al. *Telemedicine for Trauma, Emergencies, and Disaster Management*. Artech House, 2011.

Harding, Anne. "Telemedicine Improves Care for Kids Seen in Rural ERs." *MedlinePlus*, 19 Aug. 2013.

Mayo Clinic. "Telehealth: When Health Care Meets Cyberspace." *Mayo Clinic*, 13 May 2011.

MedlinePlus. "Evaluating Internet Health Information: A Tutorial from the National Library of Medicine." *MedlinePlus*, 19 Apr. 2012.

Office for the Advancement of Telehealth, www.hrsa.gov/telehealth.

Riva, Giuseppe, and B. K. Wiederhold. *Annual Review of Cybertherapy and Telemedicine 2012: Advanced Technologies in the Behavioral, Social and Neurosciences*. IOS Press, 2012.

Society of Critical Care Medicine. "What Is Telemedicine?" *My ICU Care*, 2001–2013.

"What Is Telehealth? How Is Telehealth Different from Telemedicine?" *HealthIT.gov*, www.healthit.gov/faq/what-telehealth-how-telehealth-different-telemedicine. Accessed 2 Sept. 2020.

Wootton, Richard, et al. *Telehealth in the Developing World*. Royal Society of Medicine Press, 2011.

INTERNET AND HEALTH INFORMATION

ABSTRACT

Online resources for health information are being used more and more by patients and their families. It's often difficult to determine sound advice from inaccurate information.

OVERVIEW

The internet is a global network that provides an extremely popular source of information on countless topics, including health and disease management. The World Wide Web, also referred to as the web, is a collection of sites the user can access. The internet provides current, comprehensive, and searchable information on any almost any topic providing an advantage over traditional forms of media, such as print. It is estimated that 80 percent of internet users have searched for a health-related topic on line and Google reports more than one billion health questions daily. However, because virtually anyone can publish information on the internet through personal websites and blogs, web-based information can be inaccurate, and relying on it can even be dangerous. Seeking health-related information is one of the strongest uses of internet search and nurses are uniquely positioned to assist both the consumer and patient with finding trusted sources.

The most reliable information can be obtained from sources such as the National Health Institutes and their Divisions, including the National Cancer Institute; the World Health Organization (WHO); university medical centers and comprehensive health systems; from PubMed, the public research database that includes millions of citations for biomedical literature, run by the National Center for Biotechnology Information of the National Institutes of Health (NIH); from the Centers for Disease Control and Prevention (CDC); and multiple other sites and professional organizations.

Often websites may appear as reliable and trustworthy but that may not have any relation to quality of data. While not to discourage internet research, searchers are encouraged to seek out multiple sites to cross-check information for consistency and reliability. Websites can use search engine optimization to move their site up to the front of searches, even absent quality information. Discussing information found on the internet with the healthcare provider is always recommended.

POPULAR SEARCHES

As consumers go online for health information, more than half say they go to the internet first for a specific health-related question before going to their physician. Middle-aged women with higher education and income levels are higher users of internet search than man and are often the one the family trusts to search out information. Searches for specific treatments, information about symptoms, procedures and drugs lead health-related searches. Other topics related to health information include searching for healthcare providers, complementary and alternative medicine (CAM) interventions, exercise and diet, and purchasing health-related products. The information available on the internet would have little impact if interest were lacking; in fact, interest is surging.

PURCHASING PRODUCTS ON THE WEB

A variety of products are available on the internet. There is no barrier to advertising a product on the internet whether it is safe or not. Herbal products, for example, are widely available for sale through commercial websites. Ordering prescription drugs is possible, but there is no guarantee that the quality of the product meets US Food and Drug Administration (FDA) or US Pharmacopeia (USP) standards.

Because herbal products are natural products, they do not fall under the jurisdiction of government agencies such as the FDA. The FDA requires a rigorous testing process before a drug can be made available to the general public. No such oversight occurs with herbal products. For example, the herbal product digitalis, which is used for the treatment of heart conditions, is derived from the foxglove shrub (*Digitalis lanata*). Quinine, which has a number of medicinal uses (as, for example, an antimalarial and an analgesic) is derived from the bark of the cinchona tree (*Cinchona* species). Ordering these herbal supplements can interfere with medically prescribed drugs and can lead to serious complications, including death.

Medical experts fear that some persons with serious medical conditions, such as malignant cancers, will purchase worthless products through the web and fail to seek conventional medical care for life-threatening illnesses. Before purchasing products on the internet, verify that they are from a trusted source if at all possible. Many "cures" are advertised which have no therapeutic benefit.

INTERNET RESOURCES

Much of the internet is devoted to the marketing of products or services. In addition to purchasing products, the searcher can locate medical practitioners, other practitioners such as acupuncturists and massage therapists, and instructors for yoga and meditation. The simplest method for information gathering is via a search engine. Typing a subject, for example breast cancer, into a search engine will return over 500 million results in less than a second. With this search, it would be important to look for content from the American Cancer Society or National Cancer Institute or well-known health systems. For example, searching on the phrase "prostate and saw palmetto" reveals information on the use of saw palmetto for benign prostatic hypertrophy. Search results will include links to scientific papers, but also to anecdotal accounts and commercial sites.

The sites of the following resources, however, provide focused research articles and other trustworthy information:

PubMed contains a searchable database of published scientific papers on many medical topics.

The website of the Centers for Disease Control and Prevention (CDC), a US government organization focused on maintaining and improving health, features a comprehensive list of diseases and conditions (communicable, genetic, environmental, and self-inflicted), healthy living, and traveler's health.

The WHO, the health authority within the United Nations system, "is responsible for providing leadership on global health matters, shaping the health research agenda, setting norms and standards, articulating evidence-based policy options, providing technical support to countries and monitoring and assessing health trends." The organization's website contains informative links on a variety of health topics and publications.

While most medical centers in the United States contain public information on conventional medicine, many also provide other resources through searchable databases. Medical centers with searchable databases include the Mayo Clinic (www.mayoclinic.com) and the UCLA Medical Center (www.uclahealth.org). The health system in the local area is also a good place to search for both information and available practitioners.

—*Patricia Stanfill Edens and Robin L. Wulffson*

Further Reading

Centers for Disease Control and Prevention (CDC), cdc.gov.

Edens, P. S. "How to Develop a Cancer Information Internet Strategy." *Journal of Communication in Healthcare*, www.tandfonline.com/doi/abs/10.1179/cih.2008.1.3.266. Accessed 25 Aug. 2020.

Freeman, Lyn. *Mosby's Complementary and Alternative Medicine: A Research-Based Approach*. 3rd ed., Mosby/Elsevier, 2009. Providing a comprehensive overview, this text includes practical, clinically relevant coverage of complementary and alternative medicine, with commentary by well-known experts, descriptions of medical advances, case studies, and discussion of the history and philosophy of each discipline.

"Health on the Net Foundation." United Nations, www.hon.ch.

Hock, Randolph. *The Extreme Searcher's Internet Handbook: A Guide for the Serious Searcher*. 3rd ed., CyberAge Books, 2010. A guide to internet research for librarians, teachers, students, writers, business professionals, and health consumers.

National Center for Complementary and Alternative Medicine (NCCAM), www.nccam.nih.gov.

National Institutes of Health, www.nih.gov.

PubMed. National Center for Biotechnology Information, www.ncbi.nlm.nih.gov/pubmed.

Tonsaker, T., G. Bartlett, and C. Trpkov. "Health Information on the Internet: Gold Mine or Minefield?" *Canadian family physician Medecin de famille canadien*, vol. 60, no. 5, pp. 407–8, www.ncbi.nlm.nih.gov/pmc/articles/PMC4020634/. Accessed 25 Aug. 2020.

US Food and Drug Administration, www.fda.gov.

US Pharmacopeia (USP), www.usp.org.

World Health Organization, www.who.int.

Zshorlich, B., D. Gechter, I. M. JanBen, et.al. "Health Information on the Internet: Who Is Searching for What, When and How?" *Z Evid Fortbild Qual Gesundhwes*, vol. 10, no. 2, 2015, pp. 144–52, pubmed.ncbi.nlm.nih.gov.

Office of Cancer Complementary and Alternative Medicine (OCCAM)

ABSTRACT

The Office of Cancer Complementary and Alternative Medicine (OCCAM) is the consumer hub for U.S. government information on complementary and alternative medicine for persons with cancer and those who treat them.

MISSION AND OBJECTIVES

The OCCAM works to improve the quality of cancer care through the support and advancement of research in evidence-based complementary and alternative medical (CAM) practices. OCCAM also provides quality information about CAM for healthcare professionals, researchers, and the public. The focus of the office is to coordinate CAM activities in diagnosing, preventing, and treating cancer through managing cancer-related symptoms and cancer treatment side effects. OCCAM's focus on cancer distinguishes it from the related National Center for Complementary and Alternative Medicine, part of the National Institutes of Health (NIH).

HISTORY

Before establishing a separate division for CAM, the National Cancer Institute (NCI) of the NIH was interested in using CAM to treat cancer. In the 1940s, the NCI looked at studies to treat cancer with various CAM therapies. One treatment alternative reviewed by the NCI was the chemical compound laetrile, a purified amygdalin found in the pits of fruits and nuts, lima beans, sorghum, and clover. The Gerson regimen, named for German physician Max Gerson, also was considered. This regimen used a diet of raw and fresh organic fruits, vegetables, and juices, and coffee enemas, supplements, and detoxification, to help the body heal itself of cancer. The NCI also examined the Hoxley treatment, which employed herbs and salves to treat cancer; the NCI found no evidence that this treatment was effective.

NCI's interest in CAM for cancer treatment continued during the next several decades, leading to the development of the Best Case Series in 1991. This program provided a way for CAM practitioners to use scientific approaches with rigorous research to evaluate these therapies in the treatment of cancer.

In 1998, OCCAM was founded under the leadership of Jeffrey D. White, a board-certified cancer oncologist and researcher who joined the NCI in 1990. The Best Case Series was moved from the Cancer Therapy Evaluation program at NCI to the then-new OCCAM. The following year, the CAM Cancer Research Interest Group and Invited Speaker Series was established at OCCAM.

In 2006, OCCAM published the first NCI annual report on CAM. The following year, the office moved to the Division of Cancer Treatment and Diagnosis at the NCI. In 2008, OCCAM published "Survey of Cancer Researchers Regarding Complementary and Alternative Medicine" in the *Journal of the Society of Integrative Oncology*. That same year, the NCI provided more than $121 million for CAM research in more than four hundred projects.

BEST CASE SERIES PROGRAM

One notable program coordinated through OCCAM is the NCI Best Case Series (BCS) program. Established in 1991, BCS evaluates CAM research data through independent reviews of records and review of the test results of persons with cancer who were treated with CAM therapies. With valid data supporting CAM cancer therapies, the NIH can then determine funding for further research in CAM effectiveness.

CAM practitioners are encouraged to submit their research on persons treated for tumor regression to the BCS program. To be accepted for review, the practitioner must meet specific criteria, including having a patient with a definitive diagnosis of cancer, having detailed records of cancer response, and having a chronicled treatment history.

—*Marylane Wade Koch*

Further Reading

Cassileth, B. "Gerson Regimen." *Oncology*, vol. 24, no. 2, 2010, p. 201.

Office of Cancer Complementary and Alternative Medicine, www.cam.cancer.gov. This site provides health professionals, persons with cancer, and the general public information about complementary and alternative medicine in treating cancer.

Rees, Alan M., editor. *The Complementary and Alternative Medicine Information Source Book*. Oryx Press, 2001. Defines CAM terms and the background of CAM and includes a listing of resources.

Rosenbaum, Earnest H., and Isadora Rosenbaum. *Everyone's Guide to Cancer Supportive Care: A Comprehensive Handbook for Patients and Their Families*. 4th ed., Andrews McMeel, 2005. Comprehensive guide with more than fifty chapters. Includes Web resources on CAM.

Smith, W. B., et al. "Survey of Cancer Researchers Regarding Complementary and Alternative Medicine." *Journal of the Society of Integrative Oncology*, vol. 6, no. 1, 2008, pp. 2–12. Survey results published by the NCI to assess the interest and concern of 329 research respondents in CAM.

"Thinking About Complementary and Alternative Medicine: A Guide for People with Cancer." National Cancer Institute, www.cancer.gov/publications/patient-education/thinking-about-cam. A booklet that explains CAM and what choices are available to people with cancer.

Office of Dietary Supplements (ODS)

ABSTRACT

The Office of Dietary Supplements (ODS) is a US government office formed to enhance knowledge of dietary supplements to ensure medical understanding and consumer safety.

INTRODUCTION

The ODS was established in 1995, as mandated by the Dietary Supplement Health and Education Act of 1994. ODS was formed to better understand the science behind dietary supplements, to identify useful and harmful supplements, and to disseminate reliable information to the medical community and the public. As part of the National Institutes of Health (NIH), the office collaborates with other government organizations, including the National Center for Complementary and Alternative Medicine (NCCAM) and the US Food and Drug Administration (FDA), to raise public awareness of the benefits and risks of dietary supplements. ODS, NCCAM, and the FDA evaluate the methods of action of thousands of supplements and develop tools to understand their use within given populations.

DIETARY SUPPLEMENTS

As the name suggests, dietary supplements are any tablets, pills, capsules, or liquids that are taken orally to enhance a person's diet. There are approximately thirty thousand dietary supplements available in the United States. Between 50 and 75 percent of American adults, and possibly one-third of all children in the United States, use some type of supplement, including vitamins, minerals, and weight-reduction supplements, for health promotion and disease prevention.

FDA regulation of dietary supplements, which are often complex mixtures, is less strict than it is for prescription and nonprescription pharmaceuticals, leading to an enhanced role for ODS. Manufacturers of supplements do not need to follow standard guidelines, nor do they need to back up medical claims, such as claims that a product lowers the risk of a certain disease, with scientific research. As a result, the manufacture of dietary supplements is not standardized, and some products fail to meet their health claims. To increase the authority of the ODS and to ensure public safety, the FDA, in 2009, issued an evaluation of health claims of both conventional foods and dietary supplements.

HIGHLIGHTS AND ACCOMPLISHMENTS

Since its inception, ODS has helped to fund dietary supplement research grants and projects that examine usage rates and that evaluate, for example, the science behind supplements; has developed reference databases (which cite approximately 750,000 world references); has sponsored conferences and workshops; has led campaigns to educate the public on the potential risks of supplements; and has helped establish good manufacturing practices (GMPs) to ensure the quality of dietary supplements. These efforts are supported by six Dietary Supplement Research Centers located at different universities in the United States. Ongoing research programs include studies on glucosamine and chondroitin for knee osteoarthritis, on saw palmetto as a urinary aid for males, and on the potential cardiovascular benefits of omega-3 fatty acids.

Through ODS-sponsored research, many dietary supplements have proven essential to maintaining health: Calcium is now known as effective in reducing the risk of osteoporosis; certain vitamins and antioxidant supplements have been found to help reduce the effects of macular degeneration; and iron supplements during pregnancy are now known to be essential in preventing maternal anemia and reducing the rate of premature births. Other supplements have been found to be potentially harmful. Beta-carotene, which was promoted as reducing the risk of developing cancer, was later found to increase lung cancer rates in people who smoke cigarettes. Ephedra and ephedrine-containing supplements for weight reduction are now banned in the United States because of the side effects from taking the supplements, side effects that include high blood pressure and heart damage.

—Renée Euchner

Further Reading

Betz, J. M., et al. "The NIH Analytical Methods and Reference Materials Program for Dietary Supplements." *Analytical and Bioanalytical Chemistry*, vol. 389, 2007, pp. 19–25.

Costello R. B., and P. Coates. "In the Midst of Confusion Lies Opportunity: Fostering Quality Science in Dietary

Supplement Research." *Journal of the American College of Nutrition*, vol. 20, 2001, pp. 21–25.

Dietary Supplements. U.S. Food and Drug Administration, www.fda.gov/food/dietary-supplements. Accessed 25 Aug. 2020.

Dwyer, J. T., D. B. Allison, and P. M. Coates. "Dietary Supplements in Weight Reduction." *Journal of the American Dietary Association*, vol. 105, no. 5, suppl., 2005, pp. 80–86.

Dwyer, J. T., et al. "Measuring Vitamins and Minerals in Dietary Supplements for Nutrition Studies in the USA." *Analytical and Bioanalytical Chemistry*, vol. 389, 2007, pp. 37–46.

Haggans, C., et al. "Computer Access to Research on Dietary Supplements: A Database of Federally Funded Dietary Supplement Research." *Journal of Nutrition*, vol. 135, 2005, pp. 1796–99.

Office of Dietary Supplements. National Institutes of Health, www.ods.od.nih.gov.

Timbo, B. B., et al. "Dietary Supplements in a National Survey: Prevalence of Use and Reports of Adverse Events." *Journal of the American Dietary Association*, vol. 106, 2006, pp. 1966–74.

SELF-CARE

ABSTRACT

Self-care is a type of therapy that can be performed by persons themselves, often aided by training from a practitioner or by educational materials.

OVERVIEW

A person undertakes self-care decisions and actions to address a health problem or to improve his or her health. Popular self-care therapies include relaxation, meditation, imagery, hypnosis, biofeedback, education, special diets, natural products, and nutrition supplements. In 2016, the National Center for Complementary and Integrative Health (NCCIH) announced that Americans had spent an estimated $2.7 billion on purchases related to self-care in 2012.

MECHANISM OF ACTION

It is difficult to evaluate the action of self-care therapy because, in most situations, it is not feasible to use placebo controls. For example, in one of the better-documented modalities, the Arthritis Self-Management Program, retrospective analysis shows that pain reduction was maintained four years after therapy began and that physician visits decreased by 40 percent. The program used education, cognitive restructuring, relaxation, and physical activity, but it is impossible to show what treatment was responsible for what result; also, no control group was included for comparison.

USES AND APPLICATIONS

Several healthcare trends favor the use of self-care therapies. Some persons see conventional healthcare as effective but also unaffordable for many. Studies show that those who have delayed or skipped medical care for financial reasons are highly likely to try self-care, particularly self-medication.

At the other end of the spectrum are those who distrust mainstream healthcare and want instead a type of care that promotes empowerment and personal control. Another factor leading people to try self-care is having learned about and becoming comfortable with complementary and alternative medicine (CAM) therapies over time. In addition, CAM therapies that previously could be found only through nontraditional outlets are now widely available. Likely CAM users include the elderly, those who are well educated, and those with conditions such as severe depression and panic attacks. Studies also show that people between the ages of thirty-five and fifty years are part of a fast-growing group of CAM users. The coronavirus 2019 (COVID-19) pandemic that began with an outbreak of a novel coronavirus in China in late 2019 sparked further discussion about the potential for implementing self-care. Many people around the world, including in the United States, were isolated from conventional medical care due to efforts to limit phys-

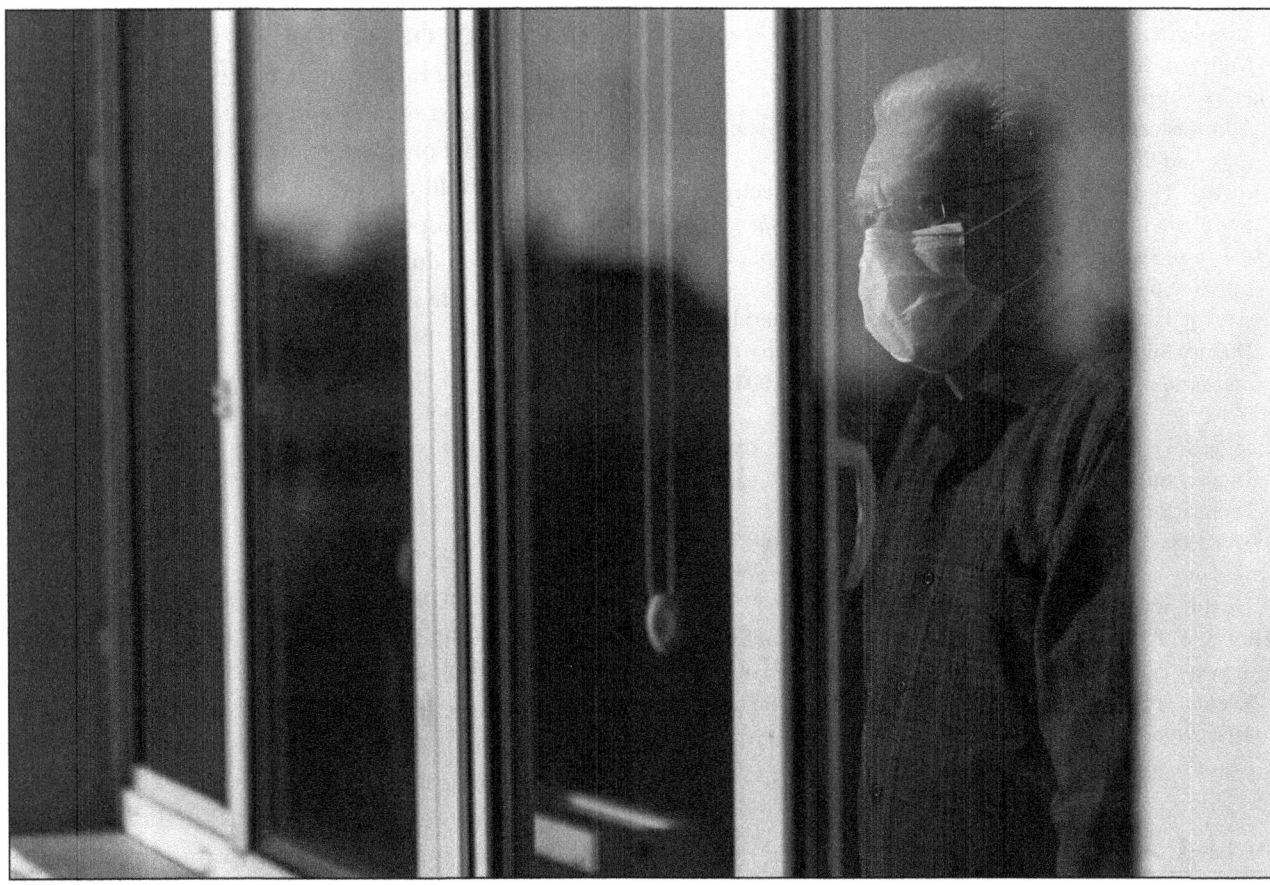

The COVID-19 pandemic sparked further discussion about implementing self-care, as many people were isolated from conventional medical care while the spread of the virus was still not under control. (Phynart Studio via iStock)

ical contact, and some expressed concern over going to medical facilities as the spread of the virus was still not under control. Therefore, some experts recommended practicing more habitual, reasonable self-care as a means of potentially maintaining physical and mental health.

Another study showed that twice as many people read self-help literature as see a CAM practitioner to learn relaxation techniques. This follows a general trend showing that the use of self-care therapies has increased at the same time that consultation with CAM providers has decreased. An analysis of persons on Medicare showed that the most frequently sought forms of CAM were those for back problems, chronic pain, general health improvement, and arthritis. Research has demonstrated the efficacy of relaxation, biofeedback therapy, cognitive strategies, and education in treating chronic pain conditions such as osteoarthritis, rheumatoid arthritis, and fibromyalgia. Persons using self-care engaged in health-affirming practices such as exercise, smoking reduction, and limiting alcohol consumption.

SCIENTIFIC EVIDENCE

Some studies used to measure self-care are flawed because the research questions depend on a person's ability to report CAM use accurately or to remember his or her use of CAM. Typically, information is collected once, so there is no opportunity to study CAM use over time.

Flawed methodology can occur if researchers do not spell out distinctions between complementary and alternative therapies versus more radical alternatives. Peer-reviewed studies of self-care have shown improvements in cancer-related pain, headache pain, and cardiovascular disease as a result of relaxation techniques, behavior modification, imagery, hypnosis, stress management, and health education. Clinical trials showed, for example, a 43 percent reduction in headache activity, improvement of chemotherapy-related symptoms such as nausea and vomiting, and a 41 percent reduction in cardiac deaths.

One study looked at changes in health status longitudinally and found no difference in health status when researchers compared therapies such as chiropractic, massage, acupuncture, and herbs with conventional medicine. However, the results of CAM therapies in general, and of self-care specifically, may take longer to manifest. Researchers have called for controlled clinical trials, including large-scale surveys, and in-depth studies of specific populations.

SAFETY ISSUES

A lack of relevant scientific studies makes it difficult to determine the safety and efficacy of self-care. Herbal remedies may interact with prescription medicines in harmful ways, with both the person seeking care and the prescribing physician unaware of the risks. Scientific literature on interactions is scarce. Existing information may be skewed, because many people do not tell their physicians that they are using a self-care modality of CAM. It is important to discuss self-care measures with the physicians involved in your care.

—Merrill Evans

Further Reading

"Americans Spent $30.2 Billion Out-of-Pocket on Complementary Health Approaches." US Department of Health and Human Services. *National Center for Complementary and Integrative Health*, 22 June 2016, www.nccih.nih.gov/news/press-releases/americans-spent-302-billion-outofpocket-on-complementary-health-approaches. Accessed 29 June 2020.

Astin, J. A., et al. "Complementary and Alternative Medicine Use Among Elderly Persons." *Journal of Gerontology: Medical Sciences*, vol. 55A, 2000, pp. M4–M9.

Astin, J. A., et al. "Mind-Body Medicine: State of the Science, Implications for Practice." *Journal of the American Board of Family Medicine*, vol. 16, 2003, pp. 131–47.

Jonas, Wayne. "When Less Means More: Less Medical Care Means More Self-Care." *Psychology Today*, 22 June 2020, www.psychologytoday.com/us/blog/how-healing-works/202006/when-less-means-more-less-medical-care-means-more-self-care. Accessed 29 June 2020.

Nahin, R. L., et al. "Costs of Complementary and Alternative Medicine (CAM) and Frequency of Visits to CAM Practitioners: United States, 2007." *National Health Statistics Reports*, vol. 18, 2009, pp. 1–15.

Pagán, J. A., and M. V. Pauly. "Access to Conventional Medical Care and the Use of Complementary and Alternative Medicine." *Health Affairs*, vol. 24, 2004, pp. 255–62.

Palinkas, L. A., and M. L. Kabongo. "The Use of Complementary and Alternative Medicine by Primary Care Patients." *Journal of Family Practice*, vol. 49, 2000, pp. 1121–30.

Sparber, A., and J. C. Wootton. "Use of Alternative and Complementary Therapies for Psychiatric and Neurologic Diseases." *Journal of Alternative and Complementary Medicine*, vol. 8, 2002, pp. 93–96.

SPIRITUALITY AND CAM

ABSTRACT

The use of spirituality, one's sense of meaning in life and relationship with the transcendent, is often used as part of healing in complementary and alternative medicine.

OVERVIEW

For many around the world, spirituality plays an integral part in complementary and alternative medicine, or CAM. Large-scale surveys conducted in the United States, Europe, and other parts of the world show that spirituality is associated with higher levels of CAM usage and with the use of a wider variety of CAM modalities to treat many illnesses, including depression, headaches, back and neck pain, gastrointestinal problems, allergies, diabetes, and cancer.

PRAYER AND OTHER MODALITIES

Spirituality is considered by some researchers and practitioners to constitute CAM practices per se. Some CAM modalities, such as prayer, are explicitly spiritual in nature, while other modalities, particularly mind/body therapies, often have a spiritual component. The most prominent example of spirituality as CAM is that of prayer, an active process of appealing to a higher spiritual power. Prayer as CAM includes solitary and group prayer on behalf of oneself or others. Based on data from the 2002 National Health Information Survey, the National Center for Complementary and Alternative Medicine (NCCAM) (later renamed as the National Center for Complementary and Integrative Health (NCCIH)) reported in 2004 that prayer for oneself was the most widely used CAM modality among Americans. (It was endorsed by more than 60 percent of survey respondents.) Prayer for others was the second most commonly used modality, and prayer in groups was the fifth most commonly used modality. Older adults, women, and ethnic and racial minorities were more likely to use prayer as CAM.

The NCCIH, however, no longer considers prayer a form of CAM, a change that has led to much contro-

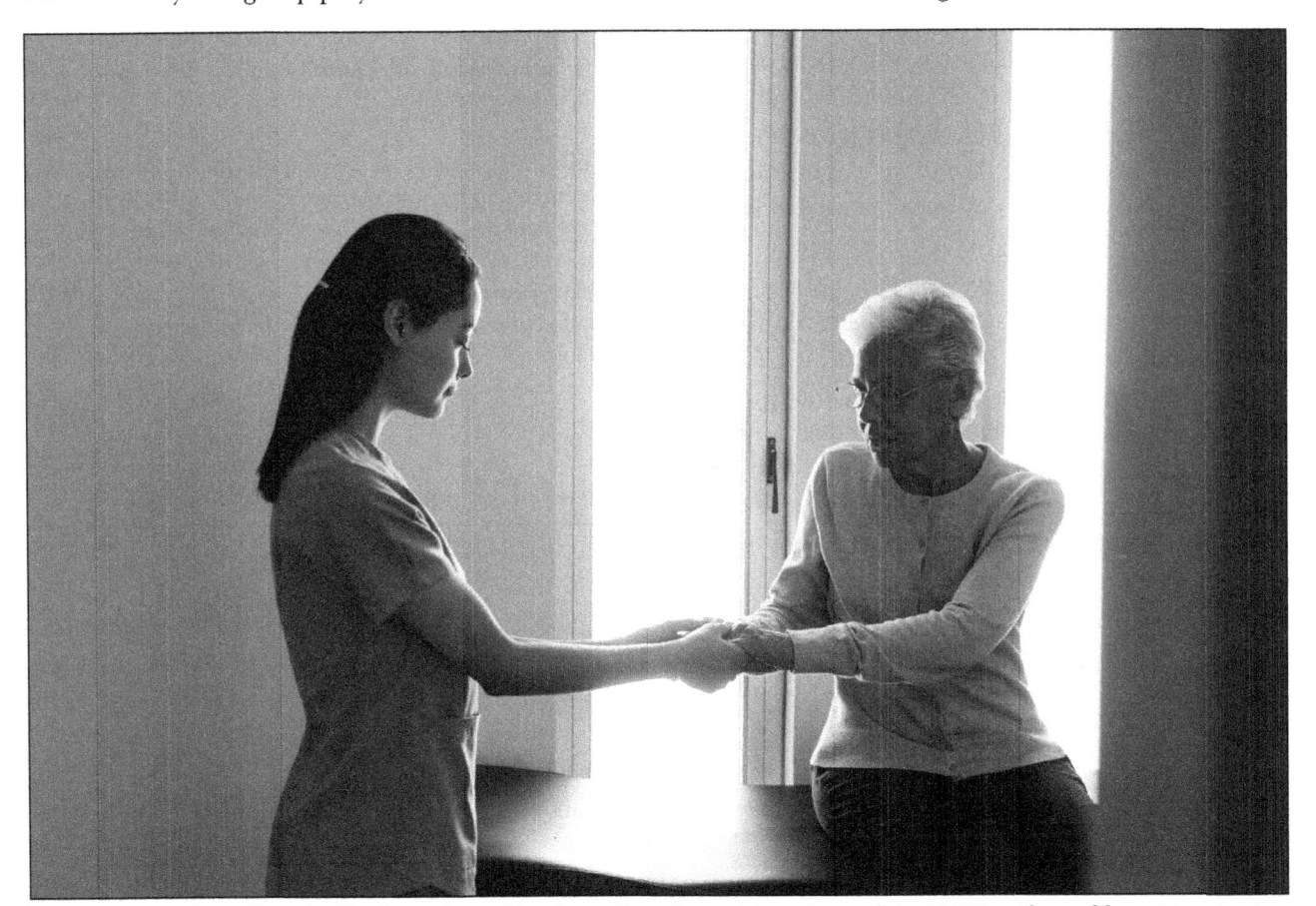

For many around the world, spirituality plays an integral part in complementary and alternative medicine (CAM), with one of the most prominent examples being prayer. (Aldo Murillo via iStock)

versy. For example, considering prayer a form of CAM leads to increased estimates of CAM usage. Excluding prayer from the definition of CAM, however, does not reflect the true numbers of CAM users.

Another spiritually based CAM is faith healing. This includes therapeutic approaches based on religious faith. Faith healing is most commonly associated with some Christian denominations and is typically conducted in religious communal settings. The therapeutic powers of faith healers are attributed to their evocation of divine or supernatural influences, which may bring about miracles. Relatedly, other cultural and religious traditions feature spiritual healers, such as shamans and curanderos, whose healing powers are largely spiritual in nature. Many traditional cultures do not draw clear distinctions among physical, mental, and spiritual health. In addition to explicitly spiritual modalities, other CAM modalities, such as meditation, yoga, Tai Chi, qigong, and Reiki, often have a spiritual component.

EFFECTIVENESS

Evidence regarding the effectiveness of spirituality-based forms of CAM is preliminary, given the many limitations of research and the complexity of the issues. For example, the most common spiritual CAM modality, prayer, is complex and can take many forms, including conversation, intercession, contemplation, and ritual; these different types of prayer may have different effects on health and well-being. Research suggests that some types of prayer can be beneficial to the person praying and can include the alleviation of emotional distress and pain. Such effects have been attributed to increased relaxation, less distraction, an increase in positive emotions, and divine intervention. Research indicates that most people who use prayer as CAM find prayer to be helpful. In a recent study, Blacks were among the highest users of CAM as compared to Whites when prayer was included as a CAM modality but more research is needed.

More controversial is distance or intercessory prayer, which involves the influence of praying for the health of another person independent of that person's knowledge of the prayer. Intercessory prayer has received much research attention, including attention from researchers using large, randomized control trials. In the aggregate, results are inconsistent and the interpretation of findings remains hotly debated.

Evidence of the effectiveness of faith healing, for example, is sparse. A small but growing body of literature suggests, however, that CAM modalities such as meditation and yoga are more effective in alleviating pain and improving functioning when they include an explicit spiritual component.

Although persons rarely discuss with healthcare providers their reliance on spirituality as part of their approach to personal health, evidence suggests that such communication may facilitate understanding and promote better care. Approaches to integrative medicine now emphasize the need to pay attention to the spiritual issues and concerns of one's patients.

—*Crystal L. Park*

Further Reading

Barnes, P. M., B. Bloom, and R. L. Nahin. "Complementary and Alternative Medicine Use Among Adults and Children: 2007 United States." *National Health Statistics Reports*, vol. 12, pp. 1–23.

Barnes, P. M., et al. "Complementary and Alternative Medicine Use Among Adults: United States, 2002." *CDC Advance Data Report*, vol. 343, 2004.

"Complementary, Alternative or Integrative Health: What's in a Name?" National Center for Complementary and Integrative Health. *National Institutes of Health*, www.nccih.nih.gov/health/complementary-alternative-or-integrative-health-whats-in-a-name. Accessed 25 Aug. 2020.

McCaffrey, A. M., et al. "Prayer for Health Concerns: Results of a National Survey on Prevalence and Patterns of Use." *Archives of Internal Medicine*, vol. 164, no. 8, 2004, pp. 858–62.

Roberts, L., et al. "Intercessory Prayer for the Alleviation of Ill Health." *Cochrane Database of Systematic Reviews*, 2009. CD000368. EBSCO DynaMed Systematic Literature Surveillance, www.ebscohost.com/dynamed. Reviews findings regarding intercessory prayer and describes the limitations of research on this topic.

Robles, B., D. M. Upchurch, and T. Kuo. "Comparing Complementary and Alternative Medicine Use with or without Including Prayer as a Modality in a Local and Diverse United States Jurisdiction." Front. *Public Health*, 21 Mar. 2017, core.ac.uk/download/pdf/82863954.pdf.

Tippens, K., K. Marsman, and H. Zwickey. "Is Prayer CAM?" *Journal of Alternative and Complementary Medicine*, vol. 15, 2009, pp. 435–38.

RELAXATION RESPONSE

ABSTRACT
The relaxation response is a self-induced, peaceful, relaxed mental state attained through various techniques.

OVERVIEW
Herbert Benson, a graduate of Harvard Medical School and director emeritus at Benson-Henry Institute for Mind Body Medicine at Massachusetts General Hospital, published the book *The Relaxation Response* in 1975. It is considered the leading text on the relaxation response. The book includes data produced from research Benson conducted at Harvard's Thorndike Memorial Laboratory and at Beth Israel Hospital in Boston. Walter B. Cannon, another researcher who was at Harvard Medical School in the 1920s, had identified what he called the fight-or-flight physical response to stress on body and mind. Cannon found that perceived and actual life-threatening situations produced a flood of stress hormones to prepare a person to fight (confront the situation) or to flee. In such situations the heart pounds, breathing accelerates, and blood flow to the muscles is increased. This response is basically a survival mechanism, a natural physical response elicited when a person's life is endangered.

Frequent situations in daily life, such as traffic jams, waiting in lines, financial difficulties, and family problems, also produce stress-related hormones that over time can take a toll on the body. The relaxation response was developed as a mechanism to counteract this hormonal response to stress. Benson's therapy was not new, and it was based on the age-old practices and philosophies of Transcendental Meditation (TM). For relaxation response, these practices are simplified and can be performed by anyone. To elicit the response, Benson offers the following instructions: Find a quiet, peaceful environment for practice; muscles should be consciously relaxed; a word such as "one" or "peace," or a phrase, possibly a prayer, should be repeated silently in the mind; any intrusive thoughts should be observed only and then passively dismissed; and breathing should be slow and deep.

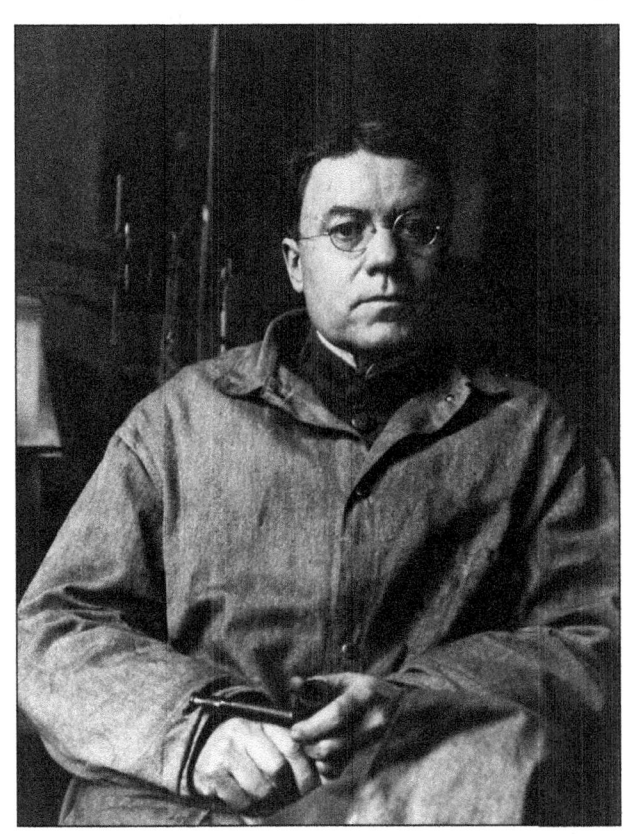

Physiologist Walter B. Cannon, who in 1915 coined the term "fight-or-flight response." (Wikimedia Commons)

Benson advises practicing this technique from ten to twenty minutes each day. The process is quite individualized, however, and no single method works for everyone. Other techniques may be equally effective, such as running, yoga, knitting, dance, or playing a musical instrument.

By studying the effects of stress on the human body and the various techniques to counteract them, Benson demonstrated the connection of mind and body and how this connection affects health and well-being. His continuing research includes the possible clinical uses of the response in medicine and psychiatry.

MECHANISM OF ACTION

The release of fight-or-flight hormones when a person is no longer threatened is counteracted through natural activation of the parasympathetic nervous system. Findings from research conducted at Harvard Medical School in the late 1960s showed that Transcendental Meditation could produce profound physiologic changes that were opposite to those produced by stress. Metabolism, blood pressure, heart rate, and rate of breathing could all be decreased. TM and the relaxation response work in essentially the same way and, when practiced, allow the practitioner to counteract stress voluntarily.

USES AND APPLICATIONS

The relaxation response may be practiced at will to counteract stress inherent in daily life, to reduce general stress levels and discomfort, to reduce levels of pain or distress in illness, and to alleviate physical symptoms of stress on the body. Continuing research has broadened possible applications to uses such as: reducing stress and improving cognition in healthy aging adults; improving productivity in workers; reducing pain in people with chronic diseases, such as human immunodeficiency virus or acquired immune deficiency syndrome (HIV/AIDS) and arthritis; and improving academic performance.

SCIENTIFIC EVIDENCE

A body of scientific evidence exists from continuing research by Benson, his associates, and others. Much of this research has been conducted at Harvard Medical School, Harvard's Thorndike Memorial Laboratory, and the Benson-Henry Institute for Mind Body Medicine.

The practice of meditation has been shown by magnetic resonance imaging to activate neural structures involved in attention and control of the autonomic nervous system. Measurably lower oxygen consumption, heart rate, respiration, and blood lactate indicate a decrease in activity of the sympathetic nervous system, resulting in a restful, or hypometabolic, state. This is the opposite of the increased activity, or hypermetabolic state, produced by stress.

Double-blind studies have been conducted with varying results. One study tried to determine if combining acupuncture treatments with the relaxation response could improve quality of life for persons with HIV infection or AIDS. Conclusions from the pilot trial confirmed the benefits of combined therapies for some measures of improved quality of life. Although skeptics remain, research is continuing on possible uses of the relaxation response in medicine and psychiatry using improved research tools and methods.

CHOOSING A PRACTITIONER

The relaxation response can be self-taught and does not require a practitioner. Classes, meditation groups, and many instruction books are available for the person who wishes to learn the technique.

SAFETY ISSUES

There are no identified safety issues with the practice of the relaxation response. Benson has warned, however, that if it is used as a medical treatment, it should be practiced only with the knowledge and approval of, and under the supervision of, a qualified physician.

—*Martha O. Loustaunau*

Further Reading

Benson, H. "The Relaxation Response: Its Subjective and Objective Historical Precedents and Physiology." *Trends in Neurosciences*, vol. 6, 1983, pp. 281–84. Discusses research at Harvard's Thorndike Memorial Laboratory in defining the physiology and in describing the subjective and objective historical precedents and clinical usefulness of the relaxation response. It is a classic text in the field.

———, and M. Klipper. *The Relaxation Response*. William Morrow, 1975. Benson's explanation and synthesis of research on the relaxation response, based on historical, religious, and literary writings, with related scientific data from research conducted by Benson and associates. This work was expanded and updated in 2000, citing additional information on updated research.

Lazar, S., et al. "Functional Brain Mapping of the Relaxation Response and Meditation." *NeuroReport*, vol. 11, 2000, pp. 1581–85. Discusses how magnetic resonance imaging shows that the practice of meditation activates neural structures affecting attention and control of the autonomic nervous system.

MacDonald, A. "Using the Relaxation Response to Reduce Stress." Harvard Medical School. *Harvard Health Publishing*, www.health.harvard.edu/blog/using-the-relaxation-response-to-reduce-stress-20101110780. Accessed 25 Aug. 2020.

RELAXATION THERAPIES

ABSTRACT

A group of stress-reduction techniques to reduce everyday stress are often called relaxation therapies. In addition to these methods, other methods that can help include yoga, Tai Chi, hypnosis, massage, and biofeedback.

OVERVIEW

Constant stress is one of the defining features of modern life and the source of many common health problems. Stress plays an obvious role in nervousness, anxiety, and insomnia, but it is also thought to contribute to a vast number of other illnesses.

In the past, most people engaged in many hours of physical exercise daily, an activity that reduces the effects of psychological stress. Life was also slower then and was more in harmony with the natural cycles of day and season. Today, however, a person is relatively sedentary, while the mind is forced to respond to the rapid pace of a society that never stops. The result is high levels of stress and a reduced ability to cope with that stress.

There are several ways to mitigate the damage caused by stress. Increased physical exercise can help, as can simple, commonsense steps such as taking relaxation breaks and vacations. If these approaches do not have adequate results, more formal methods may be helpful.

WHAT ARE RELAXATION THERAPIES?

There are many types of relaxation therapies, and they use a variety of techniques. However, most of them share certain related features.

In many relaxation techniques, one begins by either lying down or assuming a relaxed, seated posture in a quiet place and then closing the eyes. The next step differs depending on the method. In autogenic training, relaxation response, and certain forms of meditation, a person focuses his or her mind on internal sensations, such as the breath. Guided-imagery techniques employ deliberate visualization of scenes or actions, such as walking on a quiet beach. Progressive relaxation techniques involve gradual relaxation of the muscles. Finally, some schools of meditation incorporate the repetition of a phrase or sound silently or aloud.

All of these techniques are best learned with the aid of a trained practitioner. The usual format is a group class supplemented by regular home practice. If a person is diligent enough, experience suggests that he or she can develop the ability to call on a relaxed state at will, even in the middle of a very stressful situation.

USES AND APPLICATIONS

Relaxation therapies are most commonly tried in medical circumstances in which stress is believed to play a particularly large role. These circumstances include insomnia, surgery, chronic pain, and cancer chemotherapy. A specific form of guided visualization has also been used in an attempt to actually treat cancer.

SCIENTIFIC EVIDENCE

Although many studies have been performed on relaxation therapies, most of these studies are inadequately designed. To be fair, there are considerable difficulties in the path of any researcher who wishes to scientifically assess the effectiveness of a relaxation therapy such as hypnosis. There are several factors involved, but the most important is fairly fundamental: It is difficult to design a proper double-blind, placebo-controlled study of relaxation therapy. Researchers studying the herb St. John's wort, for example, can use placebo pills that are indistinguishable from the real thing. However, it is difficult to design a form of placebo relaxation therapy that cannot be detected as such by both practitioners and participants.

One clever method used by some researchers involves the use of intentionally neutral visualizations. Instead of imagining lying in bed and sleeping peacefully, participants in the placebo group might be told to visualize something like a green box. The problem here is that researchers teaching the visualization method to participants may inadvertently convey a sense of disbelief in the placebo treatment. This can be solved by using relatively untrained people who are themselves deceived by experimenters to teach the method, but the practical obstacles are significant.

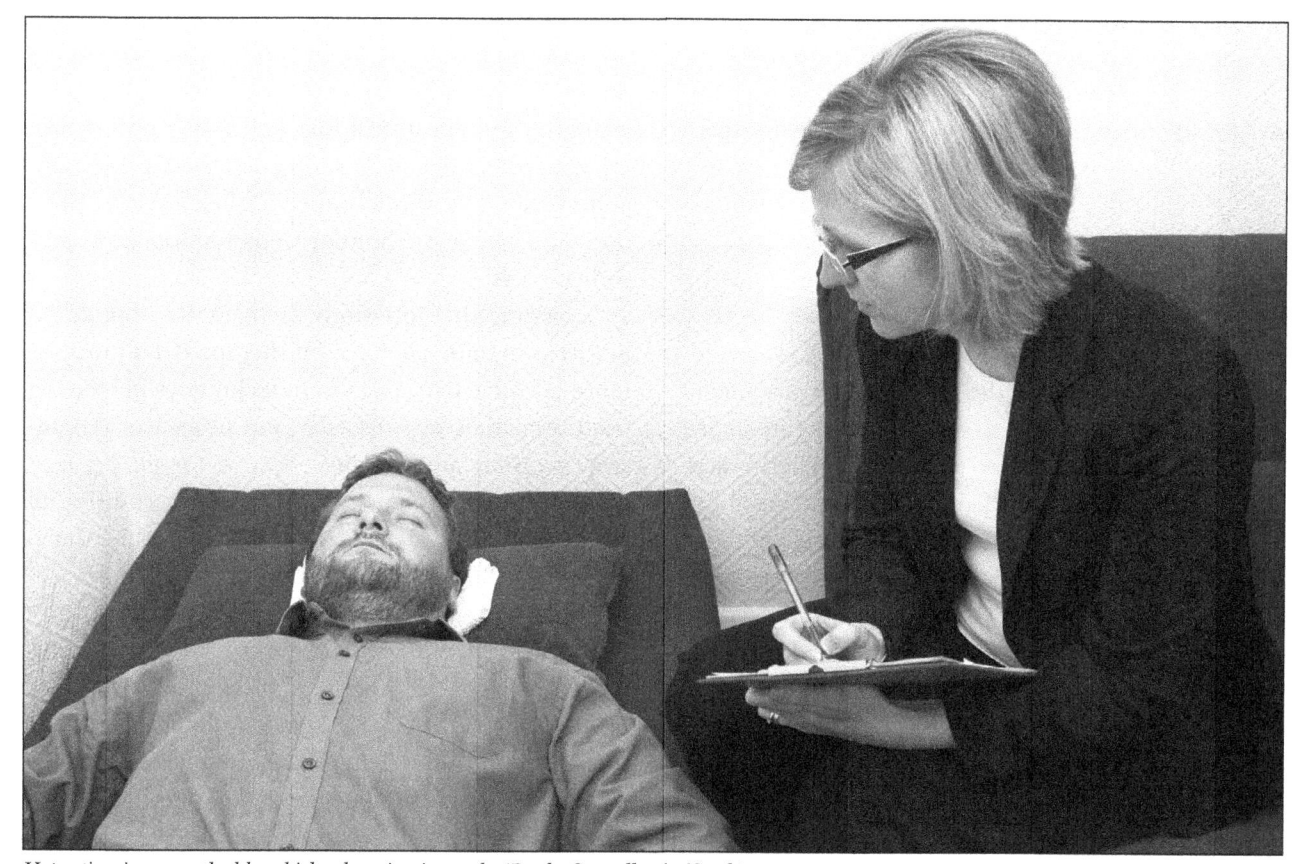

Hypnotism is one method by which relaxation is sought (Paula Connelly via iStock)

For this reason, many studies of relaxation therapy have made major compromises to the double-blind, placebo-controlled model. Some randomly assigned participants receive either relaxation therapy or no treatment. In the best of these studies, results were rated by examiners who did not know which participants were in which group (in other words, the examiners were "blinded observers"). However, it is not clear whether benefits reported in such studies come from the relaxation therapy or from less specific factors, such as mere attention.

Other studies have compared relaxation therapies to different techniques, such as hypnosis or cognitive psychotherapy. However, the same difficulties arise when trying to study these latter therapies, and the results of a study that compares an unproven treatment to one that is also imperfectly documented are not very meaningful.

Even less meaningful studies of relaxation therapies simply involved giving people the therapy and monitoring them to see whether they improved. Such open-label trials prove nothing. Given these caveats, the following is a summary of what science knows about the medical benefits of relaxation therapy.

POSSIBLE BENEFITS

Insomnia. Numerous controlled studies have evaluated relaxation therapies for the treatment of insomnia. These studies are difficult to summarize because many involved therapies combined with other methods, such as biofeedback, sleep restriction, and paradoxical intent (trying not to sleep). The type of relaxation therapy used in the majority of these trials was progressive muscle relaxation. Many of these trials used the clever form of placebo treatment described in the foregoing section; others simply compared relaxation therapy to no treatment.

Overall, the evidence indicates that relaxation therapies may be somewhat helpful for insomnia, although not dramatically so. For example, in a controlled study of seventy people with insomnia, participants using progressive relaxation showed no meaningful improvement in the time to fall asleep or the duration of sleep, but they reported feeling more rested in the morning. In another study, twenty minutes of relaxation practice was required to increase sleeping time by thirty minutes.

Asthma. A review article published in 2002 found fifteen published controlled trials that evaluated relaxation therapies for the treatment of asthma. Most of the studies were rated as very poor or poor quality. Overall, the results failed to demonstrate improvement, although a muscular relaxation technique called Jacobsen's relaxation did show some benefit. Several subsequent studies suggest breathing exercises may improve quality of life among those with asthma, as did one study involving mindfulness training.

Anxiety. A fair amount of evidence supports relaxation therapies for treating the symptoms of anxiety, at least in the short term. In a 2008 review of twenty-seven studies, researchers concluded that relaxation therapies (including Jacobson's progressive relaxation, autogenic training, applied relaxation, and meditation) were effective against anxiety. However, not all of the studies were randomized, controlled trials.

According to a fifty-study meta-analysis published in 2018, cognitive behavioral therapy (CBT) may be more effective than relaxation techniques in treating posttraumatic stress disorder and obsessive-compulsive disorder, and equally effective for generalized anxiety disorder, panic disorder, phobias, and social anxiety disorder. However, few studies have been done of specific anxiety disorders, and research biases may limit the findings.

Hypertension. It seems intuitive that relaxation should lower blood pressure. Indeed, many studies have evaluated the benefits of relaxation therapies for hypertension and related cardiovascular risks. The results, however, have been mixed at best.

In a 2008 review of twenty-five studies of various relaxation therapies for high blood pressure (with 1,198 participants), researchers found that those studies employing a control group had no significant effect on lowering blood pressure compared with sham (placebo) therapies. However, a separate review of nine randomized trials concluded that the regular use of Transcendental Meditation (TM) may significantly reduce both systolic and diastolic blood pressure compared with a control. Similarly, an analysis of seventeen randomized-controlled trials of various relaxation therapies found that only Transcendental Meditation resulted in significant reductions in blood pressure; biofeedback, progressive muscle relaxation, and stress management training produced no such benefit. In addition, a trial of eighty-six persons with hypertension suggested that daily, music-guided slow breathing reduced systolic blood pressure measured in a twenty-four-hour period.

Labor and childbirth. A 2016 systematic review of nine randomized trials involving more than 2,900 patients found that self-hypnosis or hypnotherapy reduced the use of medicinal pain relievers and anesthesia and slightly lowered the need for assisted vaginal childbirth. However, two of the largest studies evaluated found no significant differences in the reduction of pain or epidural use. Similarly, there has been mixed evidence for the use of biofeedback therapy, music therapy, and breathing technique in pain reduction.

Other conditions. Other conditions that have at least minimal supporting evidence for response to relaxation therapies include the following: angina, back pain, bulimia nervosa, cancer treatment support (including cancer pain), chronic pain, congestive heart failure, depression, fibromyalgia, interstitial cystitis, irritable bowel syndrome, menopause, nightmares, obsessive-compulsive disorder, osteoarthritis, premenstrual syndrome, pregnancy support (reducing perceived stress), psoriasis, rheumatoid arthritis, stroke rehabilitation, surgery support (primarily reducing pain and stress before or after surgery), smoking cessation, tension headaches, tinnitus, temporomandibular joint dysfunction, and ulcerative colitis. In many cases the results are marginal at best, and contradictory outcomes between trials are common.

One study suggests that the use of visualizations before surgery not only reduces the need for pain medications but also reduces the chance of developing hematomas (collections of blood under the skin). However, more study is needed to verify this somewhat difficult-to-believe result. A more easily accepted study found that either relaxation therapy or aerobic exercise can improve symptoms of fatigue after cancer surgery, and that each approach is about as effective as the other.

Another study found that persons with cancer who were exposed to empathetic care along with self-hypnotic relaxation experienced significantly less pain and anxiety during an uncomfortable, invasive procedure than similar persons receiving only empathetic or usual care. These results suggest that pain under these circumstances is more effectively relieved when the patient relies on his or her own self-coping abilities rather than on another person's kindness.

Researchers in Taiwan have also studied the role of relaxing music in reducing cancer pain. Randomly selected were 126 hospitalized persons. In one group, participants listened to music for thirty minutes and were given pain medication; participants in the other group were given the medication only. The group that listened to music experienced significantly more pain relief than the group that did not.

Numerous studies have also investigated the benefits of relaxation therapies for persons with human immunodeficiency virus (HIV) infection. A careful review of thirty-five randomized trials found that relaxation therapies may be generally helpful in improving the quality of life of HIV-positive persons and in reducing their anxiety, depression, stress, and fatigue. These interventions, though, had no significant effect on the growth of the virus, nor did they influence immunologic or hormonal activity. Subsequently, however, a small study involving forty-eight HIV-positive persons found that mindfulness meditation, a popular method for inducing the relaxation response, slowed the loss of the specific immune cells destroyed by the virus, though more research needs to be done to confirm this result.

Some studies have evaluated highly specific guided visualizations, rather than general relaxation. For example, it has been suggested that a systematic program of imagining microscopic soldiers shooting down one's cancer cells can improve the chances of surviving cancer. Despite much enthusiasm, there is still no meaningful evidence to support this appealing idea. Nonetheless, there is some evidence from a set of small trials that specific immune-oriented visualizations can provide enhanced protection against herpes flare-ups and winter colds.

Contrary to common claims, published evidence does not demonstrate that TM improves mental functioning. There is some evidence, however, that it might be helpful for improving exercise capacity and general quality of life in people with congestive heart failure.

A careful review of twenty trials found psychological interventions such as cognitive behavioral therapy, biofeedback, relaxation, and coping were associated with reduced chronic headache or migraine pain in 589 children compared with sham (placebo), standard therapies, waiting list control, or other active treatments.

CHOOSING A PRACTITIONER

There is no widely accepted license for practicing relaxation therapy. However, it is often practiced by licensed therapists and psychologists.

SAFETY ISSUES

There are few safety risks with relaxation therapies. Some adverse experiences may include intrusive thoughts, heightened anxiety, fear of losing control, and rarely, worsened symptoms from epilepsy or mood disorders. Relaxation therapies should be used in conjunction with, rather than as a substitute for, conventional medical treatment.

—*EBSCO CAM Review Board*

Further Reading

Anderson, J. W., C. Liu, and R. J. Kryscio. "Blood Pressure Response to Transcendental Meditation." *American Journal of Hypertension*, vol. 21, 2008, pp. 310–16.

"Comfort Measures (Nonpharmacologic) during Labor." *DynaMed*, 30 Nov. 2018, www.dynamed.com/topics/dmp~AN~T114734.

Eccleston, C., et al. "Psychological Therapies for the Management of Chronic and Recurrent Pain in Children and Adolescents." *Cochrane Database of Systematic Reviews*, 2009, CD003968, *EBSCO DynaMed Systematic Literature Surveillance*, www.ebscohost.com/dynamed.

Hanstede, M., Y. Gidron, and I. Nyklicek. "The Effects of a Mindfulness Intervention on Obsessive-Compulsive Symptoms in a Non-clinical Student Population." *Journal of Nervous and Mental Disease*, vol. 196, 2008, pp. 776–79.

Heather, O. D., et al. "Relaxation Therapies for the Management of Primary Hypertension in Adults." *Cochrane Database of Systematic Reviews*, 2008, CD004935, *EBSCO DynaMed Systematic Literature Surveillance*, www.ebscohost.com/dynamed.

Huang, S. T., M. Good, and J. A. Zauszniewski. "The Effectiveness of Music in Relieving Pain in Cancer Patients." *International Journal of Nursing Studies*, vol. 47, 2010, pp. 1354–62.

Jayadevappa, R., et al. "Effectiveness of Transcendental Meditation on Functional Capacity and Quality of Life of African Americans with Congestive Heart Failure." *Ethnicity and Disease*, vol. 1, 2007, pp.72–77.

Jorm, A. F., A. J. Morgan, and S. E. Hetrick. "Relaxation for Depression." *Cochrane Database of Systematic Reviews*, 2008, CD007142, *EBSCO DynaMed Systematic Literature Surveillance*, www.ebscohost.com/dynamed.

Lahmann, C., F. Röhricht, and N. Sauer. "Functional Relaxation as Complementary Therapy in Irritable Bowel Syndrome." *Journal of Alternative and Complementary Medicine*, vol. 16, 2010, pp. 47–52.

Lahmann, C., et al. "Brief Relaxation versus Music Distraction in the Treatment of Dental Anxiety." *Journal of the American Dental Association*, vol. 139, 2008, pp. 317–24.

"Mind and Body Approaches for Stress and Anxiety: What the Science Says." *NCCIH Clinical Digest for Health Professionals*, Apr. 2020, www.nccih.nih.gov/health/providers/digest/mind-and-body-approaches-for-stress-science#relaxation-techniques. Accessed 29 June 2020.

Modesti, P. A., et al. "Psychological Predictors of the Antihypertensive Effects of Music-Guided Slow Breathing." *Journal of Hypertension*, vol. 28, 2010, pp. 1097–1103.

Scott-Sheldon, L. A., et al. "Stress Management Interventions for HIV+ Adults." *Health Psychology*, vol. 27, 2008, pp. 129–39.

Trow, Terence K., editor. "Alternative Treatments for Asthma in Adults and Adolescents." *DynaMed*, 3 Dec. 2018, www.dynamed.com/topics/dmp~AN~T566085.

MEDITATION

ABSTRACT

Meditation is an awake, relaxed state characterized by decreased metabolic activity in the body.

OVERVIEW

Meditation has been practiced around the world for thousands of years. Mind and body practices focus on mind, brain, body, and behavior interactions and have four elements in common. These elements are a quiet location, a comfortable posture, a focus of attention either verbal or object or sensation, and an open mind. Physiologically, it occupies a position between wakefulness and sleep. Almost 15 percent of US adults have tried meditation and since 2012, the number of people practicing meditation has tripled. Current worldwide estimates show 200 to 500 million people meditate and it is gaining in popularity. The reasons for practicing meditation include enhancing general wellness, improving energy, decreasing anxiety, aiding memory and focus, and gaining relief from stress and depression.

Several styles of meditation are practiced, all within a continuum of two classes: concentrative and nonconcentrative. Techniques for concentrative meditation encourage the practitioner to focus on a specific stimulus (the breath or repetition of a word such as "om"), which limits incoming stimuli. Examples of this type of meditation include yogic meditation and Buddhist *samatha* meditation, both of which focus on the breath.

Nonconcentrative meditative techniques increase stimuli, encouraging the practitioner to pay attention to the thoughts, feelings, and sensations experienced, but in a nonjudgmental way. Examples of this type of meditation include Zen and mindfulness. Techniques that involve meditating while actively moving include mindful yoga, Tai Chi, and qigong. Another type of meditation, compassionate, involves meditating while feeling complete love and harmony with others.

Transcendental Meditation (TM), created by Maharishi Mahesh Yogi, encourages focusing on a specific mantra depending on the expertise level of the practitioner. The objective is to repeat the mantra without concentrative effort and to develop awareness without thought. Therefore, this type of meditation falls between the concentrative and the nonconcentrative types. Brain activity, measured by cerebral blood flow and functional magnetic resonance imaging (fMRI), has been found to have varying patterns within the same person, depending on the type of meditation being practiced.

MECHANISM OF ACTION

Meditation affects so many systems of the body it is difficult to pinpoint a mechanism of action; indeed, there would be multiple mechanisms involved with so many effects. Meditation results in lower oxygen consumption, respiration rate, and heart rate, and it impacts brain activity. These effects vary depending on the amount of time one spends meditating and the type of meditation being done.

Meditation was once thought to be a sort of hibernation or to be similar to sleep, but physiologic testing shows that neither is the case. Regular practice lowers cortisol levels, increases serotonin availability, and

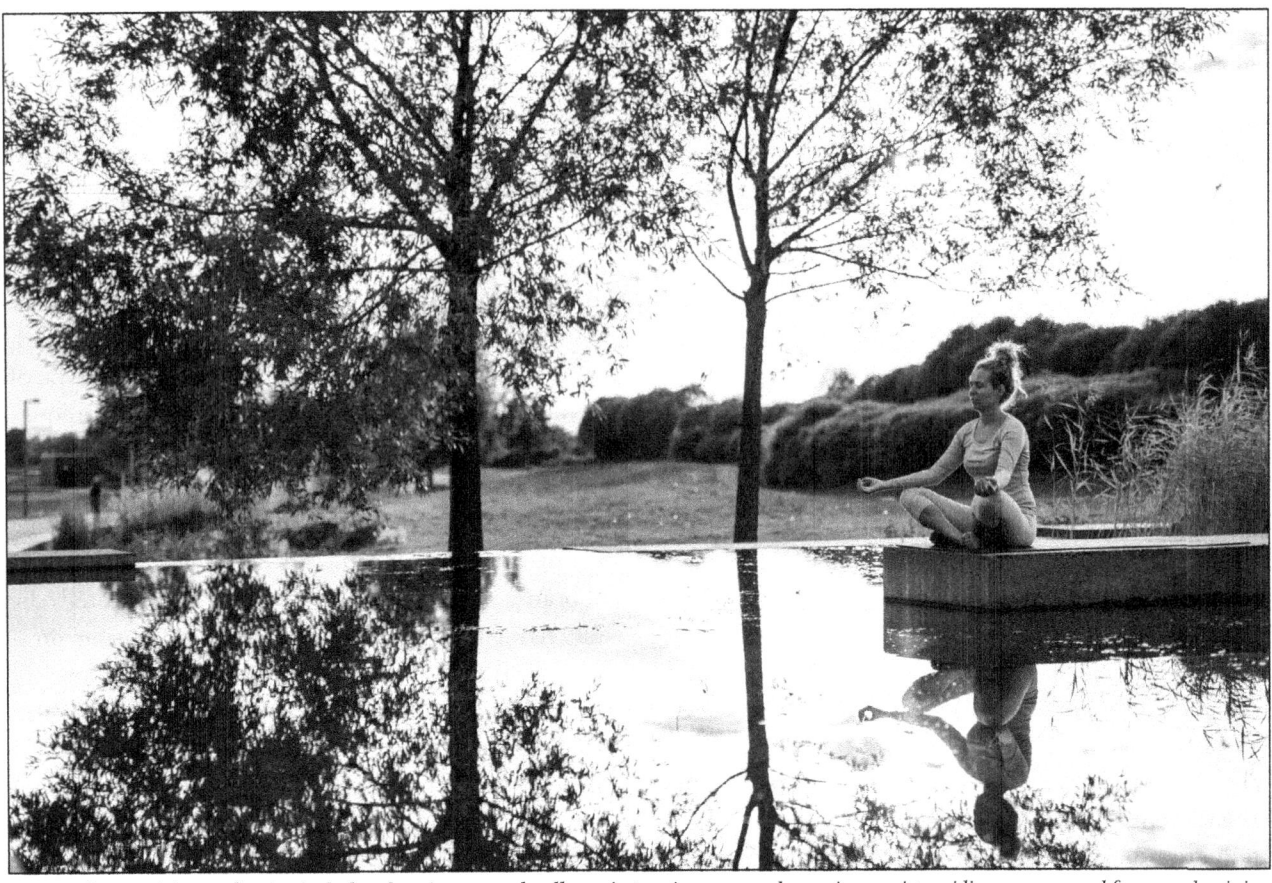

Reasons for practicing meditation include enhancing general wellness, improving energy, decreasing anxiety, aiding memory and focus, and gaining relief from stress and depression. (Marija Jovovic via iStock)

better-controls homeostasis. Meditation is generally safe for healthy people and people with limitations may need to speak with their healthcare provider to determine the best technique to use based on individual needs. People with mental health conditions need to speak with their healthcare provider before beginning a meditation program as rare reports show meditation has worsened certain psychiatric disorders.

USES AND APPLICATIONS

Meditation is used by persons worldwide. It is also prescribed by healthcare practitioners for specific conditions. Meditation has shown efficacy in treating anxiety, depression, drug addiction, fibromyalgia, and insomnia, and it is used for pain management. A randomized clinical trial of mindfulness-based stress reduction versus medication for insomnia showed comparable changes in sleep duration and quality in the two groups studied.

Meditation is useful for the elderly to assist in pain management, improve sleep quality and quantity, and decrease the need for pharmaceutical agents. In children, various types of meditation (including mindfulness, Tai Chi, and TM) have led to improvements in cognitive tasks and to decreased anxiety and distractibility. Tai Chi was associated with mood and quality of life improvements in a studied group of high school girls. TM training also has been shown to decrease blood pressure in teenagers who had high blood pressure before the training.

SCIENTIFIC EVIDENCE

It is impossible to conduct double-blind studies on meditation because participants must know they are meditating; therefore, they would not be blinded. There are some compelling studies with relatively good designs comparing physiologic measures pre- and postmeditation training. Research on persons who had magnetic resonance imaging scans before and after undergoing an eight-week mindfulness-based stress reduction course has shown that their brains are actually different. Studies show that participants have more dense gray matter in specific areas of the brain after the course. Other research has found that the specific type of meditation practiced leads to different patterns of brain activity.

Other researchers have looked at the impact of long-term meditation practice on modifying electroencephalogram (EEG) results, brain activity, and even structure of the brain, providing evidence for neural plasticity related to meditation practice. EEG alpha waves and theta waves are often found to be increased during meditation, compared with control conditions.

Comparison of the brains of longtime meditators (Western meditation practitioners) with nonpractitioners showed an increase in cortical thickness in the prefrontal cortex and right anterior insula of the brain. Scientists have studied Buddhist monks who have practiced meditation for an average of 19,000 hours in comparison with novices and found increased brain activation as measured by fMRI; those who had practiced 44,000 hours on average had lower brain activation than study controls. The researchers used distracter sounds and found that the "expert meditators" had decreased brain activity response related to the sounds, compared with study controls.

Additional research on expert Buddhist meditators versus study controls (during the meditation exercise and at rest) involved measuring brain activity during compassion meditation, when they were asked to generate an unconditional state of loving kindness. Areas of the limbic system were activated in both groups, but the response was stronger in expert meditators. When meditation was compared with rest, activation occurred in the amygdala, temporo-parietal junction, and right posterior superior temporal sulcus.

TM seems to reduce the response to pain while allowing the sensory experience of pain to remain fully activated. Research on the effect of meditating on a regular basis on the experience of pain found that meditators reported the same level of pain as those who did not meditate. However, this study was not conducted during meditation. The brains of meditators showed 40 to 50 percent decreased responsiveness by fMRI. The nonmeditators also were trained, and five months later, both groups showed the 40 to 50 percent responsiveness rate, indicating that the TM training they received had affected the brain's reaction to pain.

CHOOSING A PRACTITIONER

Before beginning a meditation program, discuss your interest with your physician who may be able to provide guidance and recommendations. Meditation can be self-taught. However, if one wants to select a teacher to learn meditation, it is important to feel comfortable with the teacher and to be aware of the various types of meditation, because one style may be better suited than another. Some types of meditation, such as TM, require specific classes taught by an approved teacher.

For persons seeking help with stress or anxiety, a program called mindfulness-based stress reduction has been shown to be effective; TM has been found to be helpful for decreasing blood pressure.

SAFETY ISSUES

Before beginning any program, consult with your physician. Meditation is generally safe for almost everyone. There have been some case reports of people with psychological illnesses such as psychosis and severe depression experiencing exacerbation of the condition in connection with meditation. Some healthy people experience repressed memories or emotions in association with meditation. Some persons may find they cannot meditate for more than a few minutes at a time, as it is too taxing for them. They can start with shorter time periods and work their way up to longer sessions gradually. For some persons who take antidepressants or thyroid medications, the dosage may actually be reduced after meditation becomes a regular daily practice. Never change any medication without your physician's input.

—Dawn M. Bielawski

Further Reading

Barinaga, Marcia. "Studying the Well-Trained Mind." *Science*, vol. 302, 2003, pp. 44–46. Discusses collaboration among scientists and Buddhist monks in a study measuring the effects of meditation on the brain.

Cormody, James, and Ruth A. Baer. "Relationships Between Mindfulness Practice and Levels of Mindfulness, Medical and Psychological Symptoms, and Well-Being in a Mindfulness-Based Stress Reduction Program." *Journal of Behavioral Medicine*, vol. 31, 2008, pp. 23–33. The researchers conducted pre- and postintervention surveys of 174 adults who participated in this mindfulness program.

"8 Things to Know about Meditation for Health." National Center for Complementary and Integrative Health. *National Institutes of Health*, www.ncch.nih.gov/health/tips/things-to-know-about-meditation-for-health. Accessed 24 Aug. 2020.

Gross, Cynthia R., et al. "Mindfulness-Based Stress Reduction Versus Pharmacotherapy for Chronic Primary Insomnia." *Explore*, vol. 7, 2011, pp. 76–87. The researchers studied thirty adults with diagnosed insomnia and randomized them to either mindfulness-based stress reduction training or pharmacotherapy, comparing various indices of sleep quality and quantity between the two treatments.

Gelles, D. "How to Meditate." *The New York Times*, www.nytimes.com/guides/well/how-to-meditate. Accessed 24 Aug. 2020.

"Meditation: In Depth." National Center for Complementary and Integrative Health. *National Institutes of Health*, www.ncch.nih.gov/health/meditation-in-depth. Accessed 24 Aug. 2020.

Sibinga, Erica M. S., and Kathi J. Kemper. "Complementary, Holistic, and Integrative Medicine: Meditation Practices for Pediatric Health." *Pediatrics in Review*, vol. 31, 2020, pp. 91–103. Directed to pediatric clinicians, this article describes cases for which meditative practices may be helpful, then provides summary tables of data from studies of various types of pediatric-focused meditation.

"22 Meditation Statistics: Data and Trends Revealed for 2019." *The Good Body*, www.thegoodbody.com/meditation-statistics/. Accessed 24 Aug. 2020.

Wang, D., et al. "Cerebral Blood Flow Changes Associated with Different Meditation Practices and Perceived Depth of Meditation." *Psychiatry Research: Neuroimaging*, Vol. 191, 2011, pp. 60–67. This study involved comparing two types of meditation (focus-based and breath-based) within subjects and looked at functional MRI and cerebral blood flow in relation to the subjects' reported experiences.

Transcendental Meditation (TM)

ABSTRACT

Transcendental meditation (TM) is a technique for relaxing the mind and body through the repetition of a mantra, or a sound without meaning.

OVERVIEW

TM has its origins in ancient Vedic tradition in India. The TM technique was revived by the Indian guru Maharishi Mahesh Yogi and has been taught since 1958. It became widely popular in the 1960s and now claims to have millions of practitioners. The technique involves fifteen to twenty minutes of quiet meditation in the morning and evening. A mantra (a sound without meaning) is used as a form of thought during the sessions.

MECHANISM OF ACTION

During TM, the mind lets go of stimuli and concentration that otherwise keep it in an agitated state. The mind enters a state of restful awareness, and the body becomes completely relaxed. The mind is then considered to be in a transcendent state beyond the normal waking, dreaming, or sleep states. The transcendent state is believed to restore normal functioning of various systems in the body, particularly those systems involved in adapting to environmental stresses. All of the alleged benefits deriving from TM can be attributed to the relaxed nonstressful state.

USES AND APPLICATIONS

Proponents of TM claim that the program can benefit anyone who wants to achieve a better quality of life by reducing stress and increasing mental alertness and memory. All the secondary benefits from the use of TM can be attributed to a reduction in stress, including lowered blood pressure, reduced metabolic disease, and reduced cardiovascular disease.

The 2010s saw a resurgence in the popularity of TM and similar meditation techniques, partly driven by endorsements by celebrity practitioners. Some businesses began programs to include meditation in the workday as a means of combating stress and improving productivity. Some schools also introduced TM practices for students across a range of ages. In 2014 reports from several California middle and high schools claimed that a version of TM known as Quiet Time was highly successful in helping to reduce suspension rates and improve attendance, grade point averages, and student happiness.

SCIENTIFIC EVIDENCE

To perform a meta-analysis, data from many trials are combined for an overall statistical analysis. This procedure is thought to add strength to research findings. The value of a meta-analysis is only as strong as the quality of the component research trials.

A 2004 review article summarized controlled research studies on the effect of TM on risk factors related to cardiovascular disease. (It should be noted that most of the review articles consulted include a minimum of one author from the Institute for Natural Medicine and Prevention, Maharishi University of Management.) Several studies showed a reduction in blood pressure in both genders and in persons at high and low risk for hypertension. Two studies showed that TM reduced carotid artery thickness, a marker of atherosclerosis. Two other studies, involving elderly persons, showed a significant reduction in all-cause mortality in the groups practicing TM.

A 2002 review paper described studies on the effect of TM to change psychological or physiological indicators or consequences of stress. Several meta-analyses showed that TM significantly reduced anxiety or other negative psychological outcomes. Several studies showed TM decreased high blood pressure, compared with controls. Other studies showed TM reduced carotid artery thickness and exercise-induced ischemia, measures of cardiovascular disease.

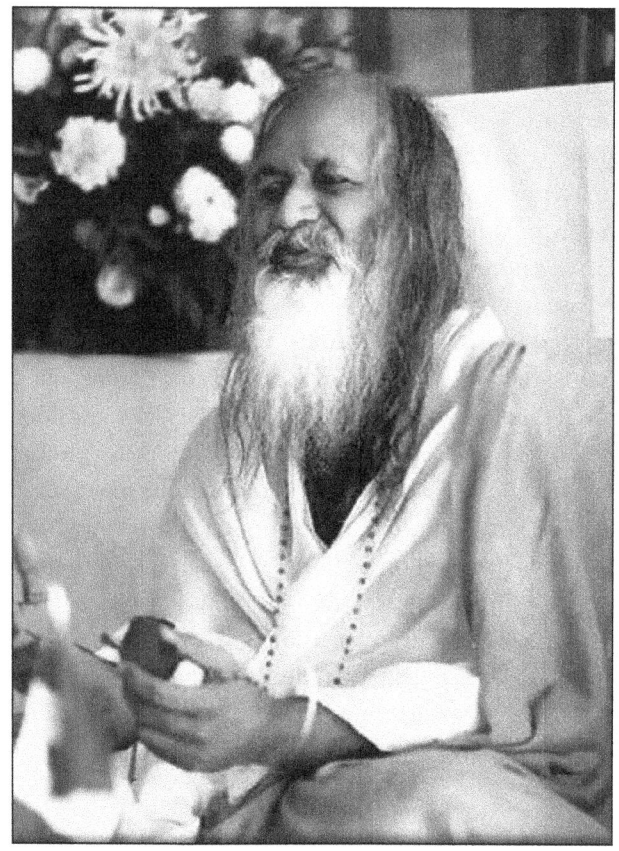

Maharishi Mahesh Yogi (Jdontfight via Wikimedia Commons)

An interesting study related TM to brain reactivity to pain. Practitioners of TM and healthy matched controls were subjected to thermally induced pain. The results indicated that TM practitioners experienced as much pain as the controls, but they were less affected by it. This was in spite of the fact that the TM mediators' brains showed a greater response to pain (reduced blood flow through certain regions).

Metabolic syndrome can be a condition of obese people, and it is thought to be a contributor to coronary heart disease. A sixteen-week study was conducted to evaluate the effect of TM on components of the syndrome. The results found that the group practicing TM, compared with the group receiving health education, showed significant reductions in blood pressure and insulin resistance and had a positive influence on cardiac autonomic tone as measured by heart rate variability.

Patient data were pooled from two studies originally designed to study the effects of TM on blood pressure. Statistical analysis of the combined data showed that the TM groups had a 23 percent decrease in all-cause mortality, compared with control groups receiving other meditation methods or no treatments. Furthermore, the TM groups showed a 30 percent decrease in cardiovascular mortality.

A 2007 review revisited previous studies and meta-analyses of the effect of relaxation techniques on reduction of high blood pressure. The authors identified 107 reports and applied rigorous criteria for selection of studies for reevaluation. Seventeen studies were selected and compiled into groups according to relaxation technique. These techniques included simple or relaxation-assisted biofeedback, progressive muscle relaxation, TM, and stress management with relaxation. Meta-analysis showed that only the TM group showed significant reductions in blood pressure.

CHOOSING A PRACTITIONER

Transcendental Meditation and TM are service marks registered in the US Patent and Trademark Office, licensed to Maharishi Vedic Education Development Corporation. Only teachers certified by the foundation are permitted to teach the TM technique. The fee for the six-step process is high, but other techniques based on mantra meditation, such as primordial sound meditation and natural stress relief, are available at more accessible prices. The effectiveness of these other mantra meditation methods apparently has not been studied in randomized trials.

SAFETY ISSUES

There are no known safety risks with the use of TM, especially when taught by certified teachers.

—*David A. Olle*

Further Reading

Kirp, David L. "Meditation Transforms Roughest San Francisco Schools." Hearst Communications. *SFGate*, 12 Jan. 2014.

"Meditation: A Simple, Fast Way to Reduce Stress." Mayo Foundation for Medical Education and Research. *Mayo Clinic*, 19 July 2014.

"Meditation: In Depth." National Center for Complementary and Integrative Health. *National Institutes of Health*, www.nccih.nih.gov/health/meditation-in-depth. Accessed 25 Aug. 2020.

Orme-Johnson, D., et al. "Neuroimaging of Meditation's Effect on Brain Reactivity." *NeuroReport*, vol. 17, no. 12, 2006, pp. 1359–1363.

Paul-Labrador, M., et al. "Effects of a Randomized Controlled Trial of Transcendental Meditation on Components of the Metabolic Syndrome in Subjects with Coronary Artery Disease." *Archives of Internal Medicine*, 2006, pp. 1218–24.

Rainforth, M., et al. "Stress Reduction Programs in Patients with Elevated Blood Pressure." *Current Hypertension Report*, vol. 9, no. 6, 2007, pp. 520–28.

Transcendental Meditation. Maharishi Foundation USA, 2015. Accessed 30 Nov. 2015.

Mind-Body Medicine

ABSTRACT
Mind-body medicine is a type of traditional healing that emphasizes the interconnectedness of the mind and the body.

OVERVIEW
According to Hippocrates, "The natural healing force within each one of us is the greatest force in getting well." Ancient civilizations and the indigenous peoples of the Americas, for example, have known and practiced mind-body medicine for centuries. These ancient healing practices include traditional Chinese medicine, Ayurvedic medicine, and various forms of indigenous medicine. This conceptual framework of interdependence of the mind-body relationship is in sharp contrast to the theory of Western medicine, which separates the mind from the body and sees no interconnection between them. Studies suggest that a variety of conditions can be helped by mind-body practices.

MODERN INTERESTS
In the early 1960s came renewed interest in the possible connection between the mind and the body in the context of healing. George Solomon, a psychiatrist, knew that persons with rheumatoid arthritis had an exacerbation of symptoms when they were depressed. From this realization he developed a new field of medicine that incorporated the knowledge of psychology, neurology, and immunology: psychoneuroimmunology. Another physician, Herbert Benson, studied the effect of meditation on blood pressure levels. Psychologist Robert Ader further illustrated the relationship of mind and body and how this interplay could be affected by mental and emotional cues. He was interested in how this relationship affected the immune system. The mind/body connection, for the most part, is no longer viewed with suspicion. Indeed, its study is now part of the curricula of many medical schools worldwide.

MIND-BODY MEDICINE
Theoretically, mind-body medicine works through reducing stress levels, thereby decreasing the overload release of hormones such as cortisol, which affect the immune system. These hormones have a major affect on the cardiovascular system, and they also increase inflammation of organs and joints. By decreasing the release of these stressors, one can manage many chronic diseases. Experiments have shown not only a reduction in blood pressure but also a reduction in body temperature.

One has only to close one's eyes and open one's mind to visualize a Hindu monk, for example, performing such physical-mental feats. These acts of will, through self-control practiced through multiple forms of relaxation, can be performed by anyone with training. Meditation, yoga, guided visualization, relaxation techniques, biofeedback, and cognitive behavioral therapy are methods employed in mind-body medicine.

Conditions that have been improved by choosing an appropriate modality include asthma, coronary heart disease, hypertension (high blood pressure), anxiety, insomnia, fibromyalgia, menopausal symptoms, and the nausea and vomiting associated with chemotherapy. By choosing the preferred modality, a participant enhances the chance for success.

Hypnosis is another form of mind-body medicine that has gained favor. It has been shown to be advantageous in multiple situations, including dental treatments, minor surgery, and treatment for phobias. Although this is a proven modality, it may not work for everybody.

David Spiegel of Stanford University School of Medicine treated eighty-six women with late-stage breast cancer; one-half received standard recommended treatments, the other half received, in addition to the standard treatment, weekly support

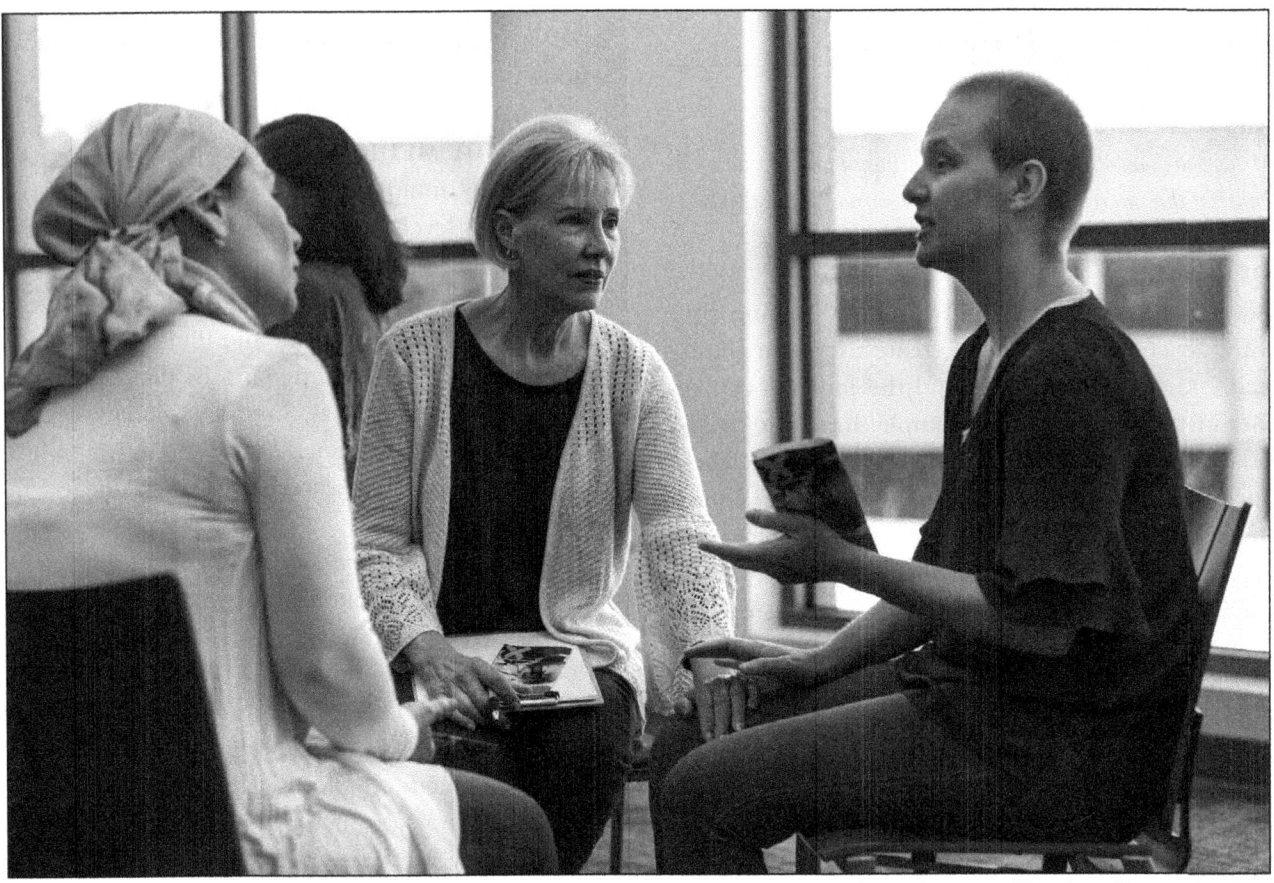

Scene from a breast cancer support group. Clinical trials have shown that such social support, as well as meditation and laughter affect mood and improve the quality and duration of one's life. (SDI Productions via iStock)

sessions in which the women shared personal triumphs and grief. The women who participated in these support groups lived twice as long as those who did not have this social support. Other clinical trials have shown that meditation and laughter affect mood and improve the quality of life.

PRACTICE

As with any form of medical therapy, treatments should be rendered by licensed professionals only. Mind/body medicine does not provide curative measures as such. It is a form of integrative medicine, complementary to well-established medical treatments.

Also, it is important to have ongoing evaluation of the success or failure of treatment. Reevaluation, which can be curative in its own right, is an ongoing process that should be incorporated into the routine activities of the person seeking care.

Motivation of the patient and the trust instilled by the practitioner are as much a part of mind-body medicine as the treatment itself. As with any form of healing, the interplay among those involved needs to be established at the start of treatment. The greatest satisfaction a practitioner can achieve is attainment of the goals set by both the practitioner and the person being treated.

—*M. Barbara Klyde*

Further Reading

Ader, R., and N. Cohen. "Psychoneuroimmunology: Conditioning and Stress." *Annual Review of Psychology*, vol. 44, 1993, pp. 53–85.

Lando, J., and S. M. Williams. "Uniting Mind and Body in Our Health Care and Public Health Systems." *Preventing Chronic Disease*, vol. 3, no. 2, 2006, p. A31.

McMillan, T. L., and S. Mark. "Complementary and Alternative Medicine and Physical Activity for Menopausal Symptoms." *Journal of the American Medical Women's Association*, vol. 59, no. 4, 2004, pp. 270–77.

"Mind and Body Practices." National Center for Complementary and Integrative Health, *National Institutes of Health*, www.nccih.nih.gov/health/mind-and-body-practices. Accessed 25 Aug. 2020.

Wheeler, C. "What Is Mind-Body Medicine?" *Psychology Today*, www.psychologytoday.com/us/blog/head-toe-happiness/201006/what-is-mind-body-medicine. Accessed 25 Aug. 2020.

Guided Imagery

ABSTRACT

Guided imagery is a therapy involving the use of imagined scenes and activities to influence the body.

OVERVIEW

Guided imagery has been used since ancient times by the Greeks and Egyptians. Normally, a person uses imagery many times each day when anticipating events or activities. Some of the imagery is negative and causes worrying. A person develops thoughts about who he or she is through mental imagery. Guided imagery channels this use of the mind to affect the body.

When initiating guided imagery, it helps to relax, because doing so makes the body more receptive to mental images. Some persons use guided imagery when they wake up in the morning and before they go to sleep at night. Guided imagery can be effective when practiced regularly, but it takes time to learn and to see its effects. Guided imagery should be practiced a minimum of twice per day.

Guided imagery is sometimes referred to as visualization or affirmations. Both visualization and affirmations apply the same principles as guided imagery.

MECHANISM OF ACTION

Guided imagery uses the mind/body connection to change the body or its functioning. The mind already has a great deal of control over the body, and this control can be increased by using guided imagery.

The brain does not "understand" words; rather it understands only pictures or images, and these mental images must be repeatedly reviewed. With enough repetition, the brain and unconscious mind will attempt to make these images real. Positive imagery can trigger the release of brain chemicals, such as serotonin and endorphins, which are natural tranquilizers.

Guided imagery is more effective if all of the senses are used in forming the images. For example, a runner imaging his or her performance in a race should imagine the smell of perspiration, feel the pain in the legs and chest, imagine the dryness of the mouth, see competitors through peripheral vision, see the finish line, feel sweat running down the neck, and hear feet beating the ground as he or she pulls ahead and crosses the finish line first. One can then imagine the joy of winning the race and receiving a trophy or medal.

USES AND APPLICATIONS

Guided imagery assists in relaxing the body, controlling some body functions, boosting the immune system, and increasing the effectiveness of performance. It can be used to treat depression, anxiety, cancer, the side effects of chemotherapy, pain, high blood pressure, obesity, diabetes, insomnia, headaches, wounds, premenstrual syndrome, asthma, spastic colon, and low white-blood-cell counts. It may be also integrated into childbirth, to control pain related to procedures and other unpleasant experiences.

SCIENTIFIC EVIDENCE

Much research has been conducted to determine the effectiveness of guided imagery. Many of the studies examined guided imagery as a complementary and alternative medicine (CAM) therapy for healing, reducing the side effects of drugs, or initiating personal change. In general, however, the effectiveness of guided imagery depends on the efforts of the individual person and cannot be controlled or measured accurately.

One study of women with breast cancer demonstrated such questionable results. The study, performed by the Oregon Health and Science University in 2002, looked at twenty-five women with either stage one or stage two breast cancer. They were taught guided imagery to see the natural killer cells of their immune system destroying the cancer cells. The initial session was taped; participants were asked to practice at home with the tape three times per week for eight weeks. Their immune function and emotional state were measured three times: before the study began, at the end of eight weeks, and three months after the study ended. Participants reported being less depressed. The measure of their immune system demonstrated higher levels of natural killer cells but no change in the physical effects of the killer cells. A study in 2019 found that cognitive behavioral strategies, including guided imagery, may be an effective therapy in advanced heart failure. Guided imagery and relaxation were shown to be a complementary approach with drug analgesia in postoperative patients.

CHOOSING A PRACTITIONER

Nurses may recommend guided imagery to ease discomfort. Guided imagery can be done without a practitioner. Audiotapes and CDs are available to provide guided imagery coaching and resources are also available online. Good books describe the process and include scripts for guided imagery. A nurse, a mental health counselor, or a physician can provide coaching in guided imagery, and trained guided imagery counselors can be consulted.

SAFETY ISSUES

There are no known safety issues with guided imagery. Intense worrying can have negative physical and emotional effects.

—*Christine M. Carroll*

Further Reading

Felix, M. M. D. S., M. B. G. Ferreira, L. F. da Cruz, and M. H. Barbosa. "Relaxation Therapy with Guided Imagery for Postoperative Pain Management: An Integrative Review." *Pain Management Nursing*, vol. 20, no. 1, 2019, pp. 3–9.

"Guided Imagery: Using Your Imagination." *Stress Management for Life: A Research-Based Experiential Approach*, edited by Michael Olpin and Margie Hesson. Wadsworth/Cengage Learning, 2010.

Kwekkeboom, K. L., and L. C. Bratzke. "A Systematic Review of Relaxation, Meditation, and Guided Imagery Strategies for Symptom Management in Heart Failure." *Journal of Cardiovascular Nursing*, vol. 31, no. 5, 2016, pp. 457–68, pubmed.ncbi.nlm.nih.gov/26065388/.

Naparstek, Belleruth. *Staying Well with Guided Imagery*. Grand Central, 1995.

Rossman, Martin L. *Guided Imagery for Self-Healing*. 2nd ed., H. J. Kramer/New World Library, 2000.

NATURAL TREATMENTS FOR STRESS

ABSTRACT

The treatment of conditions associated with emotional, mental, and physical stress can include relaxation therapies as well as nutrient and mineral supplements.

INTRODUCTION

The effects of stress on health can be far-reaching and may affect anyone. Some of the conditions often associated with stress include insomnia, high blood pressure, tension headaches, anxiety, depression, decreased mental function, and drug or alcohol abuse. Stress is known to cause changes in the body's chemistry, altering the balance of hormones in our systems in ways that can lower our resistance to disease. As a result, people can become more susceptible to colds and flu and other types of illness. Too much stress sometimes brings on outbreaks of cold sores or genital herpes for people who carry these viruses in their systems. Other chronic diseases such as irritable bowel syndrome, asthma, inflammatory bowel disease, and rheumatoid arthritis may also flare up during times of stress.

Avoiding situations that cause one to feel tense, unhappy, or worn down is beneficial. However, it is not always possible to live a stress-free existence. Work deadlines, family demands, relationship problems, traffic jams, missed appointments, forgotten birthdays, personality conflicts, college exams—all of these things, and many more, can be sources of stress. Furthermore, though most people associate stress with unpleasant events, even wonderful events, such as weddings, vacations, and holidays, can be genuinely stressful. Because of the stressful nature of nursing, stress relief should be integrated into daily life.

Not everyone responds to these situations with stress. For some persons, their pulse rate would not even go up during an earthquake, and then there are those for whom being five minutes late to an event causes panic. How one manages stress can determine its impact.

There are many different methods of dealing with stress. The basics for good health that are well known (but often forgotten) help in coping with stress: eating a balanced diet and getting adequate rest helps the body adapt and respond to life events. Ironically, stress can interfere with one's ability to take care of oneself in this way. When a person worries so much that he or she cannot sleep, getting adequate rest becomes impossible. Stress can affect eating habits too. Widely accepted stress management tools that can help a person break from a stress-induced downward spiral include exercise, meditation, and biofeedback.

For some people, stressful circumstances can trigger symptoms severe enough to warrant seeking medical attention. Conditions associated with stress, such as insomnia, anxiety, depression, and panic attacks, may become severe enough to require medication.

PRINCIPAL PROPOSED NATURAL TREATMENTS

One proposed natural approach to treating the physical consequences of stress involves the use of adaptogens. The term "adaptogen" refers to a hypothetical treatment described as follows: An adaptogen helps the body adapt to stresses of various kinds, whether heat, cold, exertion, trauma, sleep deprivation, toxic exposure, radiation, infection, or psychological stress. Furthermore, an adaptogen should cause no side effects, be effective in treating a wide variety of illnesses, and help return an organism toward balance no matter what may have gone wrong.

Relaxation techniques, including breathing techniques, guided imagery, mindfulness meditation, yoga, tai chi and qigong, and repetitive prayer are supported as invoking the relaxation response and decreasing stress. However, physical exercise is the only indubitable example of an adaptogen. There is no solid evidence that any substance functions in this way. However, there is some suggestive evidence for the herb *Panax ginseng*.

Panax ginseng. Most of the evidence cited to indicate that *Panax ginseng* has adaptogenic effects comes from animal studies involving ginseng extracts injected into the abdomen. Such studies are of questionable relevance to the oral use of ginseng by humans; furthermore, the majority of these studies were performed in the former Soviet Union and failed to reach acceptable scientific standards. However, a few potentially meaningful studies in humans have found effects that are at least consistent with the possibility of benefits in stressful situations.

According to a number of animal studies, most of which were poorly designed and reported, *P. ginseng* injections into the bloodstream or abdomen can increase stamina; improve mental function; protect against radiation, infections, toxins, exhaustion, and stress; and activate white blood cells. However, when ginseng is injected into the abdomen or bloodstream, it enters the body directly without going through the digestive tract. This mode of administration is strikingly different from taking ginseng by mouth.

A smaller number of animal studies (again, most of them poorly designed) have looked at the potential benefits of ginseng administered orally and have often reported benefit. In addition, studies in mice found that consuming ginseng before exposure to a virus significantly increased the survival rate and number of antibodies produced.

Human studies of *P. ginseng* have only indirectly examined its potential benefits as an adaptogen. For example, a double-blind, placebo-controlled study found evidence that *P. ginseng* may improve immune system response. This trial enrolled 227 participants at three medical offices in Italy. One-half were given ginseng at a dosage of 100 milligrams (mg) daily, and the other one-half received placebo. Four weeks into the study, all participants received influenza vaccine.

The results showed a significant decline in the frequency of colds and flu in the treated group, compared with the placebo group (fifteen versus forty-two cases). Also, antibody levels in response to the vaccination rose higher in the treated group than in the placebo group.

These findings have been taken by some researchers to support their belief that ginseng has an adaptogenic effect. However, the study might instead simply indicate a general form of immune support unrelated to stress.

Other studies have looked at *P. ginseng*'s effects on overall mental function, general well-being, and sports performance. While it is true that positive results in such studies might tend to hint at an adaptogenic effect, the results were, in general, too mixed to provide conclusive evidence for benefit. It is not clear that *P. ginseng* offers general benefits for stress.

OTHER PROPOSED NATURAL TREATMENTS

Multivitamins plus minerals. A treatment as simple as multivitamin-multimineral tablets may be helpful for stress. In a double-blind, placebo-controlled study, three hundred men and women were given either a multivitamin-multimineral tablet or placebo for thirty days. The results showed that people taking the nutritional supplement experienced less anxiety overall and an enhanced ability to cope with stressful circumstances. The supplement used in this study supplied the following nutrients and dosages: vitamin B_1 (10 mg), vitamin B_2 (15 mg), vitamin B_6 (10 mg), vitamin B_{12} (10 micrograms), vitamin C (1,000 mg), calcium (100 mg), and magnesium (100 mg).

Benefits were seen in another double-blind, placebo-controlled trial that enrolled eighty healthy male volunteers. The supplement used in this trial was similar but not identical.

It is not clear how these nutrients help stress. However, considering that many people would benefit from general nutritional supplementation in any case, it might be worth trying.

Eleutherococcus senticosus. In the 1940s, the same scientist who first dubbed *P. ginseng* an adaptogen decided that a much less expensive herb, *Eleutherococcus senticosus*, is also an adaptogen. A thorny bush that grows much more rapidly than true ginseng, this plant later received the misleading name of "Siberian ginseng" or "Russian ginseng." Its chemical makeup, however, is unrelated to that of *P. ginseng*.

As with *P. ginseng*, many animal studies finding adaptogenic benefits with *Eleutherococcus* have been reported, but most were relatively poorly designed and used injections rather than oral administration of the herb, making the results not particularly relevant to the normal human usage of the herb.

Numerous human trials of *Eleutherococcus* have been reported as well, some involving enormous numbers of participants. However, most of these were not double-blind and many were not even controlled, making the results nearly meaningless.

Again, as with *P. ginseng*, a few reasonably well-designed studies in humans have been reported that may have indirect bearing on the herb's potential adaptogenic properties. For example, in one double-blind trial, participants took either 10 milliliters of extract of *Eleutherococcus* or placebo three times daily for four weeks. Blood samples were analyzed to determine changes in immune cells. A statistically significant increase in numbers of cells important to immune functions was observed in the treatment group compared with the placebo group.

This study has been widely advertised as proving the *Eleutherococcus* strengthens immunity. However, mere changes in immune cell profile do not automatically translate into enhanced immunity. More meaningful data were obtained in a double-blind, placebo-controlled study involving ninety-three people who experienced recurrent flare-ups of herpes. The use of *Eleutherococcus* significantly reduced the severity, frequency, and duration of herpes outbreaks relative to placebo during the six-month trial. This study does suggest a possible immune-strengthening effect.

Like *P. ginseng*, *Eleutherococcus* has been studied for enhancing sports performance, but published studies have not been encouraging. One small, double-blind, placebo-controlled trial of endurance athletes found that the use of *Eleutherococcus* actually may increase physiologic signs of stress during intensive training.

Other possible adaptogens. Three small double-blind trials suggest that the herb rhodiola (*Rhodiola rosea*) may improve mental alertness in people undergoing sleep deprivation or other stressful circumstances. Numerous other herbs are said to be adaptogens too. These include ashwagandha, astragalus, maitake, reishi, shiitake, suma, and schisandra. However, there is little evidence that they have adaptogenic effects.

One study failed to find greater adaptogenic effects with fish oil compared with placebo.

Other options. Preliminary evidence, including small double-blind trials, suggests that the amino acid tyrosine may improve memory and mental function under conditions of sleep deprivation or other forms of stress. Another double-blind study found that the use of vitamin C at doses of 3,000 mg daily (slow release) reduced both physical and emotional responses to stress.

In small double-blind studies, theanine, a constituent of black tea, appeared to reduce the body's reaction to acute physical or psychological stress. Benefits have also been seen with a combination of lysine (2.64 grams per day) and arginine (2.64 grams per day).

One double-blind study found evidence that a processed form of casein (a protein found in milk) may reduce a variety of stress-related symptoms. According to another small double-blind trial, a mixture of soy phosphatidylserine and lecithin may decrease the physiological response to mental stress. Another study evaluated the use of phosphatidylserine for reducing stress in golfers, but the benefits seen failed to reach statistical significance.

A proprietary Ayurvedic herbal formula containing *Bacopa monniera* and almost thirty other ingredients has shown some promise for treating symptoms of stress. In a three-month, double-blind, placebo-controlled trial of forty-two people in high-stress jobs who complained of fatigue, participants using the herbal formula reported fewer stress-related problems. Also, in a three-month, double-blind, placebo-controlled study of fifty adult students, this formula appeared to improve memory and attention and to reduce other signs of stress.

In naturopathic medicine, adrenal extract is often recommended for the treatment of stress, but there is no evidence that this treatment is effective. Equivocal evidence hints that valerian, alone or with lemon balm, might reduce anxiety symptoms during stressful situations.

Many people report that they experience stress relief through the use of alternative therapies such as biofeedback, guided imagery, hypnotherapy, massage, relaxation therapy, Tai Chi, and yoga. One study failed to find regular massage more effective for controlling stress than the use of a relaxation tape. Another study failed to find either cognitive behavioral therapy or increased physical activity helpful for stress-related illnesses. Three studies failed to find Bach flower remedies helpful for situational anxiety (anxiety caused by stressful situations).

—*EBSCO CAM Review Board*

Further Reading

Ellis, J. M., and P. Reddy. "Effects of *Panax ginseng* on Quality of Life." *Annals of Pharmacotherapy*, vol. 36, 2002, pp. 375–79.

Halberstein, R., et al. "Healing with Bach Flower Essences: Testing a Complementary Therapy." *Complementary Health Practice Review*, vol. 12, 2007, pp. 3–14.

Heiden, M., et al. "Evaluation of Cognitive Behavioural Training and Physical Activity for Patients with Stress-Related Illnesses." *Journal of Rehabilitative Medicine*, vol. 39, 2007, pp. 366–73.

Jager, R., et al. "The Effect of Phosphatidylserine on Golf Performance." *Journal of the International Society of Sports Nutrition*, vol. 4, 2007, p. 23.

Kim, J. H., et al. "Efficacy of Alpha-S1-Casein Hydrolysate on Stress-Related Symptoms in Women." *European Journal of Clinical Nutrition*, vol. 61, 2007, pp. 536–41.

Kraemer, W. J., et al. "Cortitrol Supplementation Reduces Serum Cortisol Responses to Physical Stress." *Metabolism*, vol. 54, 2005, pp. 657–68.

"Six Relaxation Techniques to Reduce Stress." Harvard Medical School. *Harvard Health Publishing*, 2009, www.health.harvard.edu/mind-and-mood/six-relaxation-techniques-to-reduce-stress. Accessed 25 Aug. 2020.

Natural Treatments for Well-Being

ABSTRACT

Treatments that improve a person's overall sense of wellness through resolving specific medical conditions include vitamin and mineral supplements.

INTRODUCTION

It is one of the cardinal principles of natural medicine that treatment should aim not only to treat illness but also to enhance well-being, or wellness. According to this ideal, a proper course of treatment should improve the sense of general well-being, enhance immunity to illness, raise physical stamina, and increase mental alertness; it should also resolve specific medical conditions.

While there can be little doubt that this is a laudable goal, it is easier to laud it than to achieve it. Conventional medicine tends to focus on treating diseases rather than on increasing wellness, not as a matter of philosophical principle, but because it is easier to accomplish.

One strong force affecting wellness is genetics. Beyond this, commonsense steps endorsed by all physicians include increasing exercise, reducing stress, improving diet, getting enough sleep, and living a life of moderation without bad habits, such as smoking or overeating. However, it is difficult to make strong affirmations, and the optimum forms of diet and exercise and other aspects of lifestyle remain unclear. They may always remain unclear, as it is impossible to perform double-blind, placebo-controlled studies on most lifestyle habits. A 2012 review of national data showed that most people often use yoga and dietary supplements for wellness. Those who use complementary approaches report better overall health, higher rates of physical activity, and lower rates of obesity.

PRINCIPAL PROPOSED NATURAL TREATMENTS

Although no natural treatments have been proven effective for enhancing overall wellness, two have shown promise: multivitamin-multimineral tablets and the herb *Panax ginseng*.

Multivitamin-multimineral supplements. To function at their best, humans need good nutrition. However, the modern diet often fails to provide people with sufficient amounts of all the necessary nutrients. For this reason, the use of a multivitamin-multimineral supplement might be expected to enhance overall health and well-being, and preliminary double-blind trials generally support this view.

For example, in one double-blind study, eighty healthy men between the ages of eighteen and forty-two were given either a multivitamin-multimineral supplement or placebo and followed for twenty-eight days. The results showed that the use of the nutritional supplement improved several measures of well-being. Similarly, an eight-week, double-blind, placebo-controlled study of ninety-five people with careers in middle management also found improvements in well-being. Furthermore, several studies have found that multivitamin-multimineral supplements can improve immunity in older people. General nutritional supplements may also help improve response to stress.

Panax ginseng. The herb *Panax ginseng* has an ancient reputation as a healthful tonic. According to a more modern concept developed in the former Soviet Union, ginseng functions as an adaptogen. An adaptogen helps the body adapt to stresses of various kinds, whether heat, cold, exertion, trauma, sleep deprivation, toxic exposure, radiation, infection, or psychologic stress. In addition, an adaptogen causes no side effects, is effective in treating many illnesses, and helps return an organism toward balance no matter what may have gone wrong.

From a modern scientific perspective, it is not truly clear that such things as adaptogens actually exist. However, there is some evidence that ginseng may satisfy some of the definition's requirements.

Several studies have found that ginseng can improve the overall sense of well-being. For example, such benefits were seen in a twelve-week double-blind trial that evaluated the effects of *P. ginseng* extract in 625 people. The average age of the participants was just under forty years old. Each participant received a multivitamin supplement daily, but for one set of participants, the multivitamin also contained ginseng. Level of well-being was measured by a set of eleven questions. The results showed that people taking the ginseng-containing supplement reported significant improvement compared to those taking the supplement without ginseng.

Similarly, positive findings were reported in a double-blind, placebo-controlled study of thirty-six people newly diagnosed with diabetes. After eight weeks, participants who had been taking 200 milligrams (0.04 tsp) of ginseng daily reported improvements in mood, well-being, vigor, and psychophysical performance that were significant compared to the reports of control participants.

A twelve-week, double-blind, placebo-controlled study of 120 people found that ginseng improved general well-being among women aged thirty to sixty years and men aged forty to sixty years, but not among men aged thirty to thirty-nine years. This finding is possibly consistent with the traditional theory that ginseng is more effective for older people. Other results suggest this as well. A double-blind, placebo-controlled trial of thirty young people found marginal benefits at most, and a sixty-day, double-blind, placebo-controlled trial of eighty-three adults in their mid-twenties found no effect.

In addition, ginseng has shown some potential for enhancing immunity, mental function, and sports performance. These are all effects consistent with the adaptogen concept.

OTHER PROPOSED NATURAL TREATMENTS

Besides *P. ginseng*, certain other herbs are regarded as adaptogens, including *Eleutherococcus senticosus* (Siberian ginseng), *Rhodiola rosacea*, ashwagandha, astragalus, suma, schisandra, and the Asian mushrooms maitake, shiitake, and reishi. Meaningful supporting evidence for their benefits, however, is scant. In one of the better studies, a small, double-blind, placebo-controlled trial of *R. rosacea*, the herb seemed to improve physical and mental performance and sense of well-being in students under stress.

Although garlic is not generally regarded as an adaptogen, one study found that garlic powder (but not garlic oil) enhanced well-being. However, another study failed to find such benefits with garlic powder. So-called green juices made from such substances as spirulina and wheat grass are widely marketed for enhancing well-being. A double-blind study found that the use of one such product improved general vitality, but so did placebo, and the differences between the outcomes in the two groups were marginal.

Levels of the hormone dehydroepiandrosterone (DHEA) naturally decrease with age, and for this reason DHEA supplements have been widely hyped as a kind of fountain of youth. However, several studies have found that DHEA supplementation does not improve mood or increase the general sense of well-being in older people. A relatively large (about five hundred participants) double-blind study also failed to find selenium helpful in the elderly. Also, a smaller study failed to find evidence that vitamin B_{12} improved the general sense of well-being among elderly people with signs of mild B_{12} deficiency.

In some branches of alternative medicine, low levels of thyroid hormone are believed to be a common cause of impaired well-being. As part of this theory, it is said that the most commonly used medical form of thyroid replacement therapy (thyroxine, also called T4) is inadequate. Supposedly, better results are obtained when T4 is taken with the thyroid hormone known as T3, often in the form of "natural thyroid" extracted from animal thyroid glands. However, a double-blind study of 110 people designed to test this theory failed to find combined T3-T4 more effective than T4 alone.

Practitioners and other proponents of yoga have long claimed that its gentle stretching exercises, special breathing techniques, and deep meditative states enhance overall health. However, there is only limited evidence that yoga improves general well-being and quality of life.

Numerous other alternative therapies are claimed by their proponents to improve overall wellness, including acupuncture, Ayurveda, chiropractic, detoxification, homeopathy, massage, naturopathy, osteopathic manipulation, Reiki, Tai Chi, therapeutic touch, traditional Chinese herbal medicine, and yoga. However, there is little meaningful evidence to support these claims.

—*EBSCO CAM Review Board*

Further Reading

Dayal, M., et al. "Supplementation with DHEA: Effect on Muscle Size, Strength, Quality of Life, and Lipids." *Journal of Women's Health*, vol. 14, 2005, pp. 391–400.

Ellis, J. M., and P. Reddy. "Effects of *Panax ginseng* on Quality of Life." *Annals of Pharmacotherapy*, vol. 36, 2002, pp. 375–79.

Graat, J. M., E. G. Schouten, and F. J. Kok. "Effect of Daily Vitamin E and Multivitamin-Mineral Supplementation on Acute Respiratory Tract Infections in Elderly Persons." *Journal of the American Medical Association*, vol. 288, 2002, pp. 715–21.

Kjellgren, A., et al. "Wellness Through a Comprehensive Yogic Breathing Program." *BMC Complementary and Alternative Medicine*, vol. 7, 2007, p. 43.

Oken, B. S., et al. "Randomized, Controlled, Six-Month Trial of Yoga in Healthy Seniors: Effects on Cognition and Quality of Life." *Alternative Therapies in Health and Medicine*, vol. 12, 2006, pp. 40–47.

Rayman, M., et al. "Impact of Selenium on Mood and Quality of Life." *Biological Psychiatry*, vol. 59, 2006, pp. 147–54.

"Wellness and Well-Being." National Institutes of Health. National Center for Complementary and Integrative Health. *National Institutes of Health*, www.nccih.nih.gov/health/wellness-and-well-being. Accessed 25 Aug. 2020.

THERAPEUTIC TOUCH (TT)

ABSTRACT

Therapeutic touch (TT) is a technique in which the placement of hands just above a person's body is used for healing.

OVERVIEW

Therapeutic touch (TT) is a form of energy healing popular in nursing in the United States. In the words of its official organization, "Therapeutic Touch is an intentionally directed process of energy exchange during which the practitioner uses the hands as a focus to facilitate the healing process." TT is used by nurses in a variety of settings, from the medical office to the intensive care unit (ICU). However, there is no meaningful evidence that it is effective.

TT was developed in the early 1970s by two people: Dolores Krieger and a self-professed healer, Dora Van Gelder Kunz. Initially, TT involved setting the hands lightly on the body of the patient, but the method rapidly evolved into a noncontact energy healing method. Certified practitioners can be found in virtually all parts of the United States and in much of the world. TT is available in mainstream healthcare facilities including hospices, hospital-based alternative health programs, and even ICUs.

TT is sometimes described as a scientific version of "laying on of hands," a technique practiced by faith healers. However, there is more spirituality than science to this method; it makes use of beliefs and principles common in spiritual healing traditions but unknown to current science.

According to TT, the body has an energy field, and without physical contact, the energy field of one person can substantially affect the energy field of another. The practitioner is said to heal, balance, replenish, and improve the flow of a person's energy field, thereby leading to enhanced overall wellness. However, there is no meaningful scientific evidence for any of these beliefs.

SCIENTIFIC EVIDENCE

There has been considerable research interest in TT. However, the evidence for benefit is no more than weakly positive at best. A 1999 review of all published studies concluded that many of the studies had serious design flaws that could bias the results; in addition, the manner in which they were reported did not meet adequate scientific standards. A similar review in 2008 focusing on pain concluded that TT (along with healing touch and Reiki) may have modest effects on pain relief, particularly in the hands of more experienced practitioners, but the evidence was still fairly weak. A literature review of the use of TT in cancer patients affirmed that TT as a noninvasive intervention was a useful strategy in patients with cancer with positive effects on pain, nausea, anxiety and fatigue.

To be fair, proper study of TT presents researchers with some serious obstacles. The only truly meaningful way to determine whether a medical therapy works is to perform a double-blind, placebo-controlled trial. For hands-on therapies such as TT, however, a truly double-blind study is not possible, as the TT practitioner will inevitably know whether he or she is administering real TT or fake TT.

The best type of study that can be performed on TT is a single-blind study with "blinded" observers. In such studies, participants do not know whether they received real or fake TT, and an observer who also is blinded evaluates their medical outcome. However, such a study still has potential bias; practitioners could communicate a kind of cynicism when they use fake TT, and this problem appears to be insurmountable.

Further problems are involved in the choice of fake treatment. In most of the studies described here, sham TT involved practitioners counting backward in their heads by subtracting 7 serially from 100. The intent of this method was to avoid any possibility of projecting a healing concentration. It has been pointed out that this somewhat stressful effort would cause the practitioner to communicate tension rather than relaxation to study participants, and this too could bias results. However, it is difficult to suggest what should have been used instead as a placebo.

Some studies compared TT with no treatment. However, it has been well established that any therapy whatsoever will seem to produce benefit compared to no treatment for various nonspecific reasons; because of this, such studies say little to nothing about the specific benefits of TT. Finally, numerous trials have simply involved enrolling people with a medical problem, applying TT, and seeing whether they improve. Trials of this type prove nothing. Given these caveats, a summary of the research available thus far is presented here.

At the time of the 1999 review already noted, many published studies of TT were of unacceptably low quality and the results were quite inconsistent. For example, in one trial, thirty-one inpatients in a Veteran's Administration psychiatric facility received TT, relaxation therapy, or sham TT. The study was designed to evaluate the effectiveness of TT for reducing anxiety and stress. The results appear to indicate that TT was more effective for this purpose than the sham form. However, there are some serious design problems in this study that make the results difficult to trust. The real TT was administered by a woman in "street" clothes and the placebo treatment by a woman in a nursing uniform; to make matters more complex, the relaxation therapy was administered by a man dressed as a clergyman. These large differences in appearance could only be expected to considerably influence the results in ways that cannot be predicted.

In a better study, sixty people with tension headaches were randomly assigned to receive either TT or placebo touch. TT proved to be significantly more effective than placebo touch. However, in a reasonably well-designed study published in 1993, the use of TT in 108 people undergoing surgery failed to reduce postoperative pain to a greater extent than sham TT.

A series of studies evaluated TT for aiding wound healing. Some found TT more effective than placebo, others found no significant effect, and still others found placebo more effective than real treatment. These results suggest that the effects seen were caused by chance.

Subsequent to the 1999 review, several better-quality trials were published. One such study compared real TT and sham TT in ninety-nine men and women recovering from severe burns. Researchers hypothesized that the use of TT would decrease pain and anxiety during that arduous and traumatic process, and indeed some evidence of benefit was seen.

In a smaller study (twenty-five participants), real TT appeared to reduce the pain of knee osteoarthritis compared to sham TT. Furthermore, in a study of twenty children with human immunodeficiency virus infection, the use of TT improved anxiety while sham touch did not. Another study found that an actor pretending to perform treatment similar to TT produced significant improvements in well-being in people with advanced cancer.

Taking all these studies together, it appears that real TT may be more effective than sham TT (using the serial subtraction technique). However, whether these apparent benefits are caused by the energy-healing effects claimed by practitioners or, more simply, through emotional communication, remains unclear.

Some studies provide preliminary evidence that TT does not work in the manner practitioners believe it does. For example, in one well-designed study, TT produced no effect when conducted without eye contact. The researcher, an influential person in the history of TT, had hypothesized that TT involved a kind of energy transfer that would not need eye contact. The fact that no effects were seen without the addition of eye contact suggests that it might be focused attention that makes the difference, not energy transmitted through the hands.

Furthermore, if TT actually involves contact with a person's "energy field," it would seem that the practitioners would be able to sense the presence of such a field. However, in a widely publicized study, twenty-one practitioners who had practiced TT for one to twenty-seven years proved unable to do this. In this trial, TT practitioners placed their hands face up through holes in a barrier. The experimenter (a nine-year-old student) held a hand above one of the practitioner's hands, and the practitioner was asked to sense its presence. The practitioners' guesses proved to be no more accurate than chance would allow. This study has been strongly criticized by proponents of TT. Some said that the experimenter was in the throes of puberty, and for that reason her energy field was too disturbed to detect; others complained about the disturbing presence of video cameras. While these criticisms are potentially valid, the burden is actually on proponents of TT to prove that there really is such a thing as a human energy field.

Nonetheless, the studies already performed do indicate that, at minimum, concentrated, positive attention provided by one human being to another is consoling and calming. This is a wonderful fact, even if there is no special energy field involved.

WHAT TO EXPECT DURING TREATMENT

Therapeutic touch is generally administered in a session that lasts about twenty minutes. The patient will be asked to lie still, relax, and remain quiet. The practitioner will place his or her hands a few inches above the person's body and move them slowly and rhythmically.

Some people experience a variety of subjective sensations while receiving TT, such as heat and moving energy. Most people find TT generally relaxing, but some undergo cathartic emotional experiences.

CHOOSING A PRACTITIONER

The original and most well-established TT organization is Therapeutic Touch International Association. This organization certifies training programs in TT.

SAFETY ISSUES

There are no known or suspected safety risks with TT.

—*EBSCO CAM Review Board*

Further Reading

Coakley, A. B., and M. E. Duffy. "The Effect of Therapeutic Touch on Postoperative Patients." *Journal of Holistic Nursing*, vol. 28, 2010, pp. 193–200.

Peters, R. M. "The Effectiveness of Therapeutic Touch." *Nursing Science Quarterly*, vol. 12, 1999, pp. 52–61.

Pohl, G., et al. "'Laying on of Hands' Improves Well-Being in Patients with Advanced Cancer." *Supportive Care in Cancer*, vol. 15, 2007, pp. 143–51.

Rosa, L., et al. "A Close Look at Therapeutic Touch." *Journal of the American Medical Association*, vol. 279, 1998, pp. 1005–10.

So, P. S., Y. Jiang, and Y. Qin. "Touch Therapies for Pain Relief in Adults." *Cochrane Database of Systematic Reviews*, 2008. EBSCO DynaMed Systematic Literature Surveillance, CD006535, 2008.

Tabatabaee A., M. Z. Tafreshi, and M. Rassouli, et al. "Effect of Therapeutic Touch in Patients with Cancer: A Literature Review." *Medical Archives*, 2016, pubmed.ncbi.nlm.nih.gov/27194823/. Accessed 25 Aug. 2020.

"What Is TT: How Did Therapeutic Touch Begin?" *Therapeutic Touch International Association*, www.therapeutictouch.org/what-is-tt/. Accessed 25 Aug. 2020.

Reiki

ABSTRACT

Reiki is a form of spiritual healing that involves holding hands in certain positions over parts of the body to improve energy flow.

OVERVIEW

The Japanese word *reiki* can be translated as "life-force energy." The term refers to a form of spiritual healing that involves holding one's hands on or above another's body in order to supposedly manipulate energy fields. Many people have taken training in Reiki, and the service is provided in a variety of settings, including some hospitals. However, there is no scientific foundation in support of Reiki's effectiveness for any purpose.

History of Reiki. There are two principal stories regarding the origin of Reiki. In both versions, the method was invented in Japan by Mikao Usui. Many Reiki practitioners in the United States believe that Usui was a Christian monk who invented the technique in the mid-nineteenth century. However, according to the more traditional Japanese schools of Reiki, Usui was a member of a Japanese spiritual organization called Rei Jyutsu Ka, and he developed the technique around 1915. (The story that he was a Christian may have been invented to facilitate the acceptance of Reiki in the West.) Both versions of Reiki's history agree that Usui based his technique on methods and philosophies drawn from numerous Asian traditional healing methods.

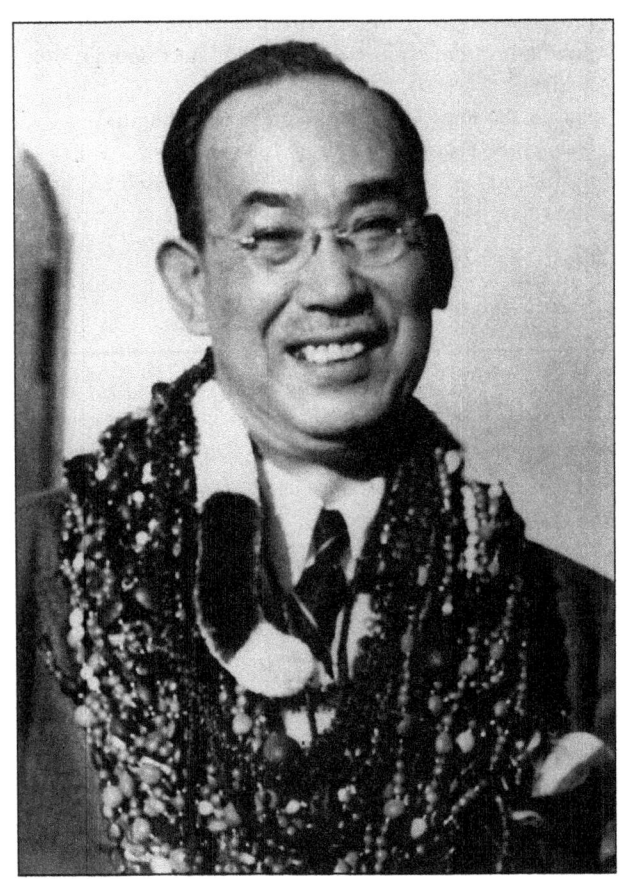

Chujiro Hayashi (Wikimedia Commons)

After Usui's death, various forms of Reiki continued to be taught by his students. One of these students, Chujiro Hayashi, systematized Reiki into three levels and added many hand movements to the technique. In turn, one of Hayashi's students, Hawayo Takata, brought Reiki to the United States.

In the early 1980s, Takata's granddaughter, Phyllis Furumoto, took on the mantle of Hayashi and Takata's line of Reiki and popularized it widely in the West. However, many other forms of Reiki continue to exist, descending through different lineages of teachers. There are considerable differences between the various approaches, and certain groups strongly challenge the validity of others.

What is Reiki? Most types of Asian traditional medicine make use of the concept of qi (also spelled ch'i and other forms), a form of vital energy that flows through the body. Free-flowing, abundant qi is said to create health, while stagnant or deficient qi is thought to lead to illness. Reiki practitioners believe that they can improve this energy by holding their hands in certain positions over parts of a person's body; advanced practitioners believe they can produce this effect from a distance. The net result, according to the theory, is accelerated healing and increased wellness.

In many ways, Reiki resembles therapeutic touch (TT), except that the instructions given to its practitioners are more specific. A certified practitioner of Reiki has spent time learning specified hand movements and positions and has also undergone an "attunement" to an already-certified Reiki practitioner. This chain of attunements goes back to Usui, the method's founder.

In its most popular Western form, Reiki is learned in three stages. The first stage involves an attunement that allegedly permits physical healing. The second stage supposedly grants the ability to carry out healing over a distance. The third degree of training is said to allow the practitioner to perform healing on a spiritual level and to give attunements to students.

Generally, each level is obtained by paying a fee and completing a weekend course.

USES AND APPLICATIONS

Reiki is promoted as a treatment that can accelerate physical, emotional, or spiritual healing in every conceivable situation. It is used as a support for conventional medical care, rather than as a replacement for it. Reiki has also been incorporated in some workplace wellness initiatives to combat stress, much like other complementary therapies such as massage and meditation.

SCIENTIFIC EVIDENCE

The only truly meaningful way to determine whether a medical therapy works is to perform a double-blind, placebo-controlled trial. For hands-on therapies such as Reiki, however, a truly double-blind study is not possible; the Reiki practitioner will inevitably know whether they are administering real Reiki rather than fake Reiki. The best that can be hoped for is a single-blind study in which participants do not know whether they received real or fake Reiki and in which the medical outcome is evaluated by an observer who also does not know who is or is not receiving real Reiki and is, therefore, "blinded."

In a 2008 review of nine randomized-controlled trials on the effectiveness of Reiki for various purposes, researchers stated that no firm conclusions could be drawn from any of these studies. In a subsequent controlled trial, one hundred persons with fibromyalgia received Reiki or direct-touch therapy from either a

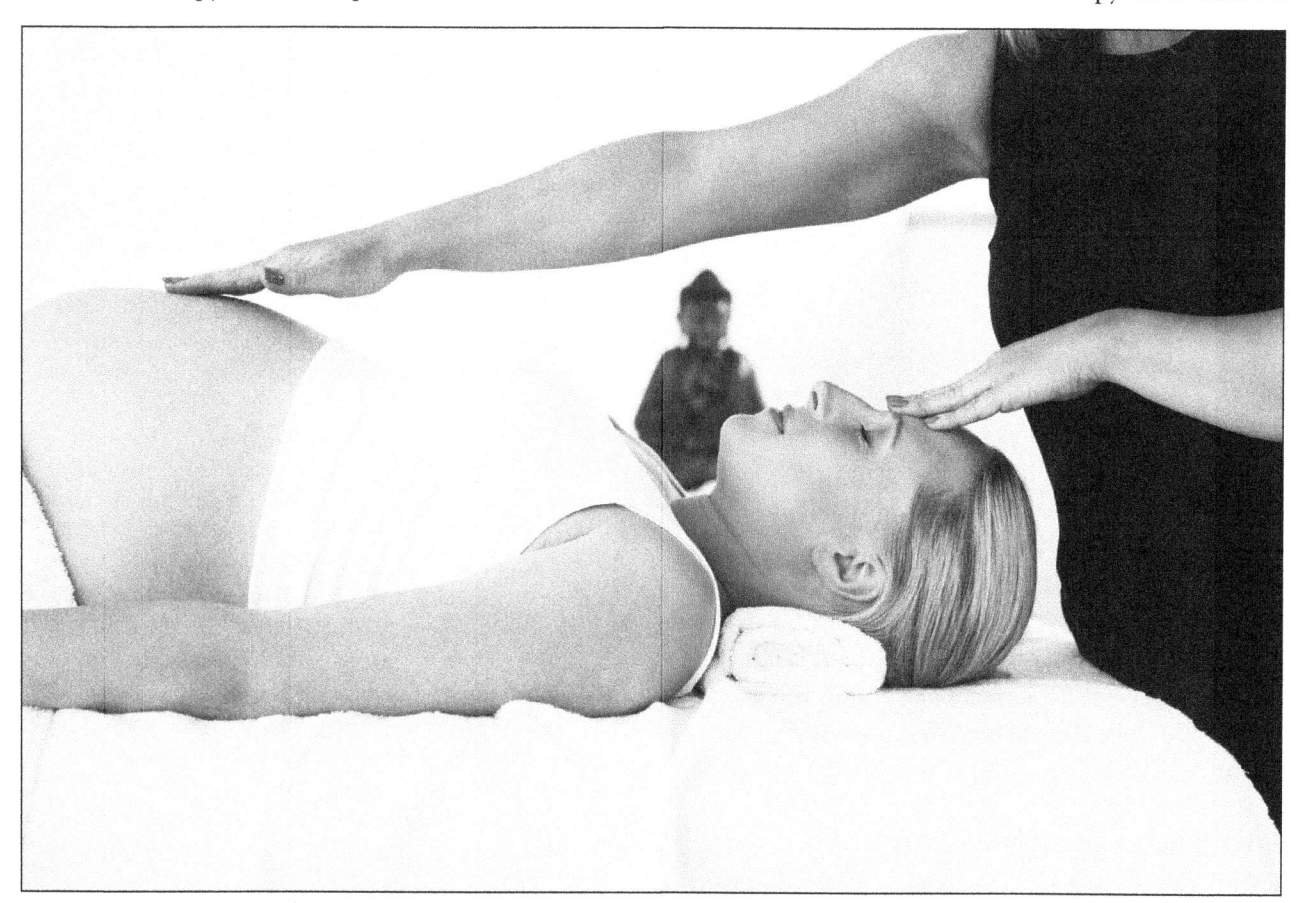

Pregnant woman getting a Reiki massage (Dean Mitchell via iStock)

true Reiki master or an actor posing as a Reiki master. There was no difference in symptom improvement between the two groups. In one review of three Reiki studies, researchers found that more experienced practitioners appeared to have a greater effect on pain reduction. This observation could not be explained.

A simpler study design compares Reiki to no treatment. However, studies of this type cannot provide reliable evidence about the efficacy of a treatment: If a benefit is seen, there is no way to determine whether it was caused by Reiki specifically or just by attention generally. (Attention alone will almost always produce some reported benefit.)

Finally, there are many case reports in which people are given Reiki and then seem to improve. Such reports do not mean anything scientifically; numerous people receiving placebo in placebo-controlled studies also seem to improve. Thus, such reports cannot say anything about whether Reiki itself offers any benefit.

In one study, female nursing students received either real Reiki or a placebo form of the treatment called mimic Reiki. Before-and-after tests failed to find any improvement in general well-being attributable to Reiki treatment.

In another study, researchers evaluated the effectiveness of Reiki (with a related technique called LeShan) in twenty-one people undergoing oral surgery for impacted wisdom teeth. Each participant received two surgeries, one with Reiki and the other without (in random order). People reported less pain when they received Reiki than when they received no treatment; however, because of the lack of a fake treatment group, the results mean little. The US National Center for Complementary and Integrative Health continues to classify Reiki as an unproven treatment with a deficiency of high-quality research.

CHOOSING A PRACTITIONER

There are several competing organizations that issue certifications to Reiki practitioners. These include the Reiki Alliance, the Reiki Foundation, and the Awareness Institute. However, as there is no official regulation of Reiki practice, medical professionals often warn that patients should use due diligence in choosing a reputable practitioner.

SAFETY ISSUES

There are no known or proposed safety risks with Reiki unless a person chooses to use Reiki instead of, rather than as a support to, standard medical care. Using any complementary or alternative medicine as the only treatment for a condition may cause the condition to persist or worsen.

—EBSCO CAM Review Board

Further Reading

Assefi, N., et al. "Reiki for the Treatment of Fibromyalgia." *Journal of Alternative and Complementary Medicine*, vol. 14, 2008, pp. 1115–22.

Lack, Caleb W., and Jacques Rousseau. *Critical Thinking, Science, and Pseudoscience: Why We Can't Trust Our Brains*. Springer, 2016.

Lee, M. S., M. H. Pittler, and E. Ernst. "Effects of Reiki in Clinical Practice." *International Journal of Clinical Practice*, vol. 62, 2008, pp. 947–54.

"Reiki." *Cancer Research UK*, 22 Jan. 2019, www.cancerresearchuk.org/about-cancer/cancer-in-general/treatment/complementary-alternative-therapies/individual-therapies/reiki.

"Reiki." *Johns Hopkins Medicine, Integrative Medicine & Digestive Center*, www.hopkinsmedicine.org/integrative_medicine_digestive_center/services/reiki.html. Accessed 1 May. 2020.

"Reiki." National Center for Complementary and Integrative Health. *US National Institutes of Health*, Dec. 2018, www.nccih.nih.gov/health/reiki. Accessed 1 May. 2020.

Richeson, N. E., et al. "Effects of Reiki on Anxiety, Depression, Pain, and Physiological Factors in Community-Dwelling Older Adults." *Research in Gerontological Nursing*, vol. 3, 2010, pp. 187–99.

So, P. S., Y. Jiang, and Y. Qin. "Touch Therapies for Pain Relief in Adults." *Cochrane Database of Systematic Reviews*, 2008. *EBSCO DynaMed Systematic Literature Surveillance*, CD006535, 2008.

Thornton, L. C. "A Study of Reiki, an Energy Field Treatment, Using Rogers' Science." *Rogerian Nursing Science News*, vol. 8, 1996, pp. 14–15.

"What Can I Expect in a Typical Reiki Session?" University of Minnesota. Taking Charge of Your Health & Wellbeing, https://www.takingcharge.csh.umn.edu/what-can-i-expect-typical-reiki-session. Accessed 1 May. 2020.

ROLFING

ABSTRACT
Rolfing is a vigorous deep tissue massage therapy designed to improve the body's overall skeletal structure and posture through collagen integration.

OVERVIEW
Rolfing is a method of deeply massaging all the connective tissue, known as fascia, between muscles, bones, ligaments, and tendons in the body in an effort to realign and restructure the overall skeletal composition. Rolfing therapy was invented in the 1930s by Ida Rolf, a biochemist, in an attempt to treat her own scoliosis and that of her two sons after being dissatisfied with the results of yoga, osteopathy, and homeopathy.

MECHANISM OF ACTION
Using hands, fingers, knuckles, elbows, and knees to apply intense pressure to inner collagen fiber, a rolfing therapist attempts to stretch and reshape the connective tissue, or fascia, between bones, tendons, muscles, and ligaments. On the theory that the skeletal structure follows the fascial makeup, rolfing therapy primarily seeks to establish increased fascial elasticity. Once tightened, fascia is unbound and lengthened through manipulation; the muscles, tendons, ligaments, and bones, which the fascia is attached to, may also then relax and realign after improper structure caused by gravity, inertia, sedentariness, repetitive movement, disease, or injury.

The first three sessions of rolfing therapy focus on massaging superficial tissue and improving breathing; the next four sessions involve deep manipulation of interior tissue structure; and the final three sessions integrate all parts of the body's skeleton through fascial redistribution and connection. After ten sessions of sixty to ninety minutes of rolfing using deep tissue reintegration, the practitioner can then rediscover proper skeletal balance, form, and posture and then release accumulated stress and energy.

USES AND APPLICATIONS
Rolfing is used primarily to reduce stress, alleviate pain, increase mobility, improve posture, and facilitate coordination. Rolfing is also frequently used in treating sports injuries and repetitive strain injuries, such as rotator cuff injuries.

SCIENTIFIC EVIDENCE
No double-blind, placebo-controlled studies of rolfing have been conducted, but there have been other scientific studies on the method. In 1963, the first major studies of rolfing being performed on children at the Foundation of Brain Injured Children concluded that after ten sessions, the impaired children improved in motor skills, muscle tone, posture, and coordination. In the 1970s, published scientific studies documented muscle tone, strength, and elasticity both before and after rolfing therapy, with empirical medical testing used to measure increased muscle performance. In 1981, a study was published that documented the improved lower body movement and mobility of persons with cerebral palsy who had been treated with rolfing therapy.

In 1988, a test revealed improved pelvic inclination in a group of women after rolfing therapy sessions, and in 1997, a study documented the decrease of low back pain in persons who had received rolfing therapy. In the late 1990s, various studies looked at rolfing to treat repetitive strain injuries, such as carpal tunnel syndrome; all showed significant improvement after rolfing therapy. Also, in the late 1990s, a study revealed that a group of elderly persons maintained improved balance after receiving rolfing therapy. Whether or not any of the above studies would have achieved the same positive results using any other therapy or technique is unknown, as no comparisons of dissimilar treatments were employed. Moreover, because no placebo or double-blind groups were implemented in any of the studies, there is no reliable scientific evidence to support these studies' claims, and the true efficacy of rolfing therapy remains unproven.

CHOOSING A PRACTITIONER

Ideally, one should choose a practitioner who is certified by the Rolf Institute of Structural Integration, headquartered in Boulder, Colorado. To achieve even basic rolfing certification, students must take advanced training of one to two years beyond traditional massage techniques. Many therapists claim to be well versed in the art of rolfing, yet these same therapists are often only superficially familiar with its specific techniques. Because rolfing involves deep tissue manipulation, treatment from a therapist who is not certified or licensed by the institute poses a risk of injury.

SAFETY ISSUES

Persons with rheumatoid arthritis and other serious inflammatory medical conditions should avoid rolfing because it may exacerbate or worsen these conditions. Likewise, all persons who are frail or fragile should abstain from rolfing, inasmuch as the intense nature of the treatments may result in subsequent bone fractures. Additionally, pregnant women, especially after the first trimester, should seek out only those certified in the use of milder, modified rolfing techniques especially designed for use during pregnancy, or they should avoid rolfing therapy altogether.

—*Mary E. Markland*

Further Reading

Anson, Briah. *Animal Healing: The Power of Rolfing*. Mill City Press, 2011.

Brecklinghaus, Hans. *Rolfing Structural Integration: What It Achieves, How It Works, and Whom It Helps*. Lightning Source, 2002.

"Complementary, Alternative or Integrative Health: What's in a Name?" National Center for Complementary and Integrative Health. National Institutes of Health, www.nccih.nih.gov/health/complementary-alternative-or-integrative-health-whats-in-a-name. Accessed 25 Aug. 2020.

Jacobson, E. E., A. L. Meleger, P. Bonato, et al. "Structural Integration as an Adjunct to Outpatient Rehabilitation for Chronic Nonspecific Low Back Pain: A Randomized Pilot Clinical Trial." *Evidence Based Complement Alternate Medicine*, 2015, pubmed.ncbi.nlm.nih.gov/25945112/. Accessed 25 Aug. 2020.

Rolf, Ida. *Rolfing: Reestablishing the Natural Alignment and Structural Integration of the Human Body for Vitality and Well-Being*. Healing Arts Press, 1989.

———, and Rosemary Feitis. *Rolfing and Physical Reality*. 2nd ed., Healing Arts Press, 1990.

Sise, Betsy. *The Rolfing Experience: Integration in the Gravity Field*. Hohm Press, 2005.

ART THERAPY

ABSTRACT

Art therapy is the combined use of psychotherapy and creative processes such as painting and drawing to enhance health and well-being.

OVERVIEW

According to the American Art Therapy Association (AATA), art therapy is based on knowledge of human developmental and psychological theories and is an effective treatment for people with developmental, medical, educational, social, or psychological problems. The theory behind art therapy is based partially on the belief that creativity and healing may come from the same place. According to experts, art therapy is not merely arts and crafts, or purely recre-

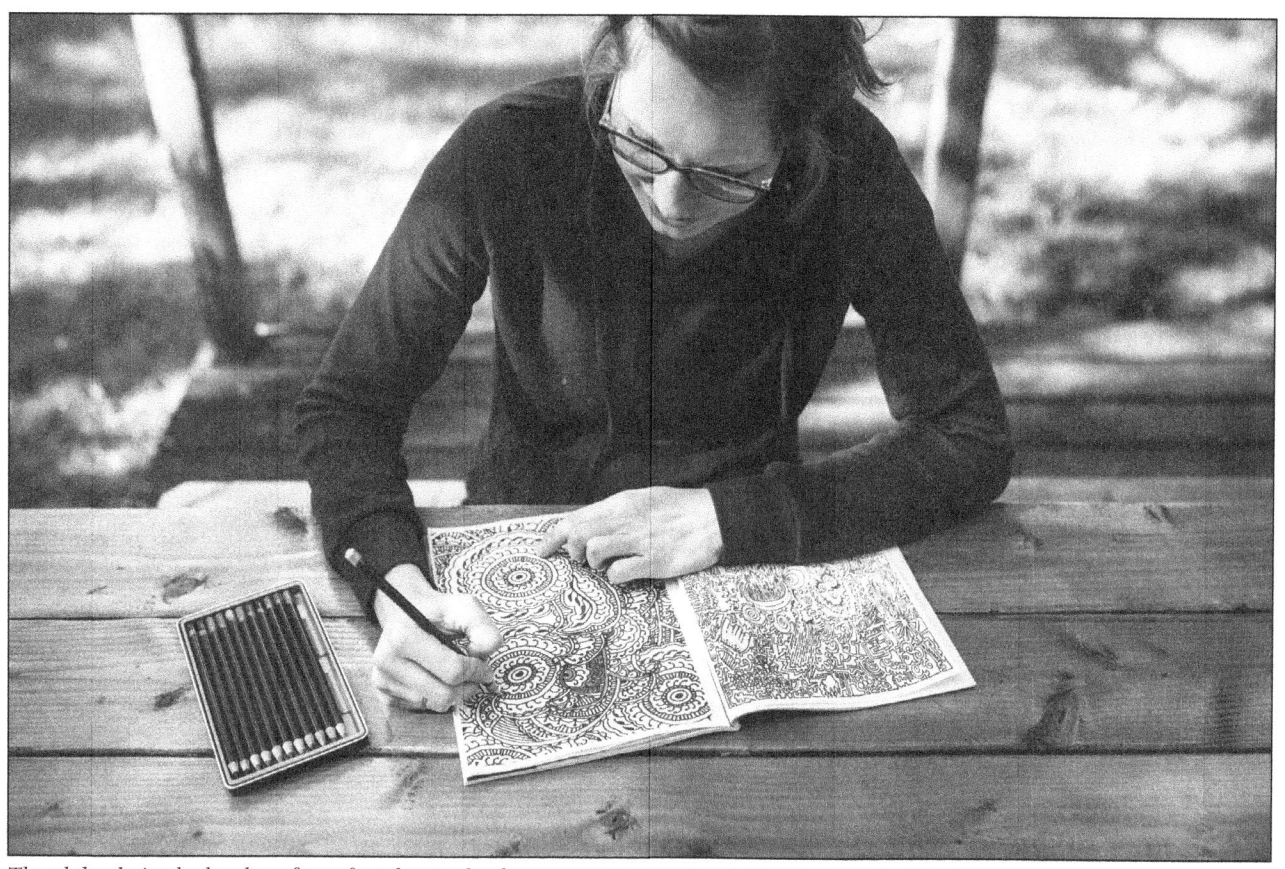

The adult coloring book, a loose form of art therapy, has become a mainstream trend (Ryan J Lane via iStock)

ational; it is multisensory and teaches people to use objects purposefully and to communicate their pain with the outside world. Often healthcare institutions may employ Art Therapists or provide referral to outside resources. The nurse is often the first to suggest art therapy for a patient and may work with the physician to obtain a physician order or referral if needed.

Although human beings have used art as a mode of expression for thousands of years, art therapy was not recognized as a distinct profession until the late 1930s, when Margaret Naumberg, now considered the founder of art therapy, advocated using art as a gateway to the subconscious in conjunction with free association and psychoanalytic interpretation.

Artist Adrian Hill took credit for inventing the term "art therapy" in 1942. While recovering from tuberculosis in a sanitarium, he felt that his own foray into art led to his emotional recovery. Introducing painting to his fellow patients, he found that they used artistic expression not only for enjoyment but also for expressing fears and emotions.

Recognizing that artwork could be useful in helping patients express internal conflicts, the psychiatric staff at the Menninger Clinic in Kansas began to employ art as therapy. The first journal in the field, *Bulletin of Art Therapy*, began publishing in 1961, and the AATA, a national professional organization that regulates educational, professional, and ethical standards for art therapists, was established in 1969.

MECHANISM OF ACTION

There are two different poles of art therapy: art psychotherapy and art as therapy. Proponents of art as therapy suggest that the process of creating art itself is curative and that verbal reflection, discussions, or interpretations about the art itself are not necessary. Advocates believe that creative activity increases brain levels of serotonin, a hormone associated with feelings of well-being, and gives rise to the alpha brainwave patterns typically seen during periods of relaxed alertness.

USES AND APPLICATIONS

Art psychotherapy proponents believe that artwork is most effective when used as a tool to elicit feelings, fears, and fantasies, which can then be worked through in traditional talk therapy. Regardless of their orientation, most contemporary art therapists integrate a variety of approaches, individualizing the treatment to best meet the needs of a specific client.

Special techniques are often particularly useful in helping people express their feelings, develop social skills, solve problems, reduce anxiety, or resolve emotional conflicts. In the unstructured approach, patients might select from a variety of materials and media (such as paint, pastels, and clay) and use them however they choose, allowing unconscious material to rise to the surface.

Then the therapist might ask the client to draw a family picture, which can help elicit complex family dynamics such as unhealthy patterns of relating or poor communication skills. Groups of people who share similar issues, such as having had cancer, might work together to create a collage or mural that can then be used to stimulate discussion of coping strategies.

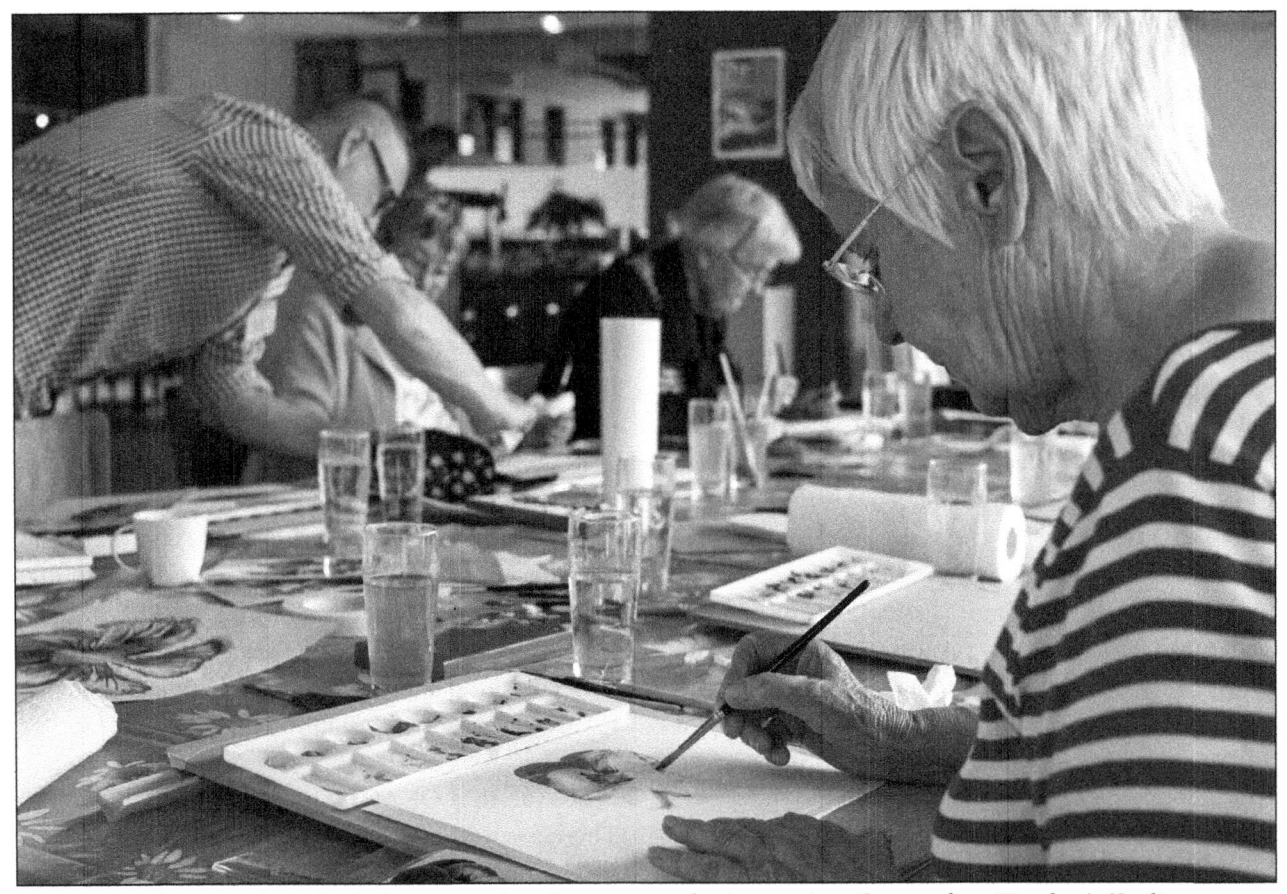

Art therapy can be conducted in individual or group sessions. Here, a group of seniors practice with watercolors. (Horsche via iStock)

Art therapists can practice alone or may be part of a treatment team that includes physicians, psychologists, nurses, social workers, counselors, and teachers. Art therapy, conducted in individual or group sessions, can be used with people of all ages, races, and ethnic backgrounds who have any one of a number of physical and emotional disorders. The adult coloring book, a loose form of art therapy, has become a mainstream trend.

CHOOSING A PRACTITIONER

Art therapists must possess a minimum of a master's degree and undergo a supervised practicum and a postgraduate internship before being certified for practice. Art therapists are registered (the credential ATR) or board certified (BC), or both, and practice in a variety of settings, including community mental health centers and psychiatric clinics; hospitals, rehabilitation facilities, and hospices; correctional facilities; nursing homes and senior centers; schools and early intervention programs; disaster relief centers; homeless shelters; and drug and alcohol rehabilitation programs.

Before referral to art therapy, determine if the service is free, requires a small fee or is reimbursable by the participant's insurance coverage. Some healthcare institutions provide art therapy as a value-added service at no charge to the patient. Some insurance plans may cover art therapy as part of comprehensive mental health or rehabilitative coverage but each plan is different and may require pre-certification. Support agencies in the community may offer art therapy free or at significantly reduced fee.

SAFETY ISSUES

There are no known safety concerns with art therapy.

—*Barbara Williams Cosentino and Brian Randall*

Further Reading

"About Art Therapy." *American Art Therapy Association*, www.arttherapy.org. Accessed 4 May 2020.
Art Therapy Credentials Board, www.atcb.org.
Canadian Art Therapy Association, canadianarttherapy.org/.
Cherry, Kendra. "How Art Therapy Is Used to Help People Heal." *Very Well Mind*, 28 Aug. 2019, www.verywellmind.com/what-is-art-therapy-2795755.
Craig, Claire. *Exploring the Self through Photography: Activities for Use in Group Work*. Jessica Kingsley, 2009.
Edwards, David. *Art Therapy*. Sage, 2004.
King, Juliet L. *Art Therapy, Trauma, and Neuroscience: Theoretical and Practical Perspectives*. Routledge, 2016.
Malchiodi, Cathy A. *The Art Therapy Sourcebook*. Rev. ed. McGraw, 2007.
Miller, Caroline. *Arts Therapists in Multidisciplinary Settings*. Jessica Kingsley, 2016.
Richardson, Carmen. *Expressive Arts Therapy for Traumatized Children and Adolescents: A Four-Phase Model*. Routledge, 2016.
Rubin, Judith Aron. *The Art of Art Therapy: What Every Art Therapist Needs to Know*. Brunner, 2011.

Music Therapy

ABSTRACT

Music therapy is the clinical and evidence-based use of music, including playing instruments and singing, in therapeutic practice.

OVERVIEW

The usefulness of music in medical settings has been recognized for more than two hundred years. It was initially used to distract patients from the monotony of a hospital stay, but the medical utility of music therapy is now being investigated as knowledge of the human brain increases. The American Music Therapy Association (AMTA) oversees professionals in the field of music therapy. In the United States, music-therapy education programs include multiple areas of study, clinical internships, and a national board certification examination.

Music therapy is frequently used in the treatment of persons with language deficits and in those persons recovering from strokes or traumatic brain injuries. Studies of healthy volunteers have identified the area of the brain that responds to and processes music; it is located within the right hemisphere. Other structures involved in experiencing music include the frontal lobe, limbic system, and imagery-related cortical regions of the temporal, parietal, and occipital lobes. The frontal lobe and the limbic system are also important structures in the formation of emotions, so the use of music may help persons with neurological conditions express themselves through means other than language.

As is well known, the left hemisphere of the brain controls language functions. Experts believe that melodic intonation therapy (MIT), which combines music with singing, may help children with autism develop language skills. (Many children with autism spectrum disorders have musical ability, so association of music with language may assist in the advancement of their language skills.) In the practice of MIT, the music component is removed after speech begins or improves; it is hoped that the child continues to develop. It is difficult, however, to determine if the development of language skills comes from music therapy or from the maturation of the child. Using the same MIT techniques, persons recovering from strokes or traumatic brain injuries who have suffered left-hemisphere damage may relearn speech using the right hemisphere of the brain. Although MIT was developed in 1973, the empirical evidence for using MIT for aphasia and apraxia of speech remains limited, as the studies conducted reported positive out-

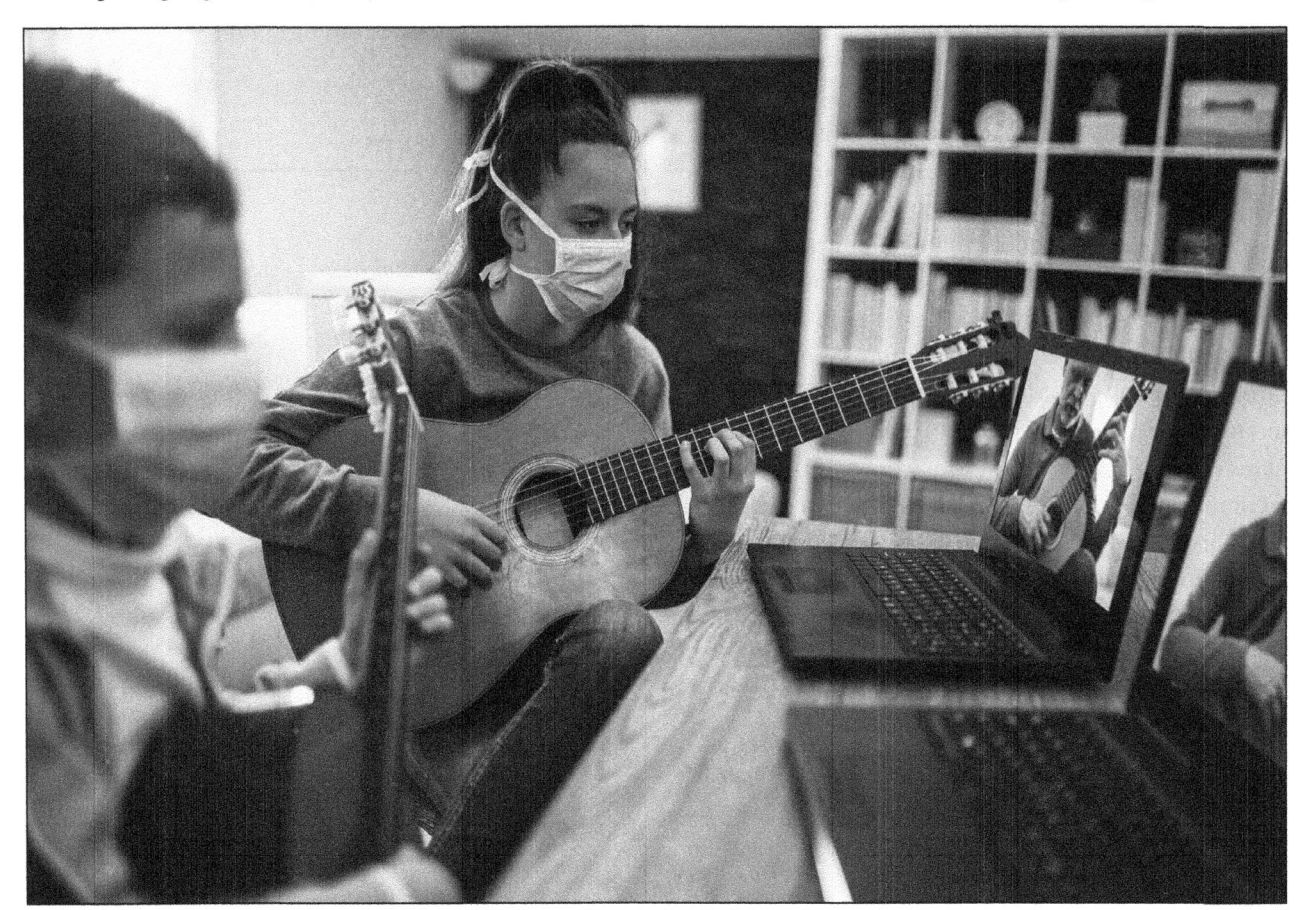

During the COVID-19 pandemic, music was a coping tool, providing emotional release and a way for people to remain connected during a difficult time. (Jovanmandic via iStock)

comes but suffered design flaws. At the same time, some studies aimed to determine whether modified forms of MIT, which could include additional techniques such as phonetic placement and tapping, could prove beneficial, particularly in use for aphasia.

Music therapy is also used with physical rehabilitation therapy and to alleviate symptoms similar to those of Parkinson's disease. During physical therapy, the rhythm of the music helps the person anticipate his or her next movement and move in a more smooth and natural manner. Persons with neurologic disorders suffering from shaking or spasms may be able to regain some control over their movements using rhythm to help them focus on regulating their movements.

Music therapy is often used as a pain management tool and in complex medical procedures in which the person must remain conscious. Music may alleviate mild to moderate pain through distraction, but it has not been effective for more painful procedures. It is unclear what, if any, effect music has on pain-detecting mechanisms in the brain. Alternative theories suggest that music therapy simply provides a distraction for a person with painful physical symptoms.

In 2014, a documentary titled *Alive Inside* premiered at the Sundance Film Festival, earning the event's Audience Award. The film highlights the increased interest in music therapy as a treatment tool for a wide range of physical and psychological issues as it presents various cases in which individuals have benefited from the experience of listening to music. In addition to these cases, the documentary also includes interviews from experts such as neurologist Oliver Sacks, who dedicated part of his career to studying the effects of music on the brain. The AMTA notes, however, that the music listening program featured in the documentary fails to meet criteria for clinical intervention.

MECHANISM OF ACTION

Although the exact mechanism of action of music therapy on the brain has yet to be elucidated, it is believed to affect areas of the brain controlling the autonomous nervous system. Music may help regulate the endocrine system and the autonomic nervous system. There is evidence that music affects areas of the temporal lobe of the brain associated with seizures, because persons with epilepsy have occasionally had seizures induced by music or have had audio hallucinations preceding a seizure.

USES AND APPLICATIONS

In active music therapy, the therapist and patient participate in playing music, such as using instruments or singing. In passive music therapy, music is played while the patient is in a relaxed state. There are five types of music therapy that may be used alone or in combination: receptive (listening to music to draw out an emotional response); compositional (the patient writes an original musical composition); improvisational (the music therapist and the patient spontaneously create music); re-creative (the patient learns to play an instrument); and activity (the patient and the therapist play musical games).

According to the AMTA, music therapy has been used to treat developmental disabilities, autism spec-

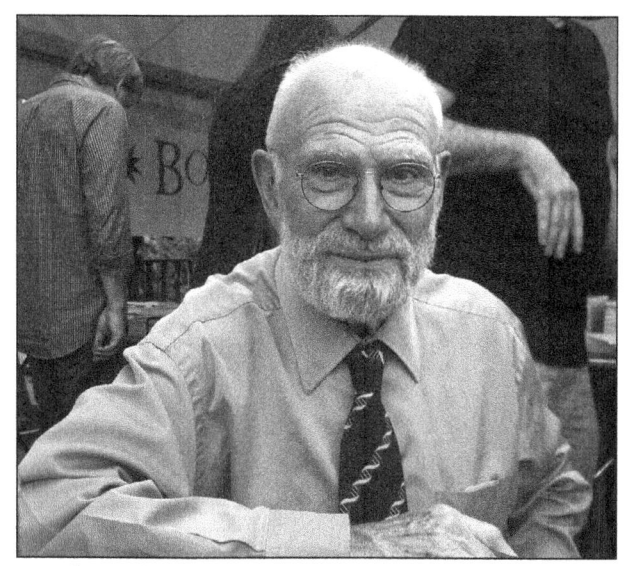

Neurologist Oliver Sacks dedicated part of his career to studying the effects of music on the brain. (Luigi Novi via Wikimedia Commons)

trum disorders, stroke, dementia and age-related conditions, psychiatric problems such as depression, substance abuse disorders, neurologic problems, and pain. It is also employed in neonatal intensive care, rehabilitation, and hospice. The psychological benefits of music were particularly discussed and highlighted during the outbreak of a novel coronavirus causing the disease COVID-19 that began in late 2019 and was declared a worldwide pandemic by March 2020. Though people in communities throughout the world suffered effects of depression and anxiety as they were compelled to isolate themselves in an effort to slow the spread of the disease, many reported that engaging with music helped to lift their spirits. While some were able to take part in virtual music therapy sessions offered through platforms such as Instagram and Zoom, others were able to listen to or take part in musical performances conducted on balconies. Often touted during the crisis as a potential coping tool, music was seen not only as a means of emotional release but also as a way for people to remain connected during a difficult time.

SCIENTIFIC EVIDENCE
The benefits of music therapy are difficult to quantify because each patient's treatment is customized based on the type and severity of disability or injury. No studies have compared the results of music therapy with other types of therapy, but there is a growing body of evidence in the form of controlled clinical studies seeming to support the effectiveness of music therapy.

In a study of forty-eight children with violent or aggressive behavior, twenty-four participated in a music intervention program and twenty-four did not take part in any therapy. The music intervention therapy comprised two music classes each week for fifteen weeks and was conducted by a certified music therapist in a group setting. At the end of the study, children who participated in the music therapy sessions demonstrated statistically significant improvements in aggressive behavior and self-esteem, as measured by questionnaires completed by parents and teachers.

Another study evaluated eighty-seven elderly, institutionalized persons with cerebrovascular disease; fifty-five persons received music therapy for forty-five minutes each week for a minimum of ten weeks, and twenty-two persons received no therapy. At the conclusion of the study, persons in the music-therapy group demonstrated statistically significant decreases in acute chronic heart failure and in plasma levels of cytokines, adrenaline, and noradrenaline. These results suggest that music therapy may be a useful tool in preventing heart failure in persons with cerebrovascular disease.

Several studies have investigated music therapy's effects in cancer treatment, with mixed results. A study of patients in hospice care suggested that pain control, the ability to relax, and overall comfort increased in those receiving music therapy compared to those that did not, although no increase in survival rate was identified. Clinical trials have also found music can reduce factors such as depression, blood pressure, insomnia, and heart rate associated with cancer. However, a 2013 survey of previous investigations of music's impact on cancer patients' levels of anxiety found that music therapy had no definite benefit.

Researchers have attempted to better understand music therapy's psychological as well as physiological effects. A study published in the journal *Music Therapy Perspectives* in 2014 examined the efficacy of group-based music therapy on men's psychological wellbeing. Using a system of outcome rating scales (ORS), the study found that such interventions were significantly effective at increasing wellbeing even among those who did not have a prior interest or ability in music.

CHOOSING A PRACTITIONER
Music therapists usually practice in conjunction with a medical or rehabilitation team. Music therapists in private practice receive clients through recommendations from either medical doctors or psychologists/

psychiatrists. In the United States, the Certification Board for Music Therapists provides national examinations to certify music therapists; choosing a certified practitioner ensures that they have met educational and training standards and can be expected to provide better therapy.

SAFETY ISSUES

No adverse events have been reported in cases using music therapy. However, attempting therapy without training or incorrectly may prove ineffective, and could potentially even increase a patient's stress level or emotional discomfort. Additionally, if a patient with a serious medical condition attempts to rely on music therapy alone, they risk complicating or worsening their condition through lack of proper treatment.

—Deborah A. Appello

Further Reading

Accordino, Robert, Ronald Comer, and Wendy B. Heller. "Searching for Music's Potential: A Critical Examination of Research on Music Therapy with Individuals with Autism." *Research in Autism Spectrum Disorders*, vol. 1, 2007, pp. 101–15.

American Music Therapy Association, 2015. Accessed 12 Feb. 2015.

Bensimon, Moshe, Dorit Armir, and Yuval Wolf. "Drumming Through Trauma: Music Therapy with Post-traumatic Soldiers." *Arts in Psychotherapy*, vol. 35, 2008, pp. 34–48.

Choi, Ae-Na, Myeong Soo Lee, and Jung-Sook Lee. "Group Music Intervention Reduces Aggression and Improves Self-Esteem in Children with Highly Aggressive Behavior." *Complementary and Alternative Medicine*, vol. 1, no. 2, 2008, pp. 213–17.

Codding, Peggy, and Suzanne Hanser. "Music Therapy." *Complementary and Integrative Medicine in Pain Management*, edited by Michael I. Weintraub, Springer, 2008.

Hurkmans, Joost, et al. "Music in the Treatment of Neurological Language and Speech Disorders: A Systematic Review." *Aphasiology*, vol. 26, no. 1, 2012, pp. 1–19. *Taylor & Francis Online*, doi.org/10.1080/02687038.2011.602514.

Irle, Kevin, and Geoff Lovell. "An Investigation into the Efficacy of a Music-Based Men's Group for Improving Psychological Wellbeing." *Music Therapy Perspectives*, vol. 32, no. 2, 2014, pp. 178–84.

"Music Therapy." American Cancer Society. *Cancer.org*, 13 Jan. 2015.

Norton, A., et al. "Melodic Intonation Therapy." *Annals of the New York Academy of Sciences*, vol. 1169, 2009, pp. 431–36. *Wiley*, doi:10.1111/j.1749-6632.2009.04859.x.

Okada, Kaoru, et al. "Effects of Music Therapy on Autonomic Nervous System Activity, Incidence of Heart Failure Events, and Plasma Cytokine and Catecholamine Levels in Elderly Patients with Cerebrovascular Disease and Dementia." *International Heart Journal*, vol. 50, 2009, pp. 95–110.

Prideaux, Ed. "Stayin' Alive! How Music Has Fought Pandemics for 2,700 Years." *The Guardian*, 6 Apr. 2020, www.theguardian.com/music/2020/apr/06/stayin-alive-how-music-fought-pandemics-2700-years-coronavirus.

Sacks, Oliver. "The Power of Music." *Brain*, vol. 129, 2006, pp. 2528–32.

Slavin, Dianne, and Renee Fabus. "A Case Study Using a Multimodal Approach to Melodic Intonation Therapy." *American Journal of Speech-Language Pathology*, vol. 27, no. 4, 2018, pp. 1352–62.

Thilman, James. "*Alive Inside* Celebrates the Healing Power of Music." *TheHuffingtonPost.com*, 10 July 2014.

Van der Meulen, Ineke, et al. "Melodic Intonation Therapy: Present Controversies and Future Opportunities." *Archives of Physical Medicine and Rehabilitation*, vol. 93, no. 1, S46–S52. *Archives of Physical Medicine and Rehabilitation*, doi.org/10.1016/j.apmr.2011.05.029.

BIOFEEDBACK

ABSTRACT

Biofeedback therapy is a mind-body approach to using auditory or visual feedback to control involuntary functions such as blood pressure, heart rate, and blood flow. The goals of biofeedback are to learn how to control their body to improve physical, mental, emotional, and spiritual health.

Biofeedback

OVERVIEW

Many of our bodily functions are involuntary, and occur without us consciously exerting control over said activities. However, the fact that these functions can occur independent of our input does not restrict us from altering or modifying some of these processes to enhance our physical and emotional well-being.

Biofeedback, which is a procedure that involves exerting conscious control over some of those autonomous bodily functions, is a method with robust empirical support for use with patients who have a myriad of clinical disorders. The methodology behind Biofeedback is fairly straightforward: a device provides "feedback" based on physiological input from the user. With this information provided, the person can bring awareness to the previously unconscious process, and learn to exert conscious control.

One common example, relevant to most, is the use of a pulse oximeter to gain basic health information at the onset of a visit to one's physician. Typically, a pulse oximeter will display the wearer's oxygen (O_2) saturation, or the extent to which a person's hemoglobin is saturated with oxygen, and their heart beats per minute (BPM). Often, when a person's BPM increase, their O_2 saturation decrease. This can lead to perceived physiological distress, such as: sweating, body tension/aches, headaches, nervousness, mood irritability, disorientation, and overall feeling unwell. These reactions are also often present during other physiological processes, such as through one's blood pressure, which is pressure of the blood as it moves through arteries following contraction from the heart.

Through principles of operant conditioning, a person is rewarded when they practice and obtain control over their physiological functions as evidenced by a reduction in one of the previously noted undesirable symptoms. For example, a person who feels dizzy related to elevated blood pressure and reduced oxygen saturation will likely experience a reduction in intensity of dizziness by utilizing a strategy (i.e., deep breathing) to attempt to return those levels to a normal range. Having a device such as a pulse oximeter or a blood pressure machine can provide information that is otherwise undetectable to the user. The devices

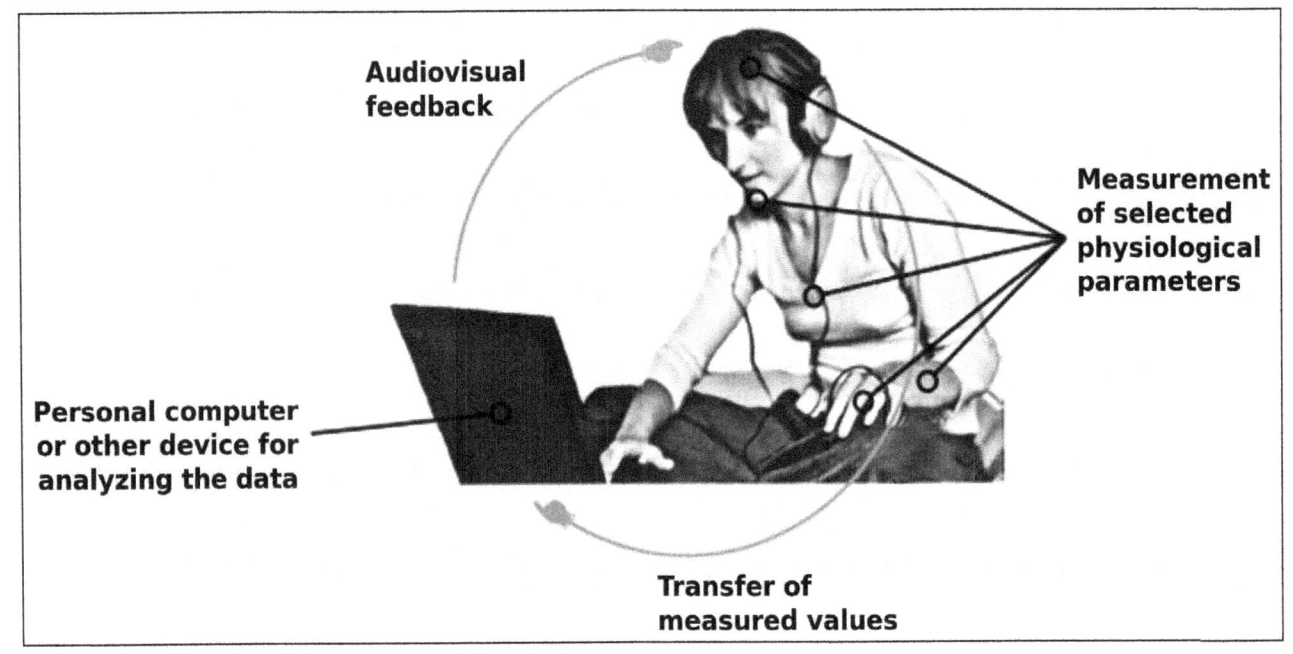

An illustration of biofeedback (Marek Jacenko via Wikimedia Commons)

298

also provide concrete, objective data which can be utilized to better assess the user's progress. In addition to measuring blood pressure, oxygen saturation and heart rate, there are biofeedback machines in fairly common use that measure muscle tension, skin temperature, skin resistance to electricity, and brain-wave activity.

USES AND APPLICATIONS

Biofeedback is commonly utilized to treat and manage stress and stress-related conditions, including but not limited to: anxiety, insomnia, high blood pressure, fibromyalgia, muscle pain, migraine headaches, and tension headaches.

MODES OF BIOFEEDBACK

A variety of modalities exist for employee biofeedback techniques. Some may be less practical for use based on added expenses and time constraints. However, many of the more readily available options provide significant and useful information for the user.

Monitoring breathing: One of the most basic and easily employed modes of employing biofeedback is through monitoring one's breathing. This can be accomplished through several methods. Often, those starting out will simply attempt to slow the intake of air, and elongate their inhale and exhale. This can be enhanced by mentally counting the seconds of inhalation and exhalation, and incrementally increasing the time so as to slow the breathing process. This technique, often referred to as deep breathing or "belly breathing," can be monitored by placing one's hand over their stomach to feel the expansion and contraction as air enters and exits the body.

Cardiac monitoring: A variety of devices, such as a pulse oximeter, blood pressure cuff, and electrocardiograph can be utilized to obtain direct physiological data of a user's cardiac functioning. Data from these sources provide direct, objective data that can provide the user with information regarding impact and progress of strategies employed (i.e., deep breathing) during biofeedback.

Glandular activity: An electrodermograph can be utilized to assess activities related to one's sweat glands. Biometric sensors are attached to a person's palms or fingers to detect the presence of perspiration. From an evolutionary perspective, perspiration is indicative of a fight or flight response. In modern times, excessive perspiration can be indicative of anxious response. Altering the user to the presence of perspiration can condition the person to being aware to the inception of anxiety or discomfort, thus cueing them to employ a relaxation technique.

Neurofeedback: By monitoring brain waves through the use of electroencephalogram (EEG), observations can be made regarding the brain's electrical activity. Using this information, the process of employing biofeedback can help the user "retrain" their brain-wave patterns. The user is able to identify feelings connected to abnormal brain-wave patterns, and can attempt to modify them in real time. Brain-wave data is supplied on a screen so that the user and clinician can discuss and explore steps the wearer can learn to alter and control brain-wave activity. This noninvasive procedure typically involves placing electrode leads on the scalp of the patient.

SCIENTIFIC EVIDENCE

Clinical use of biofeedback can be found as early as the 1960s. Since that time, and most notably since the turn of the twentieth century, robust research exists that demonstrates the efficacy of biofeedback in clinical settings for multiple disorders. Multiple studies exist that demonstrate the effective use of biofeedback for the treatment of: hypertension, headaches, gastrointestinal disorders (i.e., fecal incontinence, irritable bowel syndrome, peptic ulcer disease), chronic pain, Raynaud's disease; as well as various psychiatric disorders including: anxiety, depression, panic disorder, posttraumatic stress, Tourette's syndrome, and obsessive-compulsive disorder.

Of note, a significant proportion of recent research has been dedicated to the use of smartphone applications ("apps") designed for biofeedback purposes. The research on these "apps" is of importance and they represent an important step in the practical employment of biofeedback techniques. Having easy access to a device at low or no cost that can provide valuable and timely data is may increase the adherence to use.

The ever-expanding number of apps for various biofeedback techniques for a variety of disorders makes it difficult to validate the clinical use of each individual app. User are encouraged to conduct their own research to assess the reliability of a smartphone app. As apps continue to improve in terms of ease of use and effectiveness, their presence will become ubiquitous in the practice of biofeedback. Research into the efficacy of apps for biofeedback, in comparison with previously noted, clinician driven approaches is ongoing; however much of the research shows equivalent effectiveness for many apps, typically following introduction of biofeedback strategies and techniques with or in conjunction with clinical care.

WHAT TO EXPECT DURING TREATMENT

Clinician driven biofeedback training typically involves the use of a machine that relays information about the aspect of the body that one wishes to control. Usually, one locates a target area of the body, and that becomes the focus for the intervention. A biofeedback practitioner will teach a series of visualizations and other mental exercises (i.e. deep breathing, progressive muscle relaxation (PMR)) in order to facilitate the process.

For a patient with an anxiety disorder, common symptoms during heightened anxiety include shortness of breath, chest tightness, excessive sweating, and bodily discomfort. Targeting those symptoms utilizing biofeedback been shown to be empirically effective. For example, a clinician may ask the sufferer to wear a pulse oximeter to monitor the user's oxygen saturation and pulse rate. Typically, during times of high anxiety, a person's oxygen saturation goes down as their pulse rate increases. The physiological effects of this phenomena (i.e., shortness of breath, heart palpitations) can exacerbate an anxious response. Having the user take slow, steady, deep breaths usually helps lower their pulse rate and increase their oxygen saturation. Using the pulse oximeter allows for the user to objectively monitor their physiology, as well as make the connection between effective use of a calming strategy, and its impact on the body.

CHOOSING A PRACTITIONER

As with all medical therapies, it is best to choose a licensed, qualified and experienced practitioner. One should seek a referral from a qualified and knowledgeable healthcare provider. There are no known safety risks with biofeedback.

—*Robert S. Cavera*

Further Reading

Dillon, A., M. Kelly, I. H. Robertson, and D. A. Robertson "Smartphone Applications Utilizing Biofeedback Can Aid Stress Reduction." *Frontiers in Psychology*, vol. 7, p. 832.

Fisher, J. G., J. P. Hatch, and J. D. Rugh, editors. *Biofeedback: Studies in Clinical Efficacy*. Springer Science & Business Media, 2013.

Frank, D. L., L. Khorshid, J. F. Kiffer, C. S. Moravec, and M. G. McKee. "Biofeedback in Medicine: Who, When, Why and How?" *Mental Health in Family Medicine*, vol. 7, no. 2, 2010.

Giggins, O. M., U. M. Persson, and B. Caulfield. "Biofeedback in Rehabilitation." *Journal of Neuroengineering and Rehabilitation*, vol. 10, no. 1, p. 60.

Harvard Health, www.health.harvard.edu/medical-tests-and-procedures/biofeedback-a-to-z.

Khazan, I. Z. *The Clinical Handbook of Biofeedback: A Step-By-Step Guide for Training and Practice with Mindfulness*. John Wiley & Sons, 2013.

Peake, J. M., G. Kerr, and J. P. Sullivan. "A Critical Review of Consumer Wearables, Mobile Applications, and Equipment for Providing Biofeedback, Monitoring

Stress, and Sleep in Physically Active Populations." *Frontiers in Physiology*, vol. 9, p. 743.

Schwartz, M. S., and F. Andrasik, editors. *Biofeedback: A Practitioner's Guide*. Guilford Publications, 2017.

Yates, A. J. *Biofeedback and the Modification of Behavior*. Springer Science & Business Media, 2012.

Nursing Care Plan

ABSTRACT

A nursing care plan is a method by which medical personnel, mainly nurses, compile and share important information about patients and their treatment. Care plans record data such as a patient's detailed diagnosis, actions taken by or required of nurses, and evaluations of the patient's progress toward health goals. Nursing care plans are essential in the complex world of modern healthcare as they allow multiple healthcare personnel to easily access and update the same patient information. This helps nurses and other medical personnel work as a team. It also creates important documentation of a patient's health as well as treatments received, which can be added to health records or insurance reports.

BACKGROUND

Modern healthcare can be complicated. In most medical facilities, numerous members of the medical staff may work with an individual patient. Each staff member brings a different set of qualifications, skills, experiences, and perspectives. Scheduling and assignment changes may add further variability to the interactions between medical staff and their patients.

Without efficient communication between medical personnel, each staff member would have to start fresh with each patient, assessing all treatments and requirements. This could lead to serious delays, confusion, and potentially insufficient data, possibly inhibiting a patient's treatment.

For these reasons, careful recordkeeping and planning is essential in the healthcare environment. Nurses and other staff members involved with a patient should have access to the same vital information about that patient. They should also cooperate to carry out a shared vision of how to improve that patient's health. One fundamental means of sharing this necessary information is through nursing care plans. These plans allow medical staff to work as unified teams with shared knowledge and goals.

Nursing care plans can take several forms. The most basic is the informal care plan, which exists in the mind of the nurse. The informal care plan may be simple guidelines used for patients who do not require any ongoing or extensive treatment. For example, this kind of plan may be used for a one-time visit for a sprained ankle. It also may serve as a preliminary step toward a more comprehensive plan.

As soon as a plan is written, whether on paper or recorded digitally, it is considered a formal nursing care plan. One such type of plan is the standardized care plan, which is a relatively general plan used for patients needing a certain category of care. If a patient needs specialized help, the standardized care plan is customized into a more detailed individualized care plan tailored to more specific patient needs. Individualized care plans may grow greatly over time and include contributions from many nurses.

OVERVIEW

In general, nursing care plans are processes by which nurses and other medical personnel record and share important facts about a patient. The data in these plans include the patient's current condition, needs, and potential risks. The development of a nursing care plan begins as soon as a patient arrives for treatment, and may continue for hours, days, months, or even years, depending on the situation. The plans are constantly checked, revised, and updated to reflect the patient's changing situation. Optimal nursing care plans ensure that the level of healthcare is efficient and effective.

One of the main objectives of nursing care plans is to help the patient receive the best care possible. This involves ensuring that each patient receives individual treatment and can feel comfortable with caretakers, assured that their needs are known and understood. Care plans also help experts work with individual patients in a variety of ways, creating holistic care programs that can help patients prosper physically, mentally, and emotionally.

Nursing care plans are also helpful for healthcare institutions. These plans can help teams of medical personnel analyze cases and reach agreements on how to proceed with care. Nursing plans can also help caregivers create long-term goals and measure and evaluate the types and level of care received during treatment. The latter information is important both for the updating and accuracy of health records and for reporting to insurance companies.

Though medical needs and care can vary greatly, most nursing care plans follow a similar basic format. In general, these plans address crucial topics such as the patient's diagnosis, the anticipated outcome of the treatment, actions taken or required of nurses, and evaluations of the patient's current state.

The patient's diagnosis is a fundamental piece of information for a nursing care plan as it helps to inform and guide the rest of the planning. Medical personnel will need to understand the patient's specific situation before taking any serious course of treatment. To ensure the most accurate diagnosis, nurses may have to thoroughly assess a patient. This includes analysis of their physical and mental status. Frequently, a full diagnosis must also take into account less-tangible factors such as the patient's social, economic, cultural, and spiritual background. These factors may not seem immediately pressing, but may prove very important to successful treatment.

Assessing the anticipated outcome of the treatment in a nursing care plan is an important method of guiding nurses' choices and actions. In these plans, nurses start with a health goal and then create a map of actions most likely to lead to that goal. These actions, often referred to in planning as nursing orders or interventions, list the steps nurses should take to best care for the patient. This information may contain a high level of specificity—such as an amount of medicine to be administered at a certain time—as well as broad longer-term goals. These action plans may be revised over time according to the patient's progress.

The final main section of a nursing care plan is the evaluation, which records the actions taken and the results in regards to the patient. This evaluation helps nurses determine whether treatments are working or require alteration. It also helps nurses and other personnel decide when a patient has reached a goal and may be considered healthy enough to be discharged from care.

—*Mark Dziak*

Further Reading

Gulanick, Meg, and Judith L. Myers. *Nursing Care Plans: Nursing Diagnosis and Intervention.* 9th ed., Mosby, 2016.

"Nursing Care Plans: What You Need to Know." *Nurse.org*, nurse.org/articles/what-are-nursing-care-plans/. Accessed 3 Sept. 2020.

Papandrea, Dawn. "Nursing Care Plans: What You Need to Know." *Nurse.org*, 8 Jan. 2018, nurse.org/articles/what-are-nursing-care-plans/. Accessed 3 Sept. 2020.

Schultz, Judith M., and Sheila L. Videbeck. *Lippincott's Manual of Psychiatric Nursing Care Plans.* 9th ed., Wolters Kluwer/Lippincott, Williams, & Wilkins, 2012.

"The Nursing Process." *American Nurses Association*, www.nursingworld.org/practice-policy/workforce/what-is-nursing/the-nursing-process/. Accessed 3 Sept. 2020.

"The Ultimate Nursing Care Plan Database." *Nursing.com*, nursing.com/course/nursing-care-plans/. Accessed 3 Sept. 2020.

Vera, Matt. "Nursing Care Plans (NCP): Ultimate Guide and Database." *Nurseslabs*, 31 Jan. 2019, nurseslabs.com/nursing-care-plans/. Accessed 3 Sept. 2020.

Yazdi, Mariam. "4 Steps to Writing A Nursing Care Plan." *Nurse.org*, 23 Mar. 2018, nurse.org/articles/nursing-care-plan-how-to/.

Genetic Counseling

ABSTRACT

Genetic counseling is a form of counseling that helps patients manage having an inherited disorder or familial birth defect. Genetic counseling may be provided by physicians, medical geneticists, or advanced practice nurses or registered nurses with specialized training.

THE PROFESSION

Genetic counseling evaluates an individual's risk of an inherited medical condition such as breast cancer, assists in understanding a family's risk of an inherited medical condition such as colon cancer or determines a couple's risk of having a child with an inherited birth defect such as cystic fibrosis. There is also a need to identify individuals or families' risk factors and provide genetic testing that may involve laboratory tests or building a family history.

The reason for referral to a genetics program may vary and may include family history of disease known to be hereditary or familial in nature, a diagnosis of cancer, an abnormal ultrasound during pregnancy, or a family history of genetic disorders. Genetic counselors may have a broad practice or specialize in a field such as prenatal care, cancer, pediatrics, or other areas. The initial referral visit usually begins with an extensive family history. Once the history is complete, the genetic counselor describes the impact of the information found, potential tests available such as testing for a specific gene, and inheritance patterns.

In close communication with the referring physician, the individual and the genetic counselor will determine next steps. Genetic testing is complex, and often very expensive. Some testing is not covered by insurance plans and require an out of pocket payment by individuals being tested. Genetic counselors meet with individuals, may follow up with family meetings

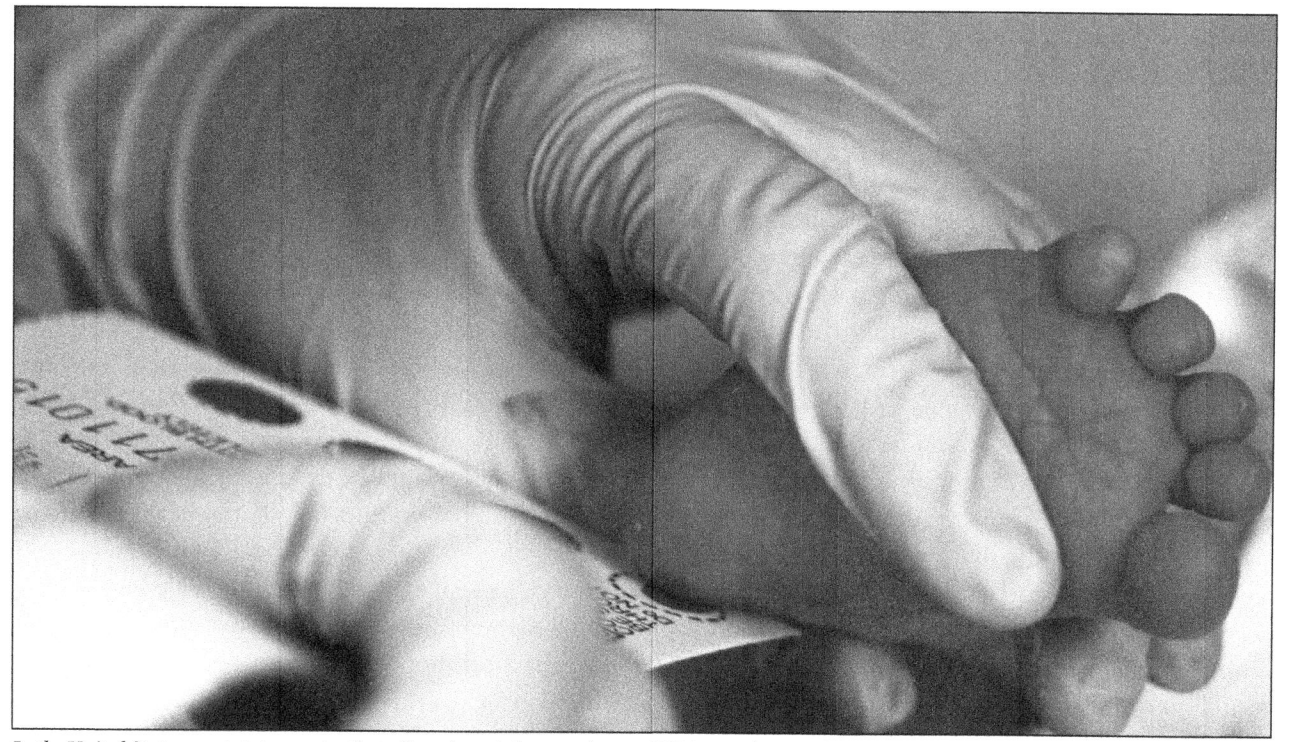

In the United States, most states require that all newborn infants undergo a PKU test. This simple test involves taking a small sample of blood by pricking the heel of the baby. (Wikimedia Commons)

if findings indicate others are at risk, provide support when information is negative, and meet with the individual to discuss test findings and ongoing steps.

GENETIC SCREENING

One of the more controversial aspects of genetic counseling is the procedure of screening. In this procedure, individuals suspected to be at risk are tested for the presence of a mutation. Screening can let people know whether they have a disease as well as whether they are carriers of the disease and therefore can pass the disease on to their children. Screening can be extended to all individuals, regardless of family or ethnic history. For example, in the United States, most states require that all newborn infants undergo a phenylketonuria (PKU) test. This simple test involves taking a small sample of blood by pricking the heel of the baby. Although the costs of this screening are not insignificant, the benefit is that those infants found to have the disease can be treated immediately by being placed on a special diet so as to avoid the debilitating effects of the disease.

Other screening procedures are targeted at specific groups. The screening program for Tay-Sachs disease focuses on ethnic Jewish populations. This successful, voluntary program has reduced the incidence of Tay-Sachs disease significantly in the United States. The key to the success of the program was the money spent to educate the targeted group. In addition, key members of the population played a leading role in designing the overall program. Because of the much larger size of the potential group at risk, similar efforts to screen African American populations for sickle cell disease have been much less successful. Ethical concerns about the motivations behind government-sponsored or government-encouraged screening of minority populations make these programs difficult to implement. In addition, in mandatory programs, concerns about confidentiality and information release become major obstacles.

Genetic testing is an individualized approach determined by medical history and family history. Single gene testing is used to test for Duchene muscular dystrophy or sickle cell disease, for example, or is used when there is a known genetic mutation in a family. Panel testing looks for changes in many genes. For example, panels may be used to look at short statue or epilepsy. Panels may also be used to examine the risk of certain kinds of cancer such as breast or colon cancers. In people with complex medical histories, exome and genome sequencing may by ordered. This type of testing may uncover other potential issues when looking for a genetic reason, for example, to explain developmental disabilities.

THE SCIENCE

Humans have between thirty thousand and thirty-five thousand genes. Genes are segments of deoxyribonucleic acid (DNA) that are arranged in linear fashion along the forty-six chromosomes. Most genes contain the information necessary for the cells to produce a specific protein, which often is involved in controlling some critical physiological function. For example, the beta globin gene produces a protein called beta globin that makes up half of the hemoglobin that carries oxygen in the red blood cells.

A genetic disease can occur when the DNA changes in structure. Such a change is also known as a mutation. A mutation can lead to the production of a defective protein that cannot carry out its normal function, thus causing a physiological defect. In the case of beta globin, changing only one of the 106 molecules that make up this protein leads to a form of hemoglobin that can produce nonfunctional protein aggregates in red blood cells. These aggregates can cause the red blood cells to collapse and take on a sickle shape. Such cells lose their function, and the tissues are starved for oxygen, a condition known as anemia. This defect, which is called sickle cell disease, is a fatal, heritable disease. As with all genetic disease, such mutations are relatively rare. Certain diseases may, however, be more prevalent within certain ethnic groups; for example, African Americans have a high incidence of sickle cell disease, and Ashkenazic Jews have a high incidence of Tay-Sachs disease.

Humans have two of each kind of chromosome; one set of twenty-three is inherited from the mother, and the other set of twenty-three is inherited from the father. Thus, each person has two copies of each gene, one located on a maternal chromosome, the other on a paternal one. Many types of defects require that both genes have mutations in order for the disease to have an effect. Individuals who have one normal gene and one with a mutation are normal but carry the disease; they can pass the mutation on to the next generation in their eggs and sperm. This type of disease is called a recessive genetic disease.

Since it is equally likely for each parent to pass on the normal gene in eggs or sperm as to pass on the mutation, the laws of probability predict that, on the average, one-fourth of such a couple's offspring should have the disease. One of the major tasks of a genetic counselor is to advise couples of these probabilities if the diagnoses and family histories suggest that they are carriers. Since the laws of genetics involve random occurrences, however, it is possible that in a family with three or four children, all the children will be normal, or that in another family, all the children will have the disease. This degree of uncertainty produces stress and anxiety in couples who seek counseling only to hear that they indeed are at risk. Discussing concepts that involve sophisticated genetic or biochemical themes or issues of probable risk with couples untrained in scientific thinking is difficult, especially considering the highly emotional atmosphere of such discussions.

Other diseases, such as Huntington's chorea, also known as Woody Guthrie's disease for the folksinger who was afflicted by it, are caused by a dominant mutation. A mutation is dominant when an individual needs to inherit only one copy of the mutation in order to have the disease. Unlike recessive diseases that can disappear from a family for generations, a dominant mutation can be inherited only from a person who has the disease. In most cases, such a person has one normal gene and one with the mutation, which means that there is a 50 percent chance that the gene will be passed on. Huntington's chorea is a particularly insidious genetic disease, because the symptoms usually begin to show only in middle age, often after childbearing decisions have been made. Thus, the children of an afflicted parent may have had children before knowing whether they have inherited the mutation from their parents.

There are no cures for the permanent physiological defects that result from genetic disease. In some cases, the disease symptoms can be controlled by supplementing the protein that is lacking. Some forms of insulin-dependent diabetes and most cases of hemophilia can be treated in this way. In other cases, as with the disease PKU, special diets can prevent the severe neurological problems that inevitably lead to childhood death if the disease is left untreated.

DNA technology and genetic engineering offer potential cures for some diseases in which the primary defect caused by the mutation is well understood. Gene therapy is a process by which an additional copy of a normal gene is inserted into the cells of an affected individual or the defective gene is replaced by a normal one. Successful experiments with animals have given scientists confidence that these techniques will provide cures for many genetic diseases. These same DNA technologies are making better diagnoses possible and, as in the case of cystic fibrosis, are helping to extend the lives and enhance the quality of life of individuals afflicted with incurable diseases.

GENETIC COUNSELOR SPECIALTIES

Genetic counseling originated in the prenatal setting as physicians recognized that birth defects and some diseases ran in families. In prenatal genetic counseling, the counselor may communicate to a couple the medical problems associated with the occurrence of an inherited disorder or birth defect in a family. About 5 to 10 percent of cancers have inherited genetic mutations in specific genes which predispose an individual to what is called a hereditary cancer syndrome. This is different than cancers that tend to "run in families" which usually is a result of shared lifestyle such as smoking or living in a polluted area. Most hospitals and health systems provide either an on-site genetics program or referral to a program in the area. Simple genetic testing may be done by physician order, but more complex issues require a counselor.

In all cases, the role of the genetic counselor is to provide unbiased information and options to the individual or couple seeking advice. The counselor must not only discuss the medical implications of a condition but also help to alleviate the emotional impact of positive diagnoses and, in particular, to assuage the guilt or denial that a diagnosis may elicit.

THE NEED FOR GENETIC COUNSELING

The need for centers specializing in genetic counseling arose when it became clear that certain diseases and birth defects had a hereditary component. Many individuals and families request the services of counselors from these centers, and the centers are also involved in both voluntary and mandatory screening programs.

Physicians have always served as counselors to families, but the rapid advances made in genetics and molecular science during the second half of the twentieth century have clearly surpassed the abilities of most physicians to keep current with treatments and diagnoses. The first formal clinic for genetic counseling was established at the University of Michigan in the 1940s. Most clinics specializing in this field were based at large medical centers; first in major metropolitan areas, and later in smaller population centers.

Genetic counseling clinics usually employ a range of specialists, including clinicians, geneticists, laboratory personnel for performing diagnostic testing, and public health and social workers. In 1969, Sarah Lawrence College instituted a master's-level program in genetic counseling to train candidates formally in the scientific, medical, and counseling skills required for this profession. Since that time, many other programs have been established in the United States. Most large counseling programs at medical centers use these specially trained personnel. In rural areas, however, family physicians are still a primary source of counseling; thus, genetic training is an important component of basic medical education.

The sophisticated medical diagnostic tools allow a counselor to provide abundant information to individuals and couples requesting counseling, but the power of DNA technology has expanded and will continue to expand the scope of current practice. Soon, counselors will not have to give advice in terms of probabilities and likelihoods of risk; molecular detection techniques will make possible the absolute identification of not only individuals with a disease but also related carriers. As these DNA tools become more widely available, counseling will become a more integral part of preventive medicine.

—*Patricia Stanfill Edens and Joseph G. Pelliccia*

Further Reading

Davis, Dena S. *Genetic Dilemmas: Reproductive Technology, Parental Choices, and Children's Futures*. 2nd ed., Routledge, 2010.

Filkins, Karen, and Joseph F. Russo, editors. *Human Prenatal Diagnosis*. 2nd rev. ed., Marcel Dekker, 1990.

"Genetic Counseling: What Is Genetic Counseling?" *Centers for Disease Control and Prevention*, www.cdc.gov/genomics/gtesting/genetic_counseling.htm. Accessed 1 Sept. 2020.

Genetics Home Reference. "Genetic Consultation." *Genetics Home Reference*, 5 Aug. 2013.

"Genetics of Cancer." National Cancer Institute. *National Institutes of Health*, www.cancer.gov/about-cancer/causes-prevention/genetics#syndromes. Accessed 1 Sept. 2020.

"Genetic Testing." *Centers for Disease Control and Prevention*, www.cdc.gov/genomics/gtesting/genetic_testing.htm. Accessed 1 Sept. 2020

Harper, Peter S. *Practical Genetic Counselling.* 7th ed., Hodder Arnold, 2010.

Jorde, Lynn B., et al. *Medical Genetics.* 4th ed., Mosby/Elsevier, 2010.

Lewis, Ricki. *Human Genetics: Concepts and Applications.* 10th ed., McGraw-Hill, 2012.

Martin, Richard J., Avroy A. Fanaroff, and Michele C. Walsh, editors. *Fanaroff and Martin's Neonatal-Perinatal Medicine: Diseases of the Fetus and Infant.* Mosby/Elsevier, 2011.

MedlinePlus. "Genetic Counseling." *MedlinePlus,* 21 June 2013.

Pritchard, D. J., and Bruce R. Korf. *Medical Genetics at a Glance.* 3rd ed., John Wiley & Sons, 2013.

"What Is Genetic Counseling?" *National Society of Genetic Counselors,* www.nsgc.org/page/frequently-asked-questions-students#whatis on September 1, 2020.

ROBOTICS IN HEALTHCARE

ABSTRACT

Constant advancements in technology have influenced the ways humans use robotics in healthcare. One of the most common applications for robotics in healthcare is using robots for minimally invasive surgeries. Yet, numerous other robotic applications—including caregiving and supply stocking—have changed healthcare around the world. As medical professionals, hospitals, and individuals rely more on robots to complete healthcare-related tasks, people have to grapple with more ethical, monetary, and technological concerns. The use of robotics in healthcare will likely increase over time, especially as a growing population strains current healthcare systems. Robotics are quickly changing the way medical professionals do their jobs and the way patients receive care.

BACKGROUND

Although researchers disagree about the exact definition of a robot, a general consensus is that a robot is a physically embodied machine that has intelligence and some ability to perform tasks autonomously. Before humans had the technology to create working robots, they imagined having mechanical assistants that could relieve humans of some of their workload. The twentieth century saw the invention of the first computers and the development of artificial intelligence. In the 1960s, a company called SRI International developed a robot called Shakey, which was most likely the first machine to fit the modern definition of a robot. Soon afterward, researchers created other types of robots, including robotic arms. People used robotic arms, which could move and lift heavy objects, in factories and manufacturing. These arms also became important in laboratories, including medical laboratories. Such machines could move samples and perform other simple functions. These were the first robots to be involved in any part of the medical field. Robotics continued to advance, although the development of useful, high-quality robots took many decades. In the 1990s, the first robots were used in surgery with a robot that guided traditional surgical tools, allowing surgeons to be more precise. In 2000, the US Food and Drug Administration (FDA) approved the robotic operating system called da Vinci, which was a large, multipart system used by surgeons. This system helped make robotic surgery even more popular. The early decades of the 2000s brought new advancements that would expand the use of robotics throughout the healthcare industry.

OVERVIEW

Robots are used in medicine and healthcare for many different reasons. Robots used for surgery are among the most common. However, the robots used in surgery are not performing the actions alone. A surgeon still performs the surgery via handheld controls that allow the surgeon to move the robotic parts. Robotic surgery has a number of benefits. One of the most important benefits is that that type of surgery is less invasive than open surgery (surgery during which a large incision is made and surgeons use cutting tools to perform the surgical functions). It is also sometimes less invasive than laparoscopic surgery (surgery con-

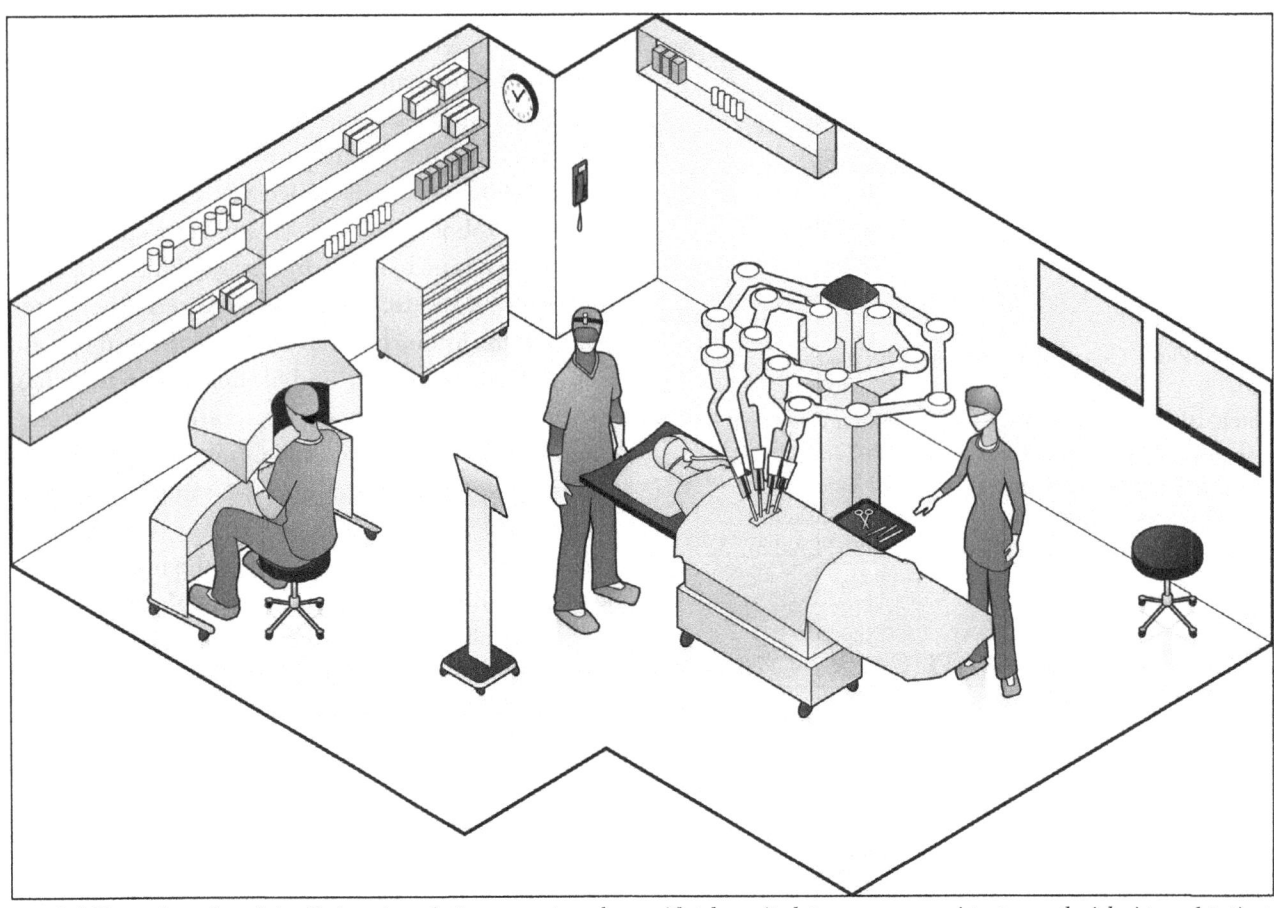

Detailed illustration of a minimally-invasive robotic surgery procedure, with telemanipulator, surgeon, assistant, anesthesiologist, and patient. (mathisworks via iStock)

ducted with small tools and a camera). Minimally invasive surgery can create better patient outcomes because it can help reduce the length of surgery, complications, patient pain, rates of infection, and recuperation times. Robotic surgery can also help doctors perform surgeries in difficult-to-reach areas where they might not have been able to operate in the past.

Modern robots used in surgery are often robotic systems with three parts. The surgeon conducts most of the surgery at the console, a large machine that controls the instruments, which are in a different part of the surgery system. The surgeon has a large screen to view the surgery as it takes place. The surgeon uses two handheld controls to move the instruments while watching the screen. The surgeon sits at the console, away from the patient, and conducts the surgery. Sometimes surgeons can control parts of the robotic system with pedals they operate with their feet. The patient cart is the second piece of the system. The cart is located at the site of the patient. The cart holds cameras and the robotic pieces that actually perform the surgical functions. This part of the system responds to the surgeon's movements at the console. The third piece of the system is the vision cart. This piece of the system facilitates communication between the other two pieces of the system. It is located between the two other pieces to make communication possible.

Surgeons use the robotic operating system in numerous different situations. Surgery systems can be used to do cardiac surgeries. Traditional open-heart surgery is very invasive, requiring a long recovery and risking numerous complications. Minimally invasive cardiac surgeries can help reduce recovery times and the risk of complications. Hysterectomies and some other gynecological surgeries can sometimes be performed by robotic surgery. Doctors can repair hernias with minimally invasive surgery. Doctors can also use robotic surgery systems to conduct colorectal, head and neck, and thoracic surgeries. In the future, more surgeries will likely take place with robotic surgery systems.

Although robotic systems for surgery have become some of the best-known uses for robotics in healthcare, they are not alone. Researchers have developed many more robots and robotic systems to use in healthcare. A number of types of robots perform functions that can help humans conduct everyday tasks that support healthcare but are not actually healthcare functions. For example, some robots clean or disinfect. Hospital-acquired infections (HAIs) are a serious threat to public health, and keeping facilities clean and sanitized is one of the biggest priorities and challenges in the field. Robots can help perform this function. One robot, called Xenex, uses full-spectrum ultraviolet (UV) rays to kill microbes, including drug-resistant bacteria. The robot can disinfect a room in a matter of minutes.

Other robots move products, including food, drugs, and supplies. around a hospital or healthcare facility. Nurses and other workers inside healthcare facilities spend much time getting patients food, blankets, drinks, and other items to make them comfortable and care for them. Robots can reduce the work humans need to do to complete these tasks. A nurse could request a particular product, such as a blanket, and have the robot deliver it. The nurse can reduce trips away from patients, increasing patient-facing time. Robots can also deliver meals and even drugs to patients. Robots that carry drugs are designed so they will open only when they arrive at a particular location, and they are locked so people cannot access the medication before it arrives at its destination.

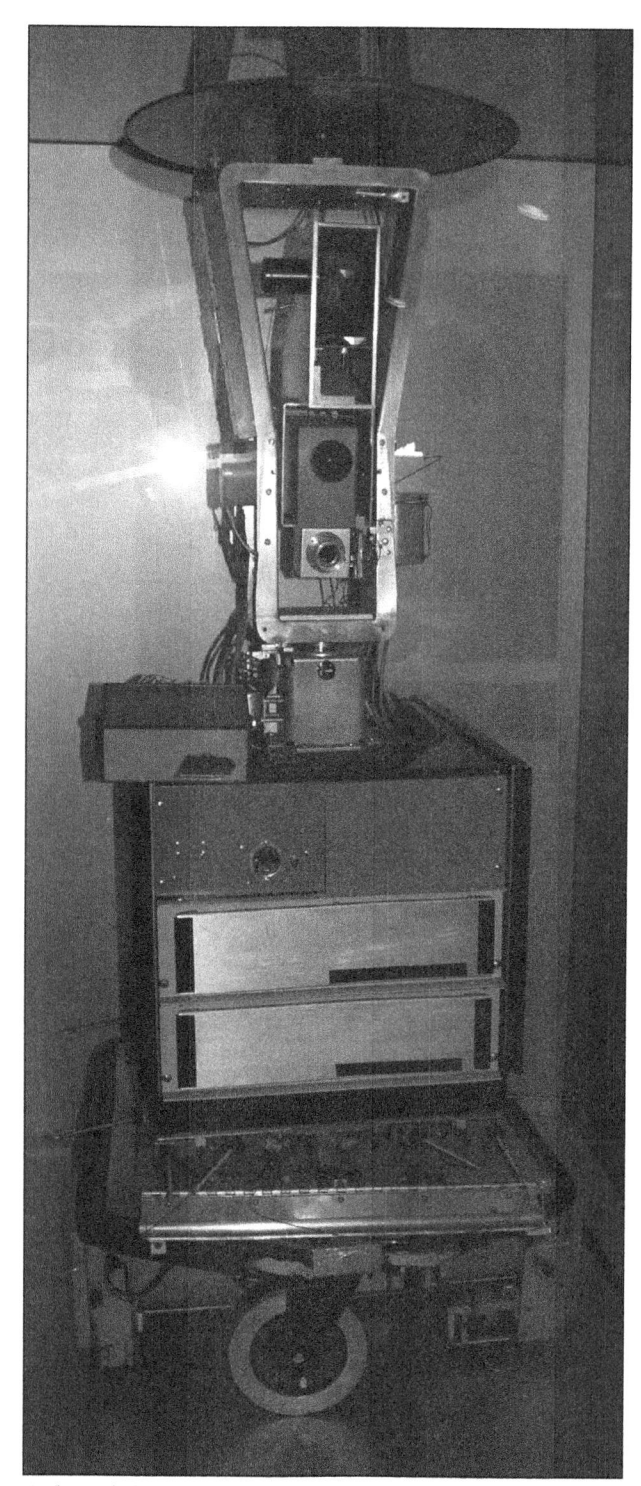

A photo of Shakey the Robot in its case at the Computer History Museum (Marshall Astor via Wikimedia Commons)

The robots that are made to run errands, clean rooms, and do other tasks in healthcare settings have specific designs that help them function. For example, the Tug robot transports food, drugs, and other items in hospitals. It was designed to make minimal sounds as to not annoy patients or workers. This robot also has special cameras and sensors that help in avoiding obstacles, including humans walking around the hospital.

Other groups of robots help care for patients. These robots do not provide direct care. Instead, they help patients communicate with medical professionals, stay connected to the outside world, support mood and mental health, and more. These types of robots have become very popular in eldercare settings. The world's population is aging. Many countries face shortages of medical professionals to care for the elderly. Humans are living longer, but many face health disorders that can impair them physically or mentally. One famous robot is called Paro, and it is meant to help patients with Alzheimer's disease and dementia. The robot is in the form of a stuffed seal. It blinks, makes facial expressions, and makes sounds. The robot helps soothe patients, giving them something to pet, talk to, and focus on. Some robots also help the elderly or other patients with their doctors, their families, and the outside world. Some robots have screens that connect patients with their loved ones for video calls. Other robots remind patients to do important tasks, such as taking medication at certain times or contacting a particular doctor.

Medical professionals can also use robots as part of a patient's treatment. For example, robotic exoskeletons have been used in limited capacities to help peo-

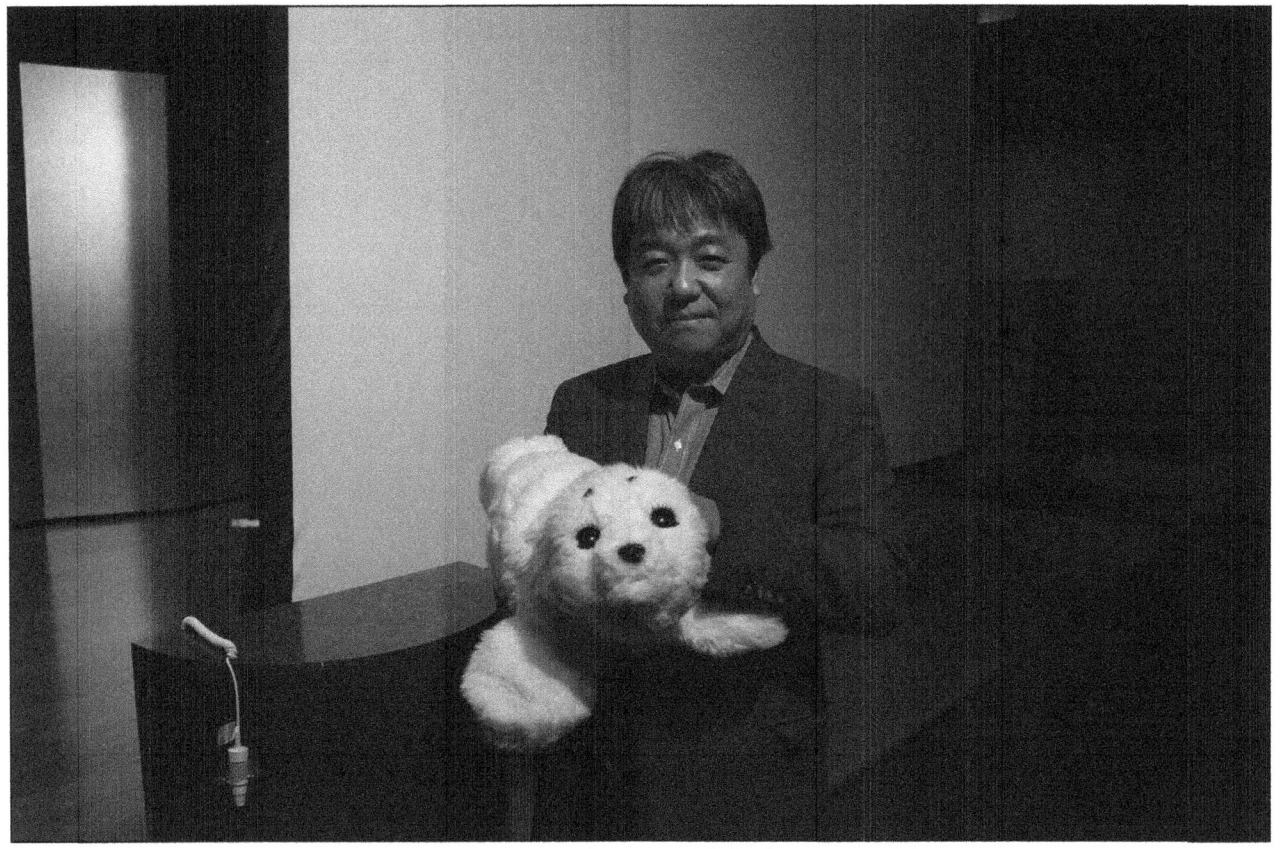

Dr Takanori Shibata holding his creation PARO, a robot therapy device. (Gerald Shields via Wikimedia Commons)

ple move body parts and even walk after an accident or illness damaged part of the body. Robotic exo- skeletons are extremely powerful and can help people walk more effectively than traditional walking aids, such as canes, crutches, or walkers. These robotic technologies are still in the early stages, but researchers hope they will help people become and remain mobile.

A positive aspect of using robots in healthcare settings is that robots cannot contract infectious diseases from patients. In 2020, the COVID-19 pandemic caused shortages of personal protective equipment (PPE) that helps reduce the rates of infection in healthcare workers. Technology advocates pointed out that increasing the number of robots in healthcare settings could help conserve PPE and could help prevent infectious diseases from spreading to as many people.

Although robots have made elements of healthcare easier or more successful, people still face ethical questions about the use of robots in medicine and healthcare. One ethical question relates to allowing robots to perform tasks that they could mismanage. Robots usually perform their tasks correctly, but one incorrect piece of code or even an incorrect input from a human could cause a robot to make a mistake. Studies show that robots actually reduce the number of mistakes made in healthcare, but humans have to decide if they comfortable with robots, not humans, making mistakes. Another ethical question is when it is proper to have a robot interact with human patients instead of other humans interacting with the patients. For example, humans have to decide if the elderly or even the dying should be comforted by robots or if only actual humans should play that role. Ideas about how humans interact with robots have created their own field of study called human-robot interactions, and people in that field consider such questions.

Another ethical question about robots faces the entire field of robotics. Robots are taking the place of humans, reducing the number of available jobs. Robots and AI will someday have the ability to complete many more human tasks. Humans could, and experts believe likely will, someday develop robots that are more intelligent than human beings. Humans have to consider if they should create technology that they could eventually lose control over.

Humans have changed and developed the ways they use robotics in healthcare, and people will continue to create new robots and find new applications for those that already exist. Currently, robots do not dispense treatment or perform medical procedures. They are currently used to augment or support the healthcare that humans provide. In the future, however, robots will continue to become more intelligent and capable. It is likely that one day humans will develop robots that could perform surgeries more skillfully than humans. Robots could also start to take the place of nurses, phlebotomists, and other health professionals for reading vital signs, taking blood samples, and more. Robots could also collect information from patients in areas with fewer doctors, allowing patients to receive information about potentially critical diagnoses (e.g., heart attack or stroke) without having to see a doctor.

Nanotechnology is a technology that is developed at the atomic or molecular level, making the technology so small that it potentially be used inside the body. Scientists could use nanotechnology to make robots that could go inside the human body and heal them. This could greatly reduce the number of patients who undergo surgery.

—*Elizabeth Mohn*

Further Reading

Adams, Tim. "The Robot Will See You Now: Could Computers Take Over Medicine Entirely?" *The Guardian,* 29 Jul. 2018, www.theguardian.com/technology/2018/jul/29/the-robot-will-see-you-now-could-computers-take-over-medicine-entirely. Accessed 6 May 2020.

Crawford, Mark. "Top 6 Robotic Applications in Medicine." *The American Society of Mechanical Engineers,* 14 Sep 2016, www.asme.org/topics-resources/content/top-6-robotic-applications-in-medicine. Accessed 6 May 2020.

Gyles, Carlton. "Robots in Medicine." *Canadian Veterinary Journal*, vol. 60, no. 8, 2019, pp. 819–20.

"Medical Robots." *Robotics Online*, www.robotics.org/service-robots/medical-robots. Accessed 6 May 2020.

Nelson, Brad. "Robotics and Medicine." *Science*, www.sciencemag.org/robotics-and-medicine. Accessed 6 May 2020.

Simon, Matt. "The WIRED Guide to Robots." *WIRED*, 13 Apr. 2020, www.wired.com/story/wired-guide-to-robots/. Accessed 6 May 2020.

Stansil, Raynetta. "What Is Robotic Surgery and How Does It Work?" *Surgical Solutions*, 31 Jul. 2019, surgical-solutions.com/blog/what-is-robotic-surgery-and-how-does-it-work/. Accessed 6 May 2020.

Williams, Andrew. "Medical Robotics Has an 'Incredibly Exciting' Future, Predict Experts." *Robotics Business Review*, 22 Nov. 2018, www.roboticsbusinessreview.com/health-medical/medical-robotics-exciting-future/. Accessed 6 May 2020.

BIOINFORMATICS

ABSTRACT

Bioinformatics is a rapidly growing area of quantitative, mathematical, and computational biology that collects and analyzes biological data, most often deoxyribonucleic acid (DNA) and amino acid sequences.

INTRODUCTION

As medicine advances, the role of bioinformatics will grow. As screening and diagnostic testing becomes more advanced and complex, storing findings in a searchable database that can be used to advance medical science is desirable. The role of genetics in healthcare is growing and bioinformatics is critical to supporting this growth.

The answer to the question "What is bioinformatics?" is not straightforward, yet in addressing this question the richness and extent of the field become clear. Part of the reason that it is difficult to give a concise definition of bioinformatics is that, as researchers publishing in the field realize, the definition is somewhat artificial and its boundaries are still expanding. This is not surprising, as bioinformatics might also be called mathematical/computational molecular biology, which points to large parts of biology taking on the aspects of a "hard" science such as physics or chemistry.

The creation of bioinformatics was triggered by a combination of factors in the 1990s. Key elements were progress in computing power, the existence of much larger data sets, and increasingly quantitative approaches to molecular biology, including molecular evolutionary studies. The large data sets came from a number of sources, including long individual DNA sequences (e.g., genomes), large between-species comparative or evolutionary alignments, microarray-generated gene expression data, proteomics data from two-dimensional (2D) gel electrophoresis and mass spectroscopy techniques, and structural information—broadly speaking, the fields of comparative, functional, and structural genomics. It was also increasingly recognized that quantitative molecular biology required vast amounts of computer power not only to assemble genomes but also to complete fundamental analyses, such as aligning related DNA sequences or building a tree from such an alignment. For example, with just twenty sequences there are more different trees relating these sequences than Avogadro's number (approximately 6 times 10_{23}), and every tree must be checked to ensure that the optimal solution has been found.

THE SCOPE OF RESEARCH

Bioinformatics itself touches on other areas of science such as biomedical informatics, computer science, statistical analysis, molecular biology, and mathematical modeling. In turn, each of these fields contributes uniquely to the progress of bioinformatics toward a mature science. Equally definitive of bioinformatics is recognizing those areas wholly or partly subsumed by an approach mixing computing power with mathematical and statistical modeling to solve biological questions based on molecular data. These areas include genomics, evolutionary biology, population genetics, structural biology, microarray gene expression analysis, proteomics, and the modeling of cellular processes plus systems biology (e.g., modeling a neurological pathway in which individual neurons respond to molecular events).

In bioinformatics, as in chemistry and physics, there is a fundamental split between empirical/experimental and theoretical science. At one extreme may be a laboratory focusing on generating large amounts of microarray data with relatively little analysis, and at the other extreme may be a mathematician working alone to solve a theorem with an application to better analyze that microarray data. It is clear that both approaches are needed for science to develop. However, it is not uncommon to find researchers actively tackling both problems (e.g., gathering large data sets and seeking better methods to analyze them). Increasingly, the scale and cost of major bioinformatics projects call for a new model of interdisciplinary biological research in which biologists, statisticians, computer scientists, chemists, mathematicians, physicians, and physicists interact closely together.

The nature of bioinformatics research highlights the need for interdisciplinary skills in modern biology. Some universities issue bioinformatics degrees based on their own formulas. A more direct approach is to require a quadruple major in statistics, computer science, mathematics, and biology. The importance of such a background is that, for example, someone who is not the best mathematician still needs to know how to ask the best mathematicians for help with the problems that inevitably crop up in research in this area. A good example of this interdependence arose in the Celera Genomics effort to complete the human genome, in which mathematicians with a specialty in tiling algorithms were essential to reassembling the millions of sequenced fragments.

In the future, bioinformatics will be increasingly involved with projects, the magnitude of which are technically and intellectually as challenging as anything previously faced in science. For example, a key problem might be a complete computer model of a single cell. Perfection would be achieved only when a biologist could not tell the difference between real and experimental data when the cell experienced a change internally or externally.

PERSPECTIVE AND PROSPECTS

The implications of bioinformatics for medicine are enormous. The strictly informatics side is already central to medical genetics. Databases of human characteristics, including detailed medical histories and biochemical profiles, are matched up with millions of genetic markers within each individual. Only through such enormous databases can statistical sleuths uncover the basis of most diseases that are caused by multiple genes. This is the population genetics of humans on a vast scale. Elsewhere, medical research such as cancer modeling is rapidly becoming a branch of bioinformatics, driven by the fact that cancer is caused by many interacting genes. Bioinformatics is key to the advancement of clinical genomic medicine and genomic technologies affecting complex diseases and disorders, drug dosing, and vaccine design.

The overall prospect is that bioinformatics will make possible a different sort of medicine in the twenty-first century in which fundamental research leads to pharmaceutical intervention, which leads to treating a disease at its root cause in a way that avoids the need for surgical intervention. Treatments of tomorrow, from diagnosis to cure, will involve processing large amounts of data via computers, with doctors remaining the key to ensuring an appropriate treatment regime, one that is personalized and precise, with the consent and comfort of the patient foremost.

In short, one answer to the question "What is bioinformatics?" is the development of virtual molecular biology. As time passes, this scientific endeavor will propagate upward and outward to meet other major areas of biology, such as physiology and ecology. Eventually, much of biology and medicine may come to rest solidly on the same principles as chemistry and physics, yet require major computational resources because of the complexity of the models needed to approximate reality reliably.

—*Peter J. Waddell*

Further Reading

"Bioinformatics." National Human Genome Research Institute. *National Institutes of Health*, www.genome.gov/genetics-glossary/Bioinformatics on Accessed 2 Sept. 2020.

Brazas, Michelle D., et al. "A Quick Guide to Genomics and Bioinformatics Training for Clinical and Public Audiences." *PLoS Computational Biology*, vol. 10, no. 4, 2014, pp. 1–6.

Campbell, A. Malcolm, and Laurie J. Heyer. *Discovering Genomics, Proteomics, and Bioinformatics*. 2nd ed., Pearson, 2007.

Davidson, Eric H. *The Regulatory Genome: Gene Regulatory Networks in Development and Evolution*. Academic, 2006.

Higgs, Paul G., and Teresa K. Attwood. *Bioinformatics and Molecular Evolution*. Wiley-Blackwell, 2013.

International Human Genome Sequencing Consortium. "Initial Sequencing and Analysis of the Human Genome." *Nature*, vol. 409, no. 6822, 2001, pp. 860–921.

Pevsner, Jonathan. *Bioinformatics and Functional Genomics*. 3rd ed., Wiley-Blackwell, 2015.

Tran, Quoc Nam, and Hamid Arabnia. *Emerging Trends in Computational Biology, Bioinformatics, and Systems Biology: Algorithms and Software Tools*. Morgan, 2015.

Vihinen, Mauno. "No More Hidden Solutions in Bioinformatics." *Nature*, 20 May 2015.

Popular Health Movement

ABSTRACT

The popular health movement was an early nineteenth-century health movement in the United States that promoted nontraditional medical treatment, in particular the use of herbal remedies, and opposed traditional medicine.

OVERVIEW

The popular health movement of the early nineteenth century led many Americans to react with skepticism to doctors and to medical practices that were common at the time. People turned instead to forms of treatment that did not involve doctors and often involved herbal remedies. Several factors led to this skepticism.

Beginning in the eighteenth century, doctors claimed knowledge, or expertise, beyond common understanding. This specialized knowledge led to a rise in status and authority for doctors and was symbolized by the increasing use of Latin terms to describe medical conditions, placing the language of doctors beyond the grasp of most people. In spite of claims to expertise, medical practice of the time was often harsh to the point of brutality, and it was still

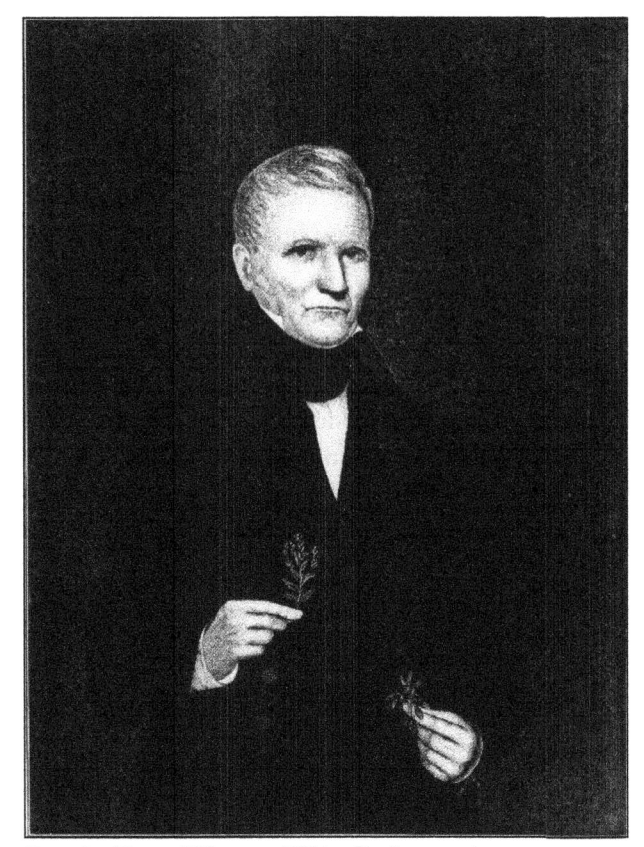

Portrait of Samuel Thomson (Wikimedia Commons)

common for a physician to use techniques such as bloodletting by cutting veins or applying leeches. One of the most common prescribed drugs was calomel (mercurous chloride), which was acknowledged to have severe toxic side effects.

A second factor influencing the popular health movement was the mood of the country with the election of Andrew Jackson to the US presidency in 1828. People denounced elitism and elites, including politicians and doctors. Just as politics during this time promoted the idea of democracy as a popular movement and expanded the vote to all white men, the country reacted against the specialized authority of doctors. One effect of this reaction was the abolition by most states of requirements that doctors be licensed.

During this time, too, the country saw philosophical and artistic movements toward nature and the idea of letting nature affect healing; this was a third factor in development of the popular health movement. Nature was embraced, especially with the wide interest in botanical remedies.

THOMSONIANISM

One of the leading figures of the popular health movement was Samuel Thomson, born in New Hampshire to a farming family. Thomson became a leading proponent of herbal cures, which he began learning from a woman who lived nearby. He had seen his mother die of measles; conventional doctors were unable to cure her. Later, after his wife grew ill and doctors had stopped treating her, Thomson called in herbal healers, who were able to help her. He later used his own cures to heal a son and a daughter, strengthening his belief in herbal cures.

Thomson's cures were largely plant-based. His book describing his system was published as *New Guide to Health: Or, Botanic Family Physician* (1822). The use of plants was part of a more complex system of belief, however.

Thomson, who believed that illness came from exposure to cold, argued that keeping the body warm would prevent illness. He applied heat to the body externally and internally with steam baths and cayenne peppers. His system also included the idea of expurgating the body of toxins, which involved the use of laxatives and emetics such as the Lobelia plant for therapeutic vomiting. Thomson's relationship with conventional physicians was not good, as he arrogantly rejected treatments not based on his own system.

ECLECTIC MEDICINE AND GRAHAMISM

Eclectic medicine. Eventually, healers who were interested in Thomson's herbal cures, but also in more conventional medicine, found themselves breaking with Thomson. The physician Wooster Beach, who used Thomson's botanical idea but disagreed with him on other issues, founded a medical school in 1829 as part of the new eclectic medicine movement. This movement argued that physicians should choose

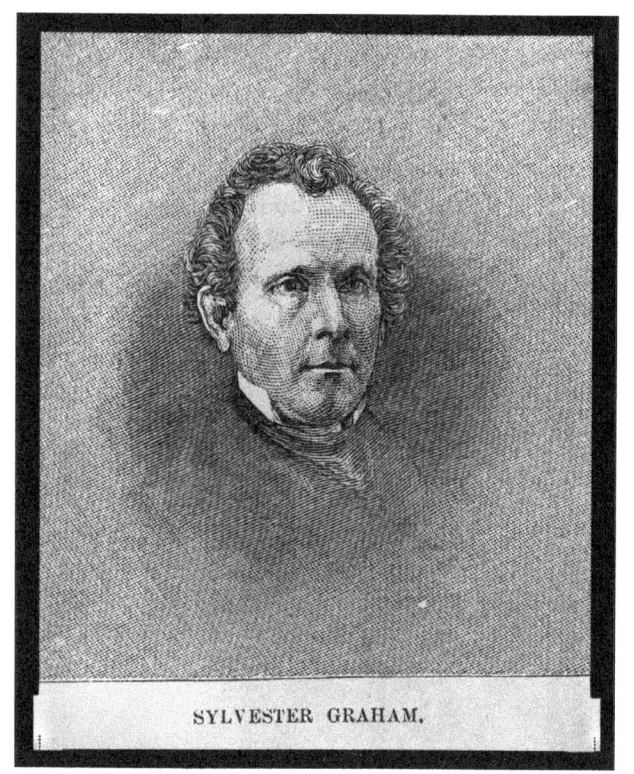

Portrait of Sylvester Graham (Wikimedia Commons)

freely from any idea or medical system they believed would help their patients. Within the eclectic movement, Thomson's ideas on the use of plants could be used without Thomson's restrictions, which included rejecting the study of physiology and anatomy. The eclectic medicine movement remained influential for a century, lasting until the 1920s.

Grahamism. Probably the most influential health reformer of the early nineteenth century after Thomson was Sylvester Graham, a Presbyterian preacher from Connecticut. Although Graham had no medical training, he had great public influence, particularly on dietary practices. His name is perhaps best known in relation to "Graham crackers," which he invented. Graham also was a strong proponent of vegetarianism and of temperance in general, advocating restrictions on alcohol consumption and sexual activity. In diet, he urged the use of dark, whole-wheat breads free of the chemical additives that were common even at that time. Other philosophies of medicine and treatment also became popular. These included hydropathy, with baths as a basic element, and homeopathy, operating from the idea that like treats like. Homeopathy opposed the methods of allopathy, or traditional medicine, which treated disease with substances unrelated to the illness.

—*David Hutto*

Further Reading

Burbick, Joan. *Healing the Republic: The Language of Health and the Culture of Nationalism in Nineteenth-Century America*. Cambridge UP, 2009.

Cabrera, Chanchal. "The History of Western Herbal Medicine." This brief but detailed history of herbal medicine is available at www.chanchalcabrera.com/articles.

"Complementary and Alternative Medicine: History." *Duquesne University*, guides.library.duq.edu/complementary_medicine/history. Accessed 16 Sept. 2020.

"Every Man His Own Physician: Thomsonianism." *Nature Cures: A History of Alternative Medicine in America*, edited by James C. Whorton, Oxford UP, 2004.

"Health Information." National Center for Complementary and Integrative Health. *National Institutes of Health*, www.nccih.nih.gov/health. Accessed 16 Sept. 2020.

Whorton, James C. "The History of Complementary and Alternative Medicine." *Essentials of Complementary and Alternative Medicine*, edited by Wayne B. Jonas and Jeffrey S. Levin, Lippincott Williams & Wilkins, 1999.

NURSING TERMINOLOGY

ACNM: The American Collage of Nurse-Midwives

ADN: Associates Degree in Nursing—the most common first step of nursing education. Takes two years to complete at a college

ADON: Assistant Director of Nursing—is there to always assist and back up the head director when not available or absent

APN: Advanced Practice Nurse—a nurse who is educationally past the post-graduate level

BCEN: Board of Certification for Emergency Nursing

BN: Bachelor in Nursing

BSN: Bachelor of Science in Nursing

CEN: Certified Emergency Nurse

CCU: Critical care unit

CDN: Certified dialysis nurse

Change nurse: Looks after the immediate functions of a specific unit

CNL: Clinical nurse leader

CNA: Certified nurse assistant

CNM: Certified nurse-midwife

CNP: Clinical nurse specialist

CPM: Certified Professional Midwifes

CPR: Cardiopulmonary resuscitation

Continuous Medical Education: An all-encompassing term within a broad spectrum of post-secondary learning activities and programs

Diploma in Nursing: Hospital based diploma program, takes about three years to complete

DNP: Doctor of Nursing Practice

DON: Director of nursing oversees that proper care is given to all individuals at their health care facility and usually reports to the CEO or COO of the company

EMT: Emergency medical technician

ENP: Emergency Nurse Practitioner

ER: Emergency room

FDA: Food and drug administration

Fight nurse: Provides pre-hospital emergency assistance, to patients aboard aircrafts and helicopters in life-threatening situations

Geriatric nurse: Focuses on the elderly or older adult patients

Graduate nurse: A nurse who has just graduated from college or a nursing program

Human Growth and Development: Involves areas related to child health

ICU: Intensive care unit

IV: Intravenous

LPN: Licensed practical nurse—needs only complete an accredited nursing program and pass a state board to practice, but must work under physicians

Mental health: Focuses on psychiatric and or child psychology nursing

Midwifery: Provides care to childbearing women during pregnancy

MRI: Magnetic resonance angiography

Neonatal nurse: Work with newborns up to 28 days old

Nephrology: Study of the kidneys

NCLEX-RN exam: National licensing exam to become a registered nurse

NCLEX-PN exam: National licensing exam to become a practical nurse

NICU: Neonatal intensive care unit

NNP: Neonatal nurse practitioner

NP: Nurse Practitioner

Nurse manager: Manages a unit on all levels and will typically report back to a service director

Nursing agency: Business that helps nurses find hospitals and other care facilities that are in need of health care professionals, like nurses

Nursing Board Certifications: These voluntary exams are offered by the board to those who would like to prove knowledge of a specific specialty and be recognized for it

Oncology: Study of cancer

OR: Operating room

Pediatric nurse: Focuses on working with children patients

Per Diem nurse: Works on a day-to-day basis with no set schedule and under no set contract

Permanent nurse: Works under contract in one location

PEN: Pediatric endocrinology nurse

Physician assistants: Licensed professionals who practice medicine under the supervision of a licensed Physician

PICU: Pediatric Intensive Care Unit

PNP: Psychiatric nurse practitioner

Post-op: After operation

Practice setting: Place where a nurse might work such as a hospital or clinic

Pre-op: Before operation

Psychiatric nurse: Also known as a mental health nurse, specially trained to care for individuals of all ages who suffer from mental illness or distress

Public health nursing: Centered on theory, practice and specializations

RN: Registered nurse is one who has graduated from college and passed the national license exam

Service director: A director will usually oversee an entire facility and have other nurse mangers reporting to them regarding the larger organization as a whole

Scope of Practice: Terminology used by state licensing boards for professions that defines the procedures, actions, and processes that are permitted for the licensed individual

SICU: Surgical Intensive Care Unit

Travel nurse: Works for short periods of time with different health care facilities

Source: Reprinted with permission from NursingJobFinder.com

General Bibliography and Further Reading

"10 Tips for Effective Networking." *University of Maryland, Baltimore County*, careers.umbc.edu/students/network/networking101/tips/. Accessed 30 Aug. 2020.

"22 Meditation Statistics: Data and Trends Revealed for 2019." *The Good Body*, www.thegoodbody.com/meditation-statistics/. Accessed 24 Aug. 2020.

"33 Common Nursing School Interview Questions." *Indeed.com*, www.indeed.com/career-advice/interviewing/nursing-school-interview-questions. Accessed 28 Aug. 2020.

"5 Leadership Skills Found in Managers." Villanova University. Updated 6 May 2009, www.villanovau.com/resources/leadership/5-leadership-skills-found-in-managers/.

"5 Places Where Public Health Nurses Work." *Nurse Journal*, 3 June 2020, nursejournal.org/public-health-nursing/5-places-where-public-health-nurses-work/.

"8 Things to Know about Meditation for Health." National Center for Complementary and Integrative Health. *National Institutes of Health*, www.ncch.nih.gov/health/tips/things-to-know-about-meditation-for-health. Accessed 24 Aug. 2020.

"A Day in the Life of an Obstetric Nurse." *City College*, www.citycollege.edu/ob-nurse/. Accessed 1 Oct. 2020.

"A Guide to Informed Consent: Guidance for Institutional Review Boards and Clinical Investigators." *US Food & Drug Administration*, www.fda.gov/regulatory-information/search-fda-guidance-documents/guide-informed-consent. Accessed 11 Sept. 2020.

"A Primer for Getting Your Nursing License in Another State." *Travel Nursing*, www.travelnursing.com/news/career-development/a-primer-for-getting-your-nursing-license-in-another-state/. Accessed 30 Sept. 2020.

Aamodt, M. G. *Industrial/Organizational Psychology: An Applied Appro*ach. 8th ed., Cengage Learning, 2016. A segment of chapter 4 describes types of employment interviews and interview questions, as well as how to conduct interviews.

"About Art Therapy." *American Art Therapy Association*, www.arttherapy.org. Accessed 4 May 2020.

"About NIH." US Department of Health and Human Services. *National Institutes of Health*, www.nih.gov/about-nih. Accessed 2 Sept. 2020.

"About the CEU." *International Association for Continuing Education and Training*, www.iacet.org/standards/ansi-iacet-2018-1-standard-for-continuing-education-and-training/continuing-education-unit-ceu/about-the-ceu/. Accessed 18 Sept. 2020.

"About the Nursing Shortage." *American Association of Colleges of Nursing*, www.aacnnursing.org/New-Information/Nursing-Shortage-Resources/About. Accessed 22 Sept. 2020.

"About U.S. Nursing Regulatory Bodies." *National Council of State Boards of Nursing*. www.ncsbn.org/ about-nursing-regulatory-bodies.htm. Accessed 7 Oct. 2020.

Academy of Medical-Surgical Nurses (AMSN), www.amsn.org. Accessed 29 Sept. 2020.

Accordino, Robert, Ronald Comer, and Wendy B. Heller. "Searching for Music's Potential: A Critical Examination of Research on Music Therapy with Individuals with Autism." *Research in Autism Spectrum Disorders*, vol. 1, 2007, pp. 101-15.

"Accreditation and Certifications." *Standards*, www.jointcommission.org. Accessed 16 Sept. 2020.

"Acute, Critical Care Nursing: The Frontlines of Patient Care." *Minority Nurse*, 30 Mar. 2013, minoritynurse.com/?s=critical+care+nursing. Accessed 4 Jan. 2017.

Adams, Caralee. "College Board Begins Redesign of SAT Exam." *Education Week*, 6 Mar. 2013, p. 4.

Adams, M. "Public Speaking 101-Become a Great Storyteller." *EDGE*, 2015, www.worldchampionsedgenet.com/resources/articles/becoming-a-great-storyteller/. This article emphasizes how learning to master the art of storytelling is integrally intertwined with becoming an exceptional public speaker. Specific strategies to increase one's storytelling abilities are outlined.

Adams, Tim. "The Robot Will See You Now: Could Computers Take Over Medicine Entirely?" *The Guardian*, 29 Jul. 2018, www.theguardian.com/technology/2018/jul/29/the-robot-will-see-you-now-could-computers-take-over-medicine-entirely. Accessed 6 May 2020.

Ader, R., and N. Cohen. "Psychoneuroimmunology: Conditioning and Stress." *Annual Review of Psychology*, vol. 44, 1993, pp. 53-85.

Aiken, Linda. "The Magnet Nursing Services Recognition Program: A Comparison of Two Groups of Magnet Hospitals." *American Journal of Nursing*, vol. 100, no. 3, 2000, pp. 26-36.

Aitken, Leanne, et al. *ACCCN's Critical Care Nursing*. 3rd ed., Elsevier Australia, 2015.

Akinsanya, Justus A. *The Roy Adaptation Model in Action.* Macmillan, 1994.

Alimohammadi, Nasrollah, et al. "The Nursing Metaparadigm Concept of Human Being in Islamic Thought." *Nursing Inquiry*, vol. 21, no. 2, 2014, pp. 121-29.

Alligood, M. R. *Nursing Theorists and their Work.* 8th ed., Mosby Elsevier, 2014, docshare01.docshare.tips/files/29843/298436680.pdf.

Alligood, M. R. *Nursing Theorists and their Work.* 9th ed., Elsevier eBook on Vital Source, 2018.

Alligood, Martha Raile, and Ann Marriner-Tomey. *Nursing Theorists and Their Work.* Mosby/Elsevier, 2010.

Alligood, Martha Raile, and Ann Marriner-Tomey. *Nursing Theory: Utilization and Application.* 5th ed., Mosby, 2013.

Alpha Iota & Xi Alpha, Perioperative Consultant, Competency and Credentialing Institute, June 2020.

American Academy of Acupuncture, medicalacupuncture.org. The American Academy of Medical Acupuncture (AAMA) is the professional society of physicians (MDs and DOs) in North America who have incorporated acupuncture into their traditional medical practice.

American Association of Integrative Medicine, www.aaimedicine.com. Promotes the development of IM.

American Association of Naturopathic Physicians, naturopathic.org.

American Association of Nurse Anesthetists (AANA), www.aana.com. Accessed 28 Sept. 2020.

American Association of Nurse Practitioners (AANP), www.aanp.org/. Accessed 25 Sept. 2020.

American Association of Occupational Health Nurses. Resources, aaohn.org. Accessed 3 Sept. 2020.

American Board of Integrative Holistic Medicine, integrativeholisticdoctors.org. Establishes and maintains standards of care.

"American Cancer Society Updates Guideline for Diet and Physical Activity." *American Cancer Society*, 9 June 2020, www.cancer.org/latest-news/american-cancer-society-updates-guideline-for-diet-and-physical-activity.html.

American Chiropractic Association, www.acatoday.org. Chiropractic is a healthcare profession that focuses on disorders of the musculoskeletal system and the nervous system, and the effects of these disorders on general health in a holistic manner.

American Holistic Medical Association, www.holisticmedicine.org. Promotes holistic and integrative principles.

American Institute for Homeopathy, homeopathyusa.org/homeopathic-medicine.html.

American Massage Therapy Association, www.amtamassage.org.

American Music Therapy Association, 2015. Accessed 12 Feb. 2015.

American Nurses Association (ANA), www.nursingworld.org/ ana/.

American Nurses Association. *Nursing: Scope and Standards of Practice.* 3rd ed. American Nurses Association, 2015.

American Nurses Credentialing Center (ANCC), www.nursingworld.org/ancc/.

American Psychological Association. "Ethical Principles of Psychologists." *American Psychologist*, vol. 36, 1981, pp. 633-38.

American Telemedicine Association. *American Telemedicine Association*, 2012.

"Americans Spent $30.2 Billion Out-of-Pocket on Complementary Health Approaches." US Department of Health and Human Services. *National Center for Complementary and Integrative Health*, 22 June 2016, www.nccih.nih.gov/news/press-releases/americans-spent-302-billion-outofpocket-on-complementary-health-approaches. Accessed 29 June 2020.

ANCC Certification General Testing and Renewal Handbook. American Nurses Credentialing Center, April 2017.

ANCC Magnet Recognition Program.(r) *American Nursing Credentialing Center*, www.nursingworld.org/organizational-programs/magnet/. Access 3 Sept. 2020.

Anderson, J. W., C. Liu, and R. J. Kryscio. "Blood Pressure Response to Transcendental Meditation." *American Journal of Hypertension*, vol. 21, 2008, pp. 310-16.

Anson, Briah. *Animal Healing: The Power of Rolfing.* Mill City Press, 2011.

Art Therapy Credentials Board, www.atcb.org.

Ashkenas, R. "Seven Mistakes Leaders Make in Setting Goals." *Forbes*, 2015, www.forbes.com/sites/ronashkenas/2012/07/09/seven-mistakes-leaders-make-in-setting-goals/.

Assefi, N., et al. "Reiki for the Treatment of Fibromyalgia." *Journal of Alternative and Complementary Medicine*, vol. 14, 2008, pp. 1115-22.

Association of periOperative Registered Nurses (AORN), www.aorn.org. Accessed 30 Sept. 2020.

Astin, J. A., et al. "Complementary and Alternative Medicine Use Among Elderly Persons." *Journal of Gerontology: Medical Sciences*, vol. 55A, 2000, pp. M4-M9.

Astin, J. A., et al. "Mind-Body Medicine: State of the Science, Implications for Practice." *Journal of the*

American Board of Family Medicine, vol. 16, 2003, pp. 131-47.

"Baby Boomer." *Investopedia*, www.investopedia.com/terms/b/baby_boomer.asp. Accessed 4 Jan. 2017.

Baer, Hans. *Toward an Integrative Medicine: Merging Alternative Therapies with Biomedicine*. Altamira Press, 2004. A comprehensive overview of the holistic movement and its journey into mainstream medicine.

Ballweg, Ruth, et al. *Physician Assistant: A Guide to Clinical Practice*. 6th ed., Elsevier, 2017.

Bankert, Marianne. *Watchful Care: A History of America's Nurse Anesthetists*. Continuum International Publishing Group, 1989.

Barclay, J. "Text Messaging: Does It Destroy Relationships?" *Snowdrift*, 2013, www.snowcollegenews.com/text-messaging-does-it-destroy-relationships/. This article discusses that while texting has benefits, the ease and frequency in which people's texts are misinterpreted can lead to significant negative outcomes. The author focuses on how texts have led to many break-ups, specifically among college students.

Barinaga, Marcia. "Studying the Well-Trained Mind." *Science*, vol. 302, 2003, pp. 44-46. Discusses collaboration among scientists and Buddhist monks in a study measuring the effects of meditation on the brain.

Barnes, P. M., B. Bloom, and R. L. Nahin. "Complementary and Alternative Medicine Use Among Adults and Children: 2007 United States." *National Health Statistics Reports*, vol. 12, pp. 1-23.

Barnes, P. M., et al. "Complementary and Alternative Medicine Use Among Adults: United States, 2002." *CDC Advance Data Report*, vol. 343, 2004.

Barnier, C. *The Big What Now Book of Learning Styles: A Fresh and Demystifying Approach*. Emerald Books, 2009. This book delivers a fresh and demystifying approach to learning styles.

Barrett, David. "Should Nurses Be at the Forefront of Telehealth?" *The Guardian*, 20 Jan. 2014, www.theguardian.com/healthcare-network/2012/jan/20/nurses-needed-at-telehealth-forefront.

Barton, P. E., and R. J. Coley. "Windows on Achievement and Inequality." *Policy Information Report*, PIC-WINDOWS. Educational Testing Service, 2008.

Becker, Ernest. *The Denial of Death*. Free Press, 1997. Written by an anthropologist and philosopher, this is an erudite and insightful analysis and synthesis of the role that the fear of death plays in motivating human activity, society, and individual actions. A profound work.

"Become a WOC Nurse." *WOCN: Wound, Ostomy, and Continence Nurses Society*, www.wocn.org/become-a-woc-nurse/. Accessed 24 Sept. 2020.

"Becoming a Geriatric Nurse." *EveryNurse.org*, everynurse.org/becoming-a-geriatric-nurse. Accessed 4 Jan. 2017.

Bell, Linda, editor. *AACN Scope and Standards for Acute Care Clinical Nurse Specialist Practice*. American Association of Critical-Care Nurses, 2014.

Bendaly, Leslie, and Nicole Bendaly. *Improving Healthcare Team Performance: The 7 Requirements for Excellence in Patient Care*. John Wiley & Sons, 2012.

Bensimon, Moshe, Dorit Armir, and Yuval Wolf. "Drumming Through Trauma: Music Therapy with Post-traumatic Soldiers." *Arts in Psychotherapy*, vol. 35, 2008, pp. 34-48.

Benson, H. "The Relaxation Response: Its Subjective and Objective Historical Precedents and Physiology." *Trends in Neurosciences*, vol. 6, 1983, pp. 281-84. Discusses research at Harvard's Thorndike Memorial Laboratory in defining the physiology and in describing the subjective and objective historical precedents and clinical usefulness of the relaxation response. It is a classic text in the field.

Benson, H.,———, and M. Klipper. *The Relaxation Response*. William Morrow, 1975. Benson's explanation and synthesis of research on the relaxation response, based on historical, religious, and literary writings, with related scientific data from research conducted by Benson and associates. This work was expanded and updated in 2000, citing additional information on updated research.

Benson, S. G., and S. P. Dundis. "Understanding and Motivating Health Care Employees: Integrating Maslow's Hierarchy of Needs, Training and Technology." *Journal of Nursing Management*, vol. 11, no. 5, 2003, pp. 315-20.

Bersoff, Donald N., Laurel P. Malson, and Donald B. Verrilli. "In the Supreme Court of the United States: Clara Watson v. Fort Worth Bank and Trust." *American Psychologist*, vol. 43, 1988, pp. 1019-28.

Betts, Joe. "2020 NCLEX Fact Sheet NCLEX Statistics." NCLEX Examinations.

Betz, J. M., et al. "The NIH Analytical Methods and Reference Materials Program for Dietary Supplements." *Analytical and Bioanalytical Chemistry*, vol. 389, 2007, pp. 19-25.

"Bioinformatics." National Human Genome Research Institute. *National Institutes of Health*, www.genome.gov/

genetics-glossary/Bioinformatics on Accessed 2 Sept. 2020.

Bisk Education. "Nursing Careers: Critical Care Nurse." *Villanova University*, www.villanovau.com/resources/nursing/icu-critical-care-nursing-job-description/#.WGw LalMrKpo. Accessed 4 Jan. 2017.

Black, Beth Perry. *Professional Nursing: Concepts and Challenges*. 7th ed., Elsevier, 2014

Boissel, J. P. "Planning of Clinical Trials." *Journal of Internal Medicine*, vol. 255, no. 4, 2004, pp. 427-38.

Bolton, R. *People Skills: How to Assert Yourself, Listen to Others, and Resolve Conflicts*. Simon and Schuster, 1986. This paperback book was published a while ago, but it is still available, and it contains additional information and specific examples of the skills mentioned in this article.

Booth, F. "30 Time Management Tips for a Work-Life Balance." *Forbes*, 28 Aug. 2014, http://www.forbes.com/sites/francesbooth/2014/08/28/30-time-management-tips. This article provides helpful tips to live a life with effective time management skills.

Bradford, Nikki. *Your Premature Baby: The First Five Years*. Firefly Books, 2003.

Bragg, Elizabeth J., and Jennie Chin Hansen. "Ensuring Care for Aging Baby Boomers: Solutions at Hand." *Generations*, 8 June 2015, www.asaging.org/blog/ensuring-care-aging-baby-boomers-solutions-hand.

Branson, R. "Richard Branson on the Art of Public Speaking." *Entrepreneur*, 4 Feb. 2013, www.entrepreneur.com/article/225627. This article discusses the author's fear of public speaking. It also describes how he learned to overcome his fear, and how his ability to do so directly led to the elevated and international success of his company.

Brazas, Michelle D., et al. "A Quick Guide to Genomics and Bioinformatics Training for Clinical and Public Audiences." *PLoS Computational Biology*, vol. 10, no. 4, 2014, pp. 1-6.

Brecklinghaus, Hans. *Rolfing Structural Integration: What It Achieves, How It Works, and Whom It Helps*. Lightning Source, 2002.

Brizee, A., and A. Olson. "What Is a Cover Letter?" *Owl Purdue*, 14 Dec. 2011, owl.english.purdue.edu/owl/resource/549/01/. This article reviews what a cover letter is and contains further links such as video instructions and sample documents.

Brizee, A., N. Jarrett, N., and K. Schmaling. "What Is an Action Verb?" *Owl Purdue*, 2 Apr. 2010, owl.english.purdue.edu/owl/resource/543/01/. This article reviews what an "action verb" is and how it should be used. A link is also included for a list of action verbs categorized by skill sets.

Brook, Marian. "Betty Neuman." *American Nursing: A Biographical Dictionary*, edited by Vern L. Bullough and Lilli Sentz, vol. 3, Springer Publishing, 2000, pp. 218-21.

Brown, Di, et al. *Lewis's Medical-Surgical Nursing: Assessment and Management of Clinical Problems*. 4th ed., Mosby, 2015.

Brown, P. C. *Make It Stick*. Harvard UP, 2014. This book offers techniques for becoming more productive learners. In addition, it cautions against counterproductive study habits.

Bulla, Sally A., and Elaine M. Scherer. "What Does 'Magnet' Have to Do with Research?" *Real Stories of Nursing Research: The Quest for Magnet Recognition*, edited by M. Maureen Kirkpatrick McLaughlin and Sally A. Bulla, Jones and Bartlett Publishers, 2010, pp. 9-13.

Bunn, Jennifer. "Telehealth—the Future of Healthcare?" *Ausmed*, 26 Oct. 2016, www.ausmed.com/cpd/articles/telehealth.

Burbick, Joan. *Healing the Republic: The Language of Health and the Culture of Nationalism in Nineteenth-Century America*. Cambridge UP, 2009.

Burger, E., and M. Starbird. *The 5 Elements of Effective Thinking*. Princeton UP, 2012. The book presents practical and inspiring techniques for learners to become more successful through better thinking strategies.

Buros Institute of Mental Measurement. *The Fourteenth Mental Measurements Yearbook*. U of Nebraska P, 2001.

Butts, Jane B. and Karen L. Rich. *Nursing Ethics: Across the Curriculum and into Practice*. 5th ed., Jones & Bartlett Learning, 2013.

Butts, Janie B., and Karen L. Rich. *Philosophies and Theories for Advanced Nursing Practice*. Jones & Bartlett Learning, 2015.

Cabrera, Chanchal. "The History of Western Herbal Medicine." This brief but detailed history of herbal medicine is available at www.chanchalcabrera.com/articles.

Caldwell, D. F., and J. M. Burger. "Personality Characteristics of Job Applicants and Success in Screening Interviews." *Personnel Psychology*, vol. 51, 1998, pp. 119-136. The paper reports the mediating functions of personality traits of conscientiousness, extraversion, and openness to experience in the associations of social preparation and background preparation to interview success.

Callaway, Barbara J. *Hildegard Peplau: Psychiatric Nurse of the Century*. Springer, 2002.

Campbell, A. Malcolm, and Laurie J. Heyer. *Discovering Genomics, Proteomics, and Bioinformatics*. 2nd ed., Pearson, 2007.

Campbell, Donald Thomas. *Manual for the Strong-Campbell Interest Inventory*. Stanford UP, 2001.

Canadian Art Therapy Association, canadianarttherapy.org/.

Caplan, Robert D., et al. *Job Demands and Worker Health: Main Effects and Occupational Differences*. U of Michigan P, 1980.

Capuzzi, David, and Mark D. Stauffer, editors. *Career Counseling: Foundations, Perspectives, and Applications*. Routledge, 2012.

"Care Management: Implications for Medical Practice, Health Policy and Health Services Research." *Agency for Healthcare Research and Quality*, www.ahrq.gov/ncepcr/care/coordination/management.html. Accessed 20 Oct. 2020.

Career Onestop." US Department of Labor. Scholarship search, www.careeronestop.org/FindTraining/Pay/scholarships.aspx. Accessed 27 Aug. 2020. This website, sponsored by the US Department of Labor, focuses on helping individuals find the job or career that is right for them. Within the website, the scholarship search tool has over 7,000 legitimate graduate, "undergraduate, and professional scholarship opportunities to explore.

Carson, C., S. Lasker-Hertz, and P. Stanfill-Edens. "Exercise for Cancer Patients." www.oumedicine.com/docs/ou-medicine/exercisecancerpatients.pdf?sfvrsn=2. Accessed 25 Aug. 2020.

Cassileth, B. "Gerson Regimen." *Oncology*, vol. 24, no. 2, 2010, p. 201.

Center to Advance Palliative Care, www.capc.org. Accessed 1 Sept. 2020. Content and tools designed to enable healthcare practitioners to provide support to patients and families living with serious or terminal illnesses.

Centers for Disease Control and Prevention (CDC), cdc.gov.

"Certification and Career Progression." CCI (The Competency and Credentialing Institute), 2019, www.cc-institute.org/why-certify/.

"Certifications." *The Association of Clinical Research Professionals*, acrpnet.org/certifications/. Accessed 11 Sept. 2020.

"Certified Registered Nurse Anesthetists Fact Sheet." *American Association of Nurse Anesthetists (AANA)*. www.aana.com/membership/become-a-crna/crna-fact-sheet. Accessed 7 Oct. 2020.

Cherry, Kendra. "How Art Therapy Is Used to Help People Heal." *Very Well Mind*, 28 Aug. 2019, www.verywellmind.com/what-is-art-therapy-2795755.

"Chief Nursing Officer." Registered Nursing.org. www.registerednursing.org/specialty/chief-nursing-officer/. Accessed 6 Oct. 2020.

Choi, Ae-Na, Myeong Soo Lee, and Jung-Sook Lee. "Group Music Intervention Reduces Aggression and Improves Self-Esteem in Children with Highly Aggressive Behavior." *Complementary and Alternative Medicine*, vol. 1, no. 2, 2008, pp. 213-17.

"Choosing a Nursing Degree? Here's What You Need to Know." *Nurse.com*, www.nurse.com/blog/2017/11/30/choosing-a-nursing-degree-heres-what-you-need-to-know/. Accessed 27 Aug. 2020.

Christian, C., and R. Bolles. *What Color Is Your Parachute for Teens: Discovering Yourself, Defining your Future*. 2nd ed., Ten Speed Press, 2010. A book about finding your strengths and interests at an early age, so that you can decide what type of schooling, job, or career is right for you. This book includes profiles of individuals who have leveraged their strengths to find their dream job.

Clarke, Pamela N., et al. "The Impact of Dorothea Orem's Life and Work: An Interview with Orem Scholars." *Nursing Science Quarterly*, vol. 22, no. 1, 2009, pp. 41-46.

"Clinical Nurse Leader (CNL) Job Description." *GraduateNursingEDU.org*, www.graduatenursingedu.org/clinical-nurse-leader/. Accessed 1 Oct. 2020.

"Clinical Nurse Specialist: Education Requirements, Career Paths, & Job Outlook." 1 Oct. 2020, www.allnursingschools.com/clinical-nurse-specialist/.

Coakley, A. B., and M. E. Duffy. "The Effect of Therapeutic Touch on Postoperative Patients." *Journal of Holistic Nursing*, vol. 28, 2010, pp. 193-200.

"Coalition Launched to Oppose Nurse Staffing Ballot Question." *Massachusetts Health & Hospital Association*, 11 Dec. 2017, www.mhalink.org/MHA/MyMHA/Communications/MondayReportItems/Content/2017/12-11/Items/Coalition-Launched-to-Oppose-Nurse-Staffing-Ballot.aspx.

Codding, Peggy, and Suzanne Hanser. "Music Therapy." *Complementary and Integrative Medicine in Pain Management*, edited by Michael I. Weintraub, Springer, 2008.

Cohen, S., A. Dwane, P. deOliveira, and M. Muska. *Getting In! The Zinch Guide to College Admissions and Financial Aid in the Digital Age*. Cliff Notes, 2011. A short, well-researched, current guide for mastering the college admissions process. Includes information on college admissions offices, application guidelines, choosing the right college, athletic recruiting, and scholarship/financial aid opportunities. This book also contains helpful sections on college essay assistance and waiting for an answer after the application process.

Coleman, E. A. "Falling Through the Cracks: Challenges and Opportunities for Improving Transitional Care for Persons with Continuous Complex Care Needs." *Journal of the American Geriatrics Society*, vol. 51, 2003, pp. 549-55.

Coleman, E. A., and R. Berenson. "Lost in Transition: Challenges and Opportunities for Improving the Quality of Transitional Care." *Annals of Internal Medicine*, vol. 140, 2004, pp. 533-36.

Colley S. "Nursing Theory: Its Importance to Practice." *Nursing Standard*, vol. 17, no. 46, 2003, pp. 33-37.

Colley, S. "Nursing Theory: Its Importance to Practice." *Nursing Standard*, vol. 17, no. 46, 2003, pp. 33-37.

"Comfort Measures (Nonpharmacologic) during Labor." *DynaMed*, 30 Nov. 2018, www.dynamed.com/topics/dmp~AN~T114734.

Committee to Develop Standards for Educational and Psychological Testing. *Standards for Educational and Psychological Testing*. American Psychological Association, 1999.

"Complementary and Alternative Medicine: History." *Duquesne University*, guides.library.duq.edu/complementary_medicine/history. Accessed 16 Sept. 2020.

"Complementary, Alternative or Integrative Health: What's in a Name?" National Center for Complementary and Integrative Health. *National Institutes of Health*, www.nccih.nih.gov/health/complementary-alternative-or-integrative-health-whats-in-a-name. Accessed 25 Aug. 2020.

"Complete History of AACN." *American Association of Critical-Care Nurses*, www.aacn.org. Accessed 3 Sept. 2020.

"Complete Job Description of a Staff Nurse." TopRNtoBSN.com. www.toprntobsn.com/job-description-staff-nurse/. Accessed 5 Oct. 2020.

"Complete List of Common Nursing Certifications." *Nurse.org*, 8 July 2017, nurse.org/articles/nursing-certifications-credentials-list/.

"Conceptual Framework." *UNC Greensboro School of Nursing*, nursing.uncg.edu/about/mission/conceptual-framework/. Accessed 14 Sept. 2020.

Consortium of Academic Health Centers for Integrative Medicine, www.imconsortium.org. Advances the principles and practice of integrative healthcare within academic institutions.

Cook, Alicia Skinner, and Daniel S. Dworkin. *Helping the Bereaved: Therapeutic Interventions for Children, Adolescents, and Adults*. Basic Books, 1992. Although not a self-help book, this work is useful to professionals and nonprofessionals alike as a review of the state of the art in grief therapy. Practical and readable. Of special interest for those becoming involved in grief counseling.

"Coping with Stress." US Department of Health and Human Services. *Centers for Disease Control and Prevention*, 2 Oct. 2015.

"Coping with the Loss of a Loved One." *American Cancer Society*, www.cancer.org/treatment/end-of-life-care/grief-and-loss.html. Accessed 1 Sept. 2020.

Cormody, James, and Ruth A. Baer. "Relationships Between Mindfulness Practice and Levels of Mindfulness, Medical and Psychological Symptoms, and Well-Being in a Mindfulness-Based Stress Reduction Program." *Journal of Behavioral Medicine*, vol. 31, 2008, pp. 23-33. The researchers conducted pre- and postintervention surveys of 174 adults who participated in this mindfulness program.

Corr, Charles A., Clyde M. Nabe, and Donna M. Corr. *Death and Dying, Life and Living*. 6th ed., Wadsworth/Cengage Learning, 2009. This book provides perspective on common issues associated with death and dying for family members and others affected by life-threatening circumstances.

Costello R. B., and P. Coates. "In the Midst of Confusion Lies Opportunity: Fostering Quality Science in Dietary Supplement Research." *Journal of the American College of Nutrition*, vol. 20, 2001, pp. 21-25.

Covey, S. *The 6 Most Important Decisions You'll Ever Make: A Guide for Teens*. Fireside, 2006. This book shows teens how to make smart choices about the six most crucial choices they'll face during these turbulent years.

Covey, S. *The 7 Habits of Highly Effective Teens: The Ultimate Teenage Success Guide*. Miniature ed. Running Press, 2002. Based on his father's bestselling book, *The 7 Habits of Highly Effective People*, Sean Covey applies the same principles to teens, using a vivacious, entertaining style.

Craig, Claire. *Exploring the Self through Photography: Activities for Use in Group Work*. Jessica Kingsley, 2009.

Cralley, Lester V., and Patrick R. Atkins, editors. *Industrial Environmental Health: The Worker and the Community*. 2nd ed., Academic, 1975.

Crawford, Mark. "Top 6 Robotic Applications in Medicine." *The American Society of Mechanical Engineers*, 14 Sep 2016, www.asme.org/topics-resources/content/

top-6-robotic-applications-in-medicine. Accessed 6 May 2020.

Creasy, Robert K., and Robert Resnik, editors. *Maternal-Fetal Medicine: Principles and Practice.* 5th ed., W. B. Saunders, 2004.

Cullen, Rowena. *Health Information on the Internet: A Study of Providers, Quality, and Users.* Praeger, 2006.

Cunningham, F. Gary, et al., editors. *Williams Obstetrics.* 23rd ed., McGraw-Hill, 2010.

Dallaire, C., and P. Krol. "Revisiting the Roots of Nursing Philosophy and Critical Theory: Past, Present and Future." *Nursing Philosophy*, vol. 19, no. 1, Jan. 2018.

D'Antonio, Patricia, et al. "The Future in the Past: Hildegard Peplau and Interpersonal Relations in Nursing." *Nursing Inquiry*, vol. 21, no. 4, 2014, pp. 311-17.

Darley, John M., Samuel Glucksberg, and Ronald A. Kinchia. *Psychology.* 5th ed., Prentice-Hall, 1991.

"DASH Diet: Healthy Eating to Lower Your Blood Pressure." *Mayo Clinic*, www.mayoclinic.org/healthy-lifestyle/nutrition-and-healthy-eating/in-depth/dash-diet/art-20048456. Accessed 24 Aug. 2020.

"DASH Ranked Best Diet Overall for Eighth Year in a Row by *U.S. News and World Report*." *National Institutes of Health*, www.nih.gov/news-events/news-releases/dash-ranked-best-diet-overall-eighth-year-row-us-news-world-report. Accessed 24 Aug. 2020.

Davidson, Eric H. *The Regulatory Genome: Gene Regulatory Networks in Development and Evolution.* Academic, 2006.

Davis, Dena S. *Genetic Dilemmas: Reproductive Technology, Parental Choices, and Children's Futures.* 2nd ed., Routledge, 2010.

Davis, James B., editor. *Health and Medicine on the Internet: A Comprehensive Guide to Medical Information on the World Wide Web.* 4th ed., Practice Management Information, 2003.

Davis, Martha, Elizabeth Robbins Eshelman, and Matthew McKay. *The Relaxation and Stress Reduction Workbook.* 6th ed., New Harbinger, 2008.

"Day in the Life of a Geriatric Nurse Practitioner". *Nurse Practitioner Schools*, www.nursepractitionerschools.com/blog/day-in-life-geriatric-np. Accessed 4 Jan. 2017.

Dayal, M., et al. "Supplementation with DHEA: Effect on Muscle Size, Strength, Quality of Life, and Lipids." *Journal of Women's Health*, vol. 14, 2005, pp. 391-400.

"Defining Health Promotion and Disease Prevention." *Rural Health Information Hub*, www.ruralhealthinfo.org/toolkits/health-promotion/1/definition. Accessed 2 Sept. 2020.

"Definition and Philosophy of Case Management." *Commission for Case Manager Certification*, ccmcertification.org/about-ccmc/about-case-management/definition-and-philosophy-case-management.

Delaune, Sue C., and Patricia K. Ladner, editors. *Fundamentals of Nursing: Standards and Practices.* 4th ed., Delmar Thomson, 2011.

Deliktas, A., O. Korukcu, R. Aydin, and K. Kabukcuoglu. "Nursing Students' Perceptions of Nursing Metaparadigms: A Phenomenological Study." *Journal of Nursing Research*, vol. 27, no. 5, Oct. 2019.

Demangone, A. "That's Not What I Meant!—Technology and Miscommunication." *National Association of Federal Credit Unions*, 2014, www.cuinsight.com/thats-not-what-i-meant-technology-and-miscommunication.html. This article focuses on how easily technology-based communication can be misinterpreted. It highlights the importance that the person writing the message take time when composing the email to increase the likelihood that the intended and received message are the same.

DeNisco, Susan M. *Advanced Practice Nursing: Essential Knowledge for the Profession.* 4th ed., Jones & Bartlett Learning, 2019.

Dietary Supplements. U.S. Food and Drug Administration, www.fda.gov/food/dietary-supplements. Accessed 25 Aug. 2020.

Dillon, A., M. Kelly, I. H. Robertson, and D. A. Robertson "Smartphone Applications Utilizing Biofeedback Can Aid Stress Reduction." *Frontiers in Psychology*, vol. 7, p. 832.

"Director of Nursing." Registered Nursing.org. www.registerednursing.org/specialty/director-of-nursing/. Accessed 6 Oct. 2020.

Dolan, Josephine A., et al. *Nursing in Society: A Historical Perspective.* 15th ed., W. B. Saunders, 1983.

Donahue, M. Patricia. *Nursing: The Finest Art.* 3rd ed., Mosby, 2011.

Donaldson, Rebecca. "Challenges of Geriatric Care Nursing." *Relias Academy*, 4 Oct. 2016, blog.reliasacademy.com/challenges-of-geriatric-care-nursing/.

"Dorothea Orem Collection." *Alan Mason Chesney Medical Archives.* Johns Hopkins Medical Inst., n.d. Accessed 28 Aug. 2016.

DoSomething.org. America's largest organization for youth volunteering opportunities. This organization provides an online resource for teenagers looking for effective and feasible volunteer and community service opportunities. There are many resources spanning a variety of opportunities and subject matters allowing students to have easy access to community service and inspiration to enact change.

Duffy, Melanie, et al. *Clinical Nurse Specialist Toolkit: A Guide for the New Clinical Nurse Specialist.* 2nd ed., Springer Publishing Company, 2016.

Dunphy, Lynne M., et al. *Primary Care: Art and Science of Advanced Practice Nursing-An Interprofessional Approach.* 5th ed., F. A. Davis Company, 2019.

Dwyer, J. T., D. B. Allison, and P. M. Coates. "Dietary Supplements in Weight Reduction." *Journal of the American Dietary Association*, vol. 105, no. 5, suppl., 2005, pp. 80-86.

Dwyer, J. T., et al. "Measuring Vitamins and Minerals in Dietary Supplements for Nutrition Studies in the USA." *Analytical and Bioanalytical Chemistry*, vol. 389, 2007, pp. 37-46.

Eccleston, C., et al. "Psychological Therapies for the Management of Chronic and Recurrent Pain in Children and Adolescents." *Cochrane Database of Systematic Reviews*, 2009, CD003968, *EBSCO DynaMed Systematic Literature Surveillance*, www.ebscohost.com/dynamed.

Edens, P. S. "How to Develop a Cancer Information Internet Strategy." *Journal of Communication in Healthcare*, www.tandfonline.com/doi/abs/10.1179/cih.2008.1.3.266. Accessed 25 Aug. 2020.

Edens, Pat Stanfill, and Catherine D. Harvey. "Developing and Financing a Palliative Care Program." *American Journal of Hospice and Palliative Medicine*, vol. 25, no. 5, Oct./Nov. 2008.

Edmunds, Marilyn W., et al. "Telehealth, Telenursing, and Advanced Practice Nurses." *Journal of Nursing Practices*, Apr. 2010, www.medscape.com/viewarticle/719335.

"Education Resources." *American Association of Colleges of Nursing*, www.aacnnursing.org/Teaching-Resources. Accessed 22 Sept. 2020.

Edwards, David. *Art Therapy.* Sage, 2004.

Ellis, J. M., and P. Reddy. "Effects of *Panax ginseng* on Quality of Life." *Annals of Pharmacotherapy*, vol. 36, 2002, pp. 375-79.

"Ethical Issues in Nursing: Explanations & Solutions." Duquesne University School of Nursing. https://onlinenursing.duq.edu/blog/ethical-issues-in-nursing/. Accessed 8 Oct. 2020.

Evans, Christina L. Sieloff. *Imogene King: A Conceptual Framework for Nursing.* Sage, 1991.

"Every Man His Own Physician: Thomsonianism." *Nature Cures: A History of Alternative Medicine in America*, edited by James C. Whorton, Oxford UP, 2004.

"Evidence-Based Practice." *Nurse.com*, www.nurse.com/evidence-based-practice. Accessed 16 Sept. 2020.

Fagin, Claire, and Patricia Franklin. "Why Choose Geriatric Nursing?" *Geriatric Nursing*, Sept./Oct. 2005, www.nsna.org/Portals/0/Skins/NSNA/pdf/Imprint_SeptOct05_geriatric_fagin.pdf.

Fairman, Julie, and Joan E. Lynaugh. *Critical Care Nursing: A History.* U of Pennsylvania P, 2000.

"FAQ: What Are the Different APRN Certification Options for NPs, CNSs, CNMs and CRNAs?" *Online FNP Programs*, www.onlinefnpprograms.com/faqs/aprn-certification-organizations/. Accessed 23 Sept. 2020.

Fawcett, Jacqueline, and Susan DeSanto-Madeya. *Contemporary Nursing Knowledge: Analysis and Evaluation of Nursing Models and Theories.* 3rd ed., Davis, 2013.

Fawcett, Jacqueline. "The Nurse Theorists: 21st Century Updates—Dorothea E. Orem." *Nursing Science Quarterly*, vol. 14, no. 1, 2001, pp. 34-38.

"Faye Glenn Abdellah." *National Women's Hall of Fame*, n.d. Accessed 19 Aug. 2016.

"Federal Agencies Partner for Military and Veteran Pain Management Research." US Department of Health and Human Services. *National Center for Complementary and Integrative Health*, 20 Sept. 2017, www.nccih.nih.gov/news/press-releases/federal-agencies-partner-for-military-and-veteran-pain-management-research.

Federal Student Aid: An Office of the US Department of Education." FASFA: Free Application for Federal Student Aid, 2020, fafsa.ed.gov/. The Office of Federal Student Aid provides scholarships, grants, loans, and work study opportunities for undergraduate and graduate students attending school in the United States. To apply for student aid, all college and university "students, or prospective students, should fill out the Free Application for Federal Student Aid (FASFA).

Felix, M. M. D. S., M. B. G. Ferreira, L. F. da Cruz, and M. H. Barbosa. "Relaxation Therapy with Guided Imagery for Postoperative Pain Management: An Integrative Review." *Pain Management Nursing*, vol. 20, no. 1, 2019, pp. 3-9.

Ferrazzi, K. "How to Avoid Virtual Miscommunication." *Harvard Business Review*, 2013, hbr.org/2013/04/how-to-avoid-virtual-miscommun/. This article discusses how simple things can be misinterpreted when communication occurs remotely versus in-person. The author outlines six techniques to help increase the accuracy and effectiveness of technology-based communication.

Filkins, Karen, and Joseph F. Russo, editors. *Human Prenatal Diagnosis.* 2nd rev. ed., Marcel Dekker, 1990.

"Find a Magnet Hospital." *American Nurses Credentialing Center*, www.nursingworld.org/organizational-programs/magnet/find-a-magnet-organization/. Accessed 3 Sept. 2020.

"Find Your Nurse Practice Act." *National Council of State Boards of Nursing*, ncsbn.org/npa.htm. Accessed 23 Sept. 2020.

"Finding Colleges That Fit." *The College Board*, parents.collegeboard.org/planning-for-college/applications-and-admission/finding-colleges-that-fit. Accessed 1 Sept. 2020.

Fisher, J. G., J. P. Hatch, and J. D. Rugh, editors. *Biofeedback: Studies in Clinical Efficacy*. Springer Science & Business Media, 2013.

Fitzpatrick, Joyce J., and Geraldine McCarthy. *Theories Guiding Nursing Research and Practice*. Springer, 2014.

Flavin, Brianna. "The Info You Need to Know About Being a Neonatal Nurse." *Rasmussen College*, 20 Jan. 2020, www.rasmussen.edu/degrees/nursing/blog/being-a-neonatal-nurse/.

Folkman, J. "The Best Gift Leaders Can Give: Honest Feedback." *Forbes*, 2013, www.forbes.com/sites/joefolkman/2013/12/19/the-best-gift-leaders-can-give-honest-feedback/.

"Food and Nutrition Information Center." US Department of Agriculture. *National Agricultural Library*, www.nal.usda.gov/fnic. Accessed 24 Aug. 2020.

Forman, Walter B., et al., editors. *Hospice and Palliative Care: Concepts and Practice*. 2nd ed., Jones and Bartlett, 2003. A classical text that examines the theoretical perspectives and practical information about hospice care. Other topics include community medical care, geriatric care, nursing care, pain management, research, counseling, and hospice management.

Frank, D. L., L. Khorshid, J. F. Kiffer, C. S. Moravec, and M. G. McKee. "Biofeedback in Medicine: Who, When, Why and How?" *Mental Health in Family Medicine*, vol. 7, no. 2, 2010.

Frederickson, Keville. "Callista Roy's Adaptation Model." *Nursing Science Quarterly*, vol. 24, no. 4, 2011, pp. 301-3.

"Free Care Plans." *RegisteredNurseRN.com*, www.registerednursern.com/free-care-plans/. Accessed 16 Sept. 2020.

Freedman, E. *Work 101: Learning the Ropes of The Workplace without Hanging Yourself*. Delta Trade Paperbacks, 2007. This book is written for people who are starting their first job and describes common workplace norms, rules of etiquette, and business know-how. It contains insights, tips, and practical advice for succeeding on the job.

Freeman, Lyn. *Mosby's Complementary and Alternative Medicine: A Research-Based Approach*. 3rd ed., Mosby/Elsevier, 2009. Providing a comprehensive overview, this text includes practical, clinically relevant coverage of complementary and alternative medicine, with commentary by well-known experts, descriptions of medical advances, case studies, and discussion of the history and philosophy of each discipline.

Freitas, F. A., and L. J. Leonard. "Maslow's Hierarchy of Needs and Student Academic Success." *Teaching and Learning in Nursing*, vol. 6, 2011, pp. 9-13, files.transtutors.com/cdn/uploadassignments/1551711-1-maslow-theory.pdf.

Frey, Maureen A., and Christina L. Sieloff, editors. *Advancing King's Systems Framework and Theory of Nursing*. Sage, 1995.

Fries. K. "8 Essential Qualities that Define Great Leadership." *Forbes*, www.forbes.com/sites/kimberlyfries/2018/02/08-essential-qualities-that-define-great-leadership/#5ad70be73b63. Accessed 24 Aug. 2020.

Fronczek, A. E. "Nursing Theory in Virtual Care." *Nursing Science Quarterly*, vol. 32, no. 1, Jan. 2019, pp. 35-38.

Fuller, C. Talkers, *Watchers, and Doers: Unlocking Your Child's Unique Learning Style*. Piñon Press, 2004. By understanding your child's basic learning style and intelligence gifts, you can craft and tailor a learning environment to their needs. These practical suggestions will change the way you approach your child's education. No matter how your child learns, you can help him or her learn better and more efficiently.

Fulton, Janet S., et al. *Foundations of Clinical Nurse Specialist Practice*. 3rd ed., Springer Publishing Company, 2020.

Garrett, Laurie. *Betrayal of Trust: The Collapse of Global Public Health*. Hyperion, 2001.

Gatchel, Robert J., and Izabela Z. Schultz. *Handbook of Occupational Health and Wellness*. Springer, 2012.

Gatlin, C. G., and L. Schulmeister. "When Medication Is Not Enough: Nonpharmacologic Management of Pain." *Clinical Journal of Oncology Nursing*, vol. 11, 2007, pp. 699-704.

Gelles, D. "How to Meditate." *The New York Times*, www.nytimes.com/guides/well/how-to-meditate. Accessed 24 Aug. 2020.

"Genetic Counseling: What Is Genetic Counseling?" *Centers for Disease Control and Prevention*, www.cdc.gov/genomics/gtesting/genetic_counseling.htm. Accessed 1 Sept. 2020.

"Genetic Testing." *Centers for Disease Control and Prevention*, www.cdc.gov/genomics/gtesting/genetic_testing.htm. Accessed 1 Sept. 2020

Genetics Home Reference. "Genetic Consultation." *Genetics Home Reference*, 5 Aug. 2013.

"Genetics of Cancer." National Cancer Institute. *National Institutes of Health*, www.cancer.gov/about-cancer/causes-prevention/genetics#syndromes. Accessed 1 Sept. 2020.

"Get Screened." US Department of Health and Human Services. *Office of Disease Prevention and Health Promotion*, health.gov/myhealthfinder/topics/doctor-visits/screening-tests/get-screened. Accessed 2 Sept. 2020.

Giang, V., and M. Stanger. "How to Write the Perfect Resume." *Business Insider*, 29 Nov. 2012, www.businessinsider.com/how-to-write-the-perfect-resume-2012-11?op=1. This article reviews the general principles of writing an effective resume, and also provides mechanical details regarding the formatting of a resume (e.g., where to put your name, how to make use of space, etc.)

Giggins, O. M., U. M. Persson, and B. Caulfield. "Biofeedback in Rehabilitation." *Journal of Neuroengineering and Rehabilitation*, vol. 10, no. 1, p. 60.

Goldberg, D., and J. Zwiebel. *The Organized Student: Teaching Children the Skills for Success in School and Beyond*. Simon & Schuster, 2005. The book presents hands-on strategies for teaching disorganized children how to organize for success. In addition, it offers special tips for children with attention deficit disorder/attention deficit/hyperactivity disorder (ADD/ADHD) and learning disorders.

Gonzalo A. "Florence Nightingale: Environmental Theory." *Nurseslabs*, Updated Aug. 2019, nurseslabs.com/florence-nightingales-environmental-theory/.

Gonzalo, A. *Betty Neuman: Neuman Systems Model*, nurseslabs.com/betty-neuman-systems-model-nursing-theory/. Accessed 24 Aug. 2020.

Graat, J. M., E. G. Schouten, and F. J. Kok. "Effect of Daily Vitamin E and Multivitamin-Mineral Supplementation on Acute Respiratory Tract Infections in Elderly Persons." *Journal of the American Medical Association*, vol. 288, 2002, pp. 715-21.

Grant, Rebecca. "The U.S. Is Running Out of Nurses." *Atlantic*, 3 Feb. 2016, www.theatlantic.com/health/archive/2016/02/nursing-shortage/459741/.

Gross, Cynthia R., et al. "Mindfulness-Based Stress Reduction Versus Pharmacotherapy for Chronic Primary Insomnia." *Explore*, vol. 7, 2011, pp. 76-87. The researchers studied thirty adults with diagnosed insomnia and randomized them to either mindfulness-based stress reduction training or pharmacotherapy, comparing various indices of sleep quality and quantity between the two treatments.

Grubisich, Kelsi, "The Relationship Between Participation in Community Service and Students Academic Success." Masters Theses 2620, 2017, thekeep.eiu.edu/cgi/viewcontent.cgi?article=3621&context=theses. Accessed 31 Aug. 2020.

Guare, R., and P. Dawson. *Smart but Scattered Teens: The "Executive Skills" Program for Helping Teens Reach Their Potential*. Guilford Press, 2013. Detailed examples demonstrate how to teach your teenager the skills needed for success. Clever strategies help address creative resistance to making necessary changes.

Guest, Charles, et al. *Oxford Handbook of Public Health Practice*. 3rd ed., Oxford UP, 2013.

"Guided Imagery: Using Your Imagination." *Stress Management for Life: A Research-Based Experiential Approach*, edited by Michael Olpin and Margie Hesson. Wadsworth/Cengage Learning, 2010.

Gulanick, Meg, and Judith L. Myers. *Nursing Care Plans: Nursing Diagnosis and Intervention*. 9th ed., Mosby, 2016.

Gutkind, Lee, editor. *I Wasn't Strong Like This When I Started Out: True Stories of Becoming a Nurse*. In Fact Books, 2013.

Guzik, Arlene. *Essentials for Occupational Health Nursing*. Wiley-Blackwell, 2013.

Gyles, Carlton. "Robots in Medicine." *Canadian Veterinary Journal*, vol. 60, no. 8, 2019, pp. 819-20.

Hadeed, George, et al. *Telemedicine for Trauma, Emergencies, and Disaster Management*. Artech House, 2011.

Haggans, C., et al. "Computer Access to Research on Dietary Supplements: A Database of Federally Funded Dietary Supplement Research." *Journal of Nutrition*, vol. 135, 2005, pp. 1796-99.

Halberstein, R., et al. "Healing with Bach Flower Essences: Testing a Complementary Therapy." *Complementary Health Practice Review*, vol. 12, 2007, pp. 3-14.

Hall, Laura J. *Autism Spectrum Disorders: From Theory to Practice*. 2nd ed., Pearson, 2012.

Hammer J. "Thou Shalt Not Underestimate Florence Nightingale." *Smithsonian*, vol. 50, no. 10, Mar. 2020, pp. 24-33, 78-79.

Hanstede, M., Y. Gidron, and I. Nyklicek. "The Effects of a Mindfulness Intervention on Obsessive-Compulsive Symptoms in a Non-clinical Student Population." *Journal of Nervous and Mental Disease*, vol. 196, 2008, pp. 776-79.

Harding, Anne. "Telemedicine Improves Care for Kids Seen in Rural ERs." *MedlinePlus*, 19 Aug. 2013.

Harper, Peter S. *Practical Genetic Counselling*. 7th ed., Hodder Arnold, 2010.

Harvard Health, www.health.harvard.edu/medical-tests-and-procedures/biofeedback-a-to-z.

Hay, William W., Jr., et al., editors. *Current Diagnosis and Treatment: Pediatrics*. 22nd ed., Lange Medical Books/McGraw-Hill, 2014.

"Health Careers Aptitude Tests." *Psychological Service Bureau*, www.psbtests.com.

"Health Information Privacy." HHS.gov, www.hhs.gov/hipaa/index.html. Accessed 27 Aug. 2020.

"Health Information." National Center for Complementary and Integrative Health. *National Institutes of Health*, www.nccih.nih.gov/health. Accessed 16 Sept. 2020.

"Health Insurance and Accountability Act of 1996 (HIPAA)." Centers for Disease Control and Prevention. https://www.cdc.gov/phlp/publications/topic/hipaa.html. Accessed 8 Oct. 2020.

"Health on the Net Foundation." United Nations, www.hon.ch.

Heather, O. D., et al. "Relaxation Therapies for the Management of Primary Hypertension in Adults." *Cochrane Database of Systematic Reviews*, 2008, CD004935, EBSCO DynaMed Systematic Literature Surveillance, www.ebscohost.com/dynamed.

Heiden, M., et al. "Evaluation of Cognitive Behavioural Training and Physical Activity for Patients with Stress-Related Illnesses." *Journal of Rehabilitative Medicine*, vol. 39, 2007, pp. 366-73.

Herbet L. "How Your Brain Perceives Time (and How to Use It to Your Advantage)." *Lifehacker*, http://lifehacker.com/how-your-brain-perceives-time-and-how-to-use-it-to-you-511184192. This article evaluates the theories many researchers hold on the perception people have of time and how they manage their time.

Herdman, T. H., and S. Kamitsuru, editors. *Nursing Diagnoses: Definitions and Classifications 2018-2020*. (NANDA International Nursing Diagnoses.) Thieme, 2017.

Higgins, P. A., and M. S. Moore. "Levels of Theoretical Thinking in Nursing." *Nursing Outlook Theory*, vol. 48, no. 4, 1 July 2000, www.nursingoutlook.org/article/S0029-6554(00)32367-3/pdf.

Higgs, Paul G., and Teresa K. Attwood. *Bioinformatics and Molecular Evolution*. Wiley-Blackwell, 2013.

Hock, Randolph. *The Extreme Searcher's Internet Handbook: A Guide for the Serious Searcher*. 3rd ed., CyberAge Books, 2010. A guide to internet research for librarians, teachers, students, writers, business professionals, and health consumers.

Holland, John L. *Manual for the Self-Directed Search*. Consulting Psychologists, 1985.

"Home Health Nurse." *Registered Nursing.org*, www.registerednursing.org/specialty/home-health-nurse/#:~:text=Home%20health%20nursing%20is%20a,unable%20to%20care%20for%20themselves. Accessed 30 Sept. 2020.

Horsager, D. "You Can't Be a Great Leader Without Trust. Here's How to Build It." *Forbes*, 2012, www.forbes.com/sites/forbesleadershipforum/2012/10/24/you-cant-be-a-great-leader-without-trust-heres-how-you-build-it/.

"Hospital Nursing vs. Clinical Nursing." *RegisteredNursing.org*, www.registerednursing.org/hospital-vs-clinic/. Accessed 2 Oct. 2020.

"How Dietary Factors Influence Disease Risk." *National Institutes of Health*, www.nih.gov/news-events/nih-research-matters/how-dietary-factors-influence-disease-risk. Accessed 24 Aug. 2020.

"How Is the Scope of Practice Determined for a Nurse?" *Registered Nursing.org*. www.registerednursing.org/answers/how-scope-practice-determined/. Accessed 7 Oct. 2020.

"How to Become a Clinic Nurse." *Study.com*, study.com/articles/How_to_Become_a_Clinic_Nurse.html#:~:text=Clinic%20nurses%20are%20usually%20licensed,and%20help%20with%20patient%20education. Accessed 2 Oct. 2020.

"How to Become a Geriatric Nurse." *All Nursing Schools*, www.allnursingschools.com/articles/geriatric-nurse. Accessed 4 Jan. 2017.

"How to Become a Home Health Nurse." *All Nursing Schools*, www.allnursingschools.com/specialties/home-health-nurse/. Accessed 30 Sept. 2020.

"How to Become a Neonatal Nurse Specialist or Practitioner." *All Nursing Schools*, www.allnursingschools.com/specialties/neonatal-nursing/. Accessed 1 Oct. 2020.

"How to Become a Perioperative Nurse." *GraduateNursingEDU.org*, www.graduatenursingedu.org/perioperative/#:~:text=Perioperative%20nurses%20help%20plan%2C%20carry,%2C%20during%2C%20and%20after%20surgery. Accessed 29, 2020.

"How to Become an RN: Begin Here." *NursingLicensure.org*, www.nursinglicensure.org/articles/how-to-become-an-rn.html. Accessed 21 Sept. 2020.

"How to Write a High School Resume for College Applications." *The Princeton Review*, www.princetonreview.com/college-advice/high-school-resume. Accessed 27 Aug. 2010.

Huang, S. T., M. Good, and J. A. Zauszniewski. "The Effectiveness of Music in Relieving Pain in Cancer Patients." *International Journal of Nursing Studies*, vol. 47, 2010, pp. 1354-62.

Huffcutt, A. I., C. H. Van Iddekinge, and P. L. Roth. "Understanding Applicant Behavior in Employment Interviews: A Theoretical Model of Interviewee Performance." *Human Resource Management Review*, vol. 21, 2011, pp. 353-367, doi:10.1016/j.hrmr.2011.05.003. The authors present a theoretical model composed of multiple factors in interviewer-interviewee dynamics and ideas for future research.

Hurkmans, Joost, et al. "Music in the Treatment of Neurological Language and Speech Disorders: A Systematic Review." *Aphasiology*, vol. 26, no. 1, 2012, pp. 1-19. *Taylor & Francis Online*, doi.org/10.1080/02687038.2011.602514.

Ignatavicius, Donna D., et al. *Clinical Companion for Medical-Surgical Nursing: Concepts for Interprofessional Collaborative Care*. 9th ed., Elsevier, 2018.

"Informed Consent: More Than Getting a Signature." *Joint Commission*, www.jointcommission.org/-/media/deprecated-unorganized/imported-assets/tjc/system-folders/joint-commission-online/quick_safety_issue_twenty-one_february_2016pdf.pdf?db=web&hash=5944307ED39088503A008A70D2C768AA. Accessed 11 Sept. 2020.

"Informed Consent-StatPearls." National Library of Medicine. National Institutes of Health. *NCBI Bookshelf*, www.ncbi.nlm.nih.gov/books/NBK430827/. Accessed 11 Sept. 2020.

"Integrative Medicine." *Psychology Today*, www.psychologytoday.com/us/basics/integrative-medicine. Accessed 24 Aug. 2020.

International Association of Clinical Research Nurses, iacrn.org. Accessed 11 Sept. 2020.

International Human Genome Sequencing Consortium. "Initial Sequencing and Analysis of the Human Genome." *Nature*, vol. 409, no. 6822, 2001, pp. 860-921.

Irle, Kevin, and Geoff Lovell. "An Investigation into the Efficacy of a Music-Based Men's Group for Improving Psychological Wellbeing." *Music Therapy Perspectives*, vol. 32, no. 2, 2014, pp. 178-84.

"Is Nursing the Right Profession for You?" *EveryNurse*, everynurse.org/blog/is-nursing-right-for-you/. Accessed 3 Sept. 2020.

Jackson, J. I. *Nursing Paradigms and Theories: A Primer*. Virginia Henderson Global Nursing e-Repository, 26 Jan. 2015, www.nursinglibrary.org/vhl/handle/10755/338888.

Jacobson, E. E., A. L. Meleger, P. Bonato, et al. "Structural Integration as an Adjunct to Outpatient Rehabilitation for Chronic Nonspecific Low Back Pain: A Randomized Pilot Clinical Trial." *Evidence Based Complement Alternate Medicine*, 2015, pubmed.ncbi.nlm.nih.gov/25945112/. Accessed 25 Aug. 2020.

Jager, R., et al. "The Effect of Phosphatidylserine on Golf Performance." *Journal of the International Society of Sports Nutrition*, vol. 4, 2007, p. 23.

Jahnke, R., et al. "A Comprehensive Review of Health Benefits of Qigong and Tai Chi." *American Journal of Health Promotion*, vol. 24, no. 6, 2010, pp. 1-25.

Jairath, N. N., et al. "Theory and Theorizing in Nursing Science: Commentary form the Nursing Research Special Issue Editorial Team." *Nursing Research*, vol. 67, no. 2, Mar./Apr. 2018, pp. 188-95.

Jarrin, Olga F. "The Integrality of Situated Caring in Nursing and the Environment." *Advances in Nursing Science*, Winter 2012, www.ncbi.nlm.nih.gov/pmc/articles/PMC3402335/. Accessed 2 Jan. 2016.

Jayadevappa, R., et al. "Effectiveness of Transcendental Meditation on Functional Capacity and Quality of Life of African Americans with Congestive Heart Failure." *Ethnicity and Disease*, vol. 1, 2007, pp.72-77.

Jennifer K. "How to Apply Maslow's Hierarchy of Needs to Nursing." Updated 18 Jan. 2018, www.theclassroom.com/how-7727994-apply-maslows-hierarchy-needs-nursing.html.

"Job Description: Clinical Research Nurse I." Human Resources. *Emory University*, apps.hr.emory.edu/JobDescriptions/class.jsp?code=PF02. Accessed 11 Sept. 2020.

Job, V., G. M. Walton, K. Bernecker, and C. S. Dweck. "Implicit Theories about Willpower Predict Self-Regulation and Grades in Everyday Life." *Journal of Personality and Social Psychology*, vol. 108, no. 4, pp. 637-47, doi:10.1037/pspp0000014. Reports a longitudinal study on how university students' limited or nonlimited view of willpower affected self-regulation behaviors.

Johnson, Betty, and Pamela Webber. *An Introduction to Theory and Reasoning in Nursing*. 4th ed., LWW, 2013.

Jonas, Wayne. "When Less Means More: Less Medical Care Means More Self-Care." *Psychology Today*, 22 June 2020, www.psychologytoday.com/us/blog/how-healing-works/202006/when-less-means-more-less-medical-care-means-more-self-care. Accessed 29 June 2020.

Jorde, Lynn B., et al. *Medical Genetics*. 4th ed., Mosby/Elsevier, 2010.

Jorm, A. F., A. J. Morgan, and S. E. Hetrick. "Relaxation for Depression." *Cochrane Database of Systematic Reviews*, 2008, CD007142, *EBSCO DynaMed Systematic Literature Surveillance*, www.ebscohost.com/dynamed.

Kadam, R. A. "Informed Consent Process: A Step Further Towards Making It Meaningful." *Perspectives in Clinical Research*, vol. 8, no. 3, 2017, pp. 107-12.

Kapes, Jerome T., Marjorie Moran Mastie, and Edwin A. Whitfeld. *A Counselor's Guide to Career Assessment Instruments*. National Career Development Association, 2008.

"Kaplan Nursing School Admissions Test." *Kaplan Nursing*, www.kaptest.com. Accessed 27 Aug. 2020.

Katz, Katy. "Everything You Need to Know about Becoming a Geriatric Nurse." *Rasmussen College*, 5 Sept. 2013, www.rasmussen.edu/degrees/nursing/blog/everything-you-need-know-about-becoming-geriatric-nurse.

Kelly, K.J., S. Doucet, and A. Luke. "Exploring the Roles, Functions, and Background of Patient Navigators and Case Managers: A Scoping Review." *International Journal of Nursing Studies*, vol. 98, Oct. 2019, pp. 27-47.

Kelly, Nora. "What's Next for the National Institutes of Health?" *The Atlantic*, 13 Jan. 2016, www.theatlantic.com/politics/archive/2016/01/national-institutes-of-health-congress-budget/423837/.

Khazan, I. Z. *The Clinical Handbook of Biofeedback: A Step-By-Step Guide for Training and Practice with Mindfulness*. John Wiley & Sons, 2013.

Kim, Hesook Suzie, and Ingrid Kollak. *Nursing Theories: Conceptual & Philosophical Foundations*. Springer, 2006.

Kim, J. H., et al. "Efficacy of Alpha-S1-Casein Hydrolysate on Stress-Related Symptoms in Women." *European Journal of Clinical Nutrition*, vol. 61, 2007, pp. 536-41.

King, Juliet L. *Art Therapy, Trauma, and Neuroscience: Theoretical and Practical Perspectives*. Routledge, 2016.

King, N. B., and V. Fraser. "Untreated Pain, Narcotics Regulation, and Global Health Ideologies." *PLoS Medicine*, vol. 10, no. 4, 2013www.ncbi.nlm.nih.gov/pmc/articles/PMC3614505.

Kirp, David L. "Meditation Transforms Roughest San Francisco Schools." Hearst Communications. *SFGate*, 12 Jan. 2014.

Kjellgren, A., et al. "Wellness Through a Comprehensive Yogic Breathing Program." *BMC Complementary and Alternative Medicine*, vol. 7, 2007, p. 43.

Kleinfield, Sonny. *Becoming a Nurse*. Simon & Schuster, 2020.

Kliegman, Robert M., and Joseph St. Geme, editors. *Nelson Textbook of Pediatrics*. 21st ed., Saunders/Elsevier, 2020.

Kokemuller, Neil. "The Pros of Being a Nurse in a Doctor's Office." *Chron*, work.chron.com/pros-being-nurse-doctors-office-1988.html. Accessed 2 Oct. 2020.

"Kolcaba's Theory of Comfort." *Nursing Theory*, www.nursing-theory.org/theories-and-models/kolbaca-theory-of-comfort.php. Accessed 19 Sept. 2020.

Koppes, Laura L., editor. *Historical Perspectives in Industrial and Organizational Psychology*. Psychology, 2014.

Koren, Herman. *Illustrated Dictionary and Resource Directory of Environmental and Occupational Health*. 2nd ed., CRC, 2005.

Kouzes, J. M., and B. Z. Posner. *The Leadership Challenge: How to Make Extraordinary Things Happen in Organizations*. Jossey Bass, 2012. A book about how individuals can create positive change within their organization by engaging in practices of modeling, shared vision, challenge, action, and heart-based encouragement. Provides information on forward moving leadership, integrating tenets of intrinsic motivation and desires in planning and doing within corporations, companies, and nonprofit organizations.

Kozier, Barbara, et al. *Fundamentals of Nursing: Concepts, Process, and Practice*. 2nd ed., Pearson, 2012.

Kraemer, W. J., et al. "Cortitrol Supplementation Reduces Serum Cortisol Responses to Physical Stress." *Metabolism*, vol. 54, 2005, pp. 657-68.

"Kristen Swanson Theory of Caring and Healing." *Psych-Mental Health NP*, pmhealthnp.com/kristen-swanson-theory-of-caring-and-healing/. Accessed 19 Sept. 2020.

Kübler-Ross, Elisabeth, editor. *Death: The Final Stage of Growth*. Reprint. Simon & Schuster, 1997. A psychiatrist by training, Kübler-Ross brings together other researchers' views of how death provides the key to how human beings make meaning in their own personal worlds. Addresses practical concerns over how people express grief and accept the death of those close to them, and how they might prepare for their own inevitable ends.

Kurn, Sidney, and Sheryl Shook. *Integrated Medicine for Neurologic Disorders*. Health Press, 2008. Review of nutritional and herbal therapies for practitioners who treat persons with neurological disorders.

Kushner, Harold. *When Bad Things Happen to Good People*. 20th anniv. ed., Schocken Books, 2001. The first of Rabbi Kushner's works on finding meaning in one's life, it was originally his personal response to make intelligible the death of his own child. It has become a highly regarded reference for those who struggle with the meaning of pain, suffering, and death in their lives.

Kutney-Lee, Ann, et al. "Changes in Patient and Nurse Outcomes Associated with Magnet Hospital Recognition." *Medical Care*, vol. 53, no. 6, 2015, pp. 550-57.

Kwekkeboom, K. L., and L. C. Bratzke. "A Systematic Review of Relaxation, Meditation, and Guided Imagery Strategies for Symptom Management in Heart Failure." *Journal of Cardiovascular Nursing*, vol. 31, no. 5, 2016, pp. 457-68, pubmed.ncbi.nlm.nih.gov/26065388/.

Lack, Caleb W., and Jacques Rousseau. *Critical Thinking, Science, and Pseudoscience: Why We Can't Trust Our Brains*. Springer, 2016.

Lahmann, C., et al. "Brief Relaxation versus Music Distraction in the Treatment of Dental Anxiety." *Journal of the American Dental Association*, vol. 139, 2008, pp. 317-24.

Lahmann, C., F. Röhricht, and N. Sauer. "Functional Relaxation as Complementary Therapy in Irritable Bowel Syndrome." *Journal of Alternative and Complementary Medicine*, vol. 16, 2010, pp. 47-52.

Lampert, Lynda. "Nurses Storm the U.S. Capitol to Demand Safe Staffing Ratios." *Daily Nurse*, 2 June 2016, dailynurse.com/nurses-storm-u-s-capitol-demand-safe-staffing-ratios/.

Lando, J., and S. M. Williams. "Uniting Mind and Body in Our Health Care and Public Health Systems." *Preventing Chronic Disease*, vol. 3, no. 2, 2006, p. A31.

LaRocque, P. *The Book on Writing: The Ultimate Guide to Writing Well*. Grey and Guvnor Press, 2013. LaRoque, a master writer, shares advice on the art and craft of composition.

Larsen, Laura. *Childhood Diseases and Disorders Sourcebook*. 3rd ed., Omnigraphics, 2012.

Law, Anica C., et al. "Patient Outcomes after the Introduction of Statewide ICU Nurse Staffing Regulations." *Critical Care Medicine*, vol. 46, no. 10, Oct. 2018, pp. 1563-69, doi:10.1097/CCM.0000000000003286, pubmed.ncbi.nlm.nih.gov/30179886/.

Lawson, Theresa G. "Betty Neuman: Systems Model." *Nursing Theorists and Their Work*, edited by Martha Raile Alligood, 8th ed., Mosby, 2014, pp. 281-302.

Lazar, S., et al. "Functional Brain Mapping of the Relaxation Response and Meditation." *NeuroReport*, vol. 11, 2000, pp. 1581-85. Discusses how magnetic resonance imaging shows that the practice of meditation activates neural structures affecting attention and control of the autonomic nervous system.

"Leadership." *Psychology Today*, www.psychologytoday.com/us/basics/leadership. Accessed 24 Aug. 2020.

Lee, H., K. Schmidt, and E. Ernst. "Acupuncture for the Relief of Cancer-Related Pain." *European Journal of Pain*, vol. 9, 2005, p. 437.

Lee, M. S., M. H. Pittler, and E. Ernst. "Effects of Reiki in Clinical Practice." *International Journal of Clinical Practice*, vol. 62, 2008, pp. 947-54.

Lee, Philip R., and Carroll L. Estes, editors. *The Nation's Health*. 7th ed., Jones and Bartlett, 2003.

Leis, A. M., L. C. Weeks, and M. J. Verhoef. "Principles to Guide Integrative Oncology and the Development of an Evidence Base." *Current Oncology*, vol. 15, suppl. 2, 2008, pp. S83-S87. Discusses the need for evidence to support the overall practice of integration and the challenges posed by the validation process.

Lenhart, A. "Teens, Social Media & Technology Overview-2015." *Pew Research Center*, www.pewinternet.org/2015/04/09/teens-social-media-technology-2015/. A review of social media and technology use in teenagers. Trends include increased use of smartphones and mobile devices, as well as continuing use of social media platforms like Facebook and Twitter. Use of Instagram, Snapchat, Tumblr, and Google+ is also discussed.

Leonard, Margaret, and Elaine Miller. *Nursing Case Management*. ANCC, Credentialing Knowledge Center, 2009.

Letham, S. "The Procrastination Problem." *Success Consciousness*, n.d., www.successconsciousness.com/guest_articles/procrastination.htm. This article examines the study of procrastination. Using scientific studies, it attempts to fully explain different concepts associated with procrastination and poor time management.

LeVeck, Danielle. "Doctorate of Nursing Practice (DNP)-What Is a DNP and Is It Worth It?" *Nurse.org*, 11 Sept. 2020, nurse.org/articles/how-to-get-a-dnp-is-it-worth-it/.

Levy, Barry S., et al., editors. *Occupational Health: Recognizing and Preventing Disease and Injury*. 5th ed., Lippincott, 2006.

Lewin, Tamar. "A New SAT Aims to Realign with Schoolwork." *New York Times*, 6 Mar. 2014, p. A1.

Lewis, N. A., and D. Oyserman. "When Does the Future Begin? Time Metrics Matter, Connecting Present and Future Selves." *Psychological Science* (OnlineFirst), 2015, doi:10.1177/0956797615572231, pss.sagepub.com/

content/early/2015/04/23/0956797615572231.full.pdf+html. Reports how time metrics affected people's connection of future and current selves, which mediated their action even the perceived importance of future events was unchanged.

Lewis, Ricki. *Human Genetics: Concepts and Applications*. 10th ed., McGraw-Hill, 2012.

"Licensed Practical and Licensed Vocational Nurses." US Bureau of Labor Statistics, *Occupational Outlook Handbook*, 13 Apr. 2018, www.bls.gov/ooh/healthcare/licensed-practical-and-licensed-vocational-nurses.htm.

"Licensed Practical Nursing: Education Requirements, Career Paths, & Job Outlook." *All Nursing Schools*, www.allnursingschools.com/licensed-practical-nurse/. Accessed 21 Sept. 2020.

"Licensed Practical/Vocational Nurses: A Place on the Team." *American Association of Occupational Health Nurses*, vol. 65, no. 4, 2017, pp. 154-57.

"List of NIH Institutes, Centers, and Offices." US Department of Health and Human Services. *National Institutes of Health*, 8 Feb. 2017, www.nih.gov/institutes-nih/list-nih-institutes-centers-offices. Accessed 2 Sept. 2020.

"List of Nursing Organizations." *Nurse.org*, nurse.org/orgs_shtml. Accessed 2 Sept. 2020. A listing of all nursing organizations, including the Academy of Neonatal Nursing, National Association of Neonatal Nurses, National Association of Pediatric Nurse Practitioners, National Association of School Nurses, and others.

Litin, Scott C., editor. *Mayo Clinic Family Health Book*. 4th ed., HarperResource, 2009.

Llewellyn, Anne. "Beyond the Bedside: The Role of Telehealth Nursing." *Nursetogether.com*, 23 June 2014, www.nursetogether.com/beyond-bedside-role-telehealth-nursing/.

"LPN Instructor Careers with BSN." *Practical Nursing.org*, www.practicalnursing.org/lpn-instructor-careers-bsn. Accessed 22 Sept. 2020.

Macarthur, Sam. "What Is a Certification in Public Health?" *MPH online*, www.mphonline.org/cph-mph-credential-explained/. Accessed 30 Sept. 2020.

MacDonald, A. "Using the Relaxation Response to Reduce Stress." Harvard Medical School. *Harvard Health Publishing*, www.health.harvard.edu/blog/using-the-relaxation-response-to-reduce-stress-20101110780. Accessed 25 Aug. 2020.

MacGregor, M. *Teambuilding with Teens: Activities for Leadership, Decision Making & Group Success*. Free Spirit Publishing, 2008. The 36 activities in this book make learning about leadership a hands-on, active experience. Young people are encouraged to recognize each other's strengths, become better listeners, communicate clearly, identify their values, build trust, set goals, and more.

"Magnet Recognition Program: Areas for Improvement." *The Truth about Nursing*, www.truthaboutnursing.org/faq/magnet.html#gsc.tab=0. Accessed 3 Sept. 2020.

Malchiodi, Cathy A. *The Art Therapy Sourcebook*. Rev. ed. McGraw, 2007.

"Manage Stress." US Department of Health and Human Services. *HealthFinder.gov*, 30 July 2015.

"Managing Employee Dress and Appearance." *Society for Human Resource Management*, www.shrm.org/resourcesandtools/tools-and-samples/toolkits/pages/employeedressandappearance.aspx. Accessed 31 Aug. 2020.

Manjlovich, Milisa. "Seeking Staffing Solutions." *American Nurse Today*, vol. 4, no. 3, Mar. 2009, www.myamericannurse.com/seeking-staffing-solutions/.

Manning, George, Kent Curtis, Steve McMillen, and Bill Attenweiler. *Stress: Living and Working in a Changing World*. 3rd ed., Savant Learning Systems, 2016.

Marrelli, Tina M. *Home Care Nursing: Surviving in an Ever-Changing Care Environment*. Sigma Theta Tau International, 2017.

Martin, Richard J., Avroy A. Fanaroff, and Michele C. Walsh, editors. *Fanaroff and Martin's Neonatal-Perinatal Medicine: Diseases of the Fetus and Infant*. 2 vols. 9th ed., Mosby/Elsevier, 2010.

Masters, Kathleen. *Nursing Theories: A Framework for Professional Practice*. 2nd ed., Jones & Bartlett Learning, 2015.

Mattern, K., W. Camara, and J. L. Kobrin. *SAT Writing: An Overview of Research and Psychometrics to Date*. College Board Research Report no. RN-32. The College Board, 2007.

Mayo Clinic. "Telehealth: When Health Care Meets Cyberspace." *Mayo Clinic*, 13 May 2011.

McCaffrey, A. M., et al. "Prayer for Health Concerns: Results of a National Survey on Prevalence and Patterns of Use." *Archives of Internal Medicine*, vol. 164, no. 8, 2004, pp. 858-62.

McEwen, Melanie. *Theoretical Basis for Nursing*. 4th ed., LWW: 2014.

McHugh, Matthew D., et al. "Lower Mortality in Magnet Hospitals." *Medical Care*, vol. 51, no. 5, 2013, pp. 382-88.

McKelvey, M. M. "Finding Meaning through Kristen Swanson's Caring Behaviors: A Cornerstone of Healing for Nursing Education." *Creative Nursing*, vol. 24, no. 1, connect.springerpub.com/content/sgrcn/24/1/6?implicit-login=true. Accessed 19 Sept. 2020.

McLeod S. "Maslow's Hierarchy of Needs." *Simply Psychology*, updated 20 Mar. 2020, www.simplypsychology.org/maslow.html.

McMillan, T. L., and S. Mark. "Complementary and Alternative Medicine and Physical Activity for Menopausal Symptoms." *Journal of the American Medical Women's Association*, vol. 59, no. 4, 2004, pp. 270-77.

"Medical Robots." *Robotics Online*, www.robotics.org/service-robots/medical-robots. Accessed 6 May 2020.

"Medical-Surgical Nurse." *Registered Nursing.org*, www.registerednursing.org/specialty/medical-surgical-nurse/. Accessed 29 Sept. 2020.

"Meditation: A Simple, Fast Way to Reduce Stress." Mayo Foundation for Medical Education and Research. *Mayo Clinic*, 19 July 2014.

"Meditation: In Depth." National Center for Complementary and Integrative Health. *National Institutes of Health*, www.nccih.nih.gov/health/meditation-in-depth. Accessed 25 Aug. 2020.

MedlinePlus. "Evaluating Internet Health Information: A Tutorial from the National Library of Medicine." *MedlinePlus*, 19 Apr. 2012.

MedlinePlus. "Genetic Counseling." *MedlinePlus*, 21 June 2013.

Meleis, Afaf Ibrahim. *Theoretical Nursing: Development and Progress*. Wolters Kluwer, 2012.

Michaels, Davida. "Nursing Care Models: Historical Review." *American Nursing History*, 22 Feb. 2020, www.americannursinghistory.org/models-nursing-care.

Miller, Caroline. *Arts Therapists in Multidisciplinary Settings*. Jessica Kingsley, 2016.

"Mind and Body Approaches for Stress and Anxiety: What the Science Says." *NCCIH Clinical Digest for Health Professionals*, Apr. 2020, www.nccih.nih.gov/health/providers/digest/mind-and-body-approaches-for-stress-science#relaxation-techniques. Accessed 29 June 2020.

"Mind and Body Practices." National Center for Complementary and Integrative Health, *National Institutes of Health*, www.nccih.nih.gov/health/mind-and-body-practices. Accessed 25 Aug. 2020.

"Mindfulness-Based Stress Reduction (MBSR) Information." *National Center for Complementary and Integrative Health*, n.d. Accessed 17 May 2016.

Mintz-Binder, R. "The Connection between Nursing Theory and Practice." *Nursing Made Incredibly Easy!*, vol. 17, no. 1, Jan.-Feb. 2019, pp. 6-9.

Modesti, P. A., et al. "Psychological Predictors of the Antihypertensive Effects of Music-Guided Slow Breathing." *Journal of Hypertension*, vol. 28, 2010, pp. 1097-1103.

Mogilner, C. "You'll Feel Less Rushed If You Give Time Away." *Harvard Business Review*, 1 Sept. 2012. This article discusses the positive benefits of volunteering. In this study, the positive correlation between committing time to service work and personal freedom, organization, and enjoyment is proven.

Moore, Keith L., and T. V. N. Persaud. *The Developing Human*. 9th ed., Saunders/Elsevier, 2013.

Morgan, Monroe T. *Environmental Health*. 3rd ed., Thomson, 2003.

Mortimer, J. T. *The Benefits and Risks of Adolescent Employment* (PMCID: PMC2936460), www.ncbi.nlm.nih.bov/PMC2936460/. This document reviewed the longitudinal Youth Development Study and identified four types of high school students who participated in employment.

Mudd, A., R. Feo, T. Conroy, and A. Kitson. "Where and How Does Fundamental Care Fit within Seminal Nursing Theories: A Narrative Review and Synthesis of Key Nursing Concepts." *Journal of Clinical Nursing*, vol. 29, Oct. 2020, pp. 19-20, www.ncbi.nlm.nih.gov/pmc/articles/PMC7540068/.

Murdaugh C. L., M. A. Parsons, and N. J. M. Pender. *Health Promotion in Nursing Practice*. 8th ed., Pearson. 2019.

Murray, Sharon, et al. *Foundations of Maternal-Newborn and Women's Health Nursing*. 7th ed., Elsevier, 2019.

"Music Therapy." American Cancer Society. *Cancer.org*, 13 Jan. 2015.

Nagel, Denise. "Health Benefits of Tai Chi and Qigong." *TheHuffingtonPost.com*, 23 June 2015.

Nagelhout, John C., and Sass Elisha. *Nurse Anesthesia*. 6th ed., Elsevier, 2018.

Nahin, R. L., et al. "Costs of Complementary and Alternative Medicine (CAM) and Frequency of Visits to CAM Practitioners: United States, 2007." *National Health Statistics Reports*, vol. 18, 2009, pp. 1-15.

Naparstek, Belleruth. *Staying Well with Guided Imagery*. Grand Central, 1995.

National Center for Complementary and Alternative Medicine, nccam.nih.gov. A comprehensive site of a leading US agency for scientific research on complementary and alternative medicine. Provides results and information on CAM obtained from clinical trials.

National Center for Complementary and Integrative Health. *National Institutes of Health*, nccih.nih.gov. Conducts and supports research and provides information about complementary health products and practices. Accessed 24 Aug. 2020.

National Institute of Child Health and Human Development, www.nichd.nih.gov/health/clinicalresearch. Provides information about clinical research and the NICHD's role in this research

National Institutes of Health, www.nih.gov.

National Institutes of Health. *ClinicalTrials.gov*, clinicaltrials.gov.

National Library of Medicine, www.pubmed.gov.

"Nationwide Survey Reveals Widespread Use of Mind and Body Practices." National Center for Complementary and Integrative Health. *National Institutes of Health*, 10 Feb. 2015.

Naylor, Mary. "A Decade of Transitional Care Research with Vulnerable Elders." *Journal of Cardiovascular Nursing*, vol. 3, 2000, pp. 88-89.

"NCSBN Welcomes You to the Nursing Profession." *New Nurse Booklet*, National Council of State Boards of Nursing, 2018, www.ncsbn.org/New_Nurse-Booklet-Web.pdf.

Nelson, Brad. "Robotics and Medicine." *Science*, www.sciencemag.org/robotics-and-medicine. Accessed 6 May 2020.

Neuman Systems Model. Neuman Systems Model Trustees Group, www.neumansystemsmodel.org/index.html. Accessed 4 Oct. 2016.

Neuman, Betty, and Jacqueline Fawcett, editors. *The Neuman Systems Model*. 5th ed., Pearson, 2011.

"NIH Clinical Research Trials and You." *National Institutes of Health*, www.nih.gov/health-information/nih-clinical-research-trials-you. Accessed 11 Sept. 2020.

"NIH Clinical Research Trials and You: The Basics." *National Institutes of Health*, www.nih.gov/health-information/nih-clinical-research-trials-you/basics. Accessed 24 Aug. 2020.

"NLC FAQs." *National Council of State Boards of Nursing*, ncsbn.org/npa.htm. Accessed 23 Sept. 2020.

"NLN PAX." *National League for Nursing*, www.nln.org. Accessed 27 Aug. 2020.

"Nola J. Pender." *School of Nursing, University of Michigan*. Regents of the University of Michigan. Accessed 29 Aug. 2016.

"Nola Pender." *WhyIWantToBeANurse.org*. WhyIWantToBeANurse.org. Accessed 29 Aug. 2016.

Norton, A., et al. "Melodic Intonation Therapy." *Annals of the New York Academy of Sciences*, vol. 1169, 2009, pp. 431-36. *Wiley*, doi:10.1111/j.1749-6632.2009.04859.x.

"Nurse Anesthetist." *Nurse.org*, nurse.org/resources/nurse-anesthetist/. Accessed 28 Sept. 2020.

"Nurse Anesthetists, Nurse Midwives, and Nurse Practitioners." US Bureau of Labor Statistics. *Occupational Outlook Handbook*, www.bls.gov/ooh/healthcare/nurse- anesthetists-nurse-midwives-and-nurse-practitioners.htm.

"Nurse Anesthetists, Nurse Midwives, and Nurse Practitioners." US Bureau of Labor Statistics, *Occupational Outlook Handbook*, www.bls.gov/ooh/healthcare/nurse-anesthetists-nurse-midwives-and-nurse-practitioners.htm. Accessed 28 Sept. 2020.

"Nurse Anesthetists, Nurse Midwives, and Nurse Practitioners: Occupational Outlook," *US Bureau of Labor Statistics*, www.bls.gov/ooh/healthcare/nurse-anesthetists-nurse-midwives-and-nurse-practitioners.htm.

"Nurse Educator." *ExploreHealthCareers.org*, explorehealthcareers.org/career/nursing/nurse-educator/. Accessed 22 Sept. 2020.

"Nurse Educators." *National League for Nursing (NLN)*, www.nln.org. Accessed 22 Sept. 2020.

"Nurse Manager." Nurse.org. 9 July 9 2020. nurse.org/resources/nurse-manager/. Accessed 6 Oct. 2020.

"Nurse Manager: Leading the Nurse Profession into the Future." Duquesne University School of Nursing. onlinenursing.duq.edu/blog/roles-nurse-manager-leading-nursing-profession-future/. Accessed 6 Oct. 2020.

"Nurse Staffing Advocacy." *American Nurses Association*, www.nursingworld.org/practice-policy/nurse-staffing/nurse-staffing-advocacy/. Accessed 3 Sept. 2020.

"Nurse Unions Continue to Push for Nurse-Patient Ratio Legislation." *Littler*, 20 Feb. 2014, www.littler.com/publication-press/publication/nurse-unions-continue-push-nurse-patient-ratio-legislation.

"Nurses Association Pushes for Federal, State Nurse-to-Patient Ratio Laws." *AHC Media*, 1 July 2015, www.reliasmedia.com/articles/135642-nurses-association-pushes-for-federal-state-nurse-to-patient-ratio-laws.

"Nursing at the Joint Commission." *The Joint Commission*, www.jointcommission.org/resources/for-nurses/. Accessed 16 Sept. 2020.

"Nursing Care Plans: What You Need to Know." *Nurse.org*, nurse.org/articles/what-are-nursing-care-plans/. Accessed 3 Sept. 2020.

"Nursing Continuing Education Requirements by State." *AACEUS: Online Continuing Education for Healthcare Professionals*, www.aaaceus.com/state_nursing_requirements.asp. Accessed 18 Sept. 2020.

"Nursing Definitions." *International Council of Nurses*, www.icn.ch/nursing-policy/nursing-definitions. Accessed 2 Sept. 2020.

"Nursing Entrance Exams: What You Can Expect." *All Nursing Schools*, www.allnursingschools.com/how-to-get-into-nursing-school/entrance-exams/. Accessed 27 Aug. 2020.

"Nursing Regulations and State Boards of Nursing." *American Nephrology Nurses Association*. www.annanurse.org/advocacy/resources-and-tools/state/nursing-regulations. Accessed 7 Oct. 2020.

"Nursing Scholarships." *Nurse.org*, nurse.org/scholarships/. Accessed 27 Aug. 2020. A comprehensive list of available nursing specific scholarships.

"Nursing Theory: Topical Overview and Research Resources for Nursing Theories." *University of Wisconsin-Milwaukee Libraries*, guides.library.uwm.edu/c.php?g+832148&p=5943165. Accessed 14 Sept. 2020.

"Nursing Vocational School Program Information." *Study.com*, 23 Apr. 2020, study.com/nursing_vocational_school.html.

O*NET Online. online.onetcenter.org, 2015. This website sponsored by the US Department of Labor provides detailed job descriptions for career exploration and job seekers. This database can be searched by job title and by occupation. It details the knowledge skills, abilities, and other characteristics required for particular jobs, the future outlook in terms of hiring potential, the typical salary range, as well as other key information.

"Obstetrics (OB) Nurse." *RegisteredNursing.org*, www.registerednursing.org/specialty/obstetrics-ob-nurse. Accessed 1 Oct. 2020.

"Occupational Health Nurse." Explore Health Careers, explorehealthcareers.org/career/nursing/occupational-health-nurse/. Accessed 3 Sept. 2020.

Occupational Health. *World Health Organization*, 2015.

Office for the Advancement of Telehealth, www.hrsa.gov/telehealth.

Office of Cancer Complementary and Alternative Medicine, www.cam.cancer.gov. This site provides health professionals, persons with cancer, and the general public information about complementary and alternative medicine in treating cancer.

Office of Dietary Supplements. National Institutes of Health, www.ods.od.nih.gov.

Okada, Kaoru, et al. "Effects of Music Therapy on Autonomic Nervous System Activity, Incidence of Heart Failure Events, and Plasma Cytokine and Catecholamine Levels in Elderly Patients with Cerebrovascular Disease and Dementia." *International Heart Journal*, vol. 50, 2009, pp. 95-110.

Oken, B. S., et al. "Randomized, Controlled, Six-Month Trial of Yoga in Healthy Seniors: Effects on Cognition and Quality of Life." *Alternative Therapies in Health and Medicine*, vol. 12, 2006, pp. 40-47.

"Opioid Misuse and Addiction." National Institutes of Health. US National Library of Medicine. *Medline Plus*, medlineplus.gov/opiodmisuseandaddiction.html. Accessed 16 Sept. 2020.

Orem, Dorothea E. "Views of Human Beings Specific to Nursing." *Nursing Science Quarterly*, vol. 10, no. 1, 1997, pp. 26-31.

"Orientation Process." Nurse Educator Resource Center. *Vanderbilt University Medical Center*, www.vumc.org/nerc/35825. Accessed 18 Sept. 2020.

Orme-Johnson, D., et al. "Neuroimaging of Meditation's Effect on Brain Reactivity." *NeuroReport*, vol. 17, no. 12, 2006, pp. 1359-1363.

Ostroff, Donna, preparer. "Betty M. Neuman Papers." Updated by Gail E. Farr. *University of Pennsylvania Finding Aids*, U of Pennsylvania, Jan. 2013, hdl.library.upenn.edu/1017/d/ead/upenn_bates_MC160. Accessed 4 Oct. 2016.

"Overview of Aging." *Geriatric Nursing*, 2018, geriatricnursing.org/overview-of-aging/. Accessed 12 Oct. 2018.

Pagán, J. A., and M. V. Pauly. "Access to Conventional Medical Care and the Use of Complementary and Alternative Medicine." *Health Affairs*, vol. 24, 2004, pp. 255-62.

"Pain Relievers." National Institutes of Health. US National Library of Medicine. *Medline Plus*, medlineplus.gov/painrelievers.html. Accessed 16 Sept. 2020.

Palinkas, L. A., and M. L. Kabongo. "The Use of Complementary and Alternative Medicine by Primary Care Patients." *Journal of Family Practice*, vol. 49, 2000, pp. 1121-30.

"Palliative Care Nurse Job Description and Salary Information." *Jacksonville University*, www.jacksonvilleu.com/blog/nursing/palliative-care-nurse-job-description-salary-information/. Accessed 11 Sept. 2020.

Papandrea, Dawn. "Nursing Care Plans: What You Need to Know." *Nurse.org*, 8 Jan. 2018, nurse.org/articles/what-are-nursing-care-plans/. Accessed 3 Sept. 2020.

Park, Melissa, et al. "Nurse Practitioners, Certified Nurse Midwives, and Physician Assistants in Physician Offices." *Centers for Disease Control and Prevention*, 17 Aug. 2011,

Parles, Karen, and J. H. Schiller. *One Hundred Questions and Answers about Lung Cancer*. 2nd ed., Jones and Bartlett, 2010. A patient-oriented guide that covers a range of topics related to lung cancer.

"Patient Education Coordinator." *Daily Nurse*, dailynurse.com/patient-education-coordinator/. Accessed 18 Sept. 2020.

Paul-Labrador, M., et al. "Effects of a Randomized Controlled Trial of Transcendental Meditation on Components of the Metabolic Syndrome in Subjects with Coronary Artery Disease." *Archives of Internal Medicine*, 2006, pp. 1218-24.

Peake, J. M., G. Kerr, and J. P. Sullivan. "A Critical Review of Consumer Wearables, Mobile Applications, and Equipment for Providing Biofeedback, Monitoring Stress, and Sleep in Physically Active Populations." *Frontiers in Physiology*, vol. 9, p. 743.

Pearson, Alan. "Dead Poets, Nursing Theorists and Contemporary Nursing Practice." *International Journal of Nursing Practice*, vol. 14, no. 1, 2008, pp. 1-2.

Pecci, Alexandra Wilson. "Nurse-Patient Ratio Law in MA Raises Cost, Quality Concerns." *HealthLeaders Media*, 23 June 2015, www.healthleadersmedia.com/nursing/nurse-patient-ratio-law-ma-raises-cost-quality-concerns.

"Pediatric Nurse." *Nurse.org*, nurse.org/resources/pediatric-nurse/#what-is-a-pediatric-nurse. Accessed 2 Sept. 2020.

"Pell Grant: Federal Student Aid." US Department of Education, studentaid.gov/understand-aid/types/grants/pell. Accessed 27 Aug. 2020.

Pender, Nola J. *Health Promotion Model (HPM): Frequent Questions and Answers*. U of Michigan, Deep Blue, 2011.

"Perinatal Nurse." *Johnson & Johnson Nursing*, nursing.jnj.com/specialty/perinatal-nurse. Accessed 3 Sept. 2020.

"Perinatal Nurse." *Nursing Explorer*, www.nursingexplorer.com/careers/perinatal-nurse. Accessed 3 Sept. 2020.

"Periop 101: A Core Curriculum(tm) OR Course Outcomes." *Association of periOperative Registered Nurses (AORN)*, www.aorn.ort/education/facility-solutions/periop-101/course-outcomes.

Peters, R. M. "The Effectiveness of Therapeutic Touch." *Nursing Science Quarterly*, vol. 12, 1999, pp. 52-61.

Peterson, Sandra J., and Timothy S. Bredow, editors. *Middle Range Theories: Application to Nursing Research*. 4th ed., Wolters, 2017.

Petiprin, Alice. "Nola Pender—Nursing Theorist." *Nursing Theory*. Alice Petiprin, Nursing-Theory.org, 2016. Accessed 29 Aug. 2016.

Pevsner, Jonathan. *Bioinformatics and Functional Genomics*. 3rd ed., Wiley-Blackwell, 2015.

"Physician Assistants." US Bureau of Labor Statistics. *Occupational Outlook Handbook*, www.bls.gov/ooh/healthcare/physician-assistants.htm#tab-1. Accessed 2 Oct. 2020

Pohl, G., et al. "'Laying on of Hands' Improves Well-Being in Patients with Advanced Cancer." *Supportive Care in Cancer*, vol. 15, 2007, pp. 143-51.

Pointer, Emma "What Is Team Nursing?" *Trusted Health*, 3 Mar. 2020, www.trustedhealth.com/blog/what-is-team-nursing.

"Policy, Data, Oversight: Assessment & Selection." *Office of Personnel Management*, www.opm.gov/policy-data-oversight/assessment-and-selection/other-assessment-methods/job-knowledge-tests/. Accessed 24 Aug. 2020.

Ponte, Patricia Reid. "Structure, Process, and Empirical Outcomes—The Magnet Journey of Continuous Improvement." *Journal of Nursing Administration*, vol. 43, no. 6, 2013, pp. 309-10.

Potter, Patricia A., Anne Griffin Perry, and Patricia Stockert. *Fundamentals of Nursing*. Mosby, 2016.

"Pregnancy and Perinatology Branch (PPB)." *National Institute of Child Health and Human Development*, 30 Nov., 2012.

Price, Debra, and Julie Gwin. *Pediatric Nursing*. 11th ed., Saunders, 2011.

Prideaux, Ed. "Stayin' Alive! How Music Has Fought Pandemics for 2,700 Years." *The Guardian*, 6 Apr. 2020, www.theguardian.com/music/2020/apr/06/stayin-alive-how-music-fought-pandemics-2700-years-coronavirus.

"Primary Care Nursing Careers & Salary Outlook." *NurseJournal*. 31 July 2020. nursejournal.org/primary-care-nursing/primary-care-nursing-careers-salary-outlook/.

Pritchard, A. *Ways of Learning: Learning Theories and Learning Styles in the Classroom*. Routledge, 2013. Provides an understanding of the ways in which learning takes place. Teachers can implement suggestions in their planning and teaching.

Pritchard, D. J., and Bruce R. Korf. *Medical Genetics at a Glance*. 3rd ed., John Wiley & Sons, 2013.

Provost, G. *100 Ways to Improve Your Writing*. New American Library, 1985. Provost provides quick, breezy, instruction on writing; in a decades-old title that has not gone out of print, or out of style.

"Public Health Nurse." *ExploreHealthCareers.org*, explorehealthcareers.org/career/nursing/public-health-nurse/#:~:text=While%20most%20nurses%20care%20for,and%20increase%20access%20to%20care. Accessed 30 Sept. 2020.

PubMed. National Center for Biotechnology Information, www.ncbi.nlm.nih.gov/pubmed.

Purnell, Larry. *Transcultural Health Care: A Culturally Competent Approach*. Davis, 2013.

Quinn, Mattie. "Should Hospitals Limit the Number of Patients Nurses Can Help?" *Governing*, 12 Sept. 2018, www.governing.com/topics/health-human-services/gov-massachusetts-ballot-nurses-patient-ratio-healthcare.html.

Quinn-Szcesuil, J. "How Can Public Speaking Help Your Career?" *Minority Nurse*, 2017, www.minoritynurse.com/how-can-public-speaking-help-your-career/. Accessed 30 Aug. 2020.

Quinn-Szcesuil, Julia. "What Does a WOC Nurse Do?" *Minority Nurse*, Apr. 2019, minoritynurse.com/what-does-a-woc-nurse-do/.

Qulehsari, M. Q., et al. "Lifelong Learning Strategies in Nursing: A Systemic Review." *Electron Physician*, vol. 9, no. 10, 2017, pp. 5541-50, www.ncbi.nlm.nih.gov/pmc/articles/PMC5718860/.

Rainforth, M., et al. "Stress Reduction Programs in Patients with Elevated Blood Pressure." *Current Hypertension Report*, vol. 9, no. 6, 2007, pp. 520-28.

Rakel, David, editor. *Integrative Medicine*. 2nd ed., Saunders/Elsevier, 2007. An authoritative textbook that discusses the philosophy and method of integrative medicine and details therapeutic modalities for numerous diseases and conditions.

Rath, T. *Strengths Finder 2.0*. Gallup Publishing, 2007. This is a classic book about finding and leveraging your strengths in the classroom, at work, during interviews, and at home. Purchase of this book in electronic or print format comes with a code that allows you to take an online assessment that highlights your five signature strengths.

Rayman, M., et al. "Impact of Selenium on Mood and Quality of Life." *Biological Psychiatry*, vol. 59, 2006, pp. 147-54.

Reed, Pamela. *Perspectives on Nursing Theory*. 6th ed., LWW, 2011.

Rees, Alan M., editor. *The Complementary and Alternative Medicine Information Source Book*. Oryx Press, 2001. Defines CAM terms and the background of CAM and includes a listing of resources.

Rees, L., and A. Weil. "Integrated Medicine [Editorial]." *British Medical Journal*, vol. 322, 2001, pp. 119-20. Defines the basic tenets of IM.

"Registered Nurse First Assistant." *Nurse.org*, nurse.org/resources/rnfa-career-guide/. Accessed 29 Sept. 2020.

"Registered Nurses." U.S. Bureau of Labor Statistics. *Occupational Outlook Handbook*. www.bls.gov/ooh/healthcare/registered-nurses.htm. Accessed 5 Oct. 2020.

"Rehabilitation." *World Health Organization*, www.who.int/health-topics/rehabilitation#tab=tab_1. Accessed 25 Aug. 2020.

"Reiki." *Cancer Research UK*, 22 Jan. 2019, www.cancerresearchuk.org/about-cancer/cancer-in-general/treatment/complementary-alternative-therapies/individual-therapies/reiki.

"Reiki." *Johns Hopkins Medicine, Integrative Medicine & Digestive Center*, www.hopkinsmedicine.org/integrative_medicine_digestive_center/services/reiki.html. Accessed 1 May. 2020.

"Reiki." National Center for Complementary and Integrative Health. *US National Institutes of Health*, Dec. 2018, www.nccih.nih.gov/health/reiki. Accessed 1 May. 2020.

Reising, Virginia A. "What Is a Nurse?" *American Journal of Nursing*, vol. 119, no. 6, June 2019.

Renpenning, Kathie McLaughlin, and Susan G. Taylor. *Self-Care Theory in Nursing: Selected Papers of Dorothea Orem*. Springer, 2003.

Reuter C., and V. Fitzsimons. "Physician Orders." *American Journal of Nursing*, vol. 113, no. 8, 2013, journals.lww.com/ajnonline/Fulltext/2013/0800/Physician_Orders.2.aspx.

Richardson, Carmen. *Expressive Arts Therapy for Traumatized Children and Adolescents: A Four-Phase Model*. Routledge, 2016.

Richeson, N. E., et al. "Effects of Reiki on Anxiety, Depression, Pain, and Physiological Factors in Community-Dwelling Older Adults." *Research in Gerontological Nursing*, vol. 3, 2010, pp. 187-99.

Riley, Julia Balzer. *Communication in Nursing*. 8th ed., Elsevier, 2017.

Riordan, C. M. "We All Need Friends at Work." *Harvard Business Review*, 3 July 2013, hbr.org/2013/07/we-all-need-friends-at-work. This describes the benefits of developing warm and friendly relationships with coworkers.

Ritti, R. R., and S. Levy. *The Ropes to Skip and The Ropes to Know: Studies in Organizational Theory and Behavior*. 8th ed., Wiley, 2009. Using a case study approach, this book highlights some of the key pitfalls that new employees make.

Riva, Giuseppe, and B. K. Wiederhold. *Annual Review of Cybertherapy and Telemedicine 2012: Advanced Technologies in the Behavioral, Social and Neurosciences*. IOS Press, 2012.

Roberts, K., S. Gelder, and H. Wild. "Clinical Research Nurse Interns: The Future Research Workforce." *Nursing Research*, vol. 24, no. 2, 18 Nov. 2016, pp. 6-7.

Roberts, L., et al. "Intercessory Prayer for the Alleviation of Ill Health." *Cochrane Database of Systematic Reviews*, 2009. CD000368. EBSCO DynaMed Systematic Literature Surveillance, www.ebscohost.com/dynamed. Reviews findings regarding intercessory prayer and describes the limitations of research on this topic.

Robles, B., D. M. Upchurch, and T. Kuo. "Comparing Complementary and Alternative Medicine Use with or without Including Prayer as a Modality in a Local and Diverse United States Jurisdiction." Front. *Public Health*, 21 Mar. 2017, core.ac.uk/download/pdf/82863954.pdf.

Rock, C. L., and C. Thomson, et al. "American Cancer Society Guideline for Diet and Physical Activity for Cancer Prevention." *CA: A Cancer Journal for Clinicians*, 9 June 2020, acsjournals.onlinelibrary.wiley.com/doi/full/103322/caac.21591. Accessed 24 Aug. 2020.

Rolf, Ida. *Rolfing: Reestablishing the Natural Alignment and Structural Integration of the Human Body for Vitality and Well-Being*. Healing Arts Press, 1989.

———, and Rosemary Feitis. *Rolfing and Physical Reality*. 2nd ed., Healing Arts Press, 1990.

Rosa, L., et al. "A Close Look at Therapeutic Touch." *Journal of the American Medical Association*, vol. 279, 1998, pp. 1005-10.

Rosenbaum, Earnest H., and Isadora Rosenbaum. *Everyone's Guide to Cancer Supportive Care: A Comprehensive Handbook for Patients and Their Families*. 4th ed., Andrews McMeel, 2005. Comprehensive guide with more than fifty chapters. Includes Web resources on CAM.

Rossman, Martin L. *Guided Imagery for Self-Healing*. 2nd ed., H. J. Kramer/New World Library, 2000.

Roussel, Linda. *Management and Leadership for Nurse Administrators*. 8th ed., Jones & Bartlett Learning, 2020.

Rubin, Judith Aron. *The Art of Art Therapy: What Every Art Therapist Needs to Know*. Brunner, 2011.

Ruesink, Megan. "What Does It Really Take to Be a Director of Nursing?" Rasmussen College. 21 June 2017. www.rasmussen.edu/degrees/nursing/blog/director-of-nursing/. Accessed 6 Oct. 2020.

Ruhlman, Michael. *Walk on Water: Inside an Elite Pediatric Surgery Unit*. Viking-Penguin, 2003.

Rydholm, M., and P. Strang. "Acupuncture for Patients in Hospital-Based Home Care Suffering from Xerostomia." *Journal of Palliative Care*, vol. 15, 1999, p. 20.

Sackett, P. R., M. J. Borneman, and B. S. Connelly. "High-Stakes Testing in Higher Education and Employment: Appraising the Evidence for Validity and Fairness." *American Psychologist*, vol. 63, no. 4, May/June 2008, pp. 215-27.

Sacks, Oliver. "The Power of Music." *Brain*, vol. 129, 2006, pp. 2528-32.

Sadhra, Steven S., and Krishna G. Rampal, editors. *Occupational Health: Risk Assessment and Management*. Blackwell Scientific, 1999.

Sadler, T. W. *Langman's Medical Embryology*. Lippincott Williams & Wilkins, 2014.

"Safe-Staffing Ratios: Benefiting Nurses and Patients." *Department for Professional Employees, AFL-CIO*, www.dpeaflcio.org/factsheets/safe-staffing-critical-for-patients-and-nurses. Accessed 3 Sept. 2020.

Saleh, U. S. "Theory Guided Practice in Nursing," www.pulsus.com/scholarly-articles/theory-guided-practice-in-nursing.pdf. Accessed 14 Sept. 2020.

Sanghavi, Darshak. *A Map of the Child: A Pediatrician's Tour of the Body*. Henry Holt, 2003.

Santana, Nadia. *The Ultimate Nurse Practitioner Guidebook: A Comprehensive Guide to Getting Into and Surviving Nurse Practitioner School, Finding a Job, and Understanding the Policy that Drives the Profession*. Peter Lang Publishing, 2018.

Schultz, David. "Nurses Fighting State by State for Minimum Staffing Laws." *Kaiser Health News*, khn.org/news/nurse-staffing-laws/. Accessed 3 Sept. 2020.

Schultz, Judith M., and Sheila L. Videbeck. *Lippincott's Manual of Psychiatric Nursing Care Plans*. 9th ed., Wolters Kluwer/Lippincott, Williams, & Wilkins, 2012.

Schwartz, M. S., and F. Andrasik, editors. *Biofeedback: A Practitioner's Guide*. Guilford Publications, 2017.

"Scope of Practice." *American Nurses Association*, www.nursingworld.org/practice-policy/scope-of-practice/. Accessed 23 Sept. 2020.

Scott-Sheldon, L. A., et al. "Stress Management Interventions for HIV+ Adults." *Health Psychology*, vol. 27, 2008, pp. 129-39.

Seaward, Brian Luke. *Managing Stress: Principles and Strategies for Health and Well-Being*. 8th ed., Jones and Bartlett Learning, 2013.

Sederstrom, Jill. "7 Specialties Lead Demand for Nurses." *Healthcare Traveler*, 22 Apr. 2013, healthcaretraveler.modernmedicine.com/healthcare-traveler/content/tags/american-association-critical-care-nurses/7-specialties-lead-demand?page=full.

Sellers, Christopher C. *Hazards of the Job: From Industrial Disease to Environmental Health Science*. U of North Carolina P, 1999.

Shih, C. Y., and C. Y. Huang. "The Association of Sociodemographic Factors and Needs of Haemodialysis

Patients According to Maslow's Hierarchy of Needs." *Journal of Clinical Nursing*, vol. 28, nos. 1-2, pp. 270-78.

Shnayerson, Michael, and Mark J. Plotkin. *The Killers Within: The Deadly Rise of Drug Resistant Bacteria*. Little, 2003.

Sibinga, Erica M. S., and Kathi J. Kemper. "Complementary, Holistic, and Integrative Medicine: Meditation Practices for Pediatric Health." *Pediatrics in Review*, vol. 31, 2020, pp. 91-103. Directed to pediatric clinicians, this article describes cases for which meditative practices may be helpful, then provides summary tables of data from studies of various types of pediatric-focused meditation.

Siegel, D., and T. Bryson. *The Whole-Brain Child: 12 Revolutionary Strategies to Nurture Your Child's Developing Mind*. Delacorte Press, 2011. Helps parents teach children about how their brain works, giving young children the self-understanding that can lead them to make better choices that ultimately lead to meaningful and joyful lives.

Silverstein, R. "Good People Make Good Leaders." *Entrepreneur*, 2010, www.entrepreneur.com/article/206832.

Simon, Matt. "The WIRED Guide to Robots." *WIRED*, 13 Apr. 2020, www.wired.com/story/wired-guide-to-robots/. Accessed 6 May 2020.

Simple Changes, Big Rewards: A Practical, Easy Guide for Healthy, Happy Living." *Harvard Health*, n.d., www.health.harvard.edu/special-health-reports/simple-changes-big-rewards-a-practical-easy-guide-for-healthy-happy-living. In this article, researchers for Harvard Health identified actual positive physical and mental benefits and an inclination towards "happiness associated with volunteering and community service.

Sise, Betsy. *The Rolfing Experience: Integration in the Gravity Field*. Hohm Press, 2005.

Sitzman, Kathleen, and Jean Watson. *Caring Science, Mindful Practice: Implementing Watson's Human Caring Theory*. Springer, 2013.

Sitzman, Kathleen, and Lisa Wright Eichelberger. *Understanding the Work of Nursing Theorists: A Creative Beginning*. 3rd ed., Jones, 2017.

"Six Relaxation Techniques to Reduce Stress." Harvard Medical School. *Harvard Health Publishing*, 2009, www.health.harvard.edu/mind-and-mood/six-relaxation-techniques-to-reduce-stress. Accessed 25 Aug. 2020.

Slavin, Dianne, and Renee Fabus. "A Case Study Using a Multimodal Approach to Melodic Intonation Therapy." *American Journal of Speech-Language Pathology*, vol. 27, no. 4, 2018, pp. 1352-62.

Smedley, Julia, et al., editors. *Oxford Handbook of Occupational Health*. 2nd ed., Oxford UP, 2012.

Smith, Marlaine C., and Marilyn E. Parker, editors. *Nursing Theories and Nursing Practices*. 4th ed., Davis, 2015.

Smith, Marlaine, and Marilyn E. Parker. *Nursing Theories and Nursing Practice*. Davis, 2015.

Smith, Mary Jane, and Patricia Liehr. *Middle Range Theory for Nursing*. Springer, 2013.

Smith, W. B., et al. "Survey of Cancer Researchers Regarding Complementary and Alternative Medicine." *Journal of the Society of Integrative Oncology*, vol. 6, no. 1, 2008, pp. 2-12. Survey results published by the NCI to assess the interest and concern of 329 research respondents in CAM.

So, P. S., Y. Jiang, and Y. Qin. "Touch Therapies for Pain Relief in Adults." *Cochrane Database of Systematic Reviews*, 2008. *EBSCO DynaMed Systematic Literature Surveillance*, CD006535, 2008.

Society of Critical Care Medicine. "What Is Telemedicine?" *My ICU Care*, 2001-2013.

"Solutions for College and Career Readiness." ACT, www.act.org. Accessed 27 Aug. 2020.

Sparber, A., and J. C. Wootton. "Use of Alternative and Complementary Therapies for Psychiatric and Neurologic Diseases." *Journal of Alternative and Complementary Medicine*, vol. 8, 2002, pp. 93-96.

Spencer, A. "The Science Behind Procrastination." *Real Simple*, n.d., www.realsimple.com/work-life/life-strategies/time-management/procrastination. This article delves further into the ideas of Dr. Pychyl and the effect of the brain's structure on time management

"Sr. Callista Roy, PhD, RN, FAAN." Trustees of Boston College. *Boston College William F. Connell School of Nursing*, 20 July 2016.

"Standards." The Joint Commission. www.jointcommission.org/standards/. Accessed 10 Oct. 2020.

Stanhope, Marcia, and Jeanette Lancaster. *Public Health Nursing: Population-Centered Health Care in the Community*. 10th ed., Elsevier, 2020.

Stansil, Raynetta. "What Is Robotic Surgery and How Does It Work?" *Surgical Solutions*, 31 Jul. 2019, surgical-solutions.com/blog/what-is-robotic-surgery-and-how-does-it-work/. Accessed 6 May 2020.

"Steps to Becoming a Clinical Trials Research Nurse—Education and Experience." *MHAOnline*, www.mhaonline.com/faq/how-do-I-become-a-clinical-trials-research-nurse. Accessed 11 Sept. 2020.

Stone, Robyn I., and Linda Barbarotta. "Caring for an Aging America in the Twenty-First Century."

Generations, 9 June 2011, www.asaging.org/blog/caring-aging-america-twenty-first-century.

"Stress Management." *American Heart Association*, n.d. Accessed 17 May 2016.

"Stress: How to Cope Better with Life's Challenges." American Academy of Family Physicians. *FamilyDoctor.org*, Nov. 2010.

Strunk, W., Jr. and White, E. B., editors. *The Elements of Style*. 4th ed., Longman, 1999. A classic, erudite practical guide to style and the basics of English composition.

Stuart, Gail Wiscarz. *Principles and Practice of Psychiatric Nursing*. 10th ed., Elsevier, 2013.

"Study Skills for Students." *Education Corner: Education that Matters*, www.educationcorner.com/study-skills.html. Accessed 30 Aug. 2010.

"Surgical Nurse." *Nurse.org*, nurse.org/resources/perioperative-surgical-nurse/. Accessed 29 Sept. 2020.

Swanson, Jane L., and Nadya A. Fouad. *Career Theory and Practice: Learning through Case Studies*. Sage, 2010.

Tabatabaee A., M. Z. Tafreshi, and M. Rassouli, et al. "Effect of Therapeutic Touch in Patients with Cancer: A Literature Review." *Medical Archives*, 2016, pubmed.ncbi.nlm.nih.gov/27194823/. Accessed 25 Aug. 2020.

Taylor, Carol, et al. *Fundamentals of Nursing: The Art and Science of Nursing Care*. 9th ed., Wolters Kluwer, 2018.

Taylor, Goldie. "The Evolution of Telehealth Nursing." *Minority Nurse*, 8 Apr. 2016, minoritynurse.com/the-evolution-of-telehealth-nursing/.

"Telehealth Nursing Practice." *American Academy of Ambulatory Care Nursing*, www.aaacn.org/telehealth.

"Telemedicine Reimbursement Guide." *eVisit*, evisit.com/resources/telemedicine-reimbursement-guide/.

"The Core Leadership Skills You Need in Every Role." *Center for Creative Leadership*, www.ccl.org/articles/leading-effectively-articles/fundamental-4-core-leadership-skills-for-every-career-stage. Accessed 30 Aug. 2020.

"The Difference Between Nurse Manager vs. Charge Nurse: Leadership Roles in Healthcare." Maryville University. online.maryville.edu/vs/nurse-manager-vs-charge-nurse/. Accessed 5 Oct. 2020.

"The Do's and Do Not's of Getting Accepted into Nursing School." *Registered Nursing*, www.registerednursing.org/dos-donts-nursing-school-acceptance/. Accessed 27 Aug. 2020.

"The History of Nursing." *Nursing School Hub*, www.nursingschoolhub.com/history-nursing/. Accessed 4 Jan. 2017.

The National Voice for Academic Nursing. American Association of Colleges of Nursing, www.aacnnursing.org. Accessed 3 Sept. 2020.

"The Nursing Process." *American Nurses Association*, www.nursingworld.org/practice-policy/workforce/what-is-nursing/the-nursing-process/. Accessed 3 Sept. 2020.

"The SAT." *College Board*, www.collegeboard.org. Accessed 27 Aug. 2020.

"The Ultimate Nursing Care Plan Database." *Nursing.com*, nursing.com/course/nursing-care-plans/. Accessed 3 Sept. 2020.

Thilman, James. "*Alive Inside* Celebrates the Healing Power of Music." *TheHuffingtonPost.com*, 10 July 2014.

"Thinking About Complementary and Alternative Medicine: A Guide for People with Cancer." National Cancer Institute, www.cancer.gov/publications/patient-education/thinking-about-cam. A booklet that explains CAM and what choices are available to people with cancer.

Thompson, Cathy J. "What Is the Nursing Metaparadigm?" *Nursing Education Expert*, 3 Oct. 2017, nursingeducationexpert.com/metaparadigm/.

Thorne, Sally, et al. "Nursing's Metaparadigm Concepts: Disimpacting the Debates." *Journal of Advanced Nursing*, vol. 27, no. 6, 1998, pp. 1257-68.

Thornton, L. C. "A Study of Reiki, an Energy Field Treatment, Using Rogers' Science." *Rogerian Nursing Science News*, vol. 8, 1996, pp. 14-15.

"Three Influential Trends in Gerontology." *Stenberg College*, 29 July 2015, www.stenbergcollege.com/blog/therapeutic-recreation/3-influential-trends-in-gerontology/.

Tierney, Gillian. *Opportunities in Holistic Health Care Careers*. Rev. ed. McGraw-Hill, 2007. This book addresses the job outlook, educational requirements, regulation, and salaries for many CAM practitioners.

Tikkanen, Roosa and Melinda K. Abrams. "U.S. Health Care from a Global Perspective, 2019: Higher Spending, Worse Outcomes?" *The Commonwealth Fund*, www.commonwealthfund.org/publications/issue-briefs/2020/jan/us-health-care-global-perspective-2019. Accessed 2 Sept. 2020.

Timbo, B. B., et al. "Dietary Supplements in a National Survey: Prevalence of Use and Reports of Adverse Events." *Journal of the American Dietary Association*, vol. 106, 2006, pp. 1966-74.

Tippens, K., K. Marsman, and H. Zwickey. "Is Prayer CAM?" *Journal of Alternative and Complementary Medicine*, vol. 15, 2009, pp. 435-38.

Toney-Butler, U. J., and J. M. Thayer. "Nursing Process." US National Library of Medicine. National Center for Biotechnology Information. *National Institutes of Health*, updated 10 July 2020, www.ncbi.nlm.nih.gov/books/NBK499937/.

Tonges, M., and J. Ray. "Translating Caring Theory into Practice." *Journal of Nursing Administration*, vol. 41, no. 9, pp. 374-81, prd-medweb-cdn.s3.amazonaws.com/documents/evidencebasedpractice/files/KS_Translating%20Caring%20Theory.pdf. Accessed 19 Sept. 2020.

Tonsaker, T., G. Bartlett, and C. Trpkov. "Health Information on the Internet: Gold Mine or Minefield?" *Canadian family physician Medecin de famille canadien*, vol. 60, no. 5, pp. 407-8, www.ncbi.nlm.nih.gov/pmc/articles/PMC4020634/. Accessed 25 Aug. 2020.

Tran, Quoc Nam, and Hamid Arabnia. *Emerging Trends in Computational Biology, Bioinformatics, and Systems Biology: Algorithms and Software Tools*. Morgan, 2015.

Transcendental Meditation. Maharishi Foundation USA, 2015. Accessed 30 Nov. 2015.

"Travel Nurse." *Registered Nursing*, www.registerednursing.org/specialty/travel-nurse/. Accessed 29 Sept. 2020.

"Treatment Options for Chronic Pain." *American Society of Regional Anesthesia and Pain Medicine*, www.asra.com/page/46/treatment-options-for-chronic-pain. Accessed 16 Sept. 2020.

Trow, Terence K., editor. "Alternative Treatments for Asthma in Adults and Adolescents." *DynaMed*, 3 Dec. 2018, www.dynamed.com/topics/dmp~AN~T566085.

Tummers, Nanette E. *Stress Management: A Wellness Approach*. Human Kinetics, 2013.

"Understanding the Healthcare Team." *Creaky Joints*, creakyjoints.org/about/what-is-the-healthcare-team/. Accessed 9 Oct. 2020.

"Understanding the Primary Nursing Care Model." *HealthStream*, 29 Aug. 2019, www.healthstream.com/resources/blog/blog/2019/08/29/understanding-the-primary-nursing-care-model.

"Understanding the Role of a Hospice Nurse." *Crossroads Hospice*, www.registerednursing.org/specialty/hospice-nurse/ on Accessed 11 Sept. 2020.

Upson, Margo. "What Are Fundamental Nursing Concepts?" *Career Trend*, careertrend.com/list-6196507-fundamental-nursing-concepts-html. Accessed 19 Oct. 2020.

Urden, Linda D., et al. *Priorities in Critical Care Nursing*. 7th ed., Elsevier Health Sciences, 2015.

US Food and Drug Administration, www.fda.gov.

US Pharmacopeia (USP), www.usp.org.

Van der Meulen, Ineke, et al. "Melodic Intonation Therapy: Present Controversies and Future Opportunities." *Archives of Physical Medicine and Rehabilitation*, vol. 93, no. 1, S46-S52. *Archives of Physical Medicine and Rehabilitation*, doi.org/10.1016/j.apmr.2011.05.029.

"Van Wicklin, Sharon Ann. "What Is the Perceived Value of Certification Among Registered Nurses? A Systematic Review,

Vera, Matt. "Nursing Care Plans (NCP): Ultimate Guide and Database." *Nurseslabs*, 31 Jan. 2019, nurseslabs.com/nursing-care-plans/. Accessed 3 Sept. 2020.

Vera, Matt. "Sister Callista L. Roy." *Nurselabs*, 18 Aug. 2014.

Vertino, K. A. "Effective Interpersonal Communication: A Practical Guide to Improve Your Life." *Online Journal of Nursing*, vol. 19, no. 3, 30 Sept. 2014, p. 1.

Vihinen, Mauno. "No More Hidden Solutions in Bioinformatics." *Nature*, 20 May 2015.

Volunteering." *Child Trends Databank*, 2014, www.childtrends.org/?indicators=volunteering; www.childtrends.org/?indicators=volunteering#sthash.BaxYKMHw.dpuf. This article outlines specific positive trends related to student's academic and vocational plans in relation to service work. Through the presentation of graphics and statistics the correlation found "through study is clearly outlined.

Waitley, D. *Psychology of Success: A Positive Approach to Lifelong Learning*. Irwin, 1990.

Waitley, D. *The Psychology of Winning*. Berkley Books, 1984. Best-selling author and speaker, Denis Waitley has painted word pictures of optimism, core values, motivation and resiliency that have become indelible and legendary in their positive impact on society. His works are easily understood and offer positive applications to living a meaningful and successful life.

Wang, D., et al. "Cerebral Blood Flow Changes Associated with Different Meditation Practices and Perceived Depth of Meditation." *Psychiatry Research: Neuroimaging*, Vol. 191, 2011, pp. 60-67. This study involved comparing two types of meditation (focus-based and breath-based) within subjects and looked at functional MRI and cerebral blood flow in relation to the subjects' reported experiences.

Watson, Jean. *Human Caring Science: A Theory of Nursing*. Jones, 2012.

Watson, Jean. *Nursing: The Philosophy and Science of Caring*. UP of Colorado, 2008.

Wayne, G. "Nursing Theories and Theorists: Your Theoretical Guide to Nursing Theories." *NursesLabs*,

nurseslabs.com/nursing-theories/#what_are_nursing_theories. Accessed 14 Sept. 2020.

Wayne, Gil. "Dorothea E. Orem." *Nurselabs*, 11 Aug. 2014.

Wayne, Gil. "Faye G. Abdellah's 21 Nursing Problems Theory." *Nurseslabs*, 29 Sept. 2014.

Wayne, Gil. "Nursing Theories and Theorists." *Nurseslabs*, nurseslabs.com/nursing-theories/. Accessed 19 Oct. 2020.

Weiss, Donna, et al. *The Interprofessional Health Care Team: Leadership and Development*. 2nd ed., Jones & Bartlett Learning, 2018.

"Wellness and Well-Being." National Institutes of Health. National Center for Complementary and Integrative Health. *National Institutes of Health*, www.nccih.nih.gov/health/wellness-and-well-being. Accessed 25 Aug. 2020.

Westendorf, Jennifer J. "Magnet Recognition Program." *Plastic Surgery Nursing*, vol. 27, no. 2, 2007, pp. 102-4.

Weston, M. J. "Strategies for Enhancing Autonomy and Control over Nursing Practice." *Online Journal of Issues in Nursing*, vol. 15, no. 1, 2010, ojin.nursingworld.org/MainMenuCategories/ANAMarketplace/ANAPeriodicals/OJIN/TableofContents/Vol152010/No1Jan2010/Enhancing-Autonomy-and-Control-and-Practice.aspx.

"What Are Clinical Trials and Studies?" US Department of Health and Human Services. *National Institute on Aging*, www.nia.nih.gov/health/what-are-clinical-trials-and-studies. Accessed 24 Aug. 2020.

"What Are Clinical Trials?" National Cancer Institute. *National Institutes of Health*, www.cancer.gov/about-cancer/treatment/clinical-trials/what-are-trials. Accessed 24 Aug. 2020.

"What Are Palliative Care and Hospice Care?" National Institute on Aging. *National Institutes of Health*, www.nia.nih.gov/health/what-are-palliative-care-and-hospice-care. Accessed 1 Sept. 2020.

"What Can I Expect in a Typical Reiki Session?" University of Minnesota. Taking Charge of Your Health & Wellbeing, https://www.takingcharge.csh.umn.edu/what-can-i-expect-typical-reiki-session. Accessed 1 May. 2020.

"What Is a Clinical Nurse Specialist (CNS)?" *MSNEDU.org*, 1 Oct. 2020, www.msnedu.org/clinical-nurse-specialist/.

"What Is a Nurse Practitioner?" *Nurse Practitioner Schools*, www.nursepractitionerschools.com/faq/what-is-np/. Accessed 25 Sept. 2020.

"What Is an Ostomy?" *United Ostomy Associations of American, Inc.*, www.ostomy.org/what-is-an-ostomy/. Accessed 25 Sept. 2020.

"What Is Cardiac Rehabilitation?" *American Heart Association*, www.heart.org/en/health-topics/cardiac-rehab/what-is-cardiac-rehabilitation. Accessed 25 Aug. 2020.

"What Is Genetic Counseling?" *National Society of Genetic Counselors*, www.nsgc.org/page/frequently-asked-questions-students#whatis on September 1, 2020.

"What Is Hospice Care?" *American Cancer Society*, www.cancer.org/treatment/end-of-life-care/hospice-care/what-is-hospice-care.html. Accessed 11 Sept. 2020.

"What Is Hospice Nursing?" *RegisteredNursing.org*, www.registerednursing.org/specialty/hospice-nurse/. Accessed 11 Sept. 2020.

"What Is Hospice?" *Hospice Foundation of America*, hospicefoundation.org/Hospice-Care/Hospice-Services. Accessed 1 Sept. 2020.

"What Is Nursing Theory? Key Concepts for DNPs." *Regis College*, online.regiscollege.edu/blog/what-is-nursing-theory/. Accessed 14 Sept. 2020.

"What Is Nursing?" *American Nurses Association*, www.nursingworld.org/practice-policy/workforce/what-is-nursing/. Accessed 2 Sept. 2020.

"What Is Palliative Care?" *International Association for Hospice and Palliative Care*, hospicecare.com/what-we-do/publications/getting-started/5-what-is-palliative-care. Accessed 11 Sept. 2020.

"What Is Telehealth? How Is Telehealth Different from Telemedicine?" *HealthIT.gov*, www.healthit.gov/faq/what-telehealth-how-telehealth-different-telemedicine. Accessed 27 Aug. 2020.

"What Is the Nursing Code of Ethics?" Nurse.org, 4 Sept. 2020. https://nurse.org/education/nursing-code-of-ethics/.

"What Is Transitional Care Management?" *Keystone Health*, keystone.health/what-is-transitional-care-management. Accessed 2 Sept. 2010.

"What Is Travel Nursing?" *Nurse.org*, nurse.org/articles/how-to-make-the-most-money-as-a-travel-nurse/. Accessed 29 Sept. 2020.

"What Is TT: How Did Therapeutic Touch Begin?" *Therapeutic Touch International Association*, www.therapeutictouch.org/what-is-tt/. Accessed 25 Aug. 2020.

"What You Need to Know about Informed Consent." *Healthline*, www.healthline.com/health/informed-consent. Accessed 11 Sept. 2020.

"What You Need to Know about Nursing Licensure and Boards of Nursing." National Council of State Boards of Nursing, 2011, www.ncsbn.org/licensure.htm.

Wheeler, C. "What Is Mind-Body Medicine?" *Psychology Today*, www.psychologytoday.com/us/blog/head-toe-happiness/201006/what-is-mind-body-medicine. Accessed 25 Aug. 2020.

White, P., and M.E. Hall. "Mapping the Literature of Case Management Nursing." *Journal of Medical Library Associations*, vol. 94, Suppl. 2, Apr. 2006, pp. E99-E106.

"WHO Definition of Palliative Care." *World Health Organization*, www.who.int/cancer/palliative/definition/en/. Accessed 11 Sept. 2020.

Whorton, James C. "The History of Complementary and Alternative Medicine." *Essentials of Complementary and Alternative Medicine*, edited by Wayne B. Jonas and Jeffrey S. Levin, Lippincott Williams & Wilkins, 1999.

"Who's Who on Your Hospital Team." *Patient Care Link*, patientcarelink.org/for-patients-families/whos-who-on-your-hospital-team/. Accessed 9 Oct. 2020.

Why Is Public Speaking Important?" *Writing Commons*, writingcommons.org/open-text/genres/public-speaking/844-why-is-public-speaking-important. Accessed 4 May 2015. This article describes the following three common types of public speaking: informative, persuasive, and entertaining. It also outlines the significant role that public speaking plays in all "individuals' lives and highlights how building one's public speaking abilities simultaneously improves one's critical thinking abilities.

Williams, Andrew. "Medical Robotics Has an 'Incredibly Exciting' Future, Predict Experts." *Robotics Business Review*, 22 Nov. 2018, www.roboticsbusinessreview.com/health-medical/medical-robotics-exciting-future/. Accessed 6 May 2020.

Winerman, L. "E-mails and Egos." *American Psychological Association*, www.apa.org/monitor/feb06/egos.aspx, 2006. This article discusses how the message intended in an email is often quite different than the actual message received. The inability to accurately convey one's tone of voice when writing an email is a key component that causes the discrepancy between the intended and received message. The authors discuss how people need to learn to see how others may perceive their message.

Winship, Gary, et al. "Collective Biography and the Legacy of Hildegard Peplau, Annie Altschul, and Eileen Skellern: The Origins of Mental Health Nursing and Its Relevance to the Current Crisis in Psychiatry." *Journal of Research in Nursing*, vol. 14, no. 6, 2009, pp. 505-17.

Winter T. "Maslow's Hierarchy: Separating Fact from Fiction." *Association for Talent Development*, www.td.org/insights/maslows-hierarchy-separating-fact-from-fiction. Accessed 16 Sept. 2020.

"WOC Nurses." *Nursing2020*, journals.lww.com/nursing/fulltext/2003/01001/woc_nurses.18.aspx. Accessed 24 Sept. 2020.

"Women's Health Perinatal Nursing Care Quality Measures." *The Association of Women's Health, Obstetric and Neonatal Nurses (AWHONN)*, awhonn.org/womens-health-perinatal-nursing-care-quality-measures/. Accessed 3 Sept. 2020.

Wood, Debra. "4 Common Nursing Ethics Dilemmas." Nurse Choice. https://www.nursechoice.com/traveler-resources/4-common-nursing-ethics-dilemmas/. Accessed 8 Oct. 2020.

Wood, J. F. *Interpersonal Communication: Everyday Encounters*. Cengage Publishing, 2016. This book can be obtained online and it expands the information in this article by including ways to deal with many of the communication issues of today's relationships.

Wootton, Richard, et al. *Telehealth in the Developing World*. Royal Society of Medicine Press, 2011.

World Health Organization, www.who.int.

Wright, L. D. "Meditation: A New Role for an Old Friend." *American Journal of Hospice and Palliative Care*, vol. 23, 2006, pp. 323-27.

"Writing Skills: Skills You Need." www.skillsyouneed.com/writing-skills.html. Accessed 1 Sept. 2020.

Writing Skills: Success in 20 Minutes a Day. 5th ed., Learning Press, 2012. This workbook contains basic advice on how to develop writing skills in an academic context.

Yang, K. "A Review of Yoga Programs for Four Leading Risk Factors of Chronic Diseases." *Evidence-Based Complementary and Alternative Medicine*, vol. 4, no. 4, 2007, pp. 487-91.

Yates, A. J. *Biofeedback and the Modification of Behavior*. Springer Science & Business Media, 2012.

Yazdi, Mariam. "4 Steps to Writing A Nursing Care Plan." *Nurse.org*, 23 Mar. 2018, nurse.org/articles/nursing-care-plan-how-to/.

"Your Health Care Team." University of Rochester Medicine, Strong Memorial Hospital, www.urmc.rochester.edu/strong-memorial/patients-families/health-care-team.aspx. Accessed 9 Oct. 2020.

Zander, Karen. *Case Management Models, Best Practices for Health Systems and ACO's*. 2nd ed., HCPro, 2017,

Zangerle, Claire, M. "What Are the Roles and Responsibilities of a Case Manager in a Hospital Setting?" *Nursing Management*, vol. 46, no. 10, Oct. 2015, pp. 27-28.

Zborowsky, T. "The Legacy of Florence Nightingale's Environmental Theory: Nursing Research Focusing on the Impact of Healthcare Environments." *HERD: Health Environments Research & Design Journal*, vol. 7, no. 4, pp. 19-24.

Zeoli, R. "Seven Principles of Effective Public Speaking." *American Management Association*, 16 Apr. 2014, www.amanet.org/training/articles/Seven-Principles-of-Effective-Public-Speaking.aspx. This article talks about how public speaking is a skill that is learned. It proceeds to outline seven key principles that help teach individuals how to improve their public speaking abilities.

Zinsser, W. *On Writing Well: The Classic Guide to Writing Nonfiction*. 30th anniversary ed., 7th ed., revised and updated. HarperCollins, and Harper Perennial, 2006. This title (like Strunk and White) is a classic guide that focuses on writing quality.

Zitelli, Basil J., Sara McIntire, and Andrew J. Nowalk. *Zitelli and Davis' Atlas of Pediatric Physical Diagnosis*. 6th ed., Saunders, 2012.

Zshorlich, B., D. Gechter, I. M. JanBen, et.al. "Health Information on the Internet: Who Is Searching for What, When and How?" *Z Evid Fortbild Qual Gesundhwes*, vol. 10, no. 2, 2015, pp. 144-52, pubmed.ncbi.nlm.nih.gov.

Zunker, Vernon. *Using Assessment Results for Career Development*. Brooks, 2006.

Index

A

Aamodt, Michael G., 84
Abdellah, Faye Glenn, 36, 49-51
Abortion, 5, 164
Academic Consortium for Integrative Medicine and Health, 242
Academy of American Nursing, 56
Academy of Medical-Surgical Nurses (AMSN), 155
Accreditation Commission for Acupuncture and Oriental Medicine, 237
Accreditation Commission for Education in Nursing (ACEN), 103
acetaminophen (Tylenol), 217
acquired immunodeficiency syndrome (AIDS), 50, 193, 206, 226
acupuncture, 218, 219, 237, 243, 244, 257, 261, 282
acupuncturist, 219, 237, 238, 251
Ader, Robert, 273
Adolescence, 83, 95, 121, 123, 127, 162, 231
Adult-Gerontology Primary Care Nurse Practitioner Certification (ACPCNP-BC), 152
Advanced Critical Care, 174
Advanced Oncology Certified Clinical Nurse Specialist (AOCNS), 177
advanced practice nurses (APNs), 104, 107
advanced practice registered nurses (APRNs), 12, 22, 151, 158, 177, 181
Advanced Public Health Certification (PHNA-BC), 186
Affordable Care Act (ACA), 202
alcohol use, 161
Alexander technique, 233, 234, 235, 236
Alive Inside, 295
Alligood, M. R., 33, 37
Allopathy, 316
Allport, Gordon, 88
Alzheimer's disease, 50, 170, 172, 225, 227, 243, 310
American Nursing Credentialing Center (ANCC), 185, 186
American Academy of Nurse Practitioners, 111, 152, 181
American Academy of Nurse Practitioners Certification Board (AAPCB), 111, 152, 181
American Academy of Nursing (AAN), 110, 111
American Academy of Pediatrics, 168, 244
American Academy of Wound Management (AAWM), 191
American Art Therapy Association (AATA), 290
American Association for Marriage and Family Therapy, 57
American Association of Cardiovascular Nurses, 174
American Association of Colleges of Nursing (AACN), 106, 180
American Association of Critical-Care Nurses (AACN), 174, 177
American Association of Directors of Nursing Services (AADNS), 154
American Association of Nurse Anesthetists (AANA), 184
American Association of Nurse Practitioners (AANP), 111, 181
American Board of Homeotherapeutics, 239-240
American Board of Medical Acupuncture, 237
American Board of Physician Specialties, 245
American Cancer Society, 126, 231, 251
American Case Management Society, 202
American Chiropractic Association, 238
American Civil War, 4, 45, 174
American College of Nurse Practitioners, 111, 181
American College of Nurse-Midwives (ACNM), 111
American College Test (ACT), 92
American Holistic Medical Association, 245
American Journal of Nursing, 4
American medical system, 111
American Midwifery Certification Board (ACMB), 111
American Music Therapy Association (AMTA), 293
American Naturopathic Certification Board, 241
American Naturopathic Medical Certificate Board, 240
American Nurse Credentialing Center, 201
American Nurses Association (ANA), 17, 109, 111, 199
American Nurses Credentialing Center (ANCC), 106, 108, 109, 110, 111, 152, 153, 155, 177, 181
American Nurses Foundation, 110
American Nursing Association, 18, 34
American Organization of Nurse Executives, 152
American Public Health Association, 185
American Red Cross, 174
ANA Membership Assembly, 109
androgens, 167
anesthesia, 5, 6, 12, 21, 23, 25, 105, 106, 181, 182, 183, 184, 204, 218, 265
anesthesia administrators, 183
anesthesiologist, 3, 10, 182
anesthesiology, 183
anxiety, 48, 50, 56, 85, 86, 129, 137, 144, 145, 221, 225, 229, 235, 243, 262, 264, 265, 266, 267, 268, 269, 271, 273, 275, 276, 277, 278, 279, 280, 283, 284, 292, 296, 299, 300, 305
Armed Services Vocational Aptitude Battery (ASVAB), 89

347

Army Nurse Corps, 47
aromatherapists, 237
art psychotherapy, 291, 292
art therapists, 291, 292, 293
art therapy, 290-293
arterial blood gas analysis (ABG), 211
Arthritis Self-Management Program, 255
artificial intelligence, 307
assessment, 15
associate degree in nursing (ADN), 172
associate of science in nursing (ASN), 172
Association of Clinical Research Professionals (ACRP), 199
Association of periOperative Registered Nurses (AORN), 157
asthma, 227, 229, 234, 243, 264, 273, 275, 277
Atlantic, The, 175
attention-deficit hyperactivity disorder (ADHD), 167
Attraction, Selection, Attrition (ASA) model, 96
autism spectrum disorder, 164, 167, 294
autonomy, 19-21

B
baby boomer, 172, 175
bachelor of science in nursing (BSN), 57, 154, 172, 183, 196
Back to Sleep campaign, 168
Barker, Phil, 39
Barnard, Kathryn, 37
Barton, Clarissa "Clara" Harlowe, 174
Basic Physiological Needs, 15, 62, 63
Beach, Wooster, 315
Beck, Cheryl Tatano, 38
Benson, Herbert, 219, 260, 273
bereavement specialists, 214
Bernard, Mary, 183
Bersoff, Donald N., 90
"Betty Neuman Health-Care Systems Model, The," 57
biochemistry, 179
biofeedback, 219, 297-301
biofeedback techniques, 299, 300
biofeedback therapy, 256, 265, 297
biofeedback training, 228, 229, 300
bioinformatics (biomedical informatics), 312-314
Board of Nursing (BONs), 21
body language, 138, 139, 140, 147
Bone Marrow Transplant Nurse, 205
Buehler, Roger, 128
Bulletin of Art Therapy, 291

C
California Medical Practice Act, 183
California Psychological Inventory (CPI), 89

California Society of Anesthesiologists v. Brown, 183
CAM practitioners, 237, 245, 252, 253
Campbell, D. T., 88
Cancer Therapy Evaluation program, 253
Cannon, Walter B., 260
cardiac nursing, 204
cardiologist, 10, 194
cardiopulmonary resuscitation (CPR), 174, 206
cardiovascular diseases, 231
cardiovascular disorders, 243
care navigation, 201-203
care navigators, 201, 202, 203
care planning, 14, 16, 63
career planning, 90
caring theory, 61
case management, 11, 197, 201-203
case management certification, 202
Case Management Society of America, 202
Cattell, Raymond, 89
Center for Nursing Research, 68
Center for Scientific Review (CSR), 224
Center to Advance Palliative Care (CAPC), 215
Centers for Disease Control and Prevention (CDC), 232, 250, 251
Centers for Medicare and Medicaid Services (CMS), 23
cerebral palsy, 164, 165, 168, 289
cerebrovascular disease, 296
Certification Board for Music Therapists, 297
Certified Critical Care Nurse, 175
Certified Director of Nursing (CDON), 154
Certified Hospice and Palliative Nursing Assistants (CHPNA), 197
Certified Medical-Surgical Registered Nurse (CMSRN), 155
certified nurse assistants (CNAs), 184
Certified Nurse Midwife (CNM) examination, 158
Certified Nurse-Midwives (CNMs), 105
Certified nursing assistants (CNAs), 102, 184
Certified Pediatric Nurse (CPN), 106
Certified Perioperative Nurse (CNOR), 157
Certified registered nurse anesthetist (CRNA), 105
Certified Registered Nurse Assistant (CRNFA), 157
Certified Wound Specialist (CWS), 191
chemotherapy, 20, 25, 107, 257, 263, 273, 275
Chief nurse executives (CNEs), 154
Chief nursing officers (CNOs), 154
Child Health Assessment Model, 37
Chinese herbal medicine, 282
chiropractors, 218, 237, 238
chronic illness, 14, 39, 63, 194, 196, 220, 242
chronic obstructive pulmonary disease (COPD), 195, 227

chronic pain, 218, 219, 220, 221, 244, 256, 263, 265, 299
chronic pain management, 220, 221
chronic pain specialist, 218
Churchill, Winston, 125
circulating nurses, 6
Civil Rights Act of 1964, 90
clinical investigators, 200
clinical nurse leader (CNL), 176
Clinical Nurse Leader Certification Program, 177
clinical nurse specialist (CNS), 176-177
clinical pharmacists, 10, 11
clinical research nurses (CRN), 199
clinical research trials, 25-28
clinical trials, 25, 26, 27, 28, 199, 200, 234, 235, 246, 257, 274, 296
cliques, 123
Coalition to Protect Patient Safety, 114
Code of Ethics for Nurses, 17
cognitive behavioral therapy (CBT), 220, 264
cognitive development, 127
cognitive functioning, 127
cognitive psychotherapy, 264
College Entrance Examination Board (College Board), 92
Commission on Nurse Certification (CNC), 177
communication skills, 4, 5, 102, 121, 131, 146, 196, 197, 220, 292
community health nursing, 185
community nurses, 184
community service, 124-127
Competency and Credentialing Institute (CCI), 157
complementary and alternative medicine (CAM), 233, 242, 250, 255, 276
computed tomography (CT) scan, 20, 160
computer science, 9, 312, 313
"Conceptual Model for Preventive Health Behavior, A," 68
Conceptual Models for Nursing Practice, 57
congestive heart failure (CHF), 195, 215
consent, 23-25
Content Expert Panel (CEP), 108
Continued Professional Certification (CPC) Program, 184
coronavirus 2019 (COVID-19), 255
Corporation for National and Community Service, 125
Council for Homeopathic Certification, 239
Council of Naturopathic Medical Education, 241
Council on Chiropractic Education (CCE), 238
Covey, Stephen R., 134
COVID-19 pandemic, 255, 311
Crimean War, 4, 34, 45, 46
Critical Care Nurse, 174
critical care nurses, 107, 108, 110, 173, 174, 175, 176, 177
critical care nursing, 173-176

Critical Care RN (Neonatal) certification, 159
cyberworld, 139
Cystic fibrosis, 165, 303, 305

D

da Vinci (robot), 307
Dawis, René, 88, 90
decision-making, 3, 5, 14, 17, 18, 22, 212
dehydroepiandrosterone (DHEA), 282
dementia, 170, 172, 296, 310
deoxyribonucleic acid (DNA), 304, 312
Department of Defense, 89, 244
Department of Health and Human Services, 221, 244, 249
Department of Veterans Affairs, 244
depression, 14, 40, 126, 214, 215, 221, 225, 226, 234, 243, 255, 258, 265, 267, 268, 269, 275, 276, 277, 296, 299
diabetes educators, 207
Diabetes Prevention Program, 231
diabetic specialist, 7
Dickens, Charles, 8
Dicklich, Kree, 57
Dietary Approaches to Stop Hypertension (DASH) diet, 231
Dietary Supplement Health and Education Act of 1994, 253
Dietary Supplement Research Centers, 254
diet-based therapies, 230-232
dietitians, 10, 11, 232
diphtheria, 165, 168
Director of Nursing, 55, 153, 154
Discipline and Teaching of Nursing Process, The, 52
disease management, 173, 176, 207, 231, 233, 250
Do Something (organization), 126
Doctor of anesthesia practice (DNAP), 106
Doctor of chiropractic (DC) program, 238
Doctor of Nursing Practice (DNP), 22, 23, 106, 152, 153, 154, 177, 181
domestic violence, 206
Down syndrome, 164, 165, 168
drug addiction, 50, 170, 268
DTP vaccine, 168
Dynamic Nurse-Patient Relationship: Function, Process, and Principles, The, 51, 52

E

electrocardiography (ECG), 211
electroencephalogram (EEG), 269, 299
electronic cigarettes, 228
elitism, 315
Emerson, Ralph Waldo, 145
empathy, 66, 136, 242

end-of-life care, 194, 211, 215
Enhanced Nursing Licensure Compact (eNLC), 199
Environmental Theory, 13, 31, 36, 40, 43, 45, 46
epidemiologists, 188
epidemiology, 199
epilepsy, 266, 295, 304
Erikson, Erik, 83
evaluation, 15, 16
evidence-based practice (EBP), 15, 152, 181, 184
exercise-based therapies, 232-237

F
face-to-face communication, 131, 133, 137, 190
Family Nurse Practitioner Certification (FNP-BC), 152
family nurse practitioners (FNPs), 179
Farr, William, 46
Fawcett, Jacqueline, 33
Federal Pell Grant, 74
Federal Student Loans, 74
federal tax, 224, 225
Federal Work Study program, 74
Feldenkrais method, 233, 234, 235, 236
fetal development, 160
fetal movement, 160
Food and Drug Administration (FDA), 26, 200, 251, 254, 307
Ford, Loretta, 179
Free Application for Federal Student Aid (FASFA), 73
Fromm, Erich, 47
Fromm-Reichmann, Frieda, 47
functional magnetic resonance imaging (fMRI), 267
Furumoto, Phyllis, 286

G
Gamp, Sairey, 8
gene therapy, 305
General Aptitude Test Battery (GATB), 89
genetic counseling, 303-307
genetic counselor, 303, 305, 306
genetic disorders, 165, 303
genetic testing, 225, 303, 304, 306
Genevro, Janice, 215
genome, 225, 304, 312, 313
gerontological nurses, 170, 171, 172, 173
gerontological nursing (geriatric nursing), 170-173
gerontology, 172, 173, 177, 180, 181, 185
Gerson, Max, 252
Glick, Ronald, 218
Gough, Harrison, 89
Graham, Sylvester, 316
Grand Nursing theories, 33, 37
Grand theory, 35

Grant, Ernest J., 110
Great Depression, 51, 115
grief process, 215, 216
Griffin, Dale, 128
Group beta strep (GBS) infections, 164
guided imagery, 243, 262, 275-276

H
Habitat for Humanity, 126
Harvard Business Review, 125
Harvard Community Health Plan, 52
Harvard Health Publications, 126
Hathaway, S. R., 89
Hayashi, Chujiro, 286
Health Belief Model, 67
health insurance agencies, 9
Health Insurance Portability and Accountability Act of 1996 (HIPAA), 18
health maintenance organization (HMO), 248
health movement, 314-316
Health Promotion in Nursing Practice, 68
Health Promotion Model (HPM), 68
Health promotion programs, 226
Health Promotion Research Program, 67
healthcare directives, 18
healthcare industry, 64, 137, 139, 172, 175, 202, 307
healthcare practitioners, 217, 268
healthcare professionals, 11, 15, 22, 94, 102, 151, 172, 187, 200, 201, 252
healthcare services, 59, 103, 176, 184, 186, 192, 246
hemophilia, 305
Henderson, Virginia, 37
hepatitis, 165, 168, 193, 226
Hepburn, Audrey, 125
herbal remedies, 7, 257, 314
Hierarchy of Needs Model, 64
high energy particulate air (HEPA) filters, 46
Hill, Adrian, 291
Hippocrates, 273
Hippocratic Oath, 17
Hofstadter, Douglas, 128
Holland, John L., 87
home care, 12, 50, 175, 195
home health agency, 6, 184
Home Health Clinical Nurse Specialist Certification (HHCNS-BC), 185
home health nurse, 184-187
home health nursing, 184
home healthcare nurses, 184, 185, 196
homeopathy, 238, 239, 240, 242, 244, 282, 289, 316
Hospice and Palliative Credentialing Center, 196-197

hospice care, 195
hospice nurse (HN), 197
Hospital-acquired infections (HAIs), 309
hospitalist physician, 10
human immunodeficiency virus (HIV), 164, 206, 226, 248, 265
human rights, 18, 91, 126
Human to Human Relationship Model, 37
hydrocephalus, 164, 168
hydropathy, 316
hypnotherapy, 221, 265, 280

I
imagery exercises, 219
immediate care, 50
immune system, 161, 234, 273, 275, 276, 278
implementation, 15, 16
industrial hygienists, 187
Industrial Revolution, 187
infancy, 165, 166, 168
Inpatient Obstetric Nursing certification, 158
insomnia, 229, 234, 235, 262, 263, 264, 268, 273, 275, 276, 277, 296, 299
Institute for Natural Medicine and Prevention, 271
Institutional Review Board (IRB), 24, 26
insulin, 6, 165, 168, 169, 206, 243, 272, 305
insulin-dependent diabetes mellitus (IDDM), 165
integrative medicine (IM), 242
intensive care unit (ICU), 34, 173, 205, 283
intensive care unit (ICU) nurse, 34, 173
International Council of Nurses (ICN), 110
International Association for Continuing Education and Training (IACET), 206
International Association of Clinical Research Nurses (IACRN), 199
International Council of Nursing, 48
International Neuman Systems Model Symposium, 58
internet medicine, 246-250
interpersonal communication, 48, 59, 131, 132, 134, 137
interpersonal skills, 52, 81, 82, 131, 132, 137, 138, 139, 140

J
Jackson, Andrew, 315
Jackson, Douglas, 89
John E. Fogarty International Center (FIC), 223
Johnson, Dorothy E., 59
Journal of the Society of Integrative Oncology, 253

K
Kaplan Admissions Test, 92, 94
Kim, Hesook, 34
King, Imogene Martina, 55-56
Kolbaca, Katharine, 65-67
Korean War, 50
Krieger, Dolores, 283
KSAO (knowledge, skills, abilities, and other), 95, 96
Kübler-Ross, Elisabeth, 212
Kuder Occupational Interest Survey (KOIS), 89

L
Lambertson, Eleanor, 115
Lancet, The, 192
Leader-Member Exchange (LMX) theory, 98
leadership skills, 81, 121-124
leukemia, 166, 169
licensed practical nurse (LPN), 11, 71, 81, 94, 102, 172, 204
licensed vocational nurse (LVN), 11, 71, 103, 172, 204
Lindquist, E. F., 93
Lofquist, Lloyd, 88, 90
Luther, Martin, 142

M
Magaw, Agnes, 183
Magnet Recognition Program, 111-112
Magnet Status, 111, 112
magnetic resonance imaging (MRI), 20
Maharishi Vedic Education Development Corporation, 272
malaria, 165, 222, 251
Manthey, Marie, 116
marijuana, 243
Marine Hospital Service (MHS), 222
Martin Chuzzlewit, 8
Maslow, Abraham, 15
Massachusetts Health & Hospital Association, 114
Massachusetts Nurses Association, 114
Massage and Bodywork Licensing Examination, 240
massage therapist, 237, 240, 251
Master of Business Administration, 154
Master of Health Administration, 154
master of science in nursing (MSN), 22, 104, 105, 154, 172, 177, 181, 185, 196
maternal identity, 38
Maternal Role Attainment, 38
Mayo Clinic Complementary and Integrative Medicine, 241
Mayo, Charles, 183
McClenahan, William, 174
McIntosh, Donald, 48
McKinley, J. C., 89
measles, 161, 164, 165, 168, 315

medical care, 6, 7, 45, 116, 170, 173, 174, 175, 215, 217, 246, 251, 255, 287, 288
medical management, 161, 215
medical practitioner, 192, 251
medical-surgical nurses, 154-157
Medical-Surgical Nursing Certification Board (MSNCB), 155
medicine, 3, 4, 6, 35, 50, 51, 314, 316
meditation, 267-270
Mehrabian, Albert, 133
melodic intonation therapy (MIT), 294
meningitis, 164, 165
Menopause (journal), 235
mental disability, 165, 168
mental health nursing, 39, 47, 52, 58, 61
mental health treatment, 7
Mercer, Ramona, 38
metaparadigm, 33-35
middle-range theories, 38-40
Midwest Nursing Research Society, 68
Mind-Body Medical Institute, 219
mind-body medicine, 273-275
Mishel, Merle, 39
MMR vaccine, 168
modern nursing, 8, 45, 51
Mogliner, Cassie, 125
molecular biology, 312, 313
Monitoring the Future, 125
mortality rates, 225
Mosaic Health Code, 7
movement therapy, 242, 244
multiculturalism, 125
mumps, 165, 168
Murdaugh, Carolyn, 68
Murray, Henry A., 89
music therapists, 296, 297
music therapy, 293-297
Music Therapy Perspectives, 296

N

NANDA International, 15
nanotechnology, 311
nasogastric tube (NGT), 206
National Center for Health Statistics, 233
National Association of Clinical Nurse Specialists (NACNS), 111
National Association of Directors of Nursing Administration in Long Term Care (NADONA LTC), 154
National Board of Certification and Recertification for Nurse Anesthetists (NBCRNA), 23

National Board of Chiropractic Examiners, 238
National Board of Public Health Examiners (NBPHE), 186
National Cancer Institute (NCI), 222
National Center for Biotechnology Information, 250
National Center for Complementary and Alternative Medicine (NCCAM), 254, 258
National Center for Complementary and Integrative Health (NCCIH), 255, 258
National Certification Corporation (NCC), 106, 158
National Certification Exam (NCE), 23, 106
National Council Licensure Examination (NCLEX), 103, 107
National Council Licensure Examination-Registered Nurse (NCLEX-RN), 107, 158, 183
National Council of State Boards of Nursing (NCSBN), 22, 107
National Health Information Survey, 258
National Healthcare Disaster Certification (NHDP-BC), 110
National Heart Act, 223
National Human Genome Research Institute, 224
National Institute of Mental Health, 48, 52
National Institute of Occupational Safety and Health (NIOSH), 189
National Institutes of Health (NIH), 221-226
National League for Nursing (NLN), 93, 110
National Library of Medicine (NLM), 223
National Student Nurses Association (NSNA), 110
natural therapeutics, 241
naturopathic physician, 240, 241
naturopathy, 241, 282
Naumberg, Margaret, 291
neonatal intensive care unit (NICU), 158
neonatal nurses, 157-159
neonatology, 163
networking, 146-148
Neuman Systems Model: Application to Nursing Education and Practice, The, 58
Neuman, Betty (Betty Maxine Reynolds), 57-58
Neuman, Richard, 57
Nevill, Doris, 90
New Guide to Health: Or, Botanic Family Physician, 315
"Nightingale Pledge," 17
Nightingale Training School for Nurses, 4, 45
Nightingale, Florence, 45-47
nonsteroidal anti-inflammatory drugs (NSAIDs), 217
nonverbal communication, 102, 131, 132, 133, 135, 147
nonverbal signals, 100
North American Nursing Diagnosis Association (NANDA), 15

Notes on Nursing, 45
nurse anesthetists, 104, 105, 106, 111, 180, 181-184
nurse care navigators, 203
nurse case managers, 201, 202
nurse directors, 153
nurse educators, 203, 204
Nurse Executive Certification (NE-BC), 153
Nurse Licensure Compact (NLC), 19, 108
nurse managers, 151, 152, 153
nurse midwives, 3, 104, 105, 106, 111, 158
nurse navigator, 202, 203
Nurse Practice Act (NPA), 19, 21, 107
nurse practitioner (NP), 179-181
nurse researcher, 5
nurse specialists, 104, 111, 176
Nurse-patient ratio, 113-115
nurse-patient relationship, 13, 37, 51, 52, 53, 61, 66
Nurses Associated Alumnae, 109
Nursing Regulatory Body (NRB), 21
nursing administration, 152, 154
nursing administrator, 108, 152-154
nursing assessment, 21, 133
nursing assistants, 115, 116, 197
nursing care, 3, 4, 5, 8, 12, 13, 14, 15, 16, 17, 21, 31, 32, 36, 37, 38, 40, 50, 56, 62, 107, 115-116
nursing care plan (NCP), 116
nursing case management, 203
nursing certification, 53, 102-104
nursing education, 4, 8, 16, 31, 32, 33, 34, 35, 45, 46, 47, 51, 52, 53, 57, 58, 110, 203, 206
Nursing Entrance Test (NET), 94
Nursing for Education and Research, 52
nursing interventions, 16, 33, 35, 39, 40, 41, 62, 64
nursing licensure, 85, 107, 108, 109, 110
Nursing Licensure Compact Commission, 108
Nursing Need Theory, 37
Nursing Outlook, 68
nursing philosophy, 37
Nursing Process Theory, 37, 51, 52
nursing professionals, 11, 12, 22, 115, 151, 152, 153, 158, 182, 198
Nursing Research, 57
nursing school, 58, 60, 62, 71, 73, 78, 83, 92, 93, 107, 144, 174
nursing theories, 31-33
Nursing: Concepts of Practice, 54

O

Obama, Barack, 225
observational studies, 25, 244
obsessive-compulsive disorder, 264, 265, 299
obstetric nurses, 157
obstetric-gynecology (OB-GYN), 157
obstetrician, 157, 158
occupational health, 187-189
occupational health nurse, 187
Occupational Safety and Health Act of 1970, 189
Occupational Safety and Health Administration (OSHA), 188
occupational therapists (OTs), 11
occupational therapy, 6
Office for Human Research Protections (OHRP), 28
Office for the Advancement of Telehealth, 249
Office of Cancer Complementary and Alternative Medicine (OCCAM), 252-253
Office of Dietary Supplements (ODS), 253-255
On Death and Dying, 212
Oncology Certified Nurse (ONCC), 106
oncology nurses, 114
Oncology Nursing Certification Corporation, 177
Oncology Nursing Society, 110
online learning, 78
operating room (OR) nurses, 155
Orem Model of nursing, 53
Orem, Dorothea Elizabeth, 53-55
Organization of Nurse Leaders, 114
organizational citizenship behaviors (OCBs), 97
Orlando, Ida Jean, 13, 15, 37, 51-53
osteoporosis, 172, 226, 227, 234, 243, 254
Otis Self-Administering Tests of Mental Ability, 89
over-the-counter (OTC) medicines, 217

P

pain management, 105, 176, 182, 183
pain relievers, 217, 218, 265
pain-management skills, 220
palliative care, 194-197
palliative care (PC) nurses, 196
paraphrasing, 135, 136, 141
parasympathetic nervous system, 261
Parkinson's disease, 225, 243, 295
Paro (robot), 310
Parsons, Mary Ann, 68
Patient Assessment of Care Evaluation (PACE), 50
patient care, 5, 11, 39, 50, 55, 59, 62, 66, 103, 105, 106, 112, 115, 116, 151, 155
patient educators, 207
patient navigators, 201
Patient Safety Act, 114
Pauk, Walter, 78
Peaceful End-of-Life Theory, 39
pediatric nurse, 106, 159, 162

pediatric nurse practitioners (PNP), 162
pediatric nursing, 59, 106, 169, 204
Pediatric Nursing Certification Board (PNCB), 106
pediatric palliative nurses, 197
pediatricians, 162, 163, 166, 167
pediatrics, 162-170
Pelletier, Robert, 52
Pender, Nola, 67-68
Peplau, Hildegard, 36, 47-49
perinatal medicine, 159
perinatal nurse, 157, 159, 160
perinatology, 159-162
perioperative nurses, 154-157
personal protective equipment (PPE), 311
personality development, 48, 89
pertussis (whooping cough), 165
pharmacists, 10, 11, 20, 171
pharmacokinetics, 200
pharmacology, 76, 103, 105, 169, 179, 181, 184, 222
phenylketonuria (PKU) test, 304
philanthropy, 45
phototherapy, 46
physical therapists (PTs), 11
physical therapy, 6, 168, 295
physician assistant (PA), 177
Physician Assistant National Certifying Exam (PANCE), 179
Physician Assistant National Recertifying Exam (PANRE), 179
Physician Assistant-Certified (PA-C), 179
physiology, 34, 204, 237, 239, 240, 300, 314, 316
pilates, 233, 234, 235, 236
Pilates Method Alliance, 236
placebo treatment, 263, 264, 284
placenta, 161
plan of care, 6, 15, 16, 19, 20, 21, 116, 206, 217, 233
Planning Fallacy, 128
PLUS loans, 74
pneumonia, 164, 165, 168
Position Statement on the Practice Doctorate of Nursing, 106, 180
postanesthesia care unit (PACU), 156
Postpartum Depression Theory, 38, 40
practice-level theories, 40-41
pregnancy, 66, 105, 157, 158, 159, 161, 162, 164, 167, 168, 169, 244, 254, 265, 290, 303
Prig, Betsey, 8
primary care clinicians, 241
primary care doctors, 247
Primary care nurses, 151, 152
primary care provider, 151, 178, 179, 190, 191
primary maternity care provider, 105, 158

primary nursing, 115, 116
procrastination, 127, 128, 129, 130, 131
Progressive Patient Care Protocol, 50
progressive muscle relaxation (PMR), 300
PSB Aptitude for Practical Nursing Exam, 92, 94
psychiatry, 47, 169, 261
psychologists, 87, 88, 91, 212, 229, 266, 293, 296
psychology, 48, 50, 58, 61, 62, 65, 67, 84, 169, 221, 273
psychotherapy, 228, 229, 243, 264, 290, 291, 292
public awareness, 91, 187, 254
public health, 49, 50, 51, 57, 110
Public Health and Marine Hospital Service (PH-MHS), 222
public health nurses, 184, 186
public health nursing, 51, 185, 186
Public Health Service (PHS), 222
Public Health Service Act of 1944, 223
public speaking, 142-146
Pubmed, 28, 250, 251
pulmonologist, 10
pulse oximeter, 298, 299, 300
Pychyl, Timothy A., 128

R
radiology, 20, 21, 25, 205
Ransdell Act of 1930, 222
Rapid Response Team (RRT) clinicians, 11
Reagan, Nancy, 50
Reed, Pamela, 39
reflexologists, 237
Reformation, the, 8
Registered Clinical Dietitian, 230, 231, 232
registered nurse (RN), 11, 19, 61, 94, 102, 103, 107, 162, 172, 181, 198
Registered Nurse Boards, 81
rehabilitation services, 233
rehabilitation therapy, 295
Rei Jyutsu Ka, 286
reiki, 285-289
Reiki Alliance, 288
Reiki Foundation, 288
reiki practitioners, 237, 286, 288
Relaxation and Biofeedback Program, 67
Relaxation Response, The, 260
relaxation techniques, 219, 229, 256, 257, 262, 264, 272, 273, 277
relaxation therapies, 262-267
relaxation training, 228, 229, 243, 244
Renaissance, the, 8
Research nurses, 199, 200
research-based theory, 52

Reserve Officers' Training Corps (ROTC), 73
Richards, Linda, 45
Richardson, Elliot, 179
Riehl, Joan P., 57
RN first assistant (RNFA), 156
RNC Certification for Neonatal Intensive Care (RNC-NIC), 159
robotic surgery, 307, 308, 309
robotics, 307-312
Rolf Institute of Structural Integration, 290
rolfing, 289-290
rolfing therapy, 289, 290
Rorschach inkblot test, 88
Ross, Michael, 128
Roy Adaptation Model, 59
Roy, Callista Lorraine, 58-60
Roy, Sr. Callista, 13
Royal Commission for the Health of the Army, 46
Royal Statistical Society, 46
rubella (German measles), 164

S

Sacks, Oliver, 295
safe-sex programs, 169
Safety and Security Needs, 62, 63
safety regulations, 189
SAT Reasoning Test, 92
scarlet fever, 165
Schneider, Benjamin, 96
Scholastic Aptitude Test (SAT), 92
Scope of Practice laws, 19, 104
scrub nurse, 156
Seinfeld, Jerry, 143
self-actualization, 15, 62, 63, 65
self-awareness skills, 120
self-care theory, 53
self-care therapy, 255
Self-Directed Search (SDS), 89
self-discipline, 123
self-hypnosis, 229, 265
self-sacrifice, 3
Self-Transcendence Theory, 39
Selye, Hans, 216
sex hormones, 167
sexually transmitted infections (STIs), 167
Shakey (robot), 307
Silver, Henry, 179
skepticism, 314
skilled nursing facility (SNF), 189
smallpox, 165, 222

Smoking, 54, 161, 192, 226, 227, 228, 229, 231, 256, 265, 280, 306
Social Learning Theory, 97
social media, 71, 97, 99, 132, 137, 139, 140, 141, 146, 147
social networking, 137, 146
Social Science Research Institute, 67
social service providers, 246
Society for Integrative Oncology, 244
sociology, 59
Solomon, George, 273
speech therapy, 6
Spiegel, David, 273
spina bifida, 164, 168
spirituality, 257-260
SQ3R Learning System, 76
SRI International, 307
staff nurse, 19, 47, 57, 71, 82, 151-152
State Board of Health, 19
stress, 228, 229
Strong Vocational Interest Blank (SVIB), 88
Strong, Edward K., Jr., 87
Strong-Campbell Interest Inventory (SCII), 88
sudden infant death syndrome (SIDS), 165
Sullivan, Harry Stack, 47
Super, Donald, 90
surgical nurses, 154-157
Swanson, Kristen, 39, 65-67
Symonds, Percival, 48

T

Tai Chi, 233, 234, 236, 259, 262, 267, 268, 277, 280, 282
Tay-Sachs disease, 304, 305
teenage pregnancy, 167
telecommunications technologies, 137
telehealth nursing (telenursing), 192-194
telehealth services, 194
telemedicine, 39, 137, 140, 155, 192, 246, 247
telenurses, 192, 194
Teresa, Mother, 126
Test of Academic Skills (TEAS), 94
thanatologists, 212, 213, 214
Theory of Caring, 62, 66
Theory of Comfort, 39, 65, 66
Theory of Goal Attainment, 13, 37, 55
Theory of Illness Trajectory, 39
Theory of Interpersonal Relations, The, 37, 48
Theory of needs, 89-90
Therapeutic touch (TT), 282-285
Therapeutic Touch International Association, 285
Thomson, Samuel, 315
thyroid replacement therapy, 282

Tidal Model of Mental Health Recovery, 39
time management, 97, 127-131
Tourette's syndrome, 299
Toward a Theory of Nursing, 56
toxicologists, 188
Trager approach, 233, 234, 235, 236
Transcendental Meditation (TM), 260, 265, 267, 270-272
Transitional Care Unit, 189
travel nurses, 198
Travelbee, Joyce, 37
Tri-Council of Nursing, 22
TT practitioners, 284
tuberculosis, 165, 291
Turk, Dennis C., 218
21 Nursing Problems Theory, 36
typhoid fever, 165, 168
typhus, 165
typology, 89, 90

U

U.S. News & World Report, 111
Uncertainty in Illness Theory, 39
UNISON, 46
US Department of Education, 74, 206, 238
US Department of Labor, 74, 89, 95, 204
US Pharmacopeia (USP), 251
Usui, Mikao, 286

V

vaccination, 25, 168, 178, 278
Van Gelder Kunz, Dora, 283
varicella (chickenpox), 165, 168
Vocational Adjustment Index, 94
vocational nurse, 71

volunteer work, 124, 125, 126
volunteering, 80, 81, 82, 86, 124-127

W

Watson Caring Science Institute, 61
Watson, Douglas, 61
Watson, Jean (Margaret Jean Harman), 60-62
Weil, Andrew, 242
Weiss, David, 90
White, Jeffrey D., 253
wireless communication, 137
Wonderlic Cognitive Ability Test, 89
Wonderlic Personnel Test (WPT), 89
World Health Organization (WHO), 172, 195, 250
World War I, 222
World War II, 4, 27, 47, 115, 172, 222
World Wide Web, 250
wound care, 6, 149, 185
Wound, Ostomy and Continence Nursing Certification Board (WOCNCB), 191
wound, ostomy, and continence (WOC) nurse, 191-192
writing skills, 140-142

X

Xenex, 309
X-ray, 160, 206

Y

yoga, 229, 233, 234, 235, 236, 242, 243, 251, 259, 261, 262, 267, 273, 277, 280, 282, 289
Yoga Alliance, 236
Yogi, Maharishi Mahesh, 267, 270
Young, Rae Jeanne, 57